The Psychological and Social Impact of Illness and Disability

Sixth Edition

Irmo Marini, PhD, is professor and PhD program director, Department of Rehabilitation in the College of Health Sciences and Human Services at University of Texas Pan-American, Edinburg, Texas. He has national certifications as a rehabilitation counselor and life-care planner. Dr. Marini is on the editorial boards of several rehabilitation counseling journals, editor of the *Journal of Life Care Planning,* and has authored over 70 journal publications, 25 book chapters, and authored and coedited two books, *The Professional Counselor's Desk Reference* (2009) and *Psychosocial Aspects of Disability: Insider Perspectives in Counseling Strategies* (2012). He is the recipient of four outstanding university faculty awards in scholarship and two in teaching. He also received the Distinguished Career Award in Rehabilitation Education from the National Council on Rehabilitation Education in 2009 and the J. F. Garrett Distinguished Career Award in Rehabilitation Research from the American Rehabilitation Counseling Association in 2010. Dr. Marini is former chair of the Commission on Rehabilitation Counselor Certification, the national certifying body of over 16,000 rehabilitation counselors in the United States and Canada and former president of the American Rehabilitation Counseling Association. Dr. Marini owns and operates Marini & Associates, forensic rehabilitation consultants specializing in vocational assessments and life-care planning in legal cases involving personal injuries, and he is a vocational expert with the Social Security Administration.

Mark A. Stebnicki, PhD, is a Professor in the graduate program in rehabilitation counseling at East Carolina University. He holds a doctorate in rehabilitation counseling and is a licensed professional counselor (LPC) in North Carolina. He has national certifications as a certified rehabilitation counselor (CRC), certified case manager (CCM), and is certified by the Washington, DC–based crisis response team—National Organization for Victim Assistance (NOVA). He is also a Reiki Master level-III practitioner in the Usui Reiki Ryoho tradition. Dr. Stebnicki is an active teacher, researcher, and practitioner who has written five books; most recently *The Professional Counselor's Desk Reference* (Springer Publishing, 2009), and *Empathy Fatigue: Healing the Mind, Body, and Spirit of Professional Counselors* (Springer Publishing, 2008; Korean translation, 2010). He has over 25 articles in peer-reviewed journals, and has presented statewide and nationally at over 70 conferences, seminars, and workshops on topics that range from youth violence, traumatic stress, empathy fatigue, and the psychosocial aspects of chronic illness and disability.

Dr. Stebnicki has over 20 years experience working with adolescents and adults that have a variety of psychological and chronic health conditions. He served on the crisis response team for the Westside Middle School shootings in Jonesboro, Arkansas (March 24, 1998) and has done many stress debriefings with private companies, schools, and government employees after incidents of workplace violence, hurricanes, tornadoes, and floods. His youth violence program, the Identification, Early Intervention, Prevention, and Preparation (IEPP) program, was awarded national recognition in 2001 by the American Counseling Association (ACA) foundation for its vision and excellence in the area of youth violence prevention. Other accolades include numerous professional service awards and consulting with former President Bill Clinton's staff on addressing the students of Columbine High School after their critical incident (April 20, 1999).

The Psychological and Social Impact of Illness and Disability

Sixth Edition

IRMO MARINI, PhD

MARK A. STEBNICKI, PhD

Editors

SPRINGER PUBLISHING COMPANY

NEW YORK

Springer Publishing Company, LLC
11 West 42nd Street
New York, NY 10036
www.springerpub.com

Acquisitions Editor: Sheri W. Sussman
Production Editor: Lindsay Claire
Composition: Newgen Imaging

ISBN: 978-0-8261-0655-1
E-book ISBN: 978-0-8261-0656-8

15 16 17/ 7 6 5

The author and the publisher of this Work have made every effort to use sources believed to be reliable to provide information that is accurate and compatible with the standards generally accepted at the time of publication. The author and publisher shall not be liable for any special, consequential, or exemplary damages resulting, in whole or in part, from the readers' use of, or reliance on, the information contained in this book. The publisher has no responsibility for the persistence or accuracy of URLs for external or third-party Internet websites referred to in this publication and does not guarantee that any content on such websites is, or will remain, accurate or appropriate.

Library of Congress Cataloging-in-Publication Data

Library of Congress Control Number: 2012932171

Printed in the United States of America by McNaughton & Gunn.

To my sisters, Connie, Carole, and Darlene, and my nine nieces—thank you for supporting me and never doubting I could do all this. I think my parents and sister, Diane, would have been equally proud. To my wife's family, whose ongoing love and support has inspired us—thank you. To my colleagues and friends, who continue to nourish rather than drain my life force— thank you for always being there. Finally, to my wife, Darlene, who has always selflessly been quietly behind the curtain, but whose shoulders from which I have always gazed further than most, I think you have earned your wings.

—Irmo

Words cannot express my gratitude for Irmo's deep friendship, collegial relationship, and awakening my mind, body, and spirit to the true meaning of resiliency and psychosocial response to disability. I would also like to thank all my mentors at the Rehabilitation Institute, Southern Illinois University, Carbondale, where it all began for me with its creator, Dr. Guy Renzaglia (1913–2005) and my closest mentor throughout my master's and doctoral program, Dr. Harry Allen (1941–2009).

—Mark

Contents

PART V NEW DIRECTIONS: ISSUES AND PERSPECTIVES

APPENDIX A: PERSPECTIVE EXERCISES

APPENDIX B: PERSONAL PERSPECTIVES

Contributors

Richard F. Antonak, PhD
University of Massachusetts
Boston, Massachusetts

Tosca Appel, MS
Newton, Massachusetts

Maria Barrera, BS
Research Assistant
Department of Rehabilitation
The University of Texas-Pan American
Edinburg, Texas

Richard L. Beaulaurier, PhD, MSW
Florida International University School
   of Social Work
Miami, Florida

Malachy Bishop, PhD, CRC
University of Kentucky
Lexington, Kentucky

Boni Boswell, PhD
East Carolina University
Greenville, North Carolina

Martin G. Brodwin, PhD, CRC
California State University
Los Angeles, California

Susanne M. Bruyère, PhD, CRC
Director of the Employment and
   Disability Institute
Cornell University
Ithaca, New York

Lydia P. Buki, PhD
University of Illinois
Champaign, Illinois

Elizabath Cardoso
Hunter College
New York, New York

Jane Case-Smith, EdD
Ohio State University
Columbus, Ohio

Mitka Chacon, MS, LPCI
San Benito, Texas

Wendy Coduti, MA, PhD
Michigan State University
East Lansing, Michigan

David Collins, MED
Montgomery College
Rochville, Maryland

Nancy M. Crewe, PhD
Michigan State University
East Lansing, Michigan

Alfred H. DeGraf, EdD
Fort Collins, Colorado

Paul Egan, MS
Dracut, Massachusetts

Albert Ellis, PhD
Albert Ellis Institute
New York, New York

Pamela Fadem, MPH
University of California
Berkeley, California

Danielle D. Fox, PhD Student
Department of Rehabilitation
The University of Texas-Pan American
Edinburg, Texas

Mary Glacoff, PhD
East Carolina University
Greenville, North Carolina

Michael Hamer, PhD
East Carolina University
Greenville, North Carolina

Debra A. Harley, PhD, CRC, LPC
Department of Special Education and
    Rehabilitation Counseling
University of Kentucky
Lexington, Kentucky

James T. Herbert, PhD, CRC
The Pennsylvania State University
University Park, Pennsylvania

Jamylah Jackson, PhD, ABPP
Staff Psychologist and Assistant Professor
VA North Texas Health Care System
The University of Texas Southwestern
    Medical Center
Dallas, Texas

Charlene M. Kampfe, PhD, CRC
University of Arizona
Tucson, Arizona

Bethanne Keen, MD
Arizona Department of Corrections
Phoenix, Arizona

Sharon Knight, PhD
East Carolina University
Greenville, North Carolina

Lori Kogan, PhD
Colorado State University
Fort Collins, Colorado

Hanoch Livneh, PhD, CRC
Portland State University
Portland, Oregon

Jon McChesney, PhD
Western Kentucky University
Bowling Green, Kentucky

Eva Miller, PhD, CRC
Department of Rehabilitation
The University of Texas-Pan American
Edinburg, Texas

Meredith Minkler, DPH
University of California
Berkeley, California

Chris Moy, MS
Scranton, Pennsylvania

Robert J. Neumann
Chicago, Illinois

Kim Nguyen-Finn, MA, LPC-S
The University of Texas-Pan American
Edinburg, Texas

Carol S. North, MD, MPE
The Nancy and Ray Hunt Professor of
    Crisis Psychiatry
VA North Texas Health Care System
UT Southwestern Medical Center
Dallas, Texas

Margaret A. Nosek, PhD
Center for Research on Women
    With Disabilities
Department of Physical Medicine and
Rehabilitation
Baylor College of Medicine
Houston, Texas

Sara Pedersen, PhD
University of Montreal
Montreal, Quebec
Canada

David B. Peterson, PhD, CRC
California State University
Los Angeles, California

Andrew A. Phemister, PhD
Minnesota State University
Mankato, Minnesota

Ora Prilleltensky, PhD
Vanderbilt University
Nashville, Tennessee

Chuck Reid, PhD, CRC
The University of Texas-Pan American
Edinburg, Texas

Tracey A. Revenson, PhD
Vanderbilt University
Nashville, Tennessee

Maria G. Romero, PhD, CRC
Department of Psychology
Texas A&M International University
Laredo, Texas

Francis W. Siu, PhD, CRC
California State University
Los Angeles, California

David W. Smart, PhD
Brigham Young University
Provo, Utah

Julie F. Smart, PhD, CRC
Department of Special Education
  and Rehabilitation
Utah State University
Logan, Utah

Linda Stacey
Framingham, Massachusetts

Alina M. Surís, PhD, ABPP
Professor of Psychiatry
Director, Division of Trauma and Disaster
VA North Texas Health Care System
The University of Texas
  Southwestern Medical Center
Dallas, Texas

Samuel H. Taylor, DSW
University of Southern California
Los Angeles, California

Judy Teplow, MSW
Canton, Massachusetts

Lisa Thoman, PhD
Staff Psychologist and Assistant
  Professor
VA North Texas Health Care System
The University of Texas Southwestern
  Medical Center
Dallas, Texas

Patti Uman, BS
Colorado State University
Fort Collins, Colorado

John S. Wadsworth, PhD
Department of Counseling, Rehabilitation,
  and Student Development
University of Iowa
Iowa City, Iowa

Dale Walsh, ScD
Cambridge, Massachusetts

Robert P. Winske, MS
Boston, Massachusetts

Beatrice Wright, PhD
University of Kansas
Lawrence, Kansas

Steve Zanskas, MS, PhD
Michigan State University
East Lansing, Michigan

Foreword

*I*n preparation for the prior five editions—1977, 1984, 1991, 1999 and 2007—the goal was to recognize the importance of the past literature, put it in a current context, introduce new and emerging themes, and address current as well as future needs of the consumers and providers of health care and rehabilitation services. From my review of the sixth edition of *The Psychological and Social Impact of Illness and Disability*, it is clear that this tradition has continued and has been expanded.

It is important to note, however, that while significant and substantial gains have been made—some of which we did not even consider or anticipate—there is more to be accomplished. We have realized that the journey does not have a final destination but rather the more that is accomplished often results in other emerging horizons, more challenging landscapes, and major climate change with all the anticipated and unanticipated fall out.

These points are put forward by Gunnar Dybwad, Irving Kenneth Zola, Harlan Hahn, and Bob Marinelli who in earlier forewords made the following statements:

Gunnar Dybwad: 1977, first edition; "The high expectations expressed in the resolution declaring 1970–1980 was fulfilled in part when in 1975 the United Nations General Assembly adopted the Declaration on the Rights of Disabled Persons" (xi).

Irving Kenneth Zola: 1984, second edition: "By the time the next edition of this book comes out we shall see how the Independent Living Movement has fared. I am sure that we will need another decade of dedicated effort ... the line between the able-bodied and the disabled is a thin and often temporary one" (ix).

Irving Kenneth Zola: 1991, third edition: "What is done in the name of disability today affects all of our tomorrows" (x).

Harlan Hahn: 1999, fourth edition: "Both personal and social improvements can be achieved by embracing rather than overcoming the valuable contributions of a life with a disability" (xvii).

Bob Marinelli: 2007, fifth edition: "Disability is increasingly viewed as an enabling experience. This has allowed for the development of personal growth in life domains and contributions to the lives of others that were previously unavailable" (xxii).

One of the most complex tasks in preparation of the prior and current edition was not to be comfortable in presenting some of the most prominent and significant literature, as reflected in the classic articles. The difficult task was to try to learn from the vision of scholars who had the ability to address futuristic needs and emerging issues that would be world-changing and have a lasting impact on the evolutions of policy, services, and the lives of those who are or will be impacted by a new reality. Talk about a climate change and the melting of some beliefs that have been frozen for years!

Reflection on the previous editions results in the conclusion that these scholars were successful in some areas but not so in others. It was not anticipated that with landmark legislation there would be complex issues that would surface. Also, that the dramatic impact of technology would create a gap between what was available to some would not be affordable or accessible to many others. That with great wealth and accumulation, there would be, for some, the most desperate poverty and what once was a hope, has become an uncertainty (e.g., jobs, health benefits, home ownership, and universal access).

Also, when the first edition was printed in 1977, domains that are an embedded part of our landscapes were not apparent or not even on the horizon for many (e.g., traumatic brain injury, mental illness, global financial concerns, AIDS, and natural disasters). All of these changes have a direct and indirect impact on *The Psychological and Social Impact of Illness and Disability,* as it is now and as it is evolving. This sixth edition has been successful in channeling the confluence of historic themes, current issues, and futuristic concerns.

This is accomplished in a most readable and cogent style and format. For the reader, the classic articles present some of the foundation constructs and principles in a meaningful context and the new material addresses issues and themes that are meaningful, timely, and most relevant. The personal statements validate the experience and perspectives of consumers and those who serve and advocate for them. The discussion questions stimulate thought and discussion on issues and topics that warrant consideration as well as action and resolution. For many of us, and our significant others, the journey of life and living are not exactly what we had hoped or planned for.

No surprise here, even though there is great value on planning for the future and trying to control and contain the realities of life that often become our tsunami. This point was made by Dr. Zola in the foreword of the second edition when he stated: "For then as we age and change, both in body and mind, we shall not see this time as one of impending doom and decline but rather as a time when we will grow and manage our resources differently" (x).

This point, in the context of persons who are temporarily able-bodied, had emerged as connecting construct, more limited in the earlier editions but much more prominent in the more recent fifth and the current sixth editions. It was not always this way. In the past, our understanding of the psychological and social impact of illness and disability was based on the world as it was known with an element of what could and should be. When I was a student in 1966 during my first graduate internship at a state vocational rehabilitation office, I met a young man who was living with, and in spite of, a C-4 spinal cord injury. When we were discussing potential services, I was told by my supervisor that the agency did not provide services for people with catastrophic injuries. I was amazed because this was a young man, very independent—he had modified his van—who was just looking for some basic services. While this occurred 46 years ago, it still has an impact on me because while there have been major changes in the philosophy and principles of health care and rehabilitation, there are still emerging needs and issues that must be addressed. This sixth edition puts these in a meaningful historical, current, and futuristic perspective.

A bedrock concept of this sixth edition as well as the previous editions is that there is an emerging, evolving, and challenging body of knowledge that attempts of grasp and understand the complexity of life and living in the context of transient health, illness, disability, loss, change, and human resilience.

A simple but profound saying is "One must appreciate where one has been in order to better understand where one is going, how to get there, and be prepared to make the requisite adjustments along the way." This is not unlike the rehabilitation process, which demands many life changes, challenges, losses, and rewards. For me, this has been quite a journey that began in early childhood when I bore witness to friends and family members who had major health issues but who maintained their bearings in life and became role models for many even though the resources and supports were limited or nonexistent—apart from family and friends. In some ways, some things have not changed.

As a graduate student, I had the privilege of attending a lecture by Dr. Howard Rusk. His message, focusing on the theme of "A World to Care For," is more meaningful today than it was then. My personal introduction to the psychological and social aspects of disability began as a student in the 1960s but began in reality when I was a child and in a class with a boy who had a deformed hand. This was not an issue for me since we had a great time together, but I was told by others not to play with him. Childhood can be most understanding or very brutal.

The beginning of this book, which clearly began in 1971, happened when my colleague, Dr. Robert Marinelli stopped by my office and asked me to review some new material he was developing for his course on the psychosocial aspects of disability. He told me that the field was rapidly developing and he wanted to keep the course current and wanted my input on what he had selected. This was most timely because we had an upcoming meeting with Dr. Tamara Dembo at Clark University. At this meeting, we had the opportunity to listen to her historical and futuristic perspectives, her work with Dr. Beatrice Wright, and the content of a lecture she would be giving at Boston University. When we left the meeting, Bob and I looked at each other and realized that we had a lot to learn. When the lecture date arrived, we had expected 40 or 50 people attending at the most. We were surprised and most pleased when there was well over 100 present. It was not only the number that pleased us but also who was in attendance to hear Dr. Dembo: famed international scholar, Gunnar Dybwad who wrote the foreword to the first edition in 1977, Irving Kenneth Zola who did the forewords to the second and third editions as well as many other consumers and rehabilitation leaders. These were giants in the field. People of great vision, passion, and sensitivities. They would not accept what was, and challenged all of us to address what should and could be. This was a very significant experience because it put the topic at hand in a much larger context than we had understood it to be. Also emphasized was the impact on the consumer of services, and not just the world needs and perspectives of the provider. In 1973, Bob and I had the opportunity to attend a national conference with Dr. Dembo. What was special about this journey was that we would have many hours in airports and on the plane with Dr. Dembo. Those who knew her would understand the content of the ongoing discussion with this master scholar and most special human being.

At the end of the return flight, Bob and I realized how much information and perspective we had gained, and with the encouragement of Dr. Dembo the idea for a book emerged, and it became reality with the first edition in 1977. The point of this is that we had the benefit and support of many mentors and role models who advised, encouraged, and challenged us to pursue the topic and address the current and emerging needs of the consumers whose lives are most directly impacted by the quality and relevance of services and the visions of policymakers and commitment of providers.

In all of the previous editions, we have attempted to have theory balanced by reality and validated by the testimony and perspectives of those living the treatment and rehabilitation process. Key to negotiation of the life and living process is the fusion of the ongoing life lessons and learning that demand ongoing adjustments to the grinding conflicts between what we want, what we need, what we expect, and what we have. The personal statements in the book address these issues and provide the reader with personalized messages from those consumers who have a unique and meaningful perspective on the issues related to

The Psychological and Social Impact of Illness and Disability. Consequent to this effort we have formed ongoing life-long relationships with many consumers who have shared their life stories.

This tradition of personal statements has continued in the sixth edition. This is not by default; in fact, the current editor, Dr. Irmo Marini, was an ongoing content specialist, advisor, and contributor to several prior editions. With his experience as a scholar, consumer, and researcher, he and Dr. Mark Stebnicki have been able to address emerging trends in the field and include some of the most timely content while retaining selected classics. I am most pleased that the sixth edition has continued this tradition.

When Bob Marinelli decided to retire, and not do a fifth edition, we discussed who we wanted to replace him. We wanted a person who could bring an expanded perspective to the book, and we were most pleased that Dr. Paul Power accepted our invitation and the content of the fifth edition is most reflective of his input and vision.

When the sixth edition request was made, Paul and I had decided also to retire. We did not want the book to end, and we called Bob to discuss our options. We were all in agreement that the person we wanted to turn over the helm to was Dr. Irmo Marini who was part of the book for many years. Along with his coeditor, Dr. Mark Stebnicki (this sixth edition has built on the content of past editions), he has expanded the scope of the book, addressed the topics of 2012, and also set the stage for future issues, concerns, and challenges.

I am most honored to have been asked to write this foreword. I also want to acknowledge the support and guidance of our role models and mentors whose spirit is reflected in this work as well as in prior editions. In particular, I like to acknowledge Gunnar and Rosemary Dybwad, Irving Kenneth Zola, Tamara Dembo, Bernard Kutner, Nancy Crew, Hanoch Livneh, Paul Corcoran, Al De Graff, Elmer Bartels, Bill Anthony, Harlan Hahn, and Irmo Marini. These are just a few. The rest, you know who you are. Thank you!

To the editors, Dr. Irmo Marini and Dr. Mark Stebnicki, congratulations on a most meaningful and relevant book. I hope that the seventh edition will note how some of the most challenging issues have been addressed and that the new realities are clearer in focus and within the reach, hopes, and aspirations of those whose lives will be impacted, enhanced, or limited by what has been accomplished by those who have the power, wisdom, and ability not only to make a difference but to do what is right.

Arthur E. Dell Orto, PhD, CRC
Professor Emeritus, Sargent College of
Health and Rehabilitation Sciences
Boston University

Preface

*I*t was indeed an honor, albeit somewhat intimidating, to receive a call from Art Dell Orto in 2010, indicating that he was not only retiring after an outstanding career at Boston University but also retiring from his many other professional projects as well. Art and I have been friends and colleagues for over a decade, and I was flattered and honored to learn that he and Paul Power had selected three of my previous publications for the 5th edition of this best-selling and historic textbook, which dates back to 1977, with Bob Marinelli who had coedited with Art on the first four editions. However, to receive the call from Art indicating that he had recommended me to Springer Publishing to carry on the torch for the sixth edition of this text was a flattering and humbling moment for which I could not decline.

The perplexing part for me, however, was that I was in the middle of coauthoring with colleagues Noreen Glover-Graf and Michael Millington my second book ironically dealing with the same topic. So the juggling act of course became one of recognition that, although there inevitably had to be some overlap between the two, they still had to be uniquely and distinctly different. As I write this preface and look at the table of contents for both books, I am confident to conclude that they are definitely different in many ways. This text, first and foremost, had to continue with the best-selling formula that Bob and Art, and finally Art and Paul, had originally conceptualized.

My first thought when accepting the project was realizing that I needed help. Unhesitatingly, I turned to my good friend and coeditor on our first book, Mark Stebnicki. Mark and I first met when I hired him straight out of Southern Illinois University at Carbondale back in 1995, and we have worked and played since that time. He is an outstanding clinician and writer, having shaped his career in a number of fascinating ways as you will read in his biography. I am blessed to be surrounded by such good friends and colleagues and get to write about the topics of which we all share a passion.

This brings us to the sixth edition where almost two-thirds of the chapters are new and/or updated. We wanted to maintain the quality of information from the previous editions while choosing special topics and issues that relate to the profession today. As such, we are confident that we have successfully balanced this objective. Specifically, we retained 11 of the 36 chapters in the fifth edition due to their importance and ongoing significance. Second, we went back to eight of the authors from the fifth edition and received significant updated revisions of their chapters. Third, we reread the classic articles from the first four editions, and reinserted two of those chapters which continue to be benchmarks some 35 years later. Finally, we found and/or solicited 11 new chapters, two of which were gleaned from the literature, and nine newly written chapters from some prolific writers in the field.

So, knowing that this sixth edition has been significantly reconstructed while maintaining the integrity of its predecessors, I ask exactly how is it different? Well, the landscape concerning the psychosocial issues of persons with disabilities has shifted somewhat in America and abroad. As the United States continues to struggle with its investment in two arguable wars battling terrorism, the implications to our citizens, military, and their families are numerous both to their physical and mental health. As such, we have updated the chapter concerning the psychological issues of survivors of major disasters as well as add a new chapter dealing with mental health preparedness for terrorist incidents and the persistent threat and stress of terrorism on Americans. In addition, working specifically with the mental health issues of trauma-related combat veterans and their families the Afghan and Iraqi conflicts are addressed.

The psychosocial issues of women with disabilities are also discussed, both in an updated chapter regarding their psychosocial issues and in a new chapter dealing with physical and sexual abuse. The epidemiology of obesity and its epidemic increase with related physical, psychosocial, vocational, and health-related implications are also addressed. Although the above topics represent just some of the contemporary issues facing persons with disabilities and rehabilitation professionals in the 21st century, we also explore some of our history. In two newly written chapters, we explore the history of treatment of persons with disabilities, and specifically psychiatric disabilities in the United States. As rehabilitation counselors and researchers continue to reframe disability as a socially constructed concept and the critical interrelationship between an individual and his or her environment, knowing where we have been to derive at where we are today requires this exploratory and often unpleasant sociological perspective.

Finally, a psychosocial text concerning disability would not be complete without the perspectives of persons with disabilities who have lived the experience. As such, Mark and I have retained the majority of these poignant personal accounts written by persons with disabilities and/or their loved ones who care for them. Each section of the book contains classroom discussion talking points and exercises regarding the topical areas as well as personal stories found after some of the chapters. These insights will continue to give students and practicing counselors a different perspective of life with a disability in the United States.

ACKNOWLEDGMENTS

We would like to most humbly and appreciably thank several key people who made this book possible. Editor extraordinaire Sheri W. Sussman, who now having guided and supported us through two Springer Publishing books, has made this experience stress-free, mostly fun, and flawlessly compiled. Thanks also to Kathryn Corasaniti for keeping us organized with old chapters, new chapters, and revised chapters. A special thank you to a most respected colleague Arthur Dell Orto, who after 35 years, entrusted us to carry on with his, Bob Marinelli, and Paul Power's best-selling textbook. Dr. Dell Orto's numerous book contributions to the field spanning his career has elevated thousands of educators and counselors alike in various disciplines. This sixth edition maintains at least a third of these scholar's previous ideas from the fifth and earlier editions. We also would like to acknowledge Darlene Marini, who once again took on the tedious task of inputting the reference lists for certain chapters. Finally and most importantly, we acknowledge the select group of authors who have contributed to this sixth edition. Their expertise and field research elevates the social consciousness on disability studies. Similarly, we would like to thank the authors for their personal stories regarding the lived experience of having a disability or sharing a life with someone who is disabled. The six editions of this textbook would not have been as successful without these personal perspectives.

Irmo and Mark

I

Historical Perspectives on Illness and Disability: Introduction

*T*he first part of this book addresses disability more from a sociological or social psychological perspective, focusing on exploring disability from the outside looking inward. A major premise for contemporary scholars in the field has been to explore the impact the environment can have on the individual with a disability and his or her family. Somatopsychology and ecological and minority models of disability emphasize the positive and all too often negative psychosocial implications societal attitudes, physical barriers, and so on can have on persons with disabilities. As such, we feel it is best to first explore where we have been in these matters before we can proceed to discuss why and how persons with disabilities and/or their families respond, react, adjust, or adapt to their situations. The empirical literature over the past 25 years has documented a fairly consistent set of conclusions on this matter. Perceived negative societal attitudes and physical barriers in many, but not all, cases do negatively impact the self-concept and mental health of persons with disabilities. Conversely, positive societal attitudes and minimal barriers in many, but not all, cases lead to better adaptation for persons with disabilities.

Chapter 1 is new and reviews an embarrassing and mostly closeted history of how primarily Americans with disabilities and "different others" were viewed, treated, and mistreated over the past century. Fox and Marini explore the stark contrast between Emma Lazarus's Statue of Liberty engravings that note: "Give me your tired, your poor, your huddled masses yearning to breathe free, the wretched refuse of your teeming shore. Send these, the homeless, tempest-tost to me, I lift my lamp beside the golden door!" In many instances, U.S. immigration laws and various state laws enacted quite the opposite by excluding, detaining, and sterilizing thousands of persons deemed unfit to become Americans.

Chapter 2 revives a second edition original by Livneh, in his chapter, "On the Origins of Negative Attitudes Toward Disability," and explores why "typically developing" others or those without disabilities perceive persons with disabilities the way they do. What are the reasons why some people are anxious or afraid of people with disabilities? What are these misperceptions and how do they originate? Livneh explores both conscious and often subconscious human psyche mechanisms at work as to what the root causes of some of these societal perceptions entail.

Chapter 3 is new and deservedly receives its own discussion by Nguyen-Finn, separately exploring the historical treatment of persons with psychiatric disabilities in America. Perhaps more so than any other diagnosed disability, persons with psychiatric disabilities or mental illness have arguably been perceived and treated more harshly. From early beliefs of demonic possession, involuntary confinement in subhumane "institutions," prefrontal lobotomies and what can be today defined as torture, to current-day homelessness and prison incarceration undoubtedly places psychiatric disability in a category by itself. Nguyen-Finn chronicles this history and what happens to individuals when they are perceived as less than human.

Chapter 4 by Beaulaurier and Taylor provides a brief synopsis of some of the atrocities and mistreatment of people with disabilities historically, but spends much of the time regarding the civil rights pushback of this population in social work practice. Specifically, the authors explore the disability rights movement, traditional approaches to disability in health care settings, and the need for advocacy and self-empowerment of this population concerning lack of accommodations, as well as negative societal attitudes. The authors stress the need for rehabilitation professionals to philosophically operate from a disability rights perspective and the need to assist by self-empowering them as opposed to helping but facilitating learning helplessness.

Chapter 5 by Smart and Smart explore the four primary models of disability: the biomedical model, the functional model, the environmental model, and the sociopolitical model. Depending on one's frame of reference regarding disability, each model presents a philosophical and treatment approach to working with persons with disabilities that not only impacts rehabilitation professionals' attitudes but also their emphasis on how they go about counseling and/or treating their patients/clients. This framework often lays the foundation for how persons with disabilities interrelate with professionals as well.

Chapter 6, Beatrice Wright's classic article regarding changes in attitudes toward people with disabilities, aptly concludes Part I by noting the affirmation of human rights, and a synthesis of seven of her original 18 value-laden beliefs and principles regarding working with this population. The essence of these values and beliefs are guidelines for rehabilitation professionals that largely take into consideration treating others with dignity and respect, advocacy for the removal of environmental barriers, fundamental civil rights for all persons, and the importance of self-help organizations. Wright's 40-plus years as a leader in the field regarding the psychosocial aspects of disability provides tangible examples of assisting persons with disabilities in practice.

1

History of Treatment Toward Persons With Disabilities in America

DANIELLE D. FOX AND IRMO MARINI

*D*espite the common ideal that the United States is the land of opportunity, the early history of the United States was not necessarily a welcoming one for everyone. The fear of diluting the American bloodlines had a huge impact on public and governmental beliefs and attitudes. This fear, combined with the eugenics movement in the early 19th century, led American lawmakers to pass laws that specifically restricted certain people or groups from entering the United States and, within some city ordinances, even kept them out of public view. Early American lawmakers believed that by doing this, they were protecting the welfare of the country and Americans as a whole. The purpose of this chapter is to review the history of treatment toward people with disabilities (PWDs) in the United States.

"Give me your tired, your poor, your huddled masses yearning to breathe free, the wretched refuse of your teeming shore. Send these, the homeless, tempest-tosst to me …" (Lazarus, 1883). This is a section of the 14-line sonnet that is engraved on the Statue of Liberty in New York City. The statue was completed in 1886 and the verse actually inscribed on her in 1945. These words symbolized an American ideal against oppression to all immigrants who entered the United States during the early 20th century. In reality, however, American immigration legislation and practice during this time was in direct opposition to the Statue of Liberty engraving's intended message.

EARLY IMMIGRATION LEGISLATION

"It is often said, and with truth, that each of the different alien peoples coming to America has something to contribute to American civilization. But what America needs is desirable additions to, and not inferior substitutions for, what it already possesses" (Ward, 1924, p. 103). Early immigration literature and the apparent attitudes and treatment toward PWDs, as well as certain other immigrant populations, were blatantly prejudiced and discriminatory. Antidisability sentiment became more evident with immigration restriction, which began as early as the development of the first North American settlements. It was after 1838, when a large influx of immigrants came to the United States, that the issue of disability became more pressing to the early American settlers (Treadway, 1925).

Antidisability legislation began in 1882 and continued through 1924, with some of the original laws in effect until the 1980s. The concept behind early immigration legislation was to prevent the immigration of people who were considered undesirable. Early Americans believed that preventing people considered "undesirable" to enter the United States was a means of protecting not only the people of the United States but also the welfare of the country as a whole (Ward, 1907). Baynton (2005) states, "disability was a crucial factor in deciding whether or not an immigrant would be allowed to enter the United States" (p. 34). The term "undesirable" was used to describe people from any race, ethnicity, or religion, and/or with a disability, that are believed to be more likely to pass on less-than-desirable traits to their offspring. The purpose of early immigration legislation was to protect the American bloodlines, and according to early lawmakers, this meant excluding people based on any trait that could be considered as undesirable. Baynton (2005) states,

> One of the driving forces behind early federal immigration law, beginning with the first major Immigration Act in 1882, was the exclusion of people with mental and physical defects (as well as those considered criminal or immoral, problems seen at the time as closely related to mental defect). (p. 32)

This marked the beginning of the exclusion of PWDs in America.

In the years after 1882, early American lawmakers became more and more concerned about the bloodlines of immigrants seeking entrance into the United States and their possible effect on the bloodlines that were already present. With the 1891 revised Immigration Act, a key wording change made restrictions even more discretionary regarding excluding PWDs. Baynton (2005, p. 33) notes that the original 1882 law wording was "any lunatic, idiot, or any person *unable* to take care of himself or herself without becoming a public charge," changing the phrase in the 1891 law from "unable" to "*likely* to become a public charge." In 1894, the Immigration Restriction League (IRL) was established in Boston. The primary focus of the IRL was to "carry on a general educational campaign for more effective restriction and selection" (Ward, 1924, p. 102). According to Ward of the IRL, the league's fears were that the United States was becoming an "asylum for the poor and the oppressed of every land" (p. 100). Ward went on to explain:

> Americans began to realize that the ideal of furnishing an asylum for all the world's oppressed was coming into conflict with changed economic and social conditions. The cold facts were that the supply of public land was practically exhausted; that acute labor problems, aggravated by the influx of ignorant and unskilled aliens, had arisen; that the large cities were becoming congested with foreigners; that large numbers of mentally and physically unfit, and of the economically undesirable, had come to the United States. (p. 102)

As such, by 1896 literacy requirements were imposed on all immigrants entering the United States, and by 1903 through 1907, immigration laws were broadened and became more restrictive in scope. It was not until the 1917 revisions to the 1907 Immigration Act occurred that more specific and harsher discriminatory language appeared in legislation. Prior to this, however, in 1903, persons with epilepsy were added to the list, as well as the 1903 wording "persons who have been insane within five years previous [or] who have had two or more attacks of insanity at any time previously" (Baynton, p. 33). Treadway (1925) cites the exclusionary language of the law in the 1907 Act:

> The insane; idiots; imbeciles; feebleminded; chronic alcoholics; constitutional psychopathic inferiors; the mentally defective whose defect would modify their ability to earn a living; those with loathsome or dangerous contagious diseases, and those over sixteen years of age who were without a reading knowledge of some language. (p. 351)

The 1907 Act also was the first act where the law required a medical certificate for persons judged to be "mentally or physically defective, such mental or physical defect being of a nature which *may affect* the ability of such alien to earn a living" (Baynton, p. 33).

Subsequent years saw increasing restrictions, including financial penalties on transport companies and ship captains for the transportation of immigrants considered "unfit" for entry into the United States (Barkan, 1991; Baynton, 2005; Treadway, 1925). In an attempt to gain better control of the immigration situation, ship captains at ports of entry were to examine prospective immigrants for "defects." Although they were neither physicians or had any medical experience, the purpose of their inspections was to medically examine immigrants. If a disability, either mental or physical, was observed or perceived, the ship captain at transit or the inspector at entry ports was authorized to either deny departure from the immigrant's country of origin or deny entry into the United States. If an immigrant was granted departure from his or her country of origin and, upon arrival, entry into the United States was denied, the immigrant was to be deported back to his or her country of origin at the expense of the transport company that brought them (Baynton, 2005). For this reason, many ship captains in all likelihood denied numerous individuals for various vague reasons in order to not be fined or potentially lose their jobs. Baynton notes:

> Inspectors prided themselves on their ability to make a "snapshot diagnosis" as immigrants streamed past them single file. For most immigrants, a normal appearance usually meant an uneventful passage through the immigration station. An abnormal appearance, however, meant a chalked letter on the back. Once chalked, a closer inspection was required—L for lameness, K for suspected hernia, G for goiter, X for suspected mental illness, and so on. (p. 37)

This process allowed for the discrimination and/or refusal of immigrants based on suspected impairments whether or not any impairment was present. The commissioner general of immigration in his 1907 report regarding the governing immigration laws essentially laid out that the primary reason for the laws was to exclude anyone with a disability or anyone perceived as having a disability. The commissioner wrote, "The exclusion from this country of the morally, mentally, and physically deficient is the principal object to be accomplished by the immigration laws" (Baynton, p. 34). In order to exclude those with physical disabilities, the regulations stated that inspectors were to observe individuals at rest and then in motion to detect any irregularities or abnormalities in gait. Again, the wording for excluding individuals was vague and granted the inspectors full discretion in excluding anyone they wished. Baynton write about an Ellis Island medical inspector who's job was to "detect poorly built, defective or broken down human beings" (p. 34). A few examples of the physical impairments listed included spinal curvature, varicose veins, poor eyesight, hernia, flat feet, bunions, deafness, arthritis, hysteria and, simply, poor physical development. Once again, as with all age-old debates on eugenics, ethnocentricity, and exactly who are the weaker species, there was never any consensus.

During this period individuals were often excluded based on size or physical stature, or lack thereof, and abnormal sexual development. In addition, the commissioner and IRL, among others, were concerned about the public charge or becoming an economic drain due to perceived discrimination from employers in hiring. The surgeon general in a letter to the commissioner noted that such persons were:

> a bad economic risk . . . known to their associates who make them the butt of coarse jokes to their own despair, and to the impairment of the work in hand. Among employers, it is difficult for these unfortunates to get or retain jobs, their facial and bodily appearance at least in adult life, furnishing a patent advertisement of their condition. (Baynton, 2005, p. 38)

In all, it is difficult to determine exactly how many immigrants were excluded either prior to or upon entering the United States. Baynton (2005) cites statistics that increased over the years and notes that the actual numbers were likely much higher. The number of individuals excluded because they were likely to become a public charge or were mentally or physically defective in 1895 was 1,720, in 1905 the number was over 8,000, and by 1910 rose to over 16,000. Individuals from certain countries in particular were denied more often than others. Individuals from Slovakia were viewed as slow witted, Jews were seen as having poor physique and being neurotic, and those of Portuguese, Greek, or Syrian ethnicity were described as undersized (Baynton, 2005).

For those individuals who were somehow allowed entry to or were born in the United States with any type of perceived or real impairment, life was not generally favorable regarding societal attitudes. Specifically, Longmore and Goldberger (2000) noted court rulings where railroads and public transit systems were essentially granted permission to deny access to transportation for these impaired people. School laws were upheld segregating PWDs, not alllowing them to attend school, or they we taught in a segregated room. Employers were also permitted to discriminate in hiring those with disabilities, and all public venues such as restaurants, theaters, and so on could deny access and frequently did so. For all intents and purposes, many of those with disabilities during the early 20th century were relegated to being shut-ins in their own homes, and when venturing out, were subject to ridicule and indignant comments.

PWDs were outraged by political and societal attitudes and the blatant efforts to prejudice and discriminate against them. For many, it was not only the negative attitudes of being devalued and dehumanized but also the discrimination of being excluded from the workforce. Longmore and Goldberger (2000) cite the historic accounts during the spring of 1935, after five years of the Great Depression, where a number of persons with physical and other disabilities demanded their voices be heard and protested against New York City's Emergency Relief Bureau demanding jobs. Forming the League of the Physically Handicapped (LPH), this group focused on discrimination issues as opposed to their medical impairments. Media coverage back then was also largely discriminatory and prejudice. Longmore and Goldberger cite how media and popular culture portrayals during the 1920s and 1930s perceived PWDs as villains, victims, sinners, charity cases, unsightly objects, dangerous denizens of society, and unworthy citizens (p. 896).

Franklin D. Roosevelt was a member of the LPH, and although he largely hid his own paralysis from polio at age 39, he strived for the rehabilitation of those with disabilities. He epitomized what persons with a disability "can" do and is arguably one of America's greatest presidents, having presided for 12 years over troubling times including the Great Depression, the signing of the 1935 Social Security Act, and being the successful Commander and Chief through World War II (Gallagher, 1994). In his book titled *FDR's Splendid Deception,* Gallagher cites how Roosevelt was intuitively aware of the negative societal attitudes toward disability and aware that if the public knew of both the extent of his disability and chronic pain, he would be perceived as a weak, ineffective leader. As such, Roosevelt had agreements with the media not to photograph or film him in his wheelchair or while ambulating with his leg braces. Ironically, he did not really have a disability agenda and in fact tried to reduce vocational rehabilitation funding by 25%, which was ultimately not supported by Congress (Gallagher, 1994).

THE EUGENICS MOVEMENT IN AMERICA

Driving the early immigration acts ideology was Charles Darwin's 1859 book *The Origin of Species by Means of Natural Selection or the Preservation of Favored Races in the Struggle of Life*, which initially set out to explain the concept of heredity in plants and animals. Darwin refrained from applying his beliefs to humans out of fear of the reaction from the ruling religions. Sir Francis Galton, a cousin of Darwin's, whose own studies primarily focused on mathematics and meteorology, was inspired by Darwin's work and the implications of it. Galton applied mathematics to the study of heredity as a whole, and through this application Galton established not only some of the techniques of modern statistics but also the basis for what he later called "eugenics" (Pearson, 1995). Galton, who coined the term "eugenics" in 1883, believed that natural selection could rid mankind of problems such as disease, criminality, alcoholism, and poverty (Farrall, 1978). Farrall states that when Galton introduced the word "eugenics" in 1883 he did so with the following explanation:

> We greatly want a brief word to express the science of improving stock, which is by no means confined to questions of judicious mating, but which, especially in the case of man, takes cognizance of all influences that tend in however remote a degree to give to the more suitable races or strains of blood a better chance of prevailing speedily over the less suitable than they otherwise would have had. The word eugenics sufficiently expresses the idea; it is at least a neater word and a more generalized one than viriculture which I once ventured to use. (p. 112)

The concept of eugenics reached America around 1900, and many prominent politicians, physicians, and academics in the United States agreed with Galton's premise of essentially restricting the promulgation of those considered the weaker of the species. The notion of protecting and preserving healthy American bloodlines for the betterment of future generations was idealistic in theory and would later prove extremely difficult to implement. The central question contemplated for these powerful and predominantly Caucasian White males was to decide who exactly was the weaker species, and how exactly could these undesirables be restricted from bearing children (Marini, 2011a). President Theodore Roosevelt also embraced eugenics in the United States along with other highly influential people such as Alexander Graham Bell, John Harvey Kellogg, and J.C. Penny to name a few (Pearson, 1995).

STERILIZATION IN THE UNITED STATES

Evidence of eugenic ideals became more obvious with the passage of sterilization laws in the early 20th century, the primary goal of which was to "improve the quality of the nation's citizenry by reducing the birth rate of individuals they considered to be 'feebleminded' " (Largent, 2002, p. 190). The term "feebleminded" was used at this time to describe anyone with any type of observed or perceived mental or physical disability. Eugenics continued to gain strength and support through the first quarter of the 20th century with 27 of the 48 states adopting sterilization laws (Farrall, 1979). The state of Indiana was at the forefront of the sterilization movement, being the first to implement eugenic sterilization laws in 1907.

Although the first sterilization law was passed in 1907, Osgood (2001) noted that unauthorized sterilization of the so-called defectives had already occurred in institutions in several states as early as the 1890s (p. 257). In 1909, the state of Oregon implemented eugenic sterilization laws, five years after Dr. Bethenia Owens-Adair had proposed sterilization in Oregon as a means of dealing with persons considered to be criminals and/or insane (Largent, 2002). Noll (2005) reports that the use of intelligence testing in the 1920s allowed medical and mental health doctors to more accurately identify "feeblemindedness." As the years progressed, more states adopted eugenic sterilization laws, and as the United States entered World War II, the nation's state mental health and prison authorities reported over 38,000 sterilizations (Largent, 2002, p. 192). In the 1920s, the most notable Supreme Court sterilization case was *Buck v. Bell*. In 1927, Carrie Buck, a 17-year-old Virginia girl became pregnant and was institutionalized by her foster parents in the

Virginia State Colony for Epileptics and Feeble-Minded. Carrie's mother had already been committed and was deemed feebleminded and subsequently sterilized. Because Carrie's mother was deemed feebleminded, Carrie was also deemed feebleminded and was sterilized as well. Carrie had a younger sister who, under the pretence that she was undergoing an appendectomy, was also sterilized as a result of her mother's perceived mental capacity. Although there was no evidence to the accusations that Carrie Buck was promiscuous, the case went to the U.S. Supreme Court where Judge Oliver Wendell Holmes, Jr. reported in an 8–1 decision, that the state of Virginia was supported by its sterilization law and further stated, "three generations of imbeciles are enough" (Carlson, 2009, p. 178). The case of Carrie Buck was not an isolated incident at the time, and although other cases similar in nature were found in other states to be unconstitutional, *Buck v. Bell* was never overturned. Despite the injustice associated with forced sterilization of people considered to be developmentally disabled, mentally ill, or simply criminals, sterilization laws lasted well into the 1980s in some states (Largent, 2002). While there was a focus on eugenic sterilization laws, other laws that specifically targeted persons with mental and physical disabilities were being passed.

THE UGLY LAWS

Any person who is diseased, maimed, mutilated or in any way deformed so as to be an unsightly or disgusting object, or an improper person to be allowed in or on the streets, highways, thoroughfares or public places in this city shall not therein or thereon expose himself or herself to public view under penalty of one dollar for each offense. On the conviction of any person for a violation of this section, if it shall seem proper and just, the fine provided for may be suspended, and such person detained at the police station, where he shall be well cared for, until he can be committed to the county poor house. (Coco, 2010)

This is a City of Chicago ordinance, originally passed in 1881. Unsightly beggar ordinances passed between the years 1867 and 1913 were otherwise known as "Ugly Laws." The first unsightly beggar ordinance was passed in San Francisco in 1867. Although these ordinances had been in place for 14 years prior to the passage of the Chicago ordinance, it is the most well known and considered "the most egregious example of discrimination against people with physical disabilities in the United States" (Coco, 2010, p. 23). The passing of these ordinances and laws allowed some insight into how disability was perceived. PWDs were generally thought of as burdens to society and lacked the ability to care for themselves or contribute in any way to society. This perception, however, was largely contingent upon one's social standing and contribution to society (Schweik, as cited in Coco, 2010). While unsightly beggar ordinances were commonplace in cities throughout the country, Chicago's unsightly beggar ordinance remained on the law books until 1973 (Coco, 2010).

Returning soldiers with various disabilities from World War II, however, was a good example of how some PWDs were perceived. For example, soldiers were often viewed with sympathy but were nevertheless respected because of their contribution, whereas a civilian born with a disability would often not be perceived in the same way. The Industrial Revolution in the United States further increased the number of Americans with disabilities, as factory workers began to sustain injuries leading to chronic conditions. Without effective workers compensation laws early on, injured workers had to sue their employers, with the vast majority often losing their suits for contributory negligence and for knowingly accepting the hazards of the job, otherwise known as "assumption of risk" (Marini, 2011b).

For some PWDs with facial or physical deformities, performing in circus freak shows became the only employment they could obtain. These PWDs appeared to be more highly regarded and were often considered to be prominent citizens despite the fact that in certain parts of the United States, where Ugly Laws were adopted, they were unable to show themselves in public.

MOVEMENT TOWARD EQUALITY

As disability discrimination and sterilization laws were being passed concerning PWDs, helpful legislation was also being passed. The 1920s brought about the Smith-Fees Act (P.L. 66–236), allowing services to PWDs such as vocational guidance, occupational adjustment, and placement services. In 1935 the Social Security Act (P.L. 74–271) was passed and the State-Federal Vocational Rehabilitation Program was established as a permanent program (Parker, Szymanski, & Patterson, 2005). Despite this early legislation and numerous additional laws over time designed to protect and employ PWDs in the workforce, the unemployment rate for PWDs has dismally held at around 70%. Yelin (1991) noted that the lowest unemployment rate for PWDs was actually during World War II since many able-bodied Americans were involved in the war and manufacturing jobs for the war effort increased dramatically. Once the war was over, however, men and women in the armed services returned home and thousands of workers with disabilities were displaced. There was a shift in who was entering the workforce in the United States (Longmore & Goldberger, 2000).

The year 1943 marked the passage of landmark legislation with the Vocational Rehabilitation Act Amendments (P.L. 113), essentially increasing the amount of state vocational services available to PWDs (Parker et al., 2005). The Vocational Rehabilitation Act Amendments also broadened the definition of disability, allowing persons with mental illness or psychiatric disabilities to be eligible for services. Disability rights continued to make progress for the next 30 years, without much fanfare, but unemployment rates remained relatively the same.

The 1973 Rehabilitation Act was also considered to be landmark legislation for PWDs, especially since President Nixon was considering abolishing the State-Federal Vocational Rehabilitation program altogether. After much debate and considerable outcry from disability groups, President Nixon signed into law what is believed to be the first civil rights laws for PWDs from which the 1990 Americans with Disabilities Act (ADA) was designed. Again, there was increased funding for public vocational rehabilitation programs and affirmative action in the hiring of federal employees (Parker et al., 2005). Sections 501–504 of the act also addressed access to transportation, removal of architectural barriers, and physical access to all newly constructed federal buildings. Perhaps, one of the most criticized aspects of the 1973 Act was the fact that there was no enforcement entity designed to check whether policies were being followed.

In 1975, the Rehabilitation Act was combined with the Education for All Handicapped Children Act (P.L. 94–142), now known as the Individuals with Disabilities Education Act or IDEA. IDEA allowed for opportunities such as equal access to public education for all children with disabilities in the least restrictive environment. IDEA also allowed for children with disabilities to be tested through multiple means, such as being tested in their native language. The law also gave parents the right to view their children's school records (Olkin, 1999). The 1986 revision of IDEA extended services to provide early intervention for children from birth to preschool, help with equipment purchases, and legal assistance to families with children with disabilities (Olkin, 1999).

Perhaps the single most important legislation to date concerning the civil rights of PWDs was the 1990 passage of the ADA by President George H. W. Bush. The act contains five titles: employment, extended access to state and federal government services including public or paratransit transportation access, public accommodations for physical access to all public venues (e.g., restaurants, theaters, sporting events), access to telecommunications (e.g., closed captioning, theater audio loops), and a miscellaneous title. The ADA has arguably been deemed a success as far as making communities more accessible; however, there continues to be complaints and lawsuits filed daily due to employers and businesses that continue to knowingly or unknowingly discriminate (Blackwell, Marini, & Chacon, 2001). Some PWDs continue to see the glass as half empty regarding physical access and societal attitudes; others see it as half full (Marini, 2001).

CURRENT PULSE ON AMERICA REGARDING DISABILITY

Attitudes, physical access, and the laws regarding PWDs have unquestionably improved in the last century. The eugenics movement essentially died down after World War II, primarily due to Social Darwinism and the Nazi extermination of an estimated 250,000 German citizens and war veterans with disabilities (Marini, 2011a). In America, many eugenicists realized that this extremist version was essentially a slippery slope and that the continued forced sterilization and forbidding those with epilepsy, mental illness, or mental retardation from marrying, could potentially lead them down a similar path.

Current attitudes of Americans without disabilities toward those with disabilities suggest contradictory sentiments of both admiration and pity (Harris, 1991). Most likely influenced by media portrayals, the admiration sentiment can be easily explained when we watch a documentary on FDR, Wilma Rudolf, Christopher Reeve, or Stephen Hawking. Conversely, the pity sentiment occurs when one watches any televised charitable event, particularly *Jerry's Kids–Muscular Dystrophy* Labor Day telethon. Although Americans generally believe that it is right to hire a qualified individual with a disability, many non-disabled persons still believe that PWDs are fundamentally "different" from those without disabilities (Harris, 1991).

As previously noted, how much better conditions and attitudes toward those with disabilities have gotten is open to debate. Although many outside observers anecdotally will argue that PWDs get free benefits and health care without making a contribution to society, others are quick to point out a different reality. Specifically, with an approximate 65% unemployment rate and two-thirds of those with disabilities indicating they would work if they could, this population has one of the highest poverty rates in America (Rubin & Roessler, 2008). Single minority females with children having a disability have the highest rate of poverty.

Although physical barriers and community access have improved exponentially since the 1990 ADA, several studies of persons with physical disabilities suggest that the United States still has a long way to go to become barrier free. Specifically, two recent studies have found that even 22 years after the ADA was signed into law, persons with physical disabilities still cite physical access barriers as the number-one frustration (Graf, Marini, & Blankenship, 2009; Marini, Bhakta, & Graf, 2009). Negative societal attitudes were not far behind in the rankings.

Eugenics has taken a different form in the twenty-first century. Today, scientists are improving medical technology to remove the so-called defective genes responsible for various neuromuscular diseases while an unborn fetus is still in the embryo stage (Marini, 2011a). Likewise, parents are now able to abort a fetus that may result in a child having a developmental disability and essentially start over. Designer babies are also on the horizon when parents will be able to select eye and hair color. In one extreme example of the quest for the perfect human, a playboy photographer auctioned off a supermodel's egg and 5 million people visited the website in one morning, offering $42,000 for the egg (Smart, 2009).

The survival-of-the-fittest concept and natural selection in the 21st century appear to have morphed into a survival of the financially fittest ideology. The ramifications of the 2008 great recession, continual middle-class decline into poverty, and historical government reaction recoil to cut social programs like Social Security, Medicare, and Medicaid, ultimately leaving those who need the most assistance to fend for themselves (Huffington, 2010; Reich, 2010). With the aging of America and millions of baby boomers moving into their golden years, their financial portfolio will dictate what the quality of their lives will entail like no time ever before in American history. Although Americans are living longer and healthier lives, those with disabilities and little income may face even greater precarious times ahead.

REFERENCES

Barkan, E. (1991). Reevaluating progressive eugenics: Herbert Spencer Jennings and the 1924 immigration legislation. *Journal of the History of Biology, 24*(1), 91–112.

Baynton, D. (2005). Defectives in the land: Disability and American immigration policy, 1882–1924. *Journal of American Ethnic History, 24*(30), 31–44.

Blackwell, T. M., Marini, I., Chacon, M. (2001). The impact of the Americans with Disabilities Act on independent living. *Rehabilitation Education, 15*(4), 395–408.

Carlson, E. (2009). Three generations, no imbeciles: Eugenics, the Supreme Court, and *Buck v. Bell. The Quarterly Review of Biology, 84*(2), 178–180.

Coco, A. (2010). Diseased, maimed, mutilated: Categorizations of disability and ugly law in late nineteenth-century Chicago. *Journal of Social History.*

Farrall, L. (1979). The history of eugenics: A bibliographical review. *Annals of Science, 36*(2), 111–123.

Gallagher, H. G. (1994). *FDR's splendid deception.* Arlington, TX: Vandamere.

Graf, N. M., Marini, I., & Blankenship, C. (2009). 100 words about disability. *Journal of Rehabilitation, 75*(2), 25–34.

Harris, L. (1991). *Public attitudes toward persons with disabilities.* New York: Lou Harris and Associates.

Huffington, A. (2010). *Third World America: How our politicians are abandoning the middle class and betraying the American dream.* New York: Crown Publishers.

Largent, M. (2002). The greatest curse of the race: Eugenic sterilization in Oregon 1909–1983. *Oregon Historical Quarterly, 103*(2), 188–209.

Lazarus, E. (1883). The New Colossus (1883). Retrieved from http://xroads.virginia.edu/~CAP/LIBERTY/lazarus.html

Longmore, P., & Goldberger, D. (2000). The league of the physically handicapped and the great depression: A case study in the new disability history. *Journal of American History* (December) 888–922.

Marini, I. (2001). ADA continues to be tested and tweaked. *SCI Psychosocial Process, 13*(2), 69–70.

Marini, I. (2011a). The history of treatment towards persons with disabilities. In I. Marini, N. M. Glover-Graf, & M. J. Millington (Eds.), *Psychosocial aspects of disability: Insider perspectives and counseling strategies* (pp. 3–32). New York: Springer.

Marini, I. (2011b). The psychosocial world of the injured worker. In I. Marini, N. M. Glover-Graf, & M. J. Millington (Eds.), *Psychosocial aspects of disability: Insider perspectives and counseling strategies* (pp. 235–255). New York: Springer.

Marini, I., Bhakta, M. V., & Graf, N. (2009). A content analysis of common concerns of persons with physical disabilities. *Journal of Applied Rehabilitation Counseling, 40*(1), 44–49.

Noll, S. (2005). The public face of southern institutions for the "feeble-minded." *The Public Historian, 27*(2), 25–41.

Olkin, R. (1999). *What psychotherapists should know about disability.* New York: The Guilford Press.

Osgood, R. (2001). The menace of the feebleminded: George Bliss, Amos Butler, and the Indiana Committee on mental defectives. *Indiana Magazine of History, 97*(4), 253–277.

Parker, R., Szymanski, E., & Patterson, B. (2005). *Rehabilitation counseling: Basics and beyond* (4th ed.). Austin, Texas: Pro.Ed.

Reich, R. B. (2010). *Aftershock: The next economy and America's future.* New York: Alfred A. Knopf.

Rubin, S. E., & Roessler, R. T. (2008). Philosophical and economic considerations in regard to disability rights and support for rehabilitation programs. In S. E. Rubin & R. T. Roessler (Eds.), *Foundations of the vocational rehabilitation process* (pp. 143–165). Austin, TX: Pro Ed.

2

On the Origins of Negative Attitudes Toward People With Disabilities

Hanoch Livneh

*I*n the past quarter of a century, several attempts have been made to categorize the different sources of negative attitudes toward individuals with disabling conditions. Among these attempts, the works of Gellman (1959), Raskin (1956), Siller, Ferguson, and Vann (1967), and Wright (1960) are often singled out. In addition, a plethora of theoretical and empirical work has been directed toward the narrower goal of advancing and supporting a specific cause (often referred to as *root* or *base*) for negative attitudes toward disability (see Goffman, 1963; Meng, 1938; Parsons, 1951; Schilder, 1935).

The main objective of the current chapter is twofold: to integrate the major approaches in the domain of attitudinal sources toward people with disabilities, and to offer a new classification system by which these attitudes can be better conceptualized and understood.

Of the four main classifications, earlier attempts by Raskin (1956) and Gellman (1959) were more narrowly conceived. Both offered a fourfold classification system for the roots of prejudicial attitudes toward those who are blind (Raskin) and those who are disabled in general (Gellman). Raskin perceived these attitudes to be determined by psychodynamic, situational, sociocultural, and historical factors. Gellman, on the other hand, viewed the prejudicial roots as stemming from social customs and norms, child-rearing practices, recrudescence of neurotic childhood fears in frustrating and anxiety-provoking situations, and discrimination-provoking behavior by persons with disabilities.

Wright (1960), in a comprehensive literature review, discussed attitudes toward atypical physique according to the following categories: general requiredness of cause–effect relations (i.e., phenomenal causality between certain "sinful behaviors" and disability as an "unavoidable punishment"), negative reaction to the different and strange, childhood experiences, and prevailing socioeconomic factors. Siller et al. (1967), based on their extensive attitudinal study, reported the existence of 13 aversive content categories toward those with disabilities, utilizing both empirical and clinical findings. Their discussion, however, often confuses components of attitudinal correlates (such as functional limitations or attribution of negative qualities) with attitudinal sources (e.g., aesthetic-sexual aversion, fear it could happen to self).

The present chapter attempts to deal exclusively with attitudinal sources. In other words, only approaches—both theoretical and empirical—that can be perceived in terms of cause (attitudinal source or root) and effect (negative or aversive reaction or attitude) relationships will be dealt with. Also, the classification system of the different attitudinal

From *Rehabilitation Literature,* 43 (11-12) (1982), 338–347. Reprinted with permission. Published by the National Easter Seal Society, Chicago, IL.

sources combines both process- (psychodynamic mechanisms) and content- (sociocultural factors) related formulations. It was felt that any attempt to separate the two would be rather arbitrary.

SOCIOCULTURAL CONDITIONING

Pervasive social and cultural norms, standards, and expectations often lead to the creation of negative attitudes toward the disabled population. Among the frequently mentioned contributing factors are:

1. Emphasis on concepts such as "body beautiful," "body whole," youth, health, athletic prowess, personal appearance, and wholeness: These highly stressed societal standards are often institutionalized into cultural customs, which are to be conformed to by members of society (Gellman, 1959; Roessler & Bolton, 1978; Wright, 1960).

2. Emphasis on personal productiveness and achievement: Individuals in most Western countries are judged on the basis of their ability to be socially and economically competitive (Hanks & Hanks, 1948; Safilios-Rothschild, 1968).

3. Prevailing socioeconomic level: The importance of socioeconomic factors in creating an atmosphere within which attitudes toward individuals with disabilities are often nourished was emphasized by Safilios-Rothschild (1968). The level of societal development (Jordan & Friesen, 1968), the rate of unemployment, beliefs concerning the origins of poverty, and the importance attached to the nation's welfare economy and security are all contributing factors affecting attitudes toward people with disabilities.

4. Society's delineation of the "sick role" phenomenon: Whereas the occupant of the "sick role" is exempt from normal societal obligations and responsibilities, the length of a disabled person's remaining in this role is associated with negative attitudes (Parsons, 1951, 1958; Thoreson & Kerr, 1978).

5. The status degradation attached to disability: The social deviance and inferred stigma of having a physical disability bear heavily on society's attitudes toward those affected (see Davis, 1961; Freidson, 1965; Goffman, 1963; Safilios-Rothschild, 1970; Wolfensberger, 1972, 1976; Worthington, 1974; Yamamato, 1971). The cultural values held by members of society are often based on the perception of any form of "imputed deviancy," including disability, as a sign of marginal status. The person with a disability is, therefore, viewed as an "outsider," an "offender," or as "different" (Barker, 1948; Gove, 1976; Kutner, 1971). Wolfensberger (1972, 1976) regards the devalued or deviant status as a negative role imposed on the stigmatized person and views the sources of this deviancy as stemming from physical, behavioral, and attribution-based characteristics. Yamamato (1971) goes as far as to suggest that society needs the deviates as a symbol of evil and intangible dangers.

CHILDHOOD INFLUENCES

The importance of infancy and early childhood experiences, in terms of both child-rearing practices and early parental influences (verbal and behavioral), is often stressed (Gellman, 1959; Wright, 1960). The impact of early experiences and their related emotions and cognitions have a major role in influencing the growing child's belief and value system. Parental and significant others' actions, words, tone of voice, gestures, and so forth are transmitted, directly or indirectly, to the child and tend to have a crucial impact on the formation of attitudes toward disability.

Rearing practices which emphasize the importance of health and normalcy, and which threaten any infringement of health rules with sickness, illness, and long-term disability, result in aversion toward individuals who are affected (Gellman, 1959; Wright, 1960). Childhood stages of development (oral, anal, phallic, and genital) are wrought with anxiety-laden premises regarding the etiology of certain illnesses; therefore, the association with ongoing disabilities and disabled persons, as past transgressors, is readily made.

PSYCHODYNAMIC MECHANISMS

Several mainly unconscious psychological processes have been advanced in the literature as explanatory mechanisms for the attitudes manifested by the "nondisabled" toward the "disabled." Although most of these mechanisms are apparently sown during early childhood (Gellman, 1959; Siller et al. 1967; Yamamato, 1971) and may, therefore, be regarded as related to childhood experiences, it was felt that due to their significance in creating and maintaining these attitudes such a separation is warranted.

1. *Requirement of mourning.* The person with a disability is expected to grieve the loss of a body part or function. He or she "ought" to suffer and slowly adjust to such a misfortune (Dembo, Leviton, & Wright, 1956, 1975; Kutner, 1971; Sussman, 1969; Thoreson & Kerr, 1978; Wright, 1960). The nondisabled individual has a need to safeguard his or her values, by wanting the disabled individual to suffer, and show the appropriate grieving, so as to protect one's own values of the importance of a functioning body (Dembo et al., 1956, 1975). Any attempt on the disabled person's part to deny or reject the "suffering role" is met with negative attitudes. The mechanism of rationalization is clearly operative in this case.

2. *Unresolved conflict over scopophilia and exhibitionism.* Psychoanalytic thought stresses the importance of vision in early psychosexual and ego development (Blank, 1957). The significance of sight, both in terms of pleasure of looking at and being looked upon in the pregenital stages, is stressed in the psychoanalytic literature. Any resolved conflicts related to these developmental stages may be triggered as a consequence of the approach/fascination–avoidance/repulsion conflict often associated with the sight of a disabled person.

3. Negative attributes resulting from the "spread phenomenon." Attributing to those with disabilities, certain negative characteristics frequently result when the mechanism of "halo effect" or "spread phenomenon" is in operation (Wright, 1960). The generalization from one perceived characteristic (e.g., physical disability) to other, unrelated characteristics (e.g., emotional or mental maladjustment) is referred to as "spread" and explains the too often pervasive negative correlates of a pure physical deviance (Kutner, 1971; Thoreson & Kerr, 1978).

4. Associating responsibility with etiology. The attribution of personal–moral accountability to the cause of a disabling condition results in negative attitudes. If an individual can be held responsible for an imputed deviance, certain social management approaches are then suggested (punishment, control, "rehabilitation," correction, etc.), which are frequently embedded with negative connotations (Freidson, 1965; Safilios-Rothschild, 1970; Yamamato, 1971). Again, the operation of a rationalization mechanism is evident here.

5. Fear of social ostracism. Siller et al. (1967) suggest this category as an extension of the "guilty by association" phenomenon. The nondisabled person fears that an association with disabled persons may be interpreted by others as implying some psychological maladjustment on his or her own part. The internalization of others' values and beliefs, which tends to weaken one's ego boundaries, coupled with projection onto others of unwanted personal attributes, is the main operating mechanism.

6. Guilt of being "able-bodied." Guilt of "enjoying" one's body intactness in addition to possible injustices directed toward persons with disabilities (e.g., the belief in the disabled person's responsibility for the condition, lack of involvement in charitable activities) may result in attempts at atonement or further dissociation from the presence of disabled individuals (Siller et al., 1967; Wright, 1960).

DISABILITY AS A PUNISHMENT FOR SIN

The triad of sin, punishment, and disability can be conceived as a component of the earlier discussion of psychodynamic mechanisms operating in the creation of aversive reactions toward disability. Due to their importance in elucidating the roots of negative attitudes toward people with disabling conditions and the various versions of their interrelatedness which are advanced in the literature, it seems justifiable to treat these concepts under a separate heading.

1. Disability as a punishment for sin. Alexander's (1938) concept of "emotional syllogism," when applied here (Siller et al., 1967; Wright, 1960), stresses the consequential appropriateness between physical deformity and a sinful person. The source of the disabled person's suffering is attributed to either a personally committed evil act or to an ancestral wrongdoing (Sigerist, 1945).

2. The individual with a disability as a dangerous person. Meng (reported in Barker, Wright, Meyerson, & Gonick, 1953) attributed fear and avoidance of those who are physically disabled to three unconscious mechanisms: (a) the belief that a disability is a punishment for a transgression and, therefore, that the disabled person is evil and dangerous; (b) the belief that a disability is an unjust punishment and that, therefore, the person is motivated to commit an evil act to balance the injustice; and (c) the projection of one's unacceptable impulses upon the disabled person, which results in perceiving the latter as evil and dangerous (see also Siller et al., 1967; Thoreson & Kerr, 1978). Thus, whereas in the previous section suffering was perceived as being a punishment for an evil deed, in the present section physical deviance is viewed as the cause, the consequence of which is felt to be a sinful and evil act ("a twisted mind in a twisted body").

3. The nondisabled person fearing imminent punishment. If the notion of disability as a punishment is warranted, then the nondisabled person who anticipates, often realistically, retribution for past personal misdeeds avoids the person with disabilities because of guilt of not being punished or the fear of imminent punishment by association (Gellman, 1959).

4. Vicarious self-punishment offered by the punished disabled person. An extension of the above formula was offered by Thurer (1980). The sinning disabled person, in fiction or reality, is perceived to be an easy target for one's own projections. Because the disabled individual was punished for the sin committed and since the nondisabled person unconsciously identifies with the sin, he or she is also punished, albeit vicariously, and the felt guilt is, therefore, lessened. The externalization of one's inner conflicts upon a punished target assists in controlling them. The result is, therefore, the repelling-gratifying conflict of feelings that ensues as a result of seeing, hearing, or reading about a disabled individual.

ANXIETY-PROVOKING UNSTRUCTURED SITUATIONS

The role of unfamiliar situations in creating anxiety and confusion was stressed by Hebb (1946) and Heider (1944). Similarly, upon initial interaction with a disabled person, the nondisabled person is often faced with an unstructured situation in which most socially accepted rules and regulations for proper interaction are not well-defined. These ambiguous situations tend to disrupt both cognitive–intellectual processes as well as the more fundamental perceptual–affective mechanisms.

1. Cognitively unstructured situations. The nondisabled person interacting with a disabled individual faces uncertain social outcomes engendered by the new and, therefore, cognitively vague situation (Heider, 1958). The unfamiliarity presents an incongruent cognitive gestalt which disrupts the established basic rules of social interaction and may cause withdrawal from such a situation (Yamamato, 1971) or create strain in this interaction (Siller et al., 1967). The often reported findings in the literature—that the lack of factual knowledge and information about disabling conditions tends to lead to negative attitudes (Anthony, 1972; English, 1971a, 1971b; English & Oberle, 1971)—also support this contention.
2. Lack of affective preparedness. There is an apparent fearful and negative reaction, on a visceral level, to the different and strange (Hebb, 1946; Heider, 1958; Siller et al., 1967). Strange and mutilated bodies trigger a conflict in the observer because of incompatible perceptions (Hebb, 1946). People tend to resist the strange because it does not fit into the structure of an expected life space (Heider, 1958) and because of a lack of affective readiness (Worthington, 1974; Yamamato, 1971). Siller et al. (1967) perceived it to exemplify their negative atypicality category, which creates in the observer a feeling of distress. Lack of experiential contact and exposure to persons with disabilities is a contributing factor to the origination of such an attitude (Anthony, 1972; English 1971a, 1971b).

AESTHETIC AVERSION

The impact of a purely aesthetic-sexual aversion, triggered by the sight of a visibly disabled person, has been stressed by several authors (Heider, 1958; Siller & Chipman, 1964; Siller et al., 1967). These feelings of repulsion and discomfort are felt when nondisabled persons come in contact with certain disabilities (such as amputations, body deformities, cerebral palsy, skin disorders [Richardson, Hastorf, Goodman, & Dornbusch, 1961; Safilios-Rothschild, 1970; Siller, 1963]). The importance of aesthetic-sexual aversion as a basis for negative attitudinal formation was also reported in Siller et al.'s (1967) study, in which the felt aversion referred to the direct and conscious reactions experienced on sensory and visceral levels. The role played by aesthetic attractiveness was also demonstrated by Napoleon, Chassin, and Young (1980) as a predisposing factor in judging a person's degree of mental illness.

THREATS TO BODY IMAGE INTEGRITY

The concept of body image, as the mental representation of one's own body, was originally coined by Schilder (1935). Several related formulations were proposed regarding the importance of the body image concept (i.e., self-image, body cathexis, and body satisfaction) as an explanatory vehicle in understanding attitudes toward people with disabilities.

1. Threat to the body image. Schilder (1935) argued that, via the mechanism of identification, seeing a person with a physical disability creates a feeling of discomfort because of the incongruence between an expected "normal" body and the actual perceived reality. The viewer's own unconscious and somatic body image may, therefore, be threatened due to the presence of the disabled individual (Menninger, 1949).
2. Reawakening of castration anxiety. The psychoanalytic concept of castration anxiety, as applied to explaining the formation of negative attitudes toward persons with disabilities, stresses the stirring up of archaic castration fears in the presence of analogous situations (such as direct loss of a leg or an eye or an indirect loss of a certain body function [Chevigny & Braverman, 1950; Fine, 1978; Maisel, 1953; Siller et al., 1967; Wright, 1960]).
3. Fear of losing one's physical integrity. Profound anxiety about becoming disabled plays a crucial part in forming prejudicial attitudes toward those who are. When faced with a disabled person, the nondisabled individual becomes highly anxious because the original fear of potential bodily harm is rekindled (Safilios-Rothschild, 1968, 1970). Roessler and Bolton (1978), capitalizing on Gellman's (1959) original discussion, believe that nondisabled persons, being fearful of disablement and loss of self-control, feel intense discomfort which arouses additional anxiety when in contact with a visibly disabled person. The result is avoidance of disabled persons and attempts at segregating and isolating them. Similar ideas were advanced by Siller et al. (1967), who viewed the fear that the disability could happen to oneself as a basis for an aversive attitude toward people who are disabled.
4. Separation anxiety. Although somewhat related to castration anxiety and fear of losing physical integrity, separation anxiety, in the sense of object loss, is another unconscious source leading to negative attitudes toward disability (Siller et al., 1967). The loss of a body part or function may trigger, in the viewer, narcissistic concerns and unresolved infantile anxieties, which often evolve around possible separation from parental figures (Siller, 1964a).
5. Fear of contamination or inheritance. The fear that social interaction with disabled people may lead to contamination provokes aversive attitudes (Siller et al., 1967). This refers to avoiding those with disabilities on both superficial interactive levels (social intercourse) and more in-depth relationships (marriage, having children, etc.).

MINORITY GROUP COMPARABILITY

The view that attitudes toward the disabled population parallel those manifested toward minority groups, in general, was advocated by Barker et al. (1953) and further elaborated on by Wright (1960). This view holds that disabled people, as a marginal group (Barker, 1948; Sussman, 1969), trigger negative reactions in the nondisabled majority. Being perceived as marginal, or as a member of a minority group, carries with it the same stereotypic reactions of occupying a devalued and inferior status shared by ethnic, racial, and religious groups (Chesler, 1965; Cowen, Bobrove, Rockway, & Stevenson, 1967; Cowen, Underberg, & Verrillo, 1958; Yuker, 1965). The resulting attitude can, therefore, be categorized as being discriminatory and prejudiced in nature, and as advocating isolation and segregation of disabled persons from the remaining population (Safilios-Rothschild, 1970; Wright, 1960).

DISABILITY AS A REMINDER OF DEATH

The parallelism between reactions toward those who are disabled and feelings associated with dying (anxiety, fear, dread) was suggested by several authors (Endres, 1979; Leviton,

Smart, J. (2009). *Disability, society, and the individual*. Austin, TX: Pro Ed.

The U.S. Equal Employment Opportunity Commission. Retrieved from http://www.eeoc.gov/policy/docs/quanda_adaaa_nprm.html

Treadway, W. (1925). Our immigration policy and the nation's mental health. *The Scientific Monthly, 21*(4), 347–354.

Ward, R. (1907). The new immigration act. *The North American Review, 185*(619) 587–593.

Ward, R. (1924). Our new immigration policy. *Foreign Affairs, 3*(1), 99–111.

Yelin, E. H. (1991). The recent history and immediate future of employment among persons with disabilities. In J. West (Ed.), *The Americans with Disabilities Act: From policy to practice* (pp. 129–149). New York: Milbank Memorial Fund.

Young, B. (nd). Emma Lazarus and her vision. Retrieved from http://www.digitalhistory.uh.edu/historyonline/lazarus.cfm

1972; Livneh, 1980; Parkes, 1975; Siller, 1976). The contention is that the loss of a body part or a physical function constitutes the death of a part, which in the past was integrally associated with one's ego (Bakan, 1968). The anxiety associated with death is, therefore, rekindled at the sight of a disabled person. The disabled groups, both literally and symbolically, serve as a denial of our primitive, infantile omnipotence (Ferenczi, 1956) and as a reminder of our mortality.

PREJUDICE-INVITING BEHAVIORS

Gellman (1959) and Wright (1960) discussed the effect of certain provoking behaviors, by persons with disabilities, on discriminatory practices toward them. These provoking behaviors may be categorized into two general classes:

1. Prejudice by invitation (Roessler & Bolton, 1978): Specific behaviors by disabled individuals (being dependent, seeking secondary gains; acting fearful, insecure, or inferior) create and strengthen certain prejudicial beliefs in the observer. Wright (1960) similarly traced these behaviors to the physically disabled person's expectations of being treated in depreciating ways, and as a result set themselves up in situations in which they will be devalued.

2. Prejudice by silence: Lack of interest on the disabled person's part or lack of effective public relations campaigns or self-help groups representing the interests and concerns of specific disability groups to combat the public's ignorance is a way of fostering stereotypic and negative attitudes on the latter's part.

THE INFLUENCE OF DISABILITY-RELATED FACTORS

Several disability-connected variables were reported in the literature as affecting attitudes toward disabled persons. The association of these variables with certain negative perceptions was both empirically studied (Barker, 1964; Siller, 1963) and theoretically discussed (Freidson, 1965; Safilios-Rothschild, 1970).

Among the major reported variables can be found:

1. Functionality versus organicity of disability: Barker (1964) found that a dichotomy exists between the public's perceptions regarding certain personality traits attached to functional (alcoholism) or organic (blindness, cancer) disabilities. Siller (1963) concluded that those disabilities having the least functional implications were also those reacted to least negatively. Similar conclusions were reached in the context of occupational settings where employers preferred physically disabled individuals (e.g., those with paraplegia) to the more functionally impaired persons (such as those who were mentally retarded or emotionally disabled [Barker, 1964; Rickard, Triandis, & Patterson, 1963; Safilios-Rothschild, 1970]).

2. Level of severity: Usually the more severe a disability is, the more negatively it is perceived (Safilios-Rothschild, 1970; Shontz, 1964; Siller, 1963). Severity is, of course, related to level of functional limitation involved.

3. Degree of visibility: Generally, the more visible a disability is, the more negative an attitude it tends to trigger (Safilios-Rothschild, 1970; Shontz, 1964; Siller, 1963).

4. Degree of cosmetic involvement: Generally, the more the cosmetic implication inherent in the disability, in terms of aesthetic characteristics (see also "Aesthetic Aversion"), the less favorably it is reacted to (Siller, 1963).

5. Contagiousness versus noncontagiousness of disability: Safilios-Rothschild (1970) discussed the influence of contagious disabilities on the degree of prejudice directed toward them. The more contagious a disability is, the more fear of personal contraction is aroused and the more negative, therefore, is the ensuing reaction.

6. Body part affected: The importance of the body part affected by the disability, in terms of both personal and social implications, was suggested by Safilios-Rothschild (1970) and Weinstein, Vetter, and Sersen (1964).

7. Degree of predictability: The factor of imputed prognosis or probability of curability was studied and discussed by Freidson (1965), Safilios-Rothschild (1970), and Yamamato (1971). On the whole, the more curable and therefore predictable the disability is, the less negatively it is perceived.

The final category to be briefly discussed includes the association of certain demographic and personality variables of the nondisabled population with negative attitudes toward disabled persons. Because this category has been the target of extensive empirical research in the past years and since most of these studies are correlational rather than causal in nature, discussion will only revolve around their main findings. It should be noted that although the conclusions drawn by the studies of the authors are only suggestive and cannot be generalized beyond their participating populations, most authors regarded the respondents' personal variables under study as determinants of attitudes toward disability due to their enduring and deeply ingrained qualities (such as sex, intelligence, self-concept, and anxiety level).

DEMOGRAPHIC VARIABLES ASSOCIATED WITH ATTITUDES

Several major reviews of studies investigating demographic correlates of negative attitudes toward people with disabilities (English, 1971a; McDaniel, 1969; Ryan, 1981) have reached these conclusions concerning the following variables:

1. Sex: Females display more favorable attitudes toward individuals who are physically disabled than males (Chesler, 1965; Freed, 1964; Siller, 1963, 1964b; Yuker, Block, & Younng, 1966).

2. Age: There appear to be two inverted U-shaped distributions when age-related differences toward persons with disabilities are measured (Ryan, 1981). Attitudes are, generally, more positive at late childhood and adulthood, and less favorable attitudes are recorded at early childhood, adolescence, and old age (Ryan, 1981; Siller, 1963; Siller & Chipman, 1964; Siller et al., 1967).

3. Socioeconomic status: Higher income groups manifest more favorable attitudes toward the emotionally and mentally disabled than lower income groups (English, 1971a; Jabin, 1966); however, no differences were found regarding physical disabilities (Dow, 1965; English, 1971a; Lukoff & Whiteman, 1964; Whiteman & Lukoff, 1965).

4. Educational level: In spite of age-confounding research difficulties, most studies concluded that educational level is positively correlated with more favorable attitudes toward persons with disabling conditions (Horowitz, Rees, & Horowitz, 1965; Jabin, 1966; Siller, 1964b; Tunick, Bowen, & Gillings, 1979).

PERSONALITY VARIABLES ASSOCIATED WITH ATTITUDES

Research on the association of several personality traits and characteristics in the nondisabled population with respect to negative attitudes toward disabled people was summarized and reported by several authors (e.g., English, 1971a; Kutner, 1971; McDaniel, 1969; Pederson & Carlson, 1981; Safilios-Rothschild, 1970). Major findings include the following:

1. Ethnocentrism: Chesler (1965), Cowen et al. (1967, 1958), Lukoff and Whiteman (1964), Noonan (1967), Whiteman and Lukoff (1965), and Yuker (1965), following Wright's (1960) formulation of the comparability between attitudes toward persons with disabilities and attitudes toward ethnic and religious minorities, in general, found that high ethnocentrism was related to the lack of acceptance of the disabled population.

2. Authoritarianism: Jabin (1966), Lukoff and Whiteman (1964), Noonan, Barry and Davis (1970), Tunick et al. (1979), and Whiteman and Lukoff (1965) reported a positive correlation between accepting attitudes toward disabled persons and low authoritarianism (see also Dembo et al.'s [1956] theoretical discussion).

3. Aggression: Meng's (1938) original hypothesis suggested that the projection of one's aggressive and hostile desires upon those with disabilities will lead to the belief that disabled persons are dangerous and, as a result, to prejudicial attitudes toward them. Jabin (1966), Siller (1964b), and Siller et al. (1967) confirmed this hypothesis in independent studies, concluding that less-aggressive individuals express more positive attitudes toward this group.

4. Self-insight: Siller (1964b) and Yuker (1962) reported findings which suggested a moderate relationship between the need for introspection, as a measure of insightfulness, and empathetic understanding of people who are disabled.

5. Anxiety: The degree of manifest anxiety was found to be associated with attitudes toward disabled persons. Jabin (1966), Kaiser and Moosbruker (1960), Marinelli and Kelz (1973), Siller (1964b), Siller et al. (1967), and Yuker, Block, and Campbell (1960) demonstrated that a high level of manifest anxiety is positively correlated with rejection of disabled individuals.

6. Self-concept: Several studies (e.g., Epstein & Shontz, 1962; Jabin, 1966; Siller, 1964b; Yuker, 1962; Yuker et al., 1966) reported a relationship between positive self-concept and a more accepting attitude toward disability. It seems that persons who are more secure and confident in their own selves also tend to feel more positive and accepting of disabled persons.

7. Ego strength: Similar to self-concept, ego strength was found to be related to attitudes toward people with disabilities. Siller (1964a, 1963) and Siller et al. (1967) reported on the relationship between ego weakness and rejection of the disabled, while Noonan et al. (1970) found a trend in this direction, albeit not statistically significant.

8. Body and self-satisfaction: Several studies (Cormack, 1967; Epstein & Shontz, 1962; Fisher & Cleveland, 1968; Leclair & Rockwell, 1980; Siller, 1964a) concluded that lack of satisfaction with one's own body (low "body-cathexis" score) is related, and probably a contributing factor, to the development of negative attitudes toward physically disabled persons. Siller (1964a), Siller et al. (1967), and Yuker et al. (1966) expanded the body-cathexis concept to successfully argue that a positive perception of one's self is related to the acceptance of disabled individuals. People with positive and secure self-concepts tend to show more positive and accepting attitudes toward those with disabilities, while people with low self-concepts often reject them (see also section on "Threats to Body Image Integrity" in this chapter).

9. Ambiguity tolerance: The ability of nondisabled persons to better tolerate ambiguity was found to be positively correlated with acceptance of physically disabled persons (Feinberg, 1971).

10. Social desirability: The need for social approval and acceptance by others was positively associated with acceptance of people having disabilities (Doob & Ecker, 1970; Feinberg, 1967; Jabin, 1966; Siller et al., 1967).

11. Alienation: Alienated individuals tend to be more hostile toward, and rejecting of, disabled persons (Jabin, 1966).
12. Intelligence level: English (1971a) tentatively concluded, from his review of related studies, that there may be a relationship between the nondisabled intellectual capacity and acceptance of disability.

SUMMARY AND CONCLUSIONS

The present chapter has attempted to outline a classification system according to which a number of sources or negative attitudes toward people with disabilities was categorized and discussed.

The major categories included were (a) conditioning by sociocultural norms that emphasize certain qualities not met by the disabled population; (b) childhood influences where early life experiences foster the formation of stereotypic adult beliefs and values; (c) psychodynamic mechanisms that may play a role in creating unrealistic expectations and unresolved conflicts when interacting with disabled persons; (d) perception of disability as a punishment for a committed sin or as a justification for committing a future evil act, which triggers unconscious fears in the nondisabled person; (e) the inherent capacity of unstructured social, emotional, and intellectual situations to provoke confusion and anxiety; (f) the impact of a basic aesthetic-sexual aversion, created by the sight of the visibly disfigured, on the development of negative attitudes; (g) the threat to the conscious body and unconscious body image triggered by the mere presence of physically disabled individuals; (h) the devaluative and stereotypical reactions fostered by the marginality associated with being a member of a minority group; (i) the unconscious and symbolic parallelism between disability and death as a reminder of man's transient existence; (j) prejudice-provoking behaviors, by persons with disabilities, which result in discriminatory practices toward them; (k) disability-related factors (e.g., levels of functionality, visibility, and severity) which may contribute to specific negative attitudes; and (l) observer-related factors, both demographic (sex, age) and personality-connected (ethnocentrism, authoritarianism), which may foster the development of negative attitudes.

The classification system suggested suffers one major drawback. There is a certain degree of overlap among several of the categories (e.g., castration anxiety, viewed here as a threat to body image, may well be conceived as belonging to the childhood influences category; or anxiety provoked by unstructured situations may be regarded as just another psychological-operated mechanism if viewed phenomenologically rather than environmentally based). It should be noted, however, that due to the often highly abstract and conjectural nature of several of these categories, at present there is no escape from resorting to a certain level of arbitrariness when attempting to adopt such a classification model.

No attempt was made in the present discussion to suggest the matching of certain attitude-changing techniques (informative, experiential, and persuasive) with the categories discussed. Several excellent articles have been written on strategies to combat negative attitudes toward people with disabilities and toward minority groups in general (see Allport, 1954; Anthony, 1972; Clore & Jeffery, 1972; English, 1971b; Evans, 1976; Finkelstein, 1980; Hafer & Narcus, 1979; Kutner, 1971; Safilios-Rothschild, 1968; Wright, 1980, 1960).

It seems to this author that due to the complexity of the interacting factors that contribute to the creation of negative attitudes toward this group, any attempt at change, in order to be successful, must first be cognizant of the fact that since attitudes are learned and conditioned over many years, any experimental study of short duration, hoping to change attitudes, is futile at best. Attempts to modify the prevailing negative attitudes have been generally unsuccessful

(Roessler & Bolton, 1978). They will probably continue to follow such an inevitable course as long as researchers and clinicians look for quick and easy results and solutions.

REFERENCES

Alexander, F. G. (1938) Remarks about the relation of inferiority feelings to guilt feelings. *International Journal of Psychoanalysis, 19,* 41-49.

Allport, G. W. (1954). *The nature of prejudice.* New York: Addison-Wesley.

Anthony, W. A. (1972). Societal rehabilitation: Changing society's attitudes toward the physically and mentally disabled. *Rehabilitation Psychology, 19,* 117-126.

Bakan, D. (1968). *Disease, pain and sacrifice: Toward a psychology of suffering.* Chicago, IL: University of Chicago Press.

Barker, R. G. (1948). The social psychology of physical disability. *Journal of Social Issues, 4,* 28-38.

Barker, R. G. (1964). Concepts of disabilities. *Personnel & Guidance Journal, 43,* 371-374.

Barker, R. G., Wright, B. A., Meyerson, L., and Gonick, M. R. (1953). *Adjustment to physical handicap and illness: A survey of the social psychology of physique and disability* (rev. ed.). New York: Social Science Research Council.

Blank, H. R. (1957). Psychoanalysis and blindness. *Psycho-Analytic Quarterly, 26,* 1-24.

Chesler, M. A. (1965). Ethnocentrism and attitudes toward the physically disabled. *Journal of Personality and Social Psychology, 2*(6), 877-882.

Chevigny, H., & Braverman, S. (1950). *The adjustment of the blind.* New Haven, CT: Yale University Press.

Clore, G. L., & Jeffery, K. M. (1972). Emotional role playing, attitude change, and attraction toward a disabled person. *Journal of Personality and Social Psychology, 23*(1), 105-111.

Cormack, P. A. (1967). The relationship between body cognition and attitudes expressed toward the visibly disabled. *Rehabilitation Counseling Bulletin, 11*(2), 106-109.

Cowen, E. L., Bobrove, P. H., Rockway, A. M., & Stevenson, J. (1967). Development and evaluation of an attitude to deafness scale. *Journal of Personality and Social Psychology, 6*(2), 183-191.

Cowen, E. L., Underberg, R. P., & Verrillo, R. T. (1958). The development and testing of an attitude to blindness scale. *Journal of Personality and Social Psychology, 48,* 297-304.

Davis, F. (1961). Deviance disavowal: The management of strained interaction by the visibly handicapped. *Social Problems, 9*(2), 121-132.

Dembo, T., Leviton, G. L., & Wright, B. A. (1956). Adjustment to misfortune—A problem of social psychological rehabilitation. *Artificial Limbs, 3*(2), 4-62.

Dembo, T., Leviton, G. L., & Wright, B. A. (1975). Adjustment to misfortune—A problem of social psychological rehabilitation. *Rehabilitation Psychology, 22,* 1-100.

Doob, A. N., & Ecker, B. P. (1970). Stigma and compliance. *Journal of Personality and Social Psychology, 14*(4), 302-304.

Dow, T. E. (1965). Social class and reaction to physical disability. *Psychological Reports, 17*(1), 39-62.

Endres, J. E. (1979). Fear of death and attitudinal dispositions toward physical disability. *Dissertation Abstracts International, 39* 7161A. (University Microfilm No. 79-11, 825)

English, R. W. (1971a) Correlates of stigma toward physically disabled persons. *Rehabilitation, Research & Practice Review, 2,* 1-17.

English, R. W. (1971b). Combating stigma toward physically disabled persons. *Rehabilitation, Research & Practice Review, 2,* 19-27.

English, R. W., & Oberle, J. B. (1971). Toward the development of new methodology for examining attitudes toward disabled persons. *Rehabilitation Counseling Bulletin, 15*(2), 88-96.

Epstein, S. J., & Shontz, F. C. (1962). Attitudes toward persons with physical disabilities as a function of attitudes towards one's own body. *Rehabilitation Counseling Bulletin, 5*(4), 196-201.

Evans, J. H. (1976). Changing attitudes toward disabled persons: An experimental study. *Rehabilitation Counseling Bulletin, 19*(4), 572-579.

Feinberg, L. B. (1967). Social desirability and attitudes toward the disabled. *Personnel & Guidance Journal, 46*(4), 375-381.

Feinberg, L. B. (1971). *Social desirability and attitudes toward the disabled.* Unpublished manuscript, Syracuse University, Syracuse, New York.

Ferenczi, S. (1956). Stages in the development of the sense of reality. In S. Ferenczi (Ed.), *Contributions to psychoanalysis* (rev. ed.). New York: Dover.

Fine, J. A. (1978). *Castration anxiety and self concept of physically normal children as related to perceptual awareness of attitudes toward physical deviance.* Unpublished doctoral dissertation, New York University, New York.

Finkelstein, V. (1980). Attitudes and disabled people: Issues for discussion. International exchange of information in rehabilitation (Monograph No. 5). New York: World Rehabilitation Fund.

Fisher, S., & Cleveland, S. E. (1968). *Body image and personality* (2nd rev. ed.). New York: Dover.

Freed, E. X. (1964). Opinions of psychiatric hospital personnel and college students toward alcoholism, mental illness, and physical disability: An exploratory study. *Psychological Reports, 15*(2), 615–618.

Freidson, E. (1965). Disability as social deviance. In M. B. Sussman (Ed.), *Sociology and rehabilitation*. Washington, DC: American Sociological Association.

Gellman, W. (1959). Roots of prejudice against the handicapped. *Journal of Rehabilitation, 40*(1), 4–6, 25.

Goffman, E. (1963). *Stigma: Notes on management of spoiled identity*. Englewood Cliffs, NJ: Prentice-Hall.

Gove, W. R. (1976). Societal reaction theory and disability. In G. L. Albrecht (Ed.), *The sociology of physical disability and rehabilitation*. Pittsburgh, PA: University of Pittsburgh Press.

Hafer, M., & Narcus, M. (1979). Information and attitude toward disability. *Rehabilitation Counseling Bulletin, 23*(2), 95–102.

Hanks, J. R., & Hanks, L. M. (1948). The physically handicapped in certain non-occidental societies. *Journal of Social Issues, 4*, 11–20.

Hebb, D. O. (1946). On the nature of fear. *Psychology Review, 53*, 259–276.

Heider, F. (1944). Social perception and phenomenal causality. *Psychological Review, 51*, 358–374.

Heider, F. (1958). *The psychology of interpersonal relations*. New York: Wiley.

Horowitz, L. S., Rees, N. S., & Horowitz, M. W. (1965). Attitudes toward deafness as a function of increasing maturity. *Journal of Social Psychology, 66*, 331–336.

Jabin, N. (1966). Attitudes towards the physically disabled as related to selected personality variables. *Dissertation Abstracts, 27*(2-B), 599.

Jordan, J. E., & Friesen, E. W. (1968). Attitudes of rehabilitation personnel toward physically disabled persons in Colombia, Peru, and the United States. *Journal of Social Psychology, 74*, 151–161.

Kaiser, P., & Moosbruker, J. (1960). *The relationship between attitudes toward disabled persons and GSR*. Unpublished manuscript, Human Resources Center, Albertson, New York.

Kutner, B. (1971). The social psychology of disability. In W. S. Neff (Ed.), *Rehabilitation psychology*. Washington, DC: American Psychological Association.

Leclair, S. W., & Rockwell, L. K. (1980). Counselor trainee body satisfaction and attitudes toward counseling the physically disabled. *Rehabilitation Counseling Bulletin, 23*(4), 258–265.

Leviton, D. (1972). *Education for death or death becomes less a stranger*. Paper presented at the American Psychological Association convention, Honolulu, Hawaii.

Livneh, H. (1980). Disability and monstrosity: Further comments. *Rehabilitation Literature, 41*(11–12), 280–283.

Lukoff, I. F., & Whiteman, M. (1964). *Attitudes toward blindness*. Paper presented at the American Federation of Catholic Workers for the Blind meeting, New York.

Maisel, E. (1953). *Meet a body*. Unpublished manuscript, Institute for the Crippled and Disabled, New York.

Marinelli, R. P., & Kelz, J. W. (1973). Anxiety and attitudes toward visibly disabled persons. *Rehabilitation Counseling Bulletin, 16*(4), 198–205.

McDaniel, J. W. (1969). *Physical disability and human behavior*. New York: Pergamon Press.

Meng, H. (1938). Zur sozialpsychologie der Krperbeschädigten: Ein beitrag zum problem der praktischen psychohygiene. *Schweizer Archives fr Neurologie und Psychiatrie, 40*, 328–344 (Reported in Barker, R. G., et al., 1953.)

Menninger, W. C. (1949). Emotional adjustments for the handicapped. *Crippled Children, 27*, 27.

Napoleon, T., Chassin, L., & Young, R. D. (1980). A replication and extension of physical attractiveness and mental illness. *Journal of Abnormal Psychology, 89*(2), 250–253.

Noonan, J. R. *Personality determinants in attitudes toward disability*. Unpublished doctoral dissertation, University of Florida, Gainesville, Florida.

Noonan, J. R., Barry, J. R. & Davis, H. C. (1970). Personality determinants in attitudes toward visible disability. *Journal of Personality, 38*(1), 1–15.

Parkes, C. M. (1975). Psychosocial transitions: Comparison between reactions to loss of limbs and loss of a spouse. *British Journal of Psychiatry, 127*, 204–210.

Parsons, T. (1951). *The social system*. Glencoe, IL: The Free Press.

Parsons, T. (1958). Definitions of health and illness in the light of American values and social structure. In E. G. Jaco (Ed.), *Patients, physicians, and illness*. Glencoe, IL: The Free Press.

Pederson, L. L., & Carlson, P. M. (1981). Rehabilitation service providers: Their attitudes towards people with physical disabilities, and their attitudes towards each other. *Rehabilitation Counseling Bulletin, 24*(4), 275–282.

Raskin, N. J. (1956). *The attitude of sighted people toward blindness*. Paper presented at the National Psychological Research Council on Blindness.

Richardson, S. A., Hastorf, A. H., Goodman, N., & Dornbusch, S. M. (1961). Cultural uniformity in reaction to physical disabilities. *American Sociological Review, 26*(2), 241-247.

Rickard, T. E., Triandis, H. C., & Patterson, C. H. (1963). Indices of employer prejudice toward disabled applicants. *Journal of Applied Psychology, 47*(1), 52-55.

Roessler, R., & Bolton, B. (1978). *Psychosocial adjustment to disability.* Baltimore: University Park Press.

Ryan, K. M. (1981). Developmental differences in reactions to the physically disabled. *Human Development, 24,* 240-256.

Safilios-Rothschild, C. (1968). Prejudice against the disabled and some means to combat it. *International Rehabilitation Review, 4* 8-10, 15.

Safilios-Rothschild, C. (1970). *The sociology and social psychology of disability and rehabilitation.* New York: Random House.

Schilder, P. (1935). *The image and appearance of the human body.* London: Kegan Paul, Trench, Trubner.

Shontz, F. C. (1964). Body-part size judgement. *VRA Project No. 814, Final Report.* Lawrence, Kansas: University of Kansas. (Reported in McDaniel, J.W. 1969.)

Sigerist, H. E. (1945). *Civilization and disease.* Ithaca, NY: Cornell University Press.

Siller, J. (1963). Reactions to physical disability. *Rehabilitation Counseling Bulletin, 7*(1), 12-16.

Siller, J. (1964a). Reactions to physical disability by the disabled and the non-disabled. *American Psychologist, Research Bulletin 7,* 27-36 (American Foundation for the Blind).

Siller, J. (1964b). Personality determinants of reaction to the physically disabled. *American Foundation for the Blind Research Bulletin, 7,* 37-52.

Siller, J. (1976). Attitudes toward disability. In H. Rusalem & D. Maliken (Eds.), *Contemporary vocational rehabilitation.* New York: New York University Press.

Siller, J., & Chipman, A. (1964). Factorial structure and correlates of the attitude towards disabled persons scale. *Educational and Psychological Measurement, 24*(4), 831-840.

Siller, J., & Chipman, A. (1964). *Perceptions of physical disability by the non-disabled.* Paper presented at the American Psychological Association Meeting, Los Angeles. (Reported in Safilios-Rothschild, C., 1970).

Siller, J., Chipman, A., Ferguson, L. T., & Vann, D. H. (1967). *Studies in reaction to disability: XI. Attitudes of the non-disabled toward the physically disabled.* New York: New York University, School of Education.

Sussman, M. B. (1969). Dependent disabled and dependent poor: Similarity of conceptual issues and research needs. *The Social Service Review, 43*(4), 383-395.

Thoreson, R. W., & Kerr, B. A. (1978). The stigmatizing aspects of severe disability: Strategies for change. *Journal of Applied Rehabilitation Counseling, 9*(2), 21-25.

Thurer, S. (1980). Disability and monstrosity: A look at literary distortions of handicapping conditions. *Rehabilitation Literature, 41* (1-2), 12-15.

Tunick, R. H., Bowen, J. & Gillings, J. L. (1979). Religiosity and authoritarianism as predictors of attitude toward the disabled: A regression analysis. *Rehabilitation Counseling Bulletin, 22*(5), 408-418.

Weinstein, S., Vetter, R., & Sersen, E. (1964). Physiological and Experiential Concomitants of the Phantom." VRA *Project No. 427, Final Report.* New York: Albert Einstein College of Medicine, 1964.

Whiteman, M. & Lukoff, I. F. (1965). Attitudes toward blindness and other physical handicaps. *Journal of Social Psychology, 66,* 135-145.

Wolfensberger, W. (1972). *The principle of normalization in human services.* Toronto, Canada: National Institute on Mental Retardation.

Wolfensberger, W. (1976). The normalization principle. In S. A. Grand (Ed.), *Severe disability and rehabilitation counseling training.* Washington, DC: National Council on Rehabilitation Education.

Worthington, M. E. (1974). Personal space as a function of the stigma effect. *Environment and Behavior, 6*(3), 289-294.

Wright, B. A. (1960). *Physical disability: A psychological approach.* NY: Harper & Row.

Wright, B. A. (1980). Developing constructive views of life with a disability. *Rehabilitation Literature, 41*(11-12), 274-279.

Yamamato, K. (1971). To be different. *Rehabilitation Counseling Bulletin, 14*(3), 180-189.

Yuker, H. E. (1962). *Yearly psycho-social research summary.* Albertson, NY: Human Resources Center.

Yuker, H. E. (1965). Attitudes as determinants of behavior. *Journal of Rehabilitation, 31*(1), 15-16.

Yuker, H. E., Block, J. R., & Campbell, W. J. (1960). *A scale to measure attitudes toward disabled persons: Human resources study no. 5.* Albertson, NY: Human Resources Center.

Yuker, H. E., Block, J. R., & Younng, J. H. (1966). *The measurement of attitudes toward disabled persons.* Albertson, NY: Human Resources Center.

3

History of Treatment Toward Persons With Psychiatric Disabilities

KIM NGUYEN-FINN

Perhaps the most stigmatized and misunderstood group of people with disabilities are those who live with a psychiatric or mental illness. People with psychiatric disabilities warrant their own historical account which differs from Fox and Marini's history in Chapter 1, primarily because throughout history those with mental illness have at times been demonized, misunderstood as witches, put in prisons, and often subjected to inhumane treatment. The purpose of this chapter is to explore this history from the Middle Ages to the present day, noting the trials and tribulations of a population that continues to remain poorly understood and misperceived by the general public.

MENTAL ILLNESS TREATMENT SINCE THE MIDDLE AGES

The premodern era and early modern period, specifically from the Middle Ages to the 1800s, saw much cruel and inhumane treatment toward people with mental illness and mental retardation. Those who were viewed as mentally ill were often labeled as witches and burned at the stake (Dix, 2010; Gilman, 1988; Rosen, 1968; Shorter, 1997). Many were accused of demonic possession and subjected to exorcism, beaten, flogged, ridiculed, chained, or otherwise treated with fear and derision (Dix, 2010; Gilman, 1988; Rosen, 1968; Shorter, 1997). However, to view the treatment of those with mental illness during the Middle Ages solely through the modern lens would be unduly harsh. One must be mindful of the historical and cultural context of the general population and their knowledge, or lack thereof, of mental illness. People during the Middle Ages knew little in terms of the causes and treatment of diseases and even less so about mental illness. Physicians of this time period viewed disease and disability as often being caused by an imbalance of humors in the body, a belief inherited from the ancient Greeks. The theory was that the body is composed of four humors— blood, phlegm, yellow bile, and black bile. For instance, "madness" and "melancholy" were often viewed as caused by an excess of black bile (Gilman, 1988; Rosen, 1968). One possible treatment for imbalanced humor was bloodletting (Rosen, 1968)—a process of drawing blood from a patient to balance the humors and restore health. That which could not be explained by an imbalance of humors was believed to be an evil brought forth by sin committed by the sufferer, demons, or Satan or a spell cast by a witch and thus requiring to be cured by the Church or with magical herbs and incantations (Obermann, 1965).

The *Canon Episcopi*, a document that received a great deal of attention in the early medieval period, asserted that a belief in witches and sorcery, especially the idea that women rode upon animals in the night, was a satanic delusion (Hansen, as cited in Rosen, 1968). A later document of the Middle Ages, the *Malleus Maleficarum* (*Hammer of Witches*), revised the notion, *a belief in* witchcraft was brought about by Satan, to assert that witches indeed carried out Satan's orders and espoused procedures for identifying, putting to trial, and forcing confessions out of witches (Rosen, 1968). These two documents show a shift in societal beliefs about mental illness. The *Canon Episcopi* asserted that those who believed in witchcraft had a mental illness; later, the *Malleus Maleficarum* stated that the accused likely were the ones with mental illness. In reality, accusations of witchcraft were often the result of petty jealousy, social or familial conflicts, spurned sexual advances, suggestion, delusions, and mental illness. Indeed, some accused witches seem to be described in accounts during the period of the Inquisition as elderly women afflicted with dementia. In cases of demonic possession, one may find symptoms of the accused that are consistent with dysthymia, paranoia, mania, compulsive disorders, epilepsy, schizophrenia, and senile dementia (Rosen, 1968).

Care for the mentally ill was essentially the responsibility of relatives so long as the individuals did not cause a disturbance or were deemed too dangerous to be cared for at home (Rosen, 1968; Shorter, 1997). If they could not be cared for, authorities would confine the person viewed as insane to an asylum, a hospital, a prison, or a workhouse (Rosen, 1968; Shorter, 1997). Cases have been noted of accused witches being recognized as actually mentally ill and transferred to hospitals (Lea, as cited in Rosen, 1968). One of the oldest hospitals to treat people with psychiatric disabilities was the Priory of Saint Mary of Bethlehem, or Bethlem, which was founded in the 13th century in Europe. As centuries passed, the institution began to focus almost entirely on those with mental illness, and its name gradually morphed from Bethlem to "Bedlam;" the hospital remained in use as an asylum until 1948 (Shorter, 1997). Institutions of this time often did little more than warehouse people with psychiatric disabilities to keep them away from the public.

Much of the treatment for this population during the Middle Ages was often moral or religious in nature and sometimes included fasting, prayer, and pilgrimages to shrines; for the latter, financial assistance was often provided by religious groups (Rosen, 1968). Two stained glass windows from this time period found in the Canterbury Cathedral illustrate a man suffering from mental illness and depict prayer as a treatment; one window caption states "Mad he comes," while the other reads "He prays. Sane he goes away" (Torrey & Miller, 2001). Ibn Sīnā, or Avicenna as he was known in the Western world, was a Persian physician who lived in the late 1st century or early 2nd century and promoted treatments for ailments such as melancholia and "lovesickness." These included moisturizing the body, assisting with good sleep hygiene, promoting good nutrition, giving laxatives to reduce the toxins accumulated in the colon (which was believed to drive a person to madness; Shorter, 1997), and assisting in focusing on other matters and activities as a healthy distraction (Ibn Sīnā, 12th c./2010). Some of these treatments are like those espoused by mental health professionals of today.

COLONIAL AMERICA

Conditions for people with psychiatric disabilities did not fare much better in the American colonies. Similar to the way it was during the Middle Ages, care for this population was the family's responsibility if they had a family to care for them (Torrey & Miller, 2001). Those less fortunate who were held in institutions were often subjected to extremely unhygienic conditions, flogged, jeered at, confined to workhouses, and manacled and chained to walls or floors. In extreme cases, people with psychiatric disabilities were shackled for years until they lost use of their limbs and gradually died due to lack of food (Shorter, 1997). Occasionally, if a family could not adequately care for or control what they deemed a "distracted person," a colonial town would construct a small house (generally approximately

5′ × 7′) to confine the individual (Shorter, 1997). Eventually, asylums began to be built in the United States to house those with psychiatric disabilities. In 1729, the Boston Almshouse became the first institution in America to separate those with mental illness in a ward dedicated to psychiatric patients (Shorter, 1997). The first psychiatric hospital was opened in 1773 in Williamsburg, Virginia, with 30 beds (Shorter, 1997; Torrey & Miller, 2001), partly modeled after Bethlem in England (Scull, 1981).

By contrast, although not a belief shared by all American Indian tribes, some looked upon those with possible mental illness with high regard, believing them to possess "special gifts," especially those with psychoses (Grandbois, 2005; Obermann, 1965; Thompson, Walker, & Silk-Walker, 1993). Other tribes viewed mental illness similarly to European Americans as resulting from supernatural possession, soul loss (the loss of part of the soul or life force due to trauma or substance abuse), or internal or external imbalance (Grandbois, 2005; Thompson et al., 1993). In other tribes, those who displayed behavior outside of their cultural norm due to a mental or physical disability were treated as if they had misbehaved and were punished accordingly (Thompson et al., 1993). Yellow Bird (2001) asserts that Indian nations do not generally have a word for "mentally ill;" but what is translated as "crazy" means a humorous person or someone too angry to think clearly. With the expansion of the territory of the "White man," Western views and standards of practice in addressing mental illness also spread. The first asylum for a specific ethnic group was established in 1899 for the Northern Plains tribes, the Hiawatha Asylum for Insane Indians in Canton, South Dakota (Yellow Bird, 2001).

MENTAL ILLNESS IN 19TH-CENTURY AMERICA

In the 1800s, there was a huge rise in the number of those confined to asylums. The number of beds in each of the institutions increased to the low hundreds (Shorter, 1997). Braslow (1997) states that as more asylums were being built, still more were needed. Physicians of this time had scant training in diagnosing and treating mental illness (Caplan, 1969) but believed that they would be able to cure 80% of all such cases (Yanni, 2003). Indeed, they were so confident in their work that in 1853, psychiatrists who formed the American Organization of Asylum Physicians refused any association with the American Medical Association as they held other physicians in lower regard (Shorter, 1997).

The asylums of the early 19th century were largely therapeutic institutions providing moral treatment (Yanni, 2003). This treatment modality emphasized a positive change in environment (including staying within the asylum), an avoidance of immoral behavior and temptations, living a healthy lifestyle through exercise and proper nutrition, and abiding by a consistent daily schedule. Attendants were also instructed to show respect to patients, refrain from chaining them, and encourage supervised vocational and leisure activities (Yanni, 2003). Proponents of moral treatment also founded the *American Journal of Insanity*, a publication that aimed to educate citizens about mental illness and disability, as well as combat stigma and the abuses of those with a psychiatric disability (Caplan, 1969). However, in reality, moral therapy in its truest form was practiced in only a few institutions.

Patients of this time period were still being treated with physical therapies, including those designed to balance the humors. Records show that even up to the 1830s blistering, by which a patient's skin was burned with caustic substances to extract poisonous humors, was still being performed (Shorter, 1997). Treatment also utilized laxatives, bleeding, opiates, and hydrotherapy, or therapeutic baths, which came into vogue during this period (Shorter, 1997; Yanni, 2003).

Physicians tried to link disorders with treatments but were limited in their scope of understanding. Phrenology became a popular diagnostic and predictive tool and was developed through the belief that a direct relationship existed between the shape and size of the skull and mental illness and disability (Gilman, 1988). Categorizing mental illness as chronic or curable was of paramount importance as it enabled physicians to focus only on the few patients they believed could be successfully treated (Caplan, 1969). Diagnosing during this period could also be viewed as a way of identifying and compartmentalizing people who appeared different from the rest of society. Common diagnoses included melancholia, mania, idiocy, and paresis (a condition with symptoms of dementia, seizures, and muscle impairment resulting from syphilis) (Braslow, 1997). Shorter (1997) writes of one doctor from Albany, New York, who described what he termed "insane ear" or bloodied blisters within the ear to be a symptom of mental illness. In reality, the blisters were the result of asylum workers clubbing patients' heads (Shorter, 1997).

MENTAL ILLNESS AND TREATMENT AT THE TURN OF THE CENTURY

Moral treatments began to decline in the second half of the 19th century in favor of somatic therapies and behavioral control techniques (Braslow, 1997). Behavior that was deemed loud, offensive, or otherwise obnoxious by hospital staff was frequently managed by restraint, punishment, or sedative. Patients were physically restrained through the use of straightjackets, strapped to their beds—sometimes for years—confined in cells, and wrapped tightly in wet sheets (Braslow, 1997; Dix, 2010; Shorter, 1997). Criticized as another form of restraint, medications were administered to sedate patients and control symptoms of mental illness (Braslow, 1997; Shorter, 1997). Drugs in use during the 19th century included narcotics and the sedatives bromide, chloral hydrate, and hyoscine (Ackerknecht, as cited by Braslow, 1997). The most popular drug in use in the majority of asylums at this time was chloral hydrate (Caplan, 1969). Chloral hydrate, an addictive sedative related to chloroform, was especially popular among women, whose families were too embarrassed to commit them to an asylum, as a home remedy for psychosis, anxiety, and sleeping difficulties (Shorter, 1997). Physicians and psychiatrists often diagnosed females with hysteria.

Forced sterilization to control reproduction began to be employed and continued through the 1940s (Braslow, 1997). The eugenics movement has been likened to Nazi Germany's efforts to control the quality of future generations and involved the mass sterilization of those deemed to have a mental illness or hereditary-linked disability (Braslow, 1997). Patients were often considered incurable and their offspring were at risk of inheriting the disease (Braslow, 1997). Originally, however, laws allowing for forced sterilization made no mention of offspring. For example, the original 1909 California law known as the "Asexualization Act" stated that patients could be involuntarily sterilized if it benefitted the physical, mental, or moral condition of any inmate (Braslow, 1997). Nearly 10 years later, an amendment was introduced that stated involuntary sterilization may be performed on persons confined to an asylum if they had a disorder or disability that might be inherited and could be transmitted to descendents. This law broadened physicians' ability to decide about patients' reproductive capabilities (Braslow, 1997). Many viewed forced sterilization as an economic issue. One such individual, Horatio M. Pollock, a statistician for the New York State Hospital Commission, wrote in 1921 that the United States loses over $200 million each year as a result of mental illness and less than a quarter of those afflicted are curable. Pollock (1921) further states that mental illness heredity is an accepted fact and thus the limitation of reproduction by "defective stock" should be employed to reduce the burden on taxpayers.

Sterilization was not only used to control the population of those with a psychiatric illness, but some physicians believed it to be therapeutic. In the case of men, physicians asserted that by severing the vas deferens, the testicles compensated by increasing the production of a hormone that was thought to make the patient feel physically and mentally invigorated (Money, 1983). For women, sterilization was often an ill-guided, but more socially acceptable, attempt at reducing the psychological strain of having more pregnancies than desired (Braslow, 1997). Research at this time also posits that genital abnormalities were seen as common among those with mental illness or disability—a way of nature ensuring that these individuals did not reproduce—while physicians believed that vasectomies could provide a cure (Gibbs, 1923; *JAMA,* 1915).

Hydrotherapy, based on the idea that water had healing properties, became a widely used mode of treatment that remained in use until 1940 (Braslow, 1997). Hydrotherapeutic techniques were modeled after hot or cold mineral spring spas, long used as a curative, and consisted mainly of wet-sheet packs and hours of hot continuous baths (Braslow, 1997; Shorter, 1997). Patients who underwent wet-sheet packs were tightly wrapped in either cold or hot water–drenched sheets where they had to remain until the treatment administration was deemed completed (Braslow, 1997). Continuous bath treatments required patients to remain in a bathtub with limbs bound until they appeared to be more tranquil (Winslow, as cited in Braslow, 1997).

THE SHIFTING PUBLIC VIEW OF PSYCHIATRY

While treatments were changing through the end of the 19th century, so was the public's perception of psychiatry. By the 1900s as therapy gave and treatment reverted back to confinement, physicians who specialized in mental illness were deemed in poor light (Shorter, 1997). The profession was considered to be dangerous, and quality entrants into the field were scarce (Caplan, 1969). There was a huge increase in the number of patients in mental hospitals in the United States (150,000 in 1904, or 2 for every 1000 in the population) (U.S. Bureau of the Census, 1975, as cited in Shorter, 1997). Psychiatrists in the United States lacked the education to address the mental health needs of their patients as less than 10% of psychiatrists graduated from a respected medical school and 20% had never attended a medical school lecture (Stevens, as cited in Shorter, 1997). Mental hospitals also struggled to hire attendants and other staff who were even minimally qualified (Caplan, 1969). Further, the negative perceptions of those with mental illness persisted. The "Us versus Them" attitude against those perceived to have a psychiatric illness increased with the rise in the number of immigrants in America and its asylums, particularly against Irish immigrants who psychiatrists claimed were prone to mental illness due to their irascibility and excessive indulgence in alcohol (Torrey & Miller, 2001).

The quality of mental health care in the United States not surprisingly had reached a new low during this time. Physicians who did not know how to treat mental illnesses and disabilities resorted to simply warehousing patients; reformers and former patients began to speak publicly about the treatment of those in mental institutions, which they viewed as little more than prisons. One early mental health reformer, Dorothea Dix, traveled throughout New England in the early 1840s investigating the treatment of the "insane poor" and prisoners (Shorter, 1997). Dix was spurred to activism in 1841 after teaching a class to female prisoners at a jail near Boston, Massachusetts, and was exposed to the unheated and squalid conditions in which the women presumed to be insane were confined (Torrey & Miller, 2001). Dix spoke in 1843 to the Massachusetts legislature and described how the "insane poor" were kept naked, chained, beaten with rods and whipped, and appeared filthy and disheveled. Dix (2010) also reported about those confined to cages, cellars, stalls or pens in stables, and closets. In her speech to the legislature, she related how she visited an almshouse and met a woman who was kept for years in a cellar and had wasted down to bone. Dix was told the woman had to be kept there due to violent tendencies. Dix's impassioned descriptions of the suffering of prisoners and those with mental illness helped raise the public's awareness of the needs of the "insane poor" and convinced states' legislatures across the country to increase funding for mental health needs (Torrey & Miller, 2001; Yanni, 2003).

Others spoke of their personal experiences in the nation's mental institutions. Elizabeth Packard (2010) wrote *The Prisoners' Hidden Life or Insane Asylums Unveiled* in 1868 after being freed from an asylum following being involuntarily committed by her husband after a disagreement with him about religious beliefs (Eghigian, 2010). Lawsuits were being successfully brought forward against asylums for false imprisonment (Caplan, 1969). A few newspapers had reporters committed in mental institutions so that they could investigate patients' treatment first-hand and report upon it (Caplan, 1969). In 1889, the *Chicago Times* sent a reporter into Jefferson Asylum in Cook County. The newspaper reported abuses ranging from verbal abuse to assault to murder, which spurred public outrage and an investigation by authorities (Caplan, 1969).

Another former patient, Clifford Beers, who wrote *A Mind That Found Itself* in 1907 (Beers, as cited in Clifford W. Beers Guidance Clinic, Inc., 2009) spent 798 days after a failed suicide attempt. Rosen (1968) argues that Beers's work played a tremendous part, if not the most important part, in the development of the modern mental health movement. Recounting his nearly 3-year confinement in a state mental institution, Beers describes witnessing beatings, days spent in cold cells wearing only underwear, and restrained so tightly that his hands went numb. The story of how a Yale-educated man could be degraded with shockingly brutal treatment resonated with the public. Beers founded the National Committee for Mental Hygiene in 1909 to improve the care of patients in mental institutions, promote research, and disseminate information on the prevention and treatment of mental illnesses (Caplan, 1969; Rosen, 1968).

The work of Beers and other reformers helped make substantive changes in the field of mental health. For example, "asylum" would no longer be used to refer to mental hospitals, a sign of the change in focus from confinement to treatment (Caplan, 1969). In addition, patients were afforded the opportunity to appeal the decision to commit them, and institutions were directed to keep up with the latest knowledge through the purchase of updated medical books and subscriptions to scientific medical journals (Caplan, 1969).

Initially, however, psychiatrists responded to critics indignantly and with charges of ignorance and hypocrisy. They accused reformers of unjustly frightening the public away from receiving care and tarnishing psychiatrists' reputations (Caplan, 1969). Reformers were dismissed as ill-educated concerning proper behavioral management techniques and treatment modalities for mental disorders, and accused of hypocritically refusing to care for those with mental illness or disability themselves (Caplan, 1969). Other physicians including neurologists were cast as jealous individuals who lacked the qualifications to work in a mental hospital (Caplan, 1969).

DEVELOPMENT OF TREATMENTS IN THE 20TH CENTURY

Although psychiatrists initially scoffed at the notion that the quality of the care they provided in mental hospitals was subpar, research was conducted in the treatment of mental illness that brought about improvements. Physicians continued to develop and work toward improvement of somatic treatments for psychiatric disabilities in the early part of the 20th century. Physicians of this time period largely believed that fevers could treat a wide range of psychiatric illnesses (Braslow, 1997). Fevers were also believed by many physicians to kill the bacteria that causes syphilis, and fever therapy for paresis was in use until the early 1960s (Braslow, 1997). Interestingly, Wagner-Juaregg (2010), a winner of the Nobel Prize for physiology and medicine for his work in the development of this treatment, states that fever alone does not destroy the spirochaetes in that sometimes it will return once the fever has passed.

Other treatments included shock therapies. In the 1930s, some physicians used insulin to induce hypoglycemic coma in patients as a treatment for mental illness after noticing that patients who were difficult to manage became sedate and more cooperative with insulin (Braslow, 1997; Shorter, 1997). Insulin had previously been used to relieve depression and stimulate the appetite, as well as relieve diabetic symptoms (Shorter, 1997). Researchers could not agree why producing physiological shock through the use of insulin seemed to produce a positive effect (Braslow, 1997), but its use gradually rose in popularity. More than 100 mental hospitals in the United States housed insulin units by the 1960s (Shorter, 1997).

Metrazol injections, which produced seizures or convulsions, began to be adminis- tered (Braslow, 1997). Thus began the start of convulsive therapies. Physician-researchers have been unable to definitively state why convulsive therapies work but continue to use the procedure in specific cases. Some theorize that fear of the treatment itself induced improvement (Braslow, 1997). Shorter (1997) reports that physician-researchers of the 1920s noted that when patients who had epilepsy developed schizophrenia, they expe- rienced fewer epileptic seizures. They posited that there must be a correlation; thus, by inducing epileptic-like seizures, symptoms of schizophrenia might be reduced (Shorter, 1997). Initially, camphor, a naturally produced chemical that was sometimes used to treat psychosis in the 18th century, was used to shock the body to convulse (Shorter, 1997). The drug metrazol was developed and used in place of camphor (Shorter, 1997). The use of metrazol was fraught with problems, however, because physicians could not predict the onset or the intensity of the convulsions, which were reported to be agonizingly painful for the patients who experienced them and the hospital staff who witnessed them (Braslow, 1997; Shorter, 1997).

Later, seizures were induced in patients by passing electrical currents through elec- trodes on each of the temples and deemed to be safe (Braslow, 1997; Shorter, 1997). The use of electroshock therapy or electroconvulsive therapy (ECT) soon expanded from treating symptoms of schizophrenia to treating a wide array of mental illnesses such as depression, senile psychosis, melancholia, and alcohol abuse (Braslow, 1997). While ECT remains in use today as an acceptable psychiatric intervention for mental illness, it is not without critics (Braslow, 1997). A large portion of the criticism lies in the fact that more women than men (50–75%) are administered ECT. Another criticism is that ECT alters the physician–patient relationship to one of control and discipline (Braslow, 1997).

Psychosurgery, based on the viewpoint that the cause of mental illness or dis- ease originated in the frontal lobe, began to gain ground in the 1930s (Braslow, 1997). Prefrontal lobotomy or leucotomy entails cutting the white matter in the frontal lobes of the brain, thought to be associated with insight, and severing its connection with the thal- amus, thought to control emotion, and thereby reducing mental pain (Freeman & Watts, 2010). Surgery initially involved pouring alcohol onto the white matter of the frontal lobe through two holes that were drilled into the skull (Braslow, 1997). The neurologist Egas Moniz developed the prefrontal leucotomy based on observations of wartime head inju- ries, autopsies, and animal experiments and for which he later received the Nobel Prize (Eghigian, 2010). Moniz's procedure utilized an instrument called a leukotome, which is a rod affixed with a steel loop at one end that was inserted into the skull through holes drilled to cut the brain's white matter (Braslow, 1997). Freeman and Watts, two American physician-researchers, developed the transorbital lobotomy in which an ice pick is inserted into the eye socket of the patient and then the brain tissue is destroyed by tapping the ice pick with a hammer (Eghigian, 2010; Shorter, 1997). Freeman and Watts (2010) assert that prefrontal lobotomy is most successful with those patients whose mental illness may be anxiety disorder, depression, or excitability with schizophrenia, but is not successful for those with substance-use disorders, epilepsy, organic brain disease, and criminality. They also relayed doubts about the benefits of lobotomy with severe schizophrenia (Grob, 1991a). Moniz also questioned the effectiveness of leucotomy on schizophrenia, believing the surgery to be most successful on those with affective disorders (Grob, 1991a). Mahli and Bartlett (as cited in Juckel, Uhl, Padberg, Brüne, & Winter, 2009) reported that of those with certain psychiatric disabilities who underwent prefrontal leucotomy or lobotomy, approximately 67% had schizophrenia and 20% had an affective disorder. Shorter (1997) notes that lobotomies did indeed tend to calm patients with management problems. Psychosurgery, however, is also not without its hazards. It is not only dangerous to perform this surgery, but side effects of this treatment include a decline in social skills and judgment, loss of mental capacity, avolition or apathy, and a change in personality, such as loss of interest in previously enjoyed activities and changes in temperament (Juckel et al., 2009).

With the advent of talk therapy, psychological practice began its shift from being solely hospital based and became office based (Shorter, 1997). Outpatient psychiatric clinics were started in the 1920s, and by 1934, the practice of group psychotherapy began to be conducted (Shorter, 1997). Psychotherapy became the preferred treatment for middle and upper socioeconomic class individuals who were relatively high functioning, while somatic therapies tended to be used more often on those of the lower classes (Grob, 1991a).

The early 20th century witnessed the development of psychoanalysis, or the "talking cure." Sigmund Freud, a Viennese psychiatrist, developed an insight-oriented method of therapy (Shorter, 1997). According to Freud, neuroses are caused by repressed childhood memories, especially those of a sexual nature, as well as subconscious conflicts (Shorter, 1997). The goal of psychoanalysis is to bring the subconscious to consciousness and have the patient address the psychic conflict in a safe environment (Freud, 2010). Freud's theory of psychoanalysis conflicted with his contemporaries' views. Freud's focus on the individual, unconscious thoughts and urges, and childhood sexual development was in direct contradiction and thus ripe for criticism (Oberndorf, 1953). Despite its criticisms and limitations, Freud's work continues to have a major influence on contemporary therapeutic theories and practices (Corey, 1996). A significant assertion of psychotherapeutic theories is that the decision to undergo treatment rests with the patient.

Psychotherapy has also continued to evolve. Carl Rogers's client-centered therapy represented a fundamental shift in working with patients from Freudian and Jungian psychoanalysis. Rogers asserted that it is the client who has the ability and insight to know his or her problems, and how to put forth the issues, thus making the client the expert. The psychotherapist is simply there to be a sounding board and reassure the client's progress (Rogers, 1961). Psychotherapy also does not discount the benefits of somatic treatments, but it affirms a combination with appropriate drug therapy as the most effective treatment modality for mental illness today (Shorter, 1997).

Gains in understanding brain chemistry and more effective psychotropic medication for the treatment of mental illness were being made as well. The first neurotransmitter was isolated in the early 1920s, and soon thereafter the chemical acetylcholine was found to have an effect on nerve impulse transmissions between neurons (Shorter, 1997). Chlorpromazine, an antihistamine that would have a major impact on psychiatry, was developed in 1951 and initially was used as a sedative for psychiatric patients but was found to also reduce psychosis. Today, chlorpromazine is more commonly known as an antipsychotic medication under the brand name Thorazine. Soon, other antipsychotic medications along with antidepressants and mood stabilizers were being developed and marketed. The success of psychotropic medications in reducing once debilitating symptoms of mental illness has allowed more and more individuals to lead productive lives outside institutions (Shorter, 1997).

THE SECOND WORLD WAR AND ITS INFLUENCE ON MENTAL HEALTH

Psychiatrists' wartime experiences expanded knowledge about mental health and the importance of the environment in both disorder development and treatment (Grob, 1991b); they applied what they learned during World War II (WWII) to their rehabilitation and therapeutic efforts (Grinker & Spiegel, as cited in Grob, 1991b). The war necessitated that those unfit for military service for physical and mental reasons be screened out, and those serving and requiring rehabilitation as psychological casualties needed treatment (Grob, 1991a). The screening out of recruits aroused controversy and was not wholly successful. Approximately 1.75 million potential recruits were rejected by the Selective Service (Grob, 1991a) and an additional 500,000 discharged for mental reasons (Pickren, 2005). These high numbers raised questions about prevalence, the screening criteria's validity, and personal privacy (Grob, 1991a). The problems with screenings, however, did successfully highlight the need for additional research in the field and the importance of prevention of mental health problems (Grob, 1991a). The U.S. government began to assist the funding of psychological research on a large scale, which further shaped public perception of mental illness and treatment (Pickren, 2005). Psychiatrists serving during the war successfully utilized a more holistic approach to treatment, providing supportive counseling in conjunction with prescribing adequate sleep, good nutrition, and rest close to the patient's unit and support system (Grob, 1991b).

The successful treatment of psychiatric issues for returning veterans helped elevate the profession, and in 1944, psychiatry was designated as a medical specialty within the Office of the Surgeon General (Grob, 1991b). Additional physicians were recruited into its ranks—at the outbreak of WWII, there were 35 psychiatrists serving in the military and the number swelled to 2400 by 1945 (Grob, 1991b). Psychiatrists who were transitioning to civilian life at the end of the war began to enter academia, government, private practice, and public service, and carried with them their unique knowledge and approaches (Grob, 1991a). Indeed, the end of WWII brought with it a renewed sense of hope within the mental health field and the intellectual and institutional means to effect substantive changes. It also produced fresh challenges that needed to be addressed. One year after the end of hostilities, 60% of the Veterans Administration (VA) hospital patients were WWII veterans presenting with mental disorders (Brand & Sapir, 1964). The rising number of those in need of quality mental health services spurred the VA along with the American Psychological Association (APA) and several universities to work together to develop a doctoral clinical psychology program (Miller, 1946). Significantly, the National Mental Health Act was passed in the same year, which assisted states in the implementation of services for the diagnosis, prevention, and treatment of mental illnesses, as well as provided for research, training, and the formation of the National Institute of Mental Health (Grob, 1991a; Pickren, 2005).

CLASSIFICATION OF MENTAL ILLNESS

The APA started to devise a standard nosology for mental disorders in 1948 (Shorter, 1997), but the first standardized nosology for mental illness, *The Statistical Manual for the Use of Institutions for the Insane*, was developed in 1918 by the American Medico-Psychological Association in collaboration with the National Committee for Mental Hygiene at the request of the U.S. Bureau of the Census (Grob, 1991b). Categorizing mental illnesses was found useful in that the public health statistical data regarding disorders could be collected and used in public policy development, to uncover future trends, and to show recidivism and recovery rates with different treatments or hospitals, while the use of diagnoses in the development of treatment plans was not as important at this time (Grob, 1991b). Over time, the inadequacy of the earlier classification systems was made increasingly apparent. In 1952, the APA published the *Diagnostic and Statistical Manual of Mental Disorders*, now referred to as the *DSM-I* (*DSM-IV-TR*, 2000), which, like previous classification systems, reflected the intellectual, cultural, and political viewpoints on mental illness of its day (Grob, 1991b). Since its initial publication, there have been several revisions and it continues to be used as the standard diagnostic tool by a wide array of mental health researchers and clinicians in a variety of settings (*DSM-IV-TR*, 2000). Critics of the *DSM,* however, have cited that the resource fails to fully capture a holistic picture of an individual's circumstances. As such, in coordination with the World Health Organization (WHO), the APA has endorsed a more holistic resource that can be cross-walked with almost any disability and that takes into account an individual's external environment and medical and psychological problems (Peterson, 2011). Specifically, the International Classification of Functioning represents the most contemporary source available to mental health professionals in holistically assessing an individual's situation (Peterson, 2011).

DEINSTITUTIONALIZATION

There were 131 state-funded mental hospitals at the turn of the 20th century to house 126,137 patients; by 1941, there were 419,374 patients, but the number of hospitals had increased by only 181 (Braslow, 1997). With the overcrowding of mental hospitals, the need for an alternative to institutions became apparent. The increase in the use of drug therapies gave rise to the notion that individuals with mental illness could integrate back into the community if their symptoms were managed (Shorter, 1997). In addition, WWII evidenced how successful treatments outside of institutions were, and psychiatrists who served worked to incorporate mental health care into community treatment and prevention efforts of mental illnesses (Grob, 1991a; Kelly, 2005). The antipsychiatry movement further drove the shift to deinstitutionalization. The movement in large part comprised mental health professionals themselves who were critical about overuse of psychotropic medications, the viewpoint that behaviors simply outside of the norm implied mental disorders, and what they considered inferior institutional practices (Eghigian, 2010; Grob & Goldman, 2006). Deinstitutionalization also appeared to be strongly influenced by financial reasons as Medicaid payments gave states impetus to move patients to nursing homes (Mechanic & Rochefort, 1990).

Programs and centers with a community health focus began to rise. The Menninger Clinic in Topeka, Kansas, was started by William and Karl Menninger, brothers who served as psychiatrists in WWII; their model became a respected form of mental health care (Kelly, 2005). In 1955, Public Law 84–182 established the Mental Health Study Act, which examined mental health care in the United States (Kelly, 2005). The final report contributed to the development of the Community Mental Health Centers Act of 1963 (Brand & Sapir, 1964; Stockdill, 2005). This act required community mental health centers to provide inpatient and outpatient services, partial hospitalizations, emergency services, training and education, and consultation services (Mechanic & Rochefort, 1990; Stockdill, 2005). Thousands of institutionalized patients were placed with their families for care at home; however, the difficulty of patient monitoring and the lack of case management and coordination of care plagued the community mental health clinics (Grob & Goldman, 2006). New York recognized that patients needed a transition period between hospitalization and reintegration into the family and community and developed aftercare clinics in 1954 (Carmichael, as cited in Grob & Goldman, 2006). Halfway houses, which were either linked to hospitals or founded by mental health professionals or laypeople, were created to also help patients' transition back into the community (Grob & Goldman, 2006). Underfunding and what many perceived as disinterest by professionals for the rehabilitation and support of the reintegration into the community of those with severe mental illness posed major problems for halfway houses (Grob & Goldman, 2006). As an alternative, independent living communities for those with mental illnesses called "Fairweather Community Lodge Programs" were developed in California in the 1960s (Kelly, 2005). George Fairweather created his lodges believing that those with severe psychiatric illnesses can remain deinstitutionalized if they live and work together collaboratively (Kelly, 2005). Other treatment facilities started and still in use today are supervised apartments, board and care facilities, and group homes (Mechanic & Rochefort, 1990). Outpatient programs such as Assertive Community Treatment (ACT) have also come into use to serve the needs of those with severe and persistent mental illness living in the community (NAMI, 2006). ACT programs provide highly intensive, multifaceted care available 24 hours/7 days per week with a low service provider to consumer ratio and have been shown to reduce the number of hospitalizations (NAMI, 2006). Between 1965 and 1975, the number of patients in state mental hospitals decreased an average of 8.6% per year (Mechanic & Rochefort, 1990). As the population in state mental hospitals reduced, general hospitals experienced a dramatic rise in the registration of patients with mental illness, necessitating the development of specialized psychiatric units as these hospitals were forced to house patients in surgical or emergency wards (Mechanic & Rochefort, 1990).

Reintegration into the community occurred on a large scale during the late 1960s and most of those released had been admitted to the hospitals in later life or had a lengthy confinement (Grob & Goldman, 2006). Disability and health insurance provided financial assistance and mental health benefits for individuals so that they may remain with their families (Mechanic & Rochefort, 1990). Moreover, the introduction of Medicaid and Medicare in 1966 gave states the incentive to transition patients from hospitals to nursing homes as these social programs provided for the care of elderly patients with mental illness or dementia in nursing homes (Mechanic & Rochefort, 1990). In addition, Medicaid often provided funds for short-term inpatient care in general hospitals (Mechanic & Rochefort, 1990).

DISILLUSIONMENT WITH THE PROMISES OF DEINSTITUTIONALIZATION

Deinstitutionalization in time, however, produced less-than-positive results. The concepts of utilizing the least restrictive method of care and that those with severe and persistent mental disorders would be treated in the community rather than the psychiatric institution meant that an increasing number would receive inadequate care as the community clinics were not poised to address their needs (Grob & Goldman, 2006; Mechanic & Rochefort, 1990). Many of those who would have been institutionalized in the past were forced to function independently in the community, and these individuals were frequently cited as being noncompliant with treatment, denying their mental illnesses, taking their medications irregularly, being aggressive, self-medicating with alcohol or drugs, and lacking social skills (Grob & Goldman, 2006).

The massive slash of funding for welfare programs in the 1980s further hindered mental health care efforts and precipitated a rise in the number of those with mental illness among the homeless and prison population (Mechanic & Rochefort, 1990). While a direct correlation with the cuts to social programs is difficult to make, roughly one-third of the nation's homeless population and 14% of county inmates in the 1980s were documented to have a psychiatric diagnosis (Torrey, as cited in Shorter, 1997). These figures contrast radically with the prevalence of severe mental illness in the general population at that time, which was about 2.8% (National Advisory Mental Health Council, 1993). According to the U.S. Department of Justice, over half of all inmates in 2005 had either a diagnosis of a mental disorder or met the criteria for one based on symptoms; these included psychotic disorders, major depressive disorders, and symptoms of mania (James & Glaze, 2006). In contrast, about 11% of adults in the general population now meet the criteria for a mental disorder according to the National Epidemiologic Survey on Alcohol and Related Conditions, 2001–2002 (James & Glaze, 2006).

MENTAL ILLNESS AND THE CRIMINAL JUSTICE SYSTEM

According to the U.S. Department of Justice (DOJ), inmates with mental health problems are more likely to have violent records and are generally given longer sentences (James & Glaze, 2006). While those with severe and persistent mental illness may and do commit criminal acts, many encounter law enforcement during mental crises or because they are exhibiting bizarre and/or disturbing behaviors in public (Lamberti & Weisman, 2004). Definite gains have been made in raising awareness of the unique needs of those with mental illness among law enforcement professionals. The Crisis Intervention Team (CIT) of the Memphis, Tennessee Police Department, is a model jail diversion program in use in other communities as well, in which officers volunteer to be educated about signs and symptoms of mental disorders and trained in de-escalation techniques, community mental health and social service resources, and empathy of those with mental illness (Slate & Johnson, 2008). CIT programs have resulted in fewer arrests of those with severe mental illness, as well as fewer officer and detainee injuries (Lamberti & Weisman, 2004). Other police departments have experimented with utilizing mental health professionals or social workers in crisis response (Lamberti & Weisman, 2004). The Law Enforcement and Mental Health Project Act of 2000 authorized funding for the development of "mental health courts" as an alternative for those with severe mental illness and to promote treatment and supervision for the accused (Lamberti & Weisman, 2004). They were also designed to curb reoffending among those with severe mental illness and divert them into community-based treatment (Redlich, Steadman, Monahan, Robbins, & Petrila, 2006).

Despite these improvements, the treatment of those with mental illness within the criminal justice system remains a concern. Suicide is the leading cause of death among inmates in jails and the third leading cause in prisons (Lamberti & Weisman, 2004). Some studies on inmates document that over half of those who died by suicide had a history of mental illness (Lamberti & Weisman, 2004). These inmates with mental illness are also more likely to have disciplinary problems and be involved in altercations with other inmates while incarcerated (Hayes, 1995). As many view prisons and jails as a source of punishment rather than treatment, psychotherapy and medication management is lacking for many inmates. Depending on the facility type (local jail, state or federal prison), only 17 to 35% of inmates with mental disorders are provided mental health services (James & Glaze, 2006). To prevent recidivism, prisons and jails face the challenging task of coordinating with community mental health and social services upon release of inmates with mental illness for employment, housing, and mental health assistance (Lamberti & Weisman, 2004).

ABUSE OF PERSONS WITH MENTAL ILLNESS

Not only do a high number of prisoners have a psychiatric disability, but those with mental illness also appear to be more vulnerable to sexual and physical abuse. Those incarcerated in prisons or jails were two to three times more likely to have been sexually or physically abused than other inmates (James & Glaze, 2006). While causality cannot be stated, O'Hare, Shen, and Sherrer (2010) found that of those they interviewed with severe mental illness, 51.8% reported physical abuse, 41.7% reported sexual abuse, and a greater number of women than men reported they were abused. Those with severe mental illness also may engage in high-risk behaviors such as running away and substance abuse, which puts them at greater risk for repeated abuse (O'Hare et al., 2010). In addition, people with severe mental illness are more likely to live in high-crime areas that can further expose them to risk of decompensation (Schwartz, Bradley, Sexton, Sherry, & Ressler, 2005). Those with severe mental illness are particularly vulnerable to revictimization from the judicial system given the difficulty in prosecuting based on a witness statement from someone with delusions, a history of engaging in multiple unprotected sex while having a manic episode, or having been severely impaired due to self-medication with drugs or alcohol (O'Hare et al., 2010). This also illustrates the negative public perceptions those with mental illness continue to face.

SOCIAL SECURITY BENEFICIARIES

Number of persons diagnosed with a psychiatric disability continue to rapidly grow, and psychiatric disability is the number one disability on social security benefit rolls (Marini, Feist, & Miller, 2004). It continues to be the fastest growing percentage of beneficiaries, currently estimated to be approximately 28% of disabled workers and 41% of those on Supplemental Security Disability Income plus those on Social Security Income (Vercillo, 2011). Of over 75% of beneficiaries with this diagnosis, half are younger than 30 years and the other half are aged between 30 and 39, thus representing the youngest population among beneficiaries (Marini et al., 2004). This is an alarming increase considering over 50 million individuals are on the social security benefit rolls, and less than 1% of them ever return to gainful employment.

CONTINUED STIGMA AGAINST PEOPLE WITH MENTAL ILLNESS

Link, Phelan, Bresnahan, Stueve, and Pescosolido (1999) studied people's perceptions of mental illness and their thoughts on causes of mental disorders, dangerousness of those with mental illness, and preferred social distance. Link et al. (1999) found that Americans continue to perceive individuals with mental illness to be dangerous and desire minimal contact with them. In terms of causality of mental illness, more people today share the views of mental health professionals that disorders are caused by a variety of complex factors including environment, biology, and social experiences (Link et al., 1999). A study by

Corrigan et al. (2000) found that among their participants, physical illness such as cancer was viewed benignly and depression was the only mental illness seen as nonthreatening and more acceptable. Those with cocaine addiction, psychotic disorders, and mental retardation were perceived negatively and were discriminated against in the study (Corrigan et al., 2000).

One classic study focused on the stigmatizing attitudes against people with mental illness among mental health professionals. Rosenhan (1973) studied normal and abnormal behaviors, noting that differences existed among cultures. From this, he wondered if the symptomatic criteria for diagnoses are met solely because they are exhibited by the individual or based on the environment or context (Rosenhan, 1973). Eight healthy individuals were admitted to 12 different mental hospitals across the United States as pseudopatients. Each pseudopatient falsely reported only their names, employment, and psychosocial histories, and proffered fake symptoms of hearing voices such as a "thud" sound (Rosenhan, 1973). Further, while in the wards, the pseudopatients behaved as they normally do, were compliant, and reported to the hospital staff that they no longer experienced symptoms when asked (Rosenhan, 1973). Although the individuals were very high functioning in their daily lives and were a graduate student in psychology, a psychiatrist, three psychologists, a pediatrician, a housewife, a painter, and Rosenhan himself, each was discharged with a diagnosis of schizophrenia in remission, implying that they were perceived as having schizophrenia throughout their hospitalization. In addition, the pseudopatients were treated dismissively by hospital staff; their questions were ignored completely, and in one instance, a nurse adjusted her bra in front of male patients as if they were not present. At other times, they were verbally and physically abused. Interestingly, it was other patients who detected the pseudopatients as being sane (Rosenhan, 1973). The Rosenhan study demonstrated that behaviors of the pseudopatients were judged in the context of the diagnostic label they were given and the hospital setting they were confined to (Hock, 2005).

CURRENT ISSUES REGARDING MENTAL ILLNESS AND ITS TREATMENT

Efforts are being made through public policy, advocacy organizations, and private individuals to raise awareness of mental illness, reduce its stigma, and combat discrimination against those with the disability. For example, more Americans are seeking treatment for mental health and emotional issues; 13.4% of adults in 2008 received inpatient, outpatient, or prescription medication treatment, a steady increase from previous years (National Institute of Mental Health [NIMH], 2011). However, the costs for mental health care have also been increasing. Between 1996 and 2006, the total expenditure for mental health care in the United States rose from $35.2 to $57.5 billion (NIMH, 2011). As a comparison, the cost of care for those with cancer was also $57.5 billion in 2006 (NIMH, 2011). The WHO estimates that in 2004, the burden of disability (the number of years lost due to the disability and measured in disability-adjusted life years) for neuropsychiatric disorders in the United States and Canada together accounted for the greatest number (49%), followed by cardiovascular diseases, the second leading contributor (NIMH, 2011; WHO, 2011).

In their effort to raise awareness and encourage help-seeking behaviors, NIMH organized the, now annual, National Depression Screening Day in 1991 (NIMH, 2011; Shorter, 1997). Each year since its inception, approximately half a million individuals are screened annually (Screening for Mental Health, Inc., 2011). The U.S. Surgeon General released a landmark publication, *Mental Health—A Report of the Surgeon General*, in 1999 (cited in Grob & Goldman, 2006), emphasizing that mental illnesses are valid conditions and treatments have been shown to be effective (Grob & Goldman, 2006). In addition, the report included the importance of reducing stigma and attitudinal barriers to help-seeking behaviors, tailoring intervention to the individual's cultural background, and the need for more clinicians to be trained in research-based treatments such as cognitive-behavioral therapy (OSG, 2011).

Another government agency, the Department of Veterans Affairs, is making promising efforts on treatment and preventative measures for mental illness. The global war on terrorism (GWT) and its fronts in Afghanistan and Iraq have highlighted the need for improved mental health services as an increasing number of psychiatric casualties are returning to civilian life. For example, the VA disseminates to health care providers and mental health clinicians evidence-based clinical practice guidelines for mental and physical health issues (Department of Veterans Affairs, 2011). Furthermore, taking into account the stigma against disclosing emotional concerns among service members and their resulting hesitancy to go to a mental health center, the VA expanded its primary care services to be better equipped to address veterans' clinical mental health needs (Committee on Veterans' Affairs, 2007). According to the U.S. Department of Defense (DOD), as of July, 2011, there were close to 45,000 servicemen wounded in action in the GWT, many of whom were diagnosed with a mental disability such as post-traumatic stress disorder (DOD, 2011). As veterans are returning to civilian life with service-related emotional disabilities, greater protections have been placed to help ensure they are provided equal treatment and opportunities.

In 1990, the Americans with Disabilities Act (ADA) was passed by Congress to provide equal opportunity and protection against discrimination on the basis of physical and mental disabilities (DOJ, 1990). For veterans and other individuals diagnosed with a mental illness, the ADA means that they have a right to reasonable accommodations such as their service dog trained to ease heightened anxiety be allowed to accompany them; flexible work schedules to attend counseling sessions, instructions provided in writing, tasks broken down to more manageable increments, extended deadlines, and additional breaks for those with memory impairments or difficulty focusing (DOJ, 2010).

Chamberlin (1993) noted that the ADA's inclusion of mental disabilities aroused controversy at the time and exposed some prejudices. Some of those who debated the bill questioned whether individuals with mental illnesses are reliable employees, or if they are dangerous, unstable, undependable, and lazy. Despite the controversy, the ADA was passed into law and individuals with mental disabilities are afforded the same protections as those with physical disabilities. Since its inception, the ADA has undergone several revisions to strengthen its language and enforceability (DOJ, 2009).

While those with mental illness still face multiple challenges such as discrimination, stigma, lack of access to treatment, and disability (Mechanic & Rochefort, 1990), barriers are being reduced and treatments are being improved. Individuals and organizations, both public and private, continue to strive to raise public awareness and lobby for the needs of those with mental illness. A growing number of treatment options are available, including psychiatric hospitals (long- or short-term inpatient), emergency services (short-term acute care), private practice psychotherapists and psychiatrists, community mental health centers (comprehensive and state funded), community support services (halfway houses, quarterway houses, day treatment centers), medication management, and self-help. Holistic treatment approaches are also being utilized as a way of improving the quality of mental health care combining skills training, a social support system, environmental and behavioral modification, vocational assistance, and medication. With the variety of options available, more Americans are receiving mental health treatment than ever before (Shorter, 1997). Although gaps remain, the definite gains in efforts to prevent and effectively treat mental illness through the years are worthy to note.

REFERENCES

American Psychiatric Association. (2000). *Diagnostic and statistical manual of mental disorders* (revised 4th ed.). Washington, DC: Author.

Brand, J., & Sapir, P. (1964). An historical perspective on the National Institute of Mental Health. In D. E. Woolridge (Ed.), *Biomedical science and Its administration*. Unpublished manuscript.

Braslow, J. (1997). *Mental ills and bodily cures: Psychiatric treatment in the first half of the twentieth century*. Berkley: University of California Press.

Caplan, R. B. (1969). *Psychiatry and the community in nineteenth-century America: The recurring concern with the environment in the prevention and treatment of mental illness*. New York: Basic Books.

Chamberlin, J. (1993). Psychiatric disabilities and the ADA: An advocate's perspective. In L. O. Gostin & H. A. Beyer (Eds.). *Implementing the Americans with Disabilities Act: Rights and responsibilities of all Americans* (pp. 223–227). Baltimore: Paul H. Brookes Publishing.

Clifford W. Beers Guidance Clinic, Inc. (2009). *Clifford Beers—His legacy*. Retrieved from http://www.cliffordbeers.org/clifford-beers-his-legacy

Committee on Veterans Affairs. (2007). *DoD/VA Collaboration and cooperation to meet the needs of returning service members*. Hearing before the Committee on Veterans Affairs, United States Senate, One Hundred Tenth Congress, First session. Washington, DC: U.S. Government Printing Office. Retrieved from http://veterans.senate.gov/hearings.cfm?action= release.display&release id= 928913cd-2426-4643-a 321-092f 664884ab

Corey, G. (1996). *Theory and practice of counseling and psychotherapy* (5th ed.). Pacific Grove, CA: Brooks/Cole Publishing Company.

Corrigan, P. W., River, L. P., Lundin, R. K., Wasowski, K. U., Campion, J., Mathisen, J., et al. (2000). Stigmatizing attributions about mental illness [Electronic version]. *Journal of Community Psychology, 28*(1), 91–102.

Dix, D. (2010). Memorial to the Legislature of Massachusetts. In G. Eghigian (Ed.), *From madness to mental health: Psychiatric disorder and its treatment in western civilization*. New Brunswick, NJ: Rutgers University Press. (Original work published 1843.)

Eghigian, G. (2010). *From madness to mental health: Psychiatric disorder and its treatment in Western Civilization*. New Brunswick, NJ: Rutgers University Press.

Freeman, W., & Watts, J. W. (2010). Psychosurgery during 1936–1946. In G. Eghigian (Ed.), *From madness to mental health: Psychiatric disorder and its treatment in western civilization*. New Brunswick, NJ: Rutgers University Press. (Original work published 1947)

Freud, S. (2010). The origin and development of psychoanalysis. In G. Eghigian (Ed.), *From madness to mental health: Psychiatric disorder and its treatment in western civilization*. New Brunswick, NJ: Rutgers University Press. (Original work published 1910)

Gibbs, C. E. (1923). Sex development and behavior in male patients with dementia praecox [Electronic version]. *Archives of Neurology & Psychiatry, 9,* 73–87.

Gilman, S. L. (1988). *Disease and representation: Images of illness from madness to AIDS*. Ithaca, NY: Cornell University Press.

Grandbois, D. (2005). Stigma of mental illness among American Indian and Alaska Native Nations: Historical and contemporary perspectives [Electronic version]. *Issues in Mental Health Nursing, 26,* 1001–1024.

Grob, G. N. (1991a). *From asylum to community: Mental health policy in modern America*. Princeton, NJ: Princeton University Press.

Grob, G. N. (1991b). Origins of DSM-I: A study in appearance and reality [Electronic version]. *American Journal of Psychiatry, 148*(4), 421–431.

Grob, G. N., & Goldman, H. H. (2006). *The dilemma of federal mental-health policy: Radical reform or incremental change?* New Brunswick, NJ: Rutgers University Press.

Hayes, L. M. (1995). *Prison suicide: An overview and guide to prevention*. Washington, DC: National Center on Institutions and Alternatives, U.S. Department of Justice.

Hock, R. R. (2005). *Forty studies that changed psychology: Explorations into the history of psychological research* (5th ed.), Upper Saddle River, NJ: Pearson Education, Prentice Hall.

Ibn Sīnā (2010). Lovesickness. In G. Eghigian (Ed.), *From madness to mental health: Psychiatric disorder and its treatment in Western Civilization*. New Brunswick, NJ: Rutgers University Press. (Original work published 12th c.)

JAMA (1915). Sex organ changes in insanity [Electronic version]. *Journal of the American Medical Association, 65,* 254–255.

James, D. J., & Glaze, L. E. (2006). Mental health problems of prison and jail inmates [Electronic version]. *Bureau of Justice Statistics Special Report.* Washington, DC: U.S. Department of Justice.

Juckel, G., Uhl, I., Padberg, F., Brüne, M., Winter, C. (2009). Psychosurgery and deep brain stimulation as *ultima ratio* treatment for refractory depression [Electronic version]. *European Archives of Psychiatry and Clinical Neuroscience, 259,* 1-7.

Kelly, J. G. (2005). The National Institute of Mental Health and the founding of the field of community psychology. In W. E. Pickren & S. F. Schneider (Eds.), *Psychology and the National Institute of Mental Health: A historical analysis of science, practice, and policy.* Washington, DC: American Psychological Association.

Lamberti, J. S., & Weisman, R. L. (2004). Persons with severe mental disorders in the criminal justice system: Challenges and opportunities [Electronic version]. *Psychiatric Quarterly, 75*(2), 151-164.

Link, B. G., Phelan, J. C., Bresnahan, M., Stueve, A., Pescosolido, B. A. (1999). Public conceptions of mental illness: Labels, causes, dangerousness, and social distance [Electronic version]. *American Journal of Public Health, 89,* 1328-1333.

Marini, I., Feist, A., Miller, E. (2004). Vocational expert testimony for the Social Security Administration: Observations from the field. *Journal of Forensic Vocational Analysts, 7*(1), 25-34.

Mechanic, D., & Rochefort, D. A. (1990). Deinstitutionalization: An appraisal of reform [Electronic version]. *Annual Review of Sociology, 16,* 301-327.

Miller, J. G. (1946). Clinical psychology in the Veterans Administration [Electronic version].*American Psychologist, 1,* 181-189.

Money, J. (1983). The genealogical descent of sexual psychoneuroendocrinology from sex and health theory: The eighteenth to the twentieth centuries [Electronic version]. *Psychoneuroendocrinology, 8,* 391-400.

National Advisory Mental Health Council. (1993). Health care reform for Americans with severe mental illness: Report of the National Advisory Mental Health Council. *American Journal of Psychiatry, 150*(10), 1447-1465.

National Alliance on Mental Illness (NAMI). (2006). *Grading the states: A report on America's health care system for serious mental illness.* Retrieved from http://www.nami.org/Content/NavigationMenu/Grading_the_States/Full_Report/GTS06_final.pdf

National Institute of Mental Health. (2011). Retrieved from http://www.nimh.nih.gov

Obermann, C. E. (1965). *A history of vocational rehabilitation in America* (2nd ed.) [Electronic version]. Minneapolis, MN: T.S. Denison.

Oberndorf, C. P. (1953). *A history of psychoanalysis in America.* New York: Harper & Row.

Office of the Surgeon General (2011). *Mental health: A report of the surgeon general.* Retrieved from http://www.surgeongeneral.gov/library/mentalhealth/home.html

O'Hare, T., Shen, C., & Sherrer, M. (2010). High-risk behaviors and drinking-to-cope as mediators of lifetime abuse and PTSD symptoms in clients with severe mental illness [Electronic version]. *Journal of Traumatic Stress, 23,* 255-263.

Packard, E. P. W. (2010). The prisoners' hidden life, or insane asylums unveiled. In G. Eghigian (Ed.), *From madness to mental health: Psychiatric disorder and its treatment in western civilization.* New Brunswick, NJ: Rutgers University Press. (Original work published 1868.)

Peterson, D. B. (2010). *Psychosocial aspects of functioning, disability, and health.* New York: Springer.

Pickren, W. E. (2005). Science, practice, and policy: An introduction to the history of psychology and the National Institute of Mental Health. In W. E. Pickren & S. F. Schneider (Eds.), *Psychology and the National Institute of Mental Health: A historical analysis of science, practice, and policy.* Washington, DC: American Psychological Association.

Pollock, H. M. (1921). Eugenics as a factor in the prevention of mental disease [Electronic version]. *The State Hospital Quarterly, 7,* 13-19.

Redlich, A. D., Steadman, H. J., Monahan, J. Robbins, P. C., & Petrila, J. (2006). Patterns of practice in mental health courts: A national survey [Electronic version]. *Law and Human Behavior, 30,* 347-362.

Rogers, C. (1961). *On becoming a person.* Boston: Houghton Mifflin Company.

Rosen, G. (1968). *Madness in society: Chapters in the historical sociology of mental illness.* Chicago, IL: The University of Chicago Press.

Rosenhan, D. L. (1973). On being sane in insane places [Electronic version]. *Science, 179,* 250-258.

Schwartz, A., Bradley, R., Sexton, M., Sherry, A., & Ressler, K. (2005). Posttraumatic stress disorder among African Americans in an inner city mental health clinic [Electronic version]. *Psychiatric Services, 56,* 212-215.

Screening for Mental Health, Inc. (2011). *National Depression Screening Day (NDSD).*Retrieved from http://www.mentalhealthscreening.org/events/national-depression-screening-day.aspx

Scull, A. (1981). The discovery of the asylum revisited: Lunacy reform in the new American republic. In A. Skull (Ed.), *Madhouses, mad-doctors, and madmen: The social history of psychiatry in the Victorian Era*. Philadelphia: University of Pennsylvania Press.

Shorter, E. (1997). *A history of psychiatry: From the era of the asylum to the age of prozac*. New York: John Wiley & Sons.

Slate, R. N., & Johnson, W. W. (2008). *The criminalization of mental illness: Crisis & opportunity for the justice system*. Durham, NC: Carolina Academic Press.

Stockdill, J. W. (2005). National mental health policy and the community mental health centers, 1963–1981. In W. E. Pickren & S. F. Schneider (Eds.), *Psychology and the National Institute of Mental Health: A historical analysis of science, practice, and policy*. Washington, DC: American Psychological Association.

Thompson, J. W., Walker, R. D., & Silk-Walker, P. (1993). Psychiatric care of American Indians and Alaska Natives. In A. C. Gaw (Ed.), *Culture, ethnicity and mental illness* (pp 189–243). Washington, DC: American Psychiatric Press.

Torrey, E. F., & Miller, J. (2001). *The invisible plague: The rise of mental illness from 1750 to present*. New Brunswick, NJ: Rutgers University Press.

U.S. Bureau of the Census. (1975). *Historical statistics of the United States, Colonial times to 1970, Bicentennial Edition, Part 2*. Washington, DC: Author, 1, 84, tab. B-427.

U.S. Department of Justice. (1990). *Americans with Disabilities Act*. Retrieved from http://www.ada.gov/archive/adastat91.htm.

U.S. Department of Justice. (2009). *Americans with Disabilities Act of 1990, as amended*. Retrieved from http://www.ada.gov/pubs/adastatute08mark.htm.

U.S. Department of Justice. (2010). *ADA: Know your rights: Returning service members with disabilities*. Retrieved from http://www.ada.gov/servicemembers_adainfo.html.

U.S. Department of Defense. (2011). *U.S. casualty status*. Retrieved from http://www.defense.gov/news/casualty.pdf.

U.S. Department of Veterans Affairs. (2011). *VA/DoD Clinical practice guidelines*. Retrieved from www.healthquality.va.gov

Vercillo, A. (2011). *Social security vocational expert testimony and psychiatric impairments*. Presentation August 3, International Association of Rehabilitation Professionals webinar.

Wagner-Jauregg, J. (2010). The treatment of dementia paralytica by malaria inoculation. In G. Eghigian (Ed.), *From madness to mental health: Psychiatric disorder and its treatment in Western Civilization*. New Brunswick, NJ: Rutgers University Press. (Original work published 1927)

World Health Organization. (2011). *Global burden of disease (GBD)*. Retrieved from http://www.who.int/healthinfo/global_burden_disease/en

Yanni, C. (2003). The linear plan for insane asylums in the United States before 1866 [Electronic version]. *Journal of the Society of Architectural Historians*, 62(1), 24–49.

Yellow Bird, P. (2001). *Wild Indians: Native perspective on the Hiawatha Asylum for Insane Indians*. Retrieved from http://www.mindfreedom.org/kb/mental-health-abuse/Racism/wild-indians/view.

4

Social Work Practice With People With Disabilities in the Era of Disability Rights

RICHARD L. BEAULAURIER AND SAMUEL H. TAYLOR

Over the years, social work practice in health care has managed to innovate and adapt many of its essential functions. Traditionally, these functions have included information and referral, counseling, resource acquisition (brokerage), and case advocacy. Such elements of practice are congruent with the norms, procedures, and interdisciplinary arrangements encountered in health and rehabilitation organizations. Increasingly, however, some people with disabilities are questioning the efficacy and assumptions inherent in social work's traditional helping role. Many individuals with disabilities are becoming increasingly interested in empowerment. In the process, some have come to distrust social workers and other professionals whom they believe often do things *to* rather than *with* people with disabilities (Kailes, 1988, p. 4; Mackelprang & Salsgiver, 1996, p. 11; Zola, 1983b, pp. 355–356).

As these attitudes emerged and gathered strength during the 1970s and 1980s, alternatives to various social work activities took shape, influenced in large measure by the disability rights movement (Frieden, 1983; Lachat, 1988; Roberts, 1989). This movement sought to gain some of the services necessary for people with disabilities to be able to live in communities outside institutions and they pressed for more formal acknowledgements of their right to do so. New associations and organizations were formed to meet the needs of people with disabilities and raise their levels of awareness about their basic civil rights as well as the possibility of achieving new levels of integration into community life. Included among these were groups that focused solely on policy, legislative change, and community organizing such as American Disabled for Assistance Programs Today (ADAPT[1]), the World Institute on Disability (WID), the American Coalition of Citizens with Disabilities (ACCD), Disabled in Action (DIA), and others. In part, because of grassroots support from these and other groups of people with disabilities, new laws, such as the Americans with Disabilities Act (ADA), were drafted to protect the rights of individuals with disabilities and to remove structural barriers hindering their integration into society.[2]

THE DISABILITY RIGHTS MOVEMENT

While intellectual and academic support for advancing the civil rights of people with disabilities began as early as the 1940s (Berkowitz, 1980, chapter 6; Meyerson, 1990), it was during the 1970s and 1980s that people with disabilities began to organize for political action. A principal purpose was to be able to gain increased opportunities for independent and self-determined lifestyles in the wider community. They founded organizations that advocated the integration of people with disabilities into mainstream communities to the maximum extent possible. Such advocacy groups were formed by consumers to benefit consumers (DeJong, 1981, chapter 2; Frieden, 1983; Lachat, 1988). With help from others, these groups were successful enough to have their conceptualizations of self-determination, consumer control, and nondiscrimination codified in a variety of laws, the most important of which are the Rehabilitation Act of 1973, its amendments (1978), the Individuals with Disabilities Education Act (IDEA) (1997), and the Americans with Disabilities Act of 1990. The acts contain mandates for the inclusion of people with disabilities into mainstream American life to the maximum extent possible.

These laws are symbolic of a dramatic shift in legislative thinking about the concept of disability. Hahn (1984) has called this change in perspective a transition from a "medical" to a "minority group" perspective. Legislation has increasingly recognized people with disabilities as a minority group subject to and/or at risk of exclusion and discrimination. Since 1973, disability laws, especially at the federal level have increasingly emphasized the need for the protection of their rights to inclusion in mainstream American life.

The emphasis on civil rights exhibited by many disabilities interest groups is partly due to a growing recognition that historically people with disabilities have been systematically persecuted, neglected, and forced into isolation. In the early part of this century in the United States, many people with disabilities were incarcerated and even sterilized against their wills. At one point, virtually every state had laws that supported the segregation or sterilization of various categories of people with physical, mental, and developmental disabilities often rationalizing this on Social Darwinist or similarly eugenic grounds (Berkowitz, 1980; Johnson, 1903; Reilly & Philip, 1991; Varela, 1983; Wolfensberger, 1969). By the late 20th century, laws in support of eugenic policies had been virtually eliminated. Even so, authors such as Goffman (1963) and Wright (1960, chapter 2) recognized the prevalent stigma and biased treatment accorded to people with disabilities. There is little doubt that all too often people with disabilities remain isolated and effectively segregated from mainstream society today, in part because of a lack of physical access, but also because of stereotypical attitudes about their capabilities. While laws no longer actively prevent people with disabilities from participating in society, a range of physical barriers and disability related discrimination has continued to result in a lack of opportunities for disabled people to become integrated into American society.

This is not so much the product of a will to discriminate on the part of the general public, but rather a failure to take the needs of people with disabilities into account. We design buildings with steps, doors that are too narrow, and floors that are too slick for many of our citizens. Educational systems continue to use timed tests in ways that bias against intelligent students who process or write what they know comparatively slowly. We forget that people of all abilities need to use public washrooms. This prompted an early pioneer of the movement to observe that decades after Rosa Parks moved to the front of the bus, many people with disabilities still could not even get on one (Roberts, 1989).

The crux of the new thinking about disability is that it is not so much a person's impairment that is disabling but rather the *lack of accommodation* for them that creates problems. Discrimination is less likely to result from open hostility than from omitting them from consideration altogether. We do not put stairs in buildings because we hate disabled people. We simply fail to take the needs of people who use wheelchairs into account. This failure to be responsive to the needs of people with disabilities has resulted in social and physical conditions that effectively bar many people with disabilities from full participation in society.

Social attitudes that have made people with disabilities the quintessentially "worthy poor" have ironically also had the reverse effect of making them the objects of pity and charity (Adler, Wright, & Ulicny, 1991). This orientation to disability emphasizes the *in*abilities (literally characterizing them as pitiful) of people with disabilities rather than their capabilities, particularly with regard to their ability to lead full and productive lives that include working, studying, maintaining social relationships, and consuming in the marketplace in much the same way as everyone else.

The main purpose of the ADA, passed in 1990, was to help eliminate impediments, whether they are physical barriers or related to stereotypical attitudes. This law does not so much overturn past legislation that served to prevent inclusion (as did prior civil rights law) but rather promotes accommodation. Physical and social accommodations of people with disabilities that had heretofore been merely hypothetically possible are now mandated by law. Failure to accommodate the needs for social and physical inclusion of people with disabilities is now considered a violation of their civil rights.

Traditional Approaches to Disability in Health and Rehabilitation Settings

Efforts to provide medical rehabilitation, particularly as it gained effectiveness and prominence following World War II, brought social workers into more frequent contact with people with disabilities. Medical rehabilitation efforts generally utilized a team approach that relied heavily on the contributions of social workers (Berkowitz, 1980, chapter 4). The professional role of preparing the family and the individual with a new disability for life outside the hospital milieu was highly compatible with social casework approaches already in use (Bartlett, 1957, p. 87; Burling, Lentz, & Wilson, 1956, p. 128; Cannon, 1930, pp. 90–96).

Historically medical rehabilitation efforts have sought to "restore" patients to their fullest levels of physical functioning (Cannon, 1952, p. 205; Wright, 1960, pp. 18–19). Originally, this was undertaken for the express purpose of encouraging patients to enter or return to remunerative occupations by *altering* patients in ways that made them more physically capable of dealing with an unaltered world (Berkowitz, 1980, pp. 109–112). This has remained an important part of the rehabilitative process, particularly in the acute stages, when it is still unknown what level of physical functioning people with new disabilities will be able to regain. However, the goal of maximizing physical functioning can also have unintended psychological consequences for the patient, particularly when carried to extreme levels. Decades ago, Wright (1960, chapter 2) observed that more narrowly focused efforts to help people maximize their physical functioning can lead to feelings of shame about their disability by emphasizing the notion that their limitations were unacceptable and needed to be removed. She noted that this stood in contrast with attitudes toward persons of various racial and ethnic groups. When people of color embraced characteristics particular to the cultural norms of their group, they were thought to have appropriate pride in their heritage. People who accepted their impairments and were ready to build lives that included them (particularly if this meant not accepting heroic or invasive corrective procedures) have often been labeled as persons with neurotic adjustment problems.

Partisans in the independent living and disability rights movements take a different approach. They accept the impairment in the person and emphasize organizing and working for environmental accommodations to physical limitations. Rather than altering the patient, they favor altering the norms and structures that limit full participation in society. Barriers, whether they are physical or attitudinal, are being challenged as discriminatory and unnecessary (Hahn, 1984; Kailes, 1988).

Advocates point out that there may be some good reasons for embracing a disability. Some are obvious. For example, a person might choose an artificial prosthetic foot made of light composite materials because of the greater range of motion it offers when engaging in sports, making it preferable to a less functional prosthesis that looks more "normal."[3]

Another example involves arranging for assistance from others. An individual with a disability may well be inclined to seek assistance from another person, such as a personal care attendant, even for things they are physically capable of doing by themselves. An acquaintance of the author uses a personal care attendant to help with getting dressed in the morning although he is physically able to dress himself without such help. The reason is that dressing by himself takes about 2 hours and leaves him physically exhausted. By contrast, the attendant enables him to get dressed him in about 10 minutes. He is then able to use the time gained for more rewarding activities related to his career as a university history professor. This is not so much an argument against achieving gains in physical functioning, but rather is an effort to call attention to alternative factors that can promote social independence.[4]

ORIENTATION TOWARD THE ROLE OF THE PATIENT: THE PATIENT-CONSUMER CONUNDRUM

Many disability rights authors maintain that many, if not most, medical and rehabilitation professionals have tended to view people with disabilities as relatively passive beneficiaries of their treatment regimes (DeJong, 1981, 1983, pp. 15–20; Kailes, 1988; Mackelprang & Salsgiver, 1996, p. 9; Nosek, Dart, & Dart, 1981, p. 1; Zola, 1983a). As medical and rehabilitative treatment strives to return the person with a disability to the most "normal" state of physical functioning possible, control of the process tends to be maintained by the technical experts (DeJong, 1981, pp. 28–31; Zola, 1979, pp. 453–454). However, since the actual functioning levels of people with disabilities cannot always fully reach "normal" standards, success is often thought of in terms of completion of the treatment regime. The goal of working to achieve actual social integration and a normalization of social relations is not emphasized and may not even be one of the principal objectives of rehabilitation (DeJong, 1983, pp. 15–20).

DeJong (1981) suggests that this makes for a rather sharp philosophical difference between the goals of *traditional* medical and rehabilitation institutions and disability rights groups. The former tend to define disability as the inability of a person to perform certain *activities of daily living* (ADL) as the working problem. In this view, problems are located within the individual, since they are seen to be *caused* by a *person's inabilities* and impairments. It is, therefore, the individual who needs changing. It follows that changing individuals to improve their performance on ADL requires that they follow a treatment plan laid out by experts in rehabilitation medicine and technology (e.g., the rehabilitation team). The exclusive focus on the impairment is often reflected in the language that professionals use to describe patients, who are often referred to by their condition (e.g., "paraplegics") rather than as *people with* a disabling condition.[5]

Conversely, disability rights groups tend to define and perceive the "disabler" as outside the person. This emerging perspective considers that some of the most important problems of people with disabilities reside in inflexible and insensitive health organizations that are more interested in maximizing profits and maintaining the status quo than in assisting them with what they believe to be their actual needs (DeJong, 1981).[6] In an era of cost cutting and cost consciousness, health administrators usually seek to set up a menu of standardized treatment options designed to maximize achievement of ADLs at the lowest possible cost. The emphasis is on medical aspects of the impairment rather than social advocacy aimed at bringing about important alterations in living and work environments.

The disability rights perspective departs radically from such viewpoints. Advocates tend to view people with disabilities as (a) experts on their particular condition and (b) the most appropriate persons to make decisions about the kind and the course of treatments they are to receive. Client self-determination is operationalized by the disability rights movement as being active and informed involvement with the key decision making processes that are central to the medical and rehabilitative treatment of the person being treated. One of the most important roles of the social worker may be to help both the team and the person with a disability to move toward this type of complementary role arrangement. During the course of medical and/or rehabilitation treatment, social workers need to be able to help the person take control of the process to the fullest extent possible. One of the ways that social workers can do this is by educating and advocating on behalf of the importance and the rights of patients to control of these decisions. Another is by helping patients to advocate on their own behalf in order to realize their wishes and goals. While some patients, due to an inability to articulate their desires or the acute nature of their condition, may not have much control over treatment processes in the beginning, social workers should be expected to work to help them achieve maximal decision-making control as soon as practicable and certainly before they are discharged. This process involves helping patients with the critical change as they move from being passive recipients of care in the medical system to active *consumers:* persons with basic rights and the capacity to understand and even control the course of their treatment.

Orientation Toward Independence

The key to comprehending how disability has been reconceptualized is to understand the term "independence" as it is used by disability advocates. Traditionally, both rehabilitation professionals and members of the disability rights movement have favored the maximization of independence as an important and desirable goal of rehabilitation. As noted earlier, many rehabilitation specialists believe the term has a very particular meaning: the ability to do things with minimal assistance either from other people or from machines. This creates a hierarchy of desirable treatment outcomes. Best is when the patient becomes able to approximate the activities of an unimpaired, robust individual without human or mechanical assistance. Next best is when the person can perform such tasks with the use of the latest assistive devices. The least desirable outcome is when, at the end of the rehabilitative process, the individual still requires human assistance to perform the activities of a robust, unimpaired individual (Zola, 1983b).

The meaning of the term "independence" is more complex and less obvious when defined and used by members of the disability rights movement. Their usage tends to emphasize *social* independence and has a meaning closer to self-determination and the ability to "call one's own shots." This meaning is clearer in some other languages. In German, for example, independent living is referred to as *"selbstbestimmtes Leben,"* literally, "self-determined living." For people in the disability rights movement, the most important determinant of independence is not whether one relies on others or devices for assistance, but the degree to which decisions about assistance and other aspects of life are determined by the individual with a disability. Zola (1983b) contended that the emphasis of medical and rehabilitation professionals was almost exclusively in relation to *physical independence* rather than *social independence*. The former is independence from devices or attendants while the latter is the ability to be fully involved in planning the course of one's own treatment and care. He contends that when these two values are at odds, gains in physical independence are almost never worth the losses in social independence (pp. 345–347).

To be sure, this does not always create a dilemma, particularly in the acute stages of the rehabilitation process when major gains can be expected in physical functioning. It becomes more of a dilemma when the expectation is for small gains in physical functioning or where "solutions" are intrusive, highly time-consuming, very fatiguing, experimental or do not really contribute to psycho-social reintegration into mainstream life. In the earlier example of the former rehabilitation patient who has given up dressing himself and now allows an attendant help him with this activity, it is not able that he initially spent many months in rehabilitation learning to dress himself, only to give up the activity when he decided on a more efficient alternative approach. Most often social workers are the only members of rehabilitation teams who have the knowledge and responsibility to focus on the *social* life and needs of patients. Therefore, it is incumbent on social workers to help the teams recognize this "new" definition of social independence and client self-determination.

It may also be necessary for social workers to more fully emphasize their role as educators in their work with patients and the teams. Social workers need to be attuned to the new realities of life with a disability, which make it far less restrictive and offer consumers more life options than were available in the past. Overemphasis on dealing with fears about life with a disability and "heroic" efforts to restore "normal" functioning are often perceived by the disability rights community as misguided. They contend that such forms of practice are based on stereotypes, on overly gloomy visions about what life with a disability will be like, or visions of life in institutionalized settings. Most of the general public are probably unaware of the many people with disabilities who are now able to live, work, and shop in mainstream communities, while also forming meaningful social relationships, in spite of severe disabilities. Social workers need to become familiar with case examples and be able to communicate this perspective (or even connect patients with such individuals) so that newly impaired individuals and their families may become aware of how life can be full and rich even with the acquisition of a severe impairment. Such an awareness may also lead them to reconsider the effort and attention they are asked to expend in order to achieve relatively minor gains in physical ability that may be less than worth the effort.[7]

Another important role for social workers is helping both the rehabilitation team and the patient with the process associated with transitioning decision making power from the professionals to the patient. By the time of discharge, and ideally even before that, people with disabilities should be able to weigh and articulate their desires and preferences with regard to the various treatment options.

On a seemingly more mundane level, it is important to remember that a sense of consumer control tends to be maximized to the extent that assistance personnel are hired and fired by the person with the disability (Haggstrom, 1995). For this reason, many people in the disability movement tend to eschew professional helpers who are not under their control, but rather answer directly to a third-party health system or payer. Disability rights advocates tend to favor the use of low cost, paraprofessional aides that they themselves are able to hire and fire rather than more skilled aides such as home health nurses (DeJong, Batavia, & McKnew, 1992). In recent years, disability activist groups have been working to create payment schemes that make personal care attendants more widely available and bring them under greater consumer control (DeJong et al., 1992). Zola (1983b) noted that such aides often contribute to the sense of "independence" of people with disabilities by helping them to perform basic tasks quickly, easily, and reliably. In many cases, these are everyday activities that more professionalized helpers do not perform since the tasks are not medical in nature. However, these are the very services that are often vital to an individual's ability to remain socially independent. One of the major priorities of the disability rights movement today is to develop political and legislative support for funding such paraprofessional helpers. To this end, the largest and most important disability activist organization, ADAPT, has shifted its activities from an emphasis on public transportation to attendant care services.[8]

Orientation Toward Technology

The development of technologies such as portable respirators, powerful but cheap computing devices, longer lasting batteries, and light-weight materials has helped make it possible for many people with disabilities to live independently. In light of these innovations and their contributions to people with disabilities, it is somewhat ironic that the disability rights community tends to favor the use of "low-technology" assistive devices whenever possible. Their reasoning is rather straightforward: the simpler the technology, the easier and cheaper it is likely to be to repair and maintain assistive devices. Space-age technologies are often high cost and are accompanied by hordes of professionals who are needed for training, servicing, and repairs. This can lead to an ironic situation in which disabled people feel controlled and limited by the devices that held promise for offering independence.[9]

However, Zola (1983b) concluded that an intervention that is profitable to build, requires periodic attention by health professionals, and is "technologically fascinating" will often be promoted as the next best thing to a "cure" when it is presented in the rehabilitation literature. "Thus does high-technology medicine pursued in a questionable manner contribute to greater dependence of those who seek its help" (Zola, 1983b, p. 346).

Disability rights advocates, more often than not, favor reliable, low-technology solutions that also allow for greater social integration. Examples of such arrangements include the construction of ramps, hiring and training of attendants and sign-interpreters, negotiated accommodations with employers, accessible housing, and other *environmental* changes that promote the person's ability to participate in mainstream life. A friend of the authors', for example, who has a mobility impairment traded in his van with an electronic lift for a car into which he could comfortably place and store his wheelchair. While this arrangement required a little more effort, it did not break down the way his electric lift often did, leaving him stranded until a technician-specialist could arrive to repair it.

Many in the deaf community would argue that the debate over cochlear implants for children is another case in point. Members of the medical community, as well as some of the more traditionally oriented deaf services organizations have advocated for the use of cochlear implants even when the level of improvement in auditory functioning is only marginal. More radically militant members of the deaf community view this as surgical "maiming" of innocent deaf children, potentially ostracizing them from their *birth right of deafness* and inclusion in the deaf community, as well as segregating them from the hearing community that will never accept them as "normal" (Barringer, 1993; D'Antonio, 1993). A part of this debate is a basic philosophical difference with regard to the nature of deafness. For most professionals in the medical community, deafness is a crippling medical condition to be conquered. For many in the deaf community, deafness is not so much a limiting handicap as a difference, one with its own culture and benefits. Deaf advocates argue that the *option* of deafness is worthy of consideration; one that may well be chosen over the alleged benefits of invasive procedures that all too often produce no more than marginal improvements in hearing ability. They favor informing potential recipients about all of the various consequences these procedures may have, as well as presenting information about other options. In the case of cochlear implants, medical professionals often prefer to perform surgery in order to gain even a marginal improvement in hearing, though this often creates social difficulties for the patient. Dependency on technical experts is fostered, not just around the technologies of the procedure and treatment, but also for its prescribed goals and criteria of success. This requires that people with disabilities (1) view the rehabilitation professional as an expert, (2) view themselves as in an undesirable state, and (3) work toward a prognosis and recovery that has been predefined for them (DeJong, 1981, p. 31). As this example suggests, the goals may be defined too narrowly in terms of function and not in terms of social costs. The former holds that *some* hearing is better than none. Activist elements of the deaf community would argue that it may well be better to be part of *their* community than not to be fully integrated into *any* community. Often a person with a cochlear implant, they reason, does not gain *enough* hearing to be seen as "normal," but may have just enough so that they no longer fit into the deaf community.[10]

Relatively low tech, nonmedical services may even be sufficient to help many individuals with severe disabilities remain in their homes. At one time, such persons would have required institutionalized care. For patients to remain at home, social workers need to become aware of some different community based resources. Volunteer or moderate-cost carpentry, plumbing, house cleaning, paraprofessional attendant care, and so on are available in many communities but they do not tend to advertise and must be sought out. Independent living centers are often well versed in these necessary services, have resource locators, and in some cases have developed independent living educational materials for both consumers and providers (Shreve & Access Living, 1993). Independent living centers can be found in most urban areas due in large part to the support they receive from federal funding as well as local resources (U. S. Congress, 1978).[11]

OPERATING OUT OF A DISABILITY RIGHTS PERSPECTIVE

Social workers may need to initiate ongoing liaisons with independent living centers and other alternative sources of information if they are to expand their knowledge to include options, resources, and services that go beyond what is currently available (Zola, 1983b, pp. 346–347). This suggests that there may be a role for social workers to engage in client and systems advocacy within their organizations, with third-party payers and with legislators, to ensure that funding and services are available for people with disabilities.

Moreover active partnerships with social workers to achieve services that promote independent living should go a long way toward ameliorating some of the resentment felt by many people with disabilities. In light of the failure of the medical and rehabilitation establishment to even recognize these relatively new perspectives that are now embraced by the disability rights movement, some activists openly question whether professionals can be counted on for help in working toward the empowerment of people with disabilities. In their view, over the years all too many rehabilitation professionals have tended to promote dependence rather than independence (Berrol, 1979; Zola, 1979). A recent study suggests, however, that social workers may be moving somewhat closer to the aspirations and goals of disabled people (Beaulaurier & Taylor, 2000). The authors conclude based on their findings that there may be an important role for social workers to perform as intermediaries between health services professionals and organizations and the people they seek to serve.

Before social workers can do that, however, they must become educated themselves and have their consciousness raised. Health and rehabilitation professionals may have the best of intentions and might be "dismayed" to be told that they are helping to foster "technological dependence" and that this is not supportive of disability rights movements' goals for empowerment, self-determination, and social integration at the community level.

It is important to recognize that up to now the disability rights movement has largely been a self-help movement, and sometimes it has taken on an adversarial role toward professionals whom they have not seen to be particularly supportive. It may be incumbent, therefore, for social workers to demonstrate to such groups that they have valuable skills and knowledge that can be beneficial to their purposes. Berrol (1979) suggests that professionals seeking to promote independent living and foster the empowerment of people with disabilities must

> provide leadership in their areas of expertise without dominance, they must provide services, they must be active advocates, they must share their unique skills, and they must provide training. They must assure that there are the same opportunities to develop positive role models as are available to the able-bodied population. (p. 457)

As social workers begin to reach out to the disability rights community, the roles that may be most valuable to and appreciated are those of educator and advocate (Zola, 1983b, p. 57). These are not new roles for social workers. However, this does suggest that community organizing, organizational practice, case management, and advocacy skills may take on heightened importance in working effectively with this population.

Empowering People With Disabilities

Managed care settings may well create even greater needs for social work mezzo and macro skills. Tower (1994, p. 191) has suggested that given increasing caseloads and service demands and decreasing social service budgets in the health services sector, client self-determination may be "the first thing to go" as social workers struggle to balance their workloads. In light of the increasing activism and assertiveness of many people with disabilities, this could put social workers at odds with clients and client groups. Effective social work practice with people with disabilities requires a refocused conceptual framework that will support and promote self-determination. This framework must be designed to enable people with disabilities to:

1. Expand their range of options and choices
2. Prepare them to be more effective in dealings with professionals, bureaucrats, and agencies that often do not understand or appreciate their heightened need for self-determination
3. Mobilize and help groups of people with disabilities to consider policy and program alternatives that can improve their situation

Direct practice with clients with disabilities will certainly remain a primary activity of health and rehabilitation social workers (with perhaps greater secondary emphasis on mezzo and macro skills). However, this practice must increasingly emphasize empowerment objectives rather than mere compliance with medically prescribed treatment plans and, our traditional psycho-social clinical interventions. Fostering the independence and empowerment of people with disabilities requires enabling them to become motivated and skilled at helping themselves. Independent living services, inspired by the disability rights movement, emphasize concepts that rely on preparing consumers to help themselves.

The staff's role is to provide only what relevant training and problem solving is needed in acquiring and using services until the consumer becomes self-reliant. The move from dependence on staff to self-direction marks the shift from "client/patient mentality" to "consumer mentality" (Kailes, 1988, p. 5).

Social workers can approach practice in a similar way in order to help negotiate the transitions that will enable people to move from the passive role of patient to the active role of informed and empowered consumers. Several authors have discussed and outlined approaches to advocacy practice that seem particularly useful for health social workers in their work with people with disabilities. These authors include Hardcastle, Wenocur, and Powers (1997, chapter 12), Herbert and Levin (1996), Herbert and Mould (1992), McGowan (1987), Mickelson (1995), Sosin and Caulum (1983), and Tesolowski, Rosenberg, and Stein (1983).

Gutiérrez (1990) has identified four psychological changes that are particularly important in empowering clients: (1) self-efficacy—the belief that one's actions can produce desired changes, (2) group consciousness—identification as a member of a class and recognition of how political, social, and physical structures effect the class, (3) reduction of self-blame for negative consequences of being a member of the class, and (4) assuming personal responsibility for change—preparing to take action to improve one's own situation. As social workers assess their practice with people with disabilities they need to focus more on helping them accomplish these person-in-context changes.[12]

The lack of control that many people with disabilities experience while they are in the treatment process is, however, not simply a psychological phenomenon. Social workers in health and rehabilitation settings must develop and demonstrate skills that will facilitate helping their clients to press for inclusion in the planning and decisions that will be made about the their treatment. Social workers will also need to consider more emphasis on their practice role as educators in order to help clients become effective advocates and negotiators for their own interests. This will require that practitioners modify customary approaches to include more emphasis on dealing with organizations and systems enabling

> people to identify issues, to partialize the sources of their problem, and to speculate about possible solutions. The worker converses about power and conflict, encourages people to challenge preconceived notions, and works to unleash [their] potential. (Grosser & Mondros, 1985, p. 162)

Emphasis on such practice includes familiarity and skill with the advocacy and negotiation modalities that focus on dealing effectively with bureaucracies, administrative structures, and centers of power that make decisions and allocate resources. In order to accomplish this, social workers may need to interact more deliberately and purposefully with practitioners engaged in both the independent living and disability rights movements. This suggests a need for more interorganizational dialogues and agency agreements for working together to identify issues and concerns, formulate agendas, and develop reciprocal understandings.

Finally, health social workers must gain increased levels of knowledge about the particular issues that are of concern to the disability community. Direct services social workers need to be responsive to issues such as the isolation and lack of group consciousness that many people with disabilities experience. These feelings often derive from limited contacts with other people with disabilities. People with recently acquired disabilities need to interact with *empowered* people with disabilities. Pinderhughes (1994, p. 23), writing from an ethnic minority perspective, encourages creating linkages with natural support systems such as family, church groups, fraternal, and social organizations. Such natural gatherings of networks of individuals who share similar characteristics and a desire for empowerment simply did not exist among people with disabilities until relatively recently. In the past quarter century, however, much progress has been made by people with disabilities who are working to develop and create more functional community supports. In some communities, independent living centers have been organized, developed, and administered by and for people with disabilities and they often collaborate with more advocacy oriented organizations such as ADAPT, ACCD, DIA, and others previously mentioned. They sponsor and produce newsletters and newspapers, electronic bulletin board services, and Internet newsgroups.[13] Social workers need to have first-hand familiarity with such functional communities in order to be able to link their clients to them. This requires more than a general awareness that such sources exist. Social workers also need to have the community liaison skills to create and maintain linkages and networks between such groups, services, and their own health services organizations (Taylor, 1985; Weil & Gamble, 1995).

CONCLUSIONS

ADA marked a turning point for people with disabilities. With its passage in 1990, the law began to favor the notion of societal integration of people with disabilities whenever practicable and to offer recourse at those times when they were excluded or the victims of discrimination. It also marked a turning point for disability activism in that some of the most important battles, such as for accessible public transportation, accessible public spaces, and protection from discrimination, were waged and won. This has not, however, resulted in complacency or a diminution of the movement's of militancy.[14] In part, this is a recognition that exercising and campaigning for *rights* is only a part of what is necessary to achieve independence and self-determination. What is also required are a range of essential community-based services. In particular, this means developing and increasing access to personal attendant care as well as related services and programs that support and complement clients' abilities to engage in remunerative work (DeJong & Brannont, 1998; DeJong et al., 1992). In fact, people with disabilities are increasingly seen as leaders in the push for consumer oriented and consumer directed services (Beaulaurier & Taylor, 2001).

This trend is especially observable when reviewing the literature on aging, developmental disability, and mental health (Ansello & Eustis, 1992; Tower, 1994; Wehmeyer, 1997; Wilk, 1994). For many, "person with a disability" has gone from meaning "person with severe limitations" to "person with rights to accommodation and inclusion" (Beaulaurier & Taylor, 2001). An interesting consequence is that the notion and concept of disability is increasingly being used as a unifying theme in the literature about developmental disabilities, mental illness, and aging. There seems to be a recognition that "disability" has a more universal meaning for many different kinds of problems that vulnerable and at-risk groups experience (Racino & Heumann, 1992; Wehmeyer, 1997; Wilk, 1994).

In spite of this activity there have been only a few exploratory studies on social work practice with people with disabilities that were guided by the assumptions, issues, and concerns of the disability rights movement (Renz-Beaulaurier, 1996). At present, the authors are not aware of any systematic research that has described or assessed practice modalities that incorporate such perspectives. Clearly research in this area is needed.[15]

Even without the benefit of extensive empirical research it is clear that people with disabilities are becoming increasingly militant about their right to be involved in planning and making decisions regarding their treatment. They are no longer content to accept the "wisdom" of experts. They are challenging predominant medical and rehabilitation treatment philosophies that tend to emphasize restoring them to relative physical "normality" all too often at the expense of their social integration. These considerations, in addition to the newly imposed budgetary constraints associated with managed health care, have and will create turbulence in the health and rehabilitation task environment.

It is incumbent upon all social workers to reconsider how they view their practice with people who have disabilities. In the coming years we need to learn to emphasize

> strengths rather than pathology, solution seeking rather than problem detecting, competence promotion rather than deficit reduction, and collaborative partnerships rather than professional expertise. (O'Melia, DuBois, & Miley, 1994, p. 164)

It is equally important for social workers in health settings to augment their practice capabilities with regard to organizational and community work, negotiating skills, and advocacy. This practice knowledge and skill must be combined with efforts to acquire clearer understandings of the administrative structures and priorities that operate in health settings and their task environments, so that this knowledge may be used to help people with disabilities develop increased self-determination in their dealings with health systems and professionals.

NOTES

1. The organization has remained one of the most important disability advocacy groups; however, the acronym has changed over time to reflect current legislative and lobbying efforts. Originally, it stood for American Disabled for Accessible Public Transportation, and for a short time American Disabled for Access Power Today before adopting its current name. Insiders typically refer to the organization simply as ADAPT.
2. Other laws include sections of the *Rehabilitation Act* of 1973, the *Education for All Handicapped Children Act* of 1975, The *Individuals with Disabilities Education Act* of 1997, and so on.
3. Less obvious is when the advantage is social rather than physical. A person might want to use a wheelchair instead of crutches, since wheelchairs are often more comfortable and less tiring to use even though the wheelchair makes the individual "look" relatively more disabled. The advantages of a wheelchair's speed and mobility may outweigh the advantages of appearing to be less disabled and more "normal."
4. Zola (1982, p. 346) has stated "… there is literally no physical circumstance in which increased physical independence is worth decreased social and psychological independence."
5. For an excellent discussion about the subtle bias that language and attitudes of professionals often convey, see the discussion by Wright (1980, 1988, 1989). Moreover, activist people with disabilities have expressed a strong preference that the word "people" always appear when describing them, as in "diabetic person," or "person with a disability." This chapter also follows the "person first" rule, as in "person with a disability" which emphasizes the humanity of a person before referring to the person's condition. This symbolically highlights the fact that the person has a condition rather than suggesting that the condition characterizes the person. Perhaps the best reference on how to talk to and about people with disabilities is available from the Eastern Paralyzed Veterans Association at www.epva.org (Cohen, 1998).
6. As an example, the Southern California Chapter of ADAPT—a militant disability rights organization—chose a prominent health organization as the target of its annual social action in 1994.
7. Akin to overly bleak fantasies about life with a disability are overly rosy imaginings about the benefits of new or experimental treatments. Such prognostications about treatment approaches have made Christopher Reeve and the team working with him something of a lightning rod for criticism by the disability rights movement. Many advocates feel that (a) the chances for a "cure" for spinal cord injury are minimal, and (b) what gains from experimental approaches are actually on the horizon are minimal and expensive. Many people in the disability rights movement feel that the cause of people with disabilities would be far better served by efforts to adapt environments to people with disabilities than to seek rather minimal gains in functioning at enormous expense. Media treatments of the actor generally note how this vital and healthy man in his prime was "struck down," and is now heroically working to overcome his "terrible affliction." Rarely do media reports note that he continues to have a full life, maintains a career as an actor, is still relatively healthy, has a warm and supportive family, lives in a non institutionalized setting, and heads major charitable enterprises. Some might argue that he has gained far more fame and prominence as a person with a disability than he ever had prior to his injury. In short, he continues to have a life that in some ways may be more full and meaningful by virtue of his impairments. There are many more mundane cases where this is so, and many individuals now appear to be more conscious of how their lives have continued to be full and rewarding after the onset of disability.

8. The most comprehensive list of such centers is available at www.ilru.org.
9. Again, the controversy appears to center around differing notions of "independence." Rehabilitation professionals tend to view independence as the ability of persons with disabilities to function with minimal assistance from other people.
10. This is particularly the case when there is just enough hearing so that patients (and families) focus on normal speech (which they may well *not* master) and do not learn sign language.
11. See the list maintained at www.ilru.org.
12. Such client change and development is critical in that it helps people with disabilities begin to constructively deal with their own feelings of powerlessness and their all too frequent exclusion from treatment planning and decision making.
13. These include such electronic media such as "Dimenet" and other resources with links at www.ilru. org. The SERIES electronic bulletin board dates back to the late 1980s and allowed disability advocates to communicate about progress on the ADA well before the Internet made computerized communication ubiquitous. Many individual independent living centers also have publications and newsletters in conventional print form.
14. Hahn and Beaulaurier (2001) have recently reported on current militant activities of ADAPT.
15. This may require advocacy targeted toward organizations and institutes that fund research. J. I. Kailes (personal communication, Los Angeles, 1990), a prominent independent living consultant, contends that "... the Rehabilitation Services Administration would still rather fund a program to teach paraplegics to walk on their hands than to fund programs that promote real independent living options for people with disabilities."

REFERENCES

Adler, A. B., Wright, B. A., & Ulicny, G. R. (1991). Fund raising portrayals of people with disabilities: Donations and attitudes. *Rehabilitation Psychology, 36*(4), 231–240.
Ansello, E. F., & Eustis, N. N. (1992). (Eds.). Special issue: Aging and disability. *Gerontologist, 16*(1), entire issue.
Barringer, F. (1993). Pride in a soundless world: Deaf oppose a hearing aid. *New York Times.*
Bartlett, H. M. (1957). Influence of the medical setting on social case work services. In D. Goldstine (Ed.), *Readings in the theory and practice of medical social work* (pp. 85–96). Chicago, IL: University of Chicago Press.
Beaulaurier, R. L., & Taylor, S. H. (2000). Challenges and inconsistencies in providing effective advocacy for disabled people in today's health services environment: An exploratory descriptive study. *SCI Psychosocial Process, 13*(3).
Beaulaurier, R. L., & Taylor, S. H. (2001). Dispelling fears about aging with a disability: Lessons from the disability rights community. *Journal of Gerontological Social Work, 35*(2).
Berkowitz, E. D. (1980). *Rehabilitation: The federal government's response to disability 1935–1954.* New York: Arno Press.
Berrol, S. (1979). Independent living programs: The role of the able-bodied professional. *Archives of Physical Medicine and Rehabilitation, 60,* 456–457.
Burling, T., Lentz, E. M., & Wilson, R. N. (1956). *The give and take in hospitals.* New York: G. P. Putnam's Sons.
Cannon, I. M. (1930). *Social work in hospitals: A contribution to progressive medicine.* (Revised ed.). New York: Russell Sage Foundation.
Cannon, I. M. (1952). *On the social frontier of medicine: Pioneering in medical social service.* Cambridge, MA: Harvard University Press.
Cohen, J. (1998). *Disability etiquette: Tips on interacting with people with disabilities.* New York: Eastern Paralyzed Veterans Association.
D'Antonio, M. (1993). Sound and fury. *Los Angeles Times Magazine.*
DeJong, G. (1981). *Environmental accessibility and independent living out-comes: Directions for disability policy and research.* East Lansing, MI: University Center for International Rehabilitation, Michigan State University.
DeJong, G. (1983). Defining and implementing the independent living concept. In N. M. Crewe & I. K. Zola (Eds.), *Independent living for physically disabled people* (pp. 4–27). San Francisco, CA: Jossey-Bass.
DeJong, G., Batavia, A. I., & McKnew, L. B. (1992). The independent living model of personal assistance in national long term-care policy. *Generations, 16*(1), 43–47.
DeJong, G., & Brannont, R. (1998). Trends in services to working-age people with disabilities. In S. M. Allen & V. Mor (Eds.), *Living in the community with disability* (pp. 168–196). New York: Springer.

Frieden, L. (1983). Understanding alternative program models. In N. M. Crewe & I. K. Zola (Eds.), *Independent living for physically disabled people* (pp. 62-72). San Francisco, CA: Jossey-Bass.

Goffman, E. (1963). *Stigma: Notes on the management of spoiled identity.* Englewood Cliffs, NJ: Prentice-Hall.

Grosser, C. F., & Mondros, J. (1985). Pluralism and participation: The political action approach. In S. H. Taylor & R. W. Roberts (Eds.), *Theory and practice of community social work* (pp. 154-178). New York: Columbia University Press.

Gutiérrez, L. M. (1990). Working with women of color: An empowerment perspective. *Social Work, 35*(2), 149-161.

Haggstrom, W. C. (1995). For a democratic revolution: The grassroots perspective. In J. E. Tropman, J. L. Erlich, & J. Rothman (Eds.), *Tactics and techniques of community intervention* (3rd ed., pp. 134-142). Itasca, IL: F. E. Peacock.

Hahn, H. (1984). Reconceptualizing disability: A political science perspective. *Rehabilitation lLiterature, 45* (11-12), 362-374.

Hahn, H., & Beaulaurier, R. L. (2001). Attitudes toward disabilities: A research note on "adapters" and "consumers" with disabilities. *Journal of Disability Policy Studies, 12*(1).

Hardcastle, D. A., Wenocur, S., & Powers, P. (1997). *Community practice: Theories and skills for social workers.* New York: Oxford University Press.

Herbert, M., & Levin, R. (1996). The advocacy role in hospital social work. *Social Work in Health Care, 22*(3), 71-83.

Herbert, M. D., & Mould, J. W. (1992). The advocacy role in public child welfare. *Child Welfare, 71,* 114-130.

Johnson, A. (1903). Report of committee on colonies for segregation of defectives In *Proceedings of the National Conference of Charities and Correction at the Thirtieth Annual Session Held in the City of Atlanta, May 6-12, 1903* (pp. 245-252): Fred J. Heer.

Kailes, J. I. (1988). *Putting advocacy rhetoric into practice: The role of the independent living center.* Houston, TX: Independent Living Research Utilization.

Lachat, M. A. (1988). *The independent living service model: Historical roots, core elements, and current practice.* Hampton, NH: Center for Resource Management.

Mackelprang, R. W., & Salsgiver, R. O. (1996). People with disabilities and social work: Historical and contemporary issues. *Social Work, 41*(1), 7-14.

McGowan, B. G. (1987). Advocacy. In *Encyclopedia of social work* (18th ed., Vol. 1, pp. 89-95). Silver Spring, MD: National Association of Social Workers.

Meyerson, L. (1990). The social psychology of physical disability: 1948 and 1988. In M. Nagler (Ed.), *Perspectives on disability* (pp. 13-23). Palo Alto, CA: Health Markets Research.

Mickelson, J. S. (1995). Advocacy, In R. L. Edwards (Ed.), *Encyclopedia of social work* (19th ed., Vol. 1, pp. 95-100). Silver Spring, MD: National Association of Social Workers.

Nosek, P., Dart, J., Jr., & Dart, Y. (1981). *Independent living programs: A management perspective.* Unpublished document.

O'Melia, M., DuBois, B., & Miley, K. (1994). The role of choice in empowering people with disabilities: Reconceptualizing the role of social work practice in health and rehabilitation settings. In L. Gutiérrez & P. Nurius (Eds.), *Education and research for empowerment practice* (pp. 161-170). Seattle, WA: Center for Policy and Practice Research.

Pinderhughes, E. (1994). Empowerment as an intervention goal: Early ideas. In L. Gutiérrez & P. Nurius (Eds.), *Education and research for empowerment practice* (pp. 17-30). Seattle, WA: Center for Policy and Practice Research.

Racino, J. A., & Heumann, J. E. (1992). Independent living and community life: Building coalitions among elders, people with disabilities, and our allies. *Generations, 16*(1), 43-47.

Reilly, M. D., & Philip R. (1991). *The surgical solution: A history of involuntary sterilization in the United States.* Baltimore, MD: Johns Hopkins University Press.

Renz-Beaulaurier, R. L. (1996). *Health social workers' perspectives on practice with people with disabilities in the era of the Americans with Disabilities Act: An exploratory-descriptive study.* Unpublished doctoral dissertation, University of Southern California, Los Angeles, CA.

Roberts, E. V. (1989). A history of the independent living movement: A founder's perspective. In B. W. F. Heller, M. Louis, & L. S. Zegens (Eds.), *Psychosocial interventions with physically disabled persons* (pp. 231-244). New Brunswick, NJ: Rutgers University Press.

Shreve, M., & Access Living. (1993). *Access living's independent living skills training curricula* (2nd ed.). Chicago, IL: Access Living.

Sosin, M., & Caulum, S. (1983). Advocacy: A conceptualization for social work practice. *Social Work, 28,* 12-17.

Taylor, S. H. (1985). Community work and social work: The community Liaison approach. In S. H. Taylor & R. W. Roberts (Eds.), *Theory and practice of community social work* (pp. 179-214). New York: Columbia University Press.

Tesolowski, D. G., Rosenberg, H., & Stein, R. J. (1983). Advocacy intervention: A responsibility of human service professionals. *Journal of Rehabilitation, 49*, 35–38.

Tower, K. D. (1994). Consumer-centered social work practice: Restoring client self-determination. *Social Work, 39*(2), 191–196.

U.S. Congress. (1973). *Rehabilitation Act of 1973, PL 93–112*. Washington, DC: U.S. Government Printing Office.

U.S. Congress. (1978). *Rehabilitation, Comprehensive Services and Developmental Disabilities Amendments of 1978, PL 95–602*. Washington, DC: Government Printing Office.

U.S. Congress. (1990). *Americans with Disabilities Act of 1990, PL 101–336*. Washington, DC: Government Publishing Office.

Varela, R. A. (1983). Changing social attitudes and legislation regarding disability. In N. M. Crewe & I. K. Zola (Eds.), *Independent living for physically disabled people* (pp. 28–48). San Francisco, CA: Jossey-Bass.

Wehmeyer, M. (1997). Self-determination as an educational outcome: A definitional framework and implications for intervention. *Journal of Developmental and Physical Aisabilities, 9*(3), 175–209.

Weil, M. O., & Gamble, D. N. (1995). Community practice models. In *Encyclopedia of social work* (19th ed., Vol. 1, pp. 577–594). Silver Spring, MD: National Association of Social Workers.

Wilk, R. J. (1994). Are the rights of people with mental illness still important? *Social Work, 39*(2), 167–175.

Wolfensberger, W. (1969). The origin and nature of our institutional models. In R. B. Kugel & W. Wolfensberger (Eds.), *Changing patterns in residential services for the mentally retarded* (pp. 59–172). Washington, DC: President's Committee on Mental Retardation.

Wright, B. A. (1960). *Physical disability: A psychological approach*. New York: Harper and Row.

Wright, B. A. (1980). Developing constructive views of life with a disability. *Rehabilitation Literature, 41*(11–12), 274–279.

Wright, B. A. (1988). Attitudes and the fundamental negative bias: Conditions and corrections. In H. E. Yuker (Ed.), *Attitudes toward persons with disabilities*. New York: Springer.

Wright, B. A. (1989). Extension of Heider's ideas to rehabilitation psychology. *Rehabilitation Literature, 44*(3), 525–528.

Zola, I. K. (1979). Helping one another: A speculative history of the self help movement. *Archives of Physical Medicine and Rehabilitation, 60*, 452–456.

Zola, I. K. (1982). Social and cultural disincentives to independent living. *Archives of Physical Medicine and Rehabilitation, 63*, 394–397.

Zola, I. K. (1983a). Developing new self-images and interdependence. In N. M. Crewe & I. K. Zola (Eds.), *Independent living for physically disabled people* (pp. 49–59). San Francisco, CA: Jossey-Bass.

Zola, I. K. (1983b). Toward independent living: Goals and dilemmas. In N. M. Crewe & I. K. Zola (Eds.), *Independent living for physically disabled people* (pp. 344–356). San Francisco, CA: Jossey-Bass.

5

Models of Disability: Implications for the Counseling Profession

JULIE F. SMART AND DAVID W. SMART

*D*isability is a natural part of human existence and is growing more common as a larger proportion of the U.S. population experiences some type of disability (Americans with Disabilities Act [ADA], 1990; Bowe, 1980; Employment and Disability Institute, 1996; Pope & Tarlov, 1991; Trieschmann, 1987; U.S. Department of Education, Office of Special Education and Rehabilitation Services, National Institute on Disability and Rehabilitation Research, 2000). Due to medical advances and technology, wider availability of health insurance, and a generally higher standard of living that provides more services and support, people who would have died in the past now survive with a disability. In the same way that the viewpoints, experiences, and history of various ethnic/linguistic/cultural groups have been incorporated into the broader American culture, people with disabilities wish to have their social context and experiences become a valued and acknowledged part of American life. These contributions will strengthen and enrich the lives of those who do not experience disability (Akabas, 2000). In the past, clients with disabilities were served primarily by rehabilitation counselors, probably because of the misconception that the client's disability was the sole or, at minimum, the most important concern. However, because disability is both a common and a natural fact of life and because all individuals, including people with disabilities, have multiple identities, roles, functions, and environments, clients with disabilities require the services of counselors in all specialty areas: aging and adult development; gay, lesbian, bisexual, and transsexual issues; multicultural concerns; community mental health; school counseling; group counseling; marriage and family counseling; career counseling; and spiritual, ethical, and religious values.

To meet minimum standards of practice, therefore, counselors will be required to become proficient in disability issues (Hayes, 2001; Hulnick & Hulnick, 1989). Indeed, Humes, Szymanski, and Hohenshil (1989) suggested that counselors have not facilitated the personal growth and development of their clients with disabilities: "The literature includes many testimonies of persons with disabilities ... who have achieved successful careers despite roadblocks they perceived to have been imposed by counselors" (p. 145). However, in spite of this need, which continues to grow, very few university counseling programs provide adequate training about disability issues (Kemp & Mallinckrodt, 1996; Olkin, 1999; Pledger, 2003).

This lack of training and the resulting failure to provide services may be due to the powerful influence of models of disability, because these models determine in which academic disciplines the experience of disability is studied and taught. Thomas (2004) made the point that only rehabilitation counselors are trained in disability issues. A growing interest in models of disability has emerged in recent years, led by a variety of counseling practitioners, educators, and policy makers (Bickenbach, Somnath, Badley, & Ustun, 1999; Humes et al., 1989; Melia, Pledger, & Wilson, 2003; Olkin & Pledger, 2003; J. F. Smart, 2001, 2004; Tate & Pledger, 2003). Examining these changing models can assist the counseling profession, and individual practitioners, to reorient service provision. Counselor educators and counseling practitioners, regardless of specialty, theoretical orientation, or professional setting, should recognize that disability is never entirely a personal, subjective, and idiosyncratic experience, nor is disability a completely objective, standardized, and universal experience.

The conceptualization of disability as an attribute located solely within an individual is changing to a paradigm in which disability is thought to be an interaction among the individual, the disability, and the environment (both social and physical; Dembo, 1982; Higgins, 1992). Typically, the disability is not the single defining characteristic of the individual; rather the disability is one of several important parts of the individual's self-identity. When counselors dismiss or ignore the disability, a critical part of the client's self-identity must remain unexplored. On the other hand, counselors may tend to overemphasize the salience of the disability and automatically assume that the disability is the "presenting problem" or the cause and source of all the client's concerns. Indeed, the "roadblocks" referred to by Humes et al. (1989) may be due to a lack of understanding, training, and experience with disability issues. Many individuals with disabilities view their disability as a valued part of their self-identity, see positive aspects in the disability, and would choose not to eliminate the disability if they had this option. In contrast, few counselors conceptualize the client's disability as a source of self-actualization.

In this chapter, we draw both theoretical and practice implications, which may assist practitioners and educators in gaining a clearer understanding of counseling clients who have disabilities, from four broad models of disability. Intended as a broad overview of the major models and an introductory discussion of ways in which these models can affect the profession of counseling, we present several different ways of conceptualizing the experience of disability. The four broad models discussed here are (a) the Biomedical Model, (b) the Functional Model, (c) the Environmental Model, and (d) the Sociopolitical Model. In this chapter, the Functional Model and the Environmental Model are presented together because both are interactive models, or stated differently, these two models define disability as an interaction between the individual and his or her environment and functions. Furthermore, it is these two models, the Functional and Environmental, that are most closely related to the practice of counseling. The Sociopolitical Model is considered separately because it is the newest of the models and, more important, this model conceptualizes people with disabilities as belonging to a minority group of individuals who have not yet received their full civil rights.

THE BIOMEDICAL MODEL

The Biomedical Model of disability has a long history, is the most well-known to the general public, and carries with it the power and prestige of the well-established medical profession. This model, rooted in the scientific method and the benefactor of a long tradition, has had dominance in shaping the understanding of disability. The strength of the Biomedical Model lies in its strong explanatory power, which far exceeds the explanatory power of other models. Moreover, this model defines disability in the language of medicine, lending scientific credibility to the idea that disabilities are wholly an individual experience. Due to this "individualization," "privatization," and "medicalization" of disability, the Biomedical Model has remained silent on issues of social justice. Indeed, this model is not considered to be an interactional model because the definition, the "problem," and the treatment of the disability are all considered to lie within the individual with the disability. In addition, interprofessional collaboration is rarely implemented when the disability is medicalized.

Underlying the Biomedical Model is the assumption that pathology is present, and, in addition, disabilities are objective conditions that exist in and of themselves. This "objectification" process opens the door to the possibility of dehumanizing the person because attention is focused on the supposed pathology (Albrecht, 1992; Longmore, 1995). Bickenbach (1993) described this definition of disability as deviance:

> The most commonly held belief about [this model of] disablement is that it involves a defect, deficiency, dysfunction, abnormality, failing, or medical "problem" that is located in an individual. We think it is so obvious as to be beyond serious dispute that disablement is a characteristic of a defective person, someone who is functionally limited or anatomically abnormal, diseased, or pathoanatomical, someone who is neither whole nor healthy, fit nor flourishing, someone who is biologically inferior or subnormal. The essence of disablement, in this view, is that there are things wrong with people with disabilities. (p. 61)

It is interesting that Bickenbach considered the Biomedical Model to have roots in the religious model of disability, in which biological wholeness was viewed as virtue and righteousness. The combination of religion and science in the Biomedical Model has had a formidable influence.

Furthermore, there is a clear-cut normative aspect to the Biomedical Model in that the disability is considered to be biological inferiority, malfunction, pathology, and deviance when compared with (or normed on) individuals without disabilities (McCarthy, 1993). Thus, the individual with a disability, regardless of personal qualities and assets, understands that he or she belongs to a devalued group. Frequently when clients with an identified disability seek professional services, such as counseling, they understand that, in the view of others, a life with a disability is worth less investment (McCarthy, 2003). Joanne Wilson, the commissioner for the Rehabilitation Services Administration from 2002 to 2005, is blind. She summarized the devaluation and the normative aspect of having a disability when she stated, "It's not quite respectable to have a disability" (Wilson, 2003). Furthermore, many individuals with disabilities may see no value in trying to integrate into a society that automatically discounts and pathologizes them. Taken to its extreme, the normative aspect of this model views a perfect world as a world without disabilities, and the possibility exists of providing the medical profession the mandate with which to eliminate disabilities and the people who experience them (Singer, 2000).

The Biomedical Model places people with disabilities in stigmatizing categories, therefore allowing the "general public" to view them as their category—"the blind," "quads" (individuals with quadriplegia), or "the mentally ill" (Nagi, 1969). Regardless of the category, categorized people are viewed as their category and not as individuals. Schur (1971) described the effects of categorization:

> Others respond to devalued persons in terms of their membership in the stigma-laden category. Individual qualities and actions become secondary. ... Individuals of devalued categories are treated as being ... substitutable for each other. ... Stigmatized persons, then, are little valued as persons. Classificatory status tends to displace alternative criteria of personal worth. ... Others may claim license—implicitly, if not explicitly—to treat stigmatized individuals in exploitative and degrading ways. (pp. 30–31)

This categorization according to disability type has had many pervasive, institutional, and systematic consequences, some of which have resulted in inferior services or a lack of services from the counseling professions. In addition, this categorization has fragmented people with disabilities from their own community and robbed them of a collective history (Hahn, 1985, 1988, 1993). Categorization has also successfully taught society to focus on the disability category rather than the universal problems and challenges faced by people with all types of disabilities. Because of the strength and prestige of the Biomedical Model, both the general public and individuals with disabilities have come to see people with disabilities as categories.

In the Biomedical Model, the disability exists totally within the individual, and, accordingly, the individual responsible for the "problem" should also be totally responsible for the solution (Kiesler, 1999). This view, therefore, has the authority to relieve society of any responsibility to accord civil rights to individuals with disabilities. After all, the disability is the individual's flaw and tragedy. A disability is thought to be bad luck, but it is the individual's bad luck. Society often communicates to people with disabilities: "This is how the world is. Take it or leave it." Not only does the Biomedical Model legitimatize prejudice and discrimination, but to the general public, its treatment of people with disabilities often does not appear to be prejudicial and stigmatizing. For example, when individuals with disabilities are not integrated into the workplace, schools, and other social institutions, their absence is usually not noticed. After all, according to this attribution theory, individuals with disabilities are thought to be responsible for their stigmatization. Clinicians have attempted to include environmental issues in their classification/diagnostic systems; however, the degree of prejudice and discrimination experienced or the lack of accommodations is typically not considered when medical professionals determine the level of severity of the disability or render a percentage of impairment.

In the traditional view of the Biomedical Model, both the cause of the disability and the solution and treatment rest with the individual. Liachowitz (1988) described an additional responsibility placed on individuals with disabilities: "Recent medical textbooks go further and construe disability as a variable dependent upon characteristics of motivation and adaptability as well as the limiting residue of disease and injury" (p. 12). Individuals concerned with the rights of people with disabilities derisively refer to this as the "Try Harder" syndrome. One hundred years ago, people with disabilities were often given moral and religious education in an attempt to "rehabilitate" them (Byrom, 2004).

These aspects of the Biomedical Model—the pathologizing, the objectification, the categorization, and the individualization of a disability—are dependent on the diagnosis and classification systems used by the medical professions. Certainly, the diagnostic systems of the medical professions are the most objective, standardized, reliable, and morally neutral assessments compared with those of the other models (American Psychiatric Association, 2000; Peterson, 2002; World Health Organization, 1980, 2001). Medical diagnoses are, however, only as valid as the classification systems used, and further, medical diagnoses can be subjective, impressionistic, value-laden judgments of individuals (Clendinen & Nagourney, 1999; Kirk & Kutchins, 1992; D. W. Smart & Smart, 1997a). L. Eisenberg (1996) stated, "Diagnostic categories and classification schemes are acts of the imagination rather than real things in the world ... We must not mistake this for reality itself" (p. xv), whereas Stone (1984), in a chapter titled "Disability as a Clinical Concept," referred to these systems as "false precision" and stated that medical diagnoses are not the product of "a scientific procedure of unquestionable validity, free from error" (p. 111). Stone concluded by pronouncing the determination of a diagnosis as "an unattainable quest for neutrality" (p. 111). Disability scholars (Albrecht, 1992; Reno, Mashaw, & Gradison, 1997) have posited that all diagnoses are based on the dual concepts of clinical neutrality and clear-cut measures of "normality" and that neither complete clinical neutrality nor absolutely clear-cut measures exist.

The Biomedical Model of disability does not provide a strong basis for the treatment and policy considerations of chronic conditions, which include most disabilities (J. F. Smart,

2005a, 2005b). Because of the long history of the two-outcome paradigm of medicine—total cure or the death of the individual—medical professionals work best with acute injuries rather than chronic, long-term disabilities. Vestiges of this two-outcome paradigm remain in insurance payment policies, which dictate that payments for services—such as counseling—are withdrawn once medical stabilization has been achieved and progress toward a full recovery has terminated. This has a kind of reasonableness, because the business of medical insurance was originally based on the Biomedical Model, with physicians acting as gatekeepers and policy makers.

Furthermore, due to the Biomedical Model's lack of attention to the individual's environment and its focus on the individual, this model is less useful for mental and psychiatric disabilities, which are episodic and very responsive to context and environment (Stefan, 2001). In short, the Biomedical Model is much stronger, in both diagnosis and treatment, when dealing with physical disabilities. This narrow emphasis presents difficulties because the definition of disability is enlarging and evolving beyond that of only physical disabilities to include such impairments as learning disabilities, mental illness, and other disorders.

The Biomedical Model is often conceived to be a model of experts in control (J. F. Smart, 2001, 2004), therefore reducing individuals with disabilities to the role of passive and compliant patients. Because most individuals with disabilities do not possess the expertise, knowledge, education, and experience of physicians, they may not be accorded respect as decision makers. For example, many individuals with disabilities have consistently reported that "doctors always underestimate the quality of my life." Thus, the subordinate, dependent, and inferior status of people with disabilities is reinforced by the power differential inherent in the Biomedical Model. Conrad (2004) described another result of the use of medical experts:

> Because of the way the medical profession is organized and the mandate it receives from society, decisions related to medical diagnoses and treatment are virtually controlled by the medical professions. … By defining a problem as medical, it is removed from the public realm where there can be discussion by ordinary people and put on a plane where only medical people can discuss it. (p. 22)

As would be expected, much of the current conceptualization of disability is a reaction against the Biomedical Model (Brant & Pope, 1997; Gill, Kewman, & Brannon, 2003; Pope & Tarlov, 1991; Scotch, 1988). In spite of its shortcomings, no one, including proponents of the other models, suggests totally abandoning the Biomedical Model, nor is any intentional harm on the part of the medical profession implied. Indeed, the medical profession itself is moving away from many of the assumptions of this model. Furthermore, in the final analysis, it is the broader society that has endowed the medical professions and the Biomedical Model of disability with the appearance of reality, science, and objectivity.

FUNCTIONAL AND ENVIRONMENTAL MODELS

The Functional and Environmental models are considered together in this chapter because both are interactional models. In these two models, it makes no sense to discuss the definition of disability, or the ways in which to intervene, without first considering the functions of both the individual and the individual's environment. Therefore, biology becomes less important. Disability is defined in relation to the skills, abilities, and achievements of the individual in addition to biological/organic factors. Thus, these models do recognize the biological factors of a disability. Disadvantages or limitations such as poverty or a lack of education, although social ills, are not considered to be disabilities. Also, although everyone is required to successfully negotiate difficult environments, to undertake demanding functions, and to experience disadvantages, not everyone has a disability.

These two models are considered to be interactive models because the disability (of the individual) interacts with functions and environment (Dembo, 1982; Tanenbaum, 1986; Thomason, Burton, & Hyatt, 1998). Therefore, the definition of disability, the causal attribution, and the solution attribution are not found wholly within the individual (or his or her disability). Instead, adherents of these models of disability recognize the importance of biology but also posit that the environment can cause, contribute to, and exaggerate disability. Furthermore, these models do not view the "problem" of disability as located totally within the individual, suggesting that many of the difficulties of disability are also located outside the individual, specifically within the environment and its functional requirements (Wolfensberger, 1972). If the location of the problem shifts, the onus for the solution of the problem also shifts. By viewing the definition, the cause, and the difficulties of disability as interactional, helping professionals can aim interventions at adapting the environment and functional demands to the needs of the individual with a disability in addition to "rehabilitating" the individual.

Causal attribution differs also, but it is safe to state that for most individuals, the Biomedical Model's conception of causation is much easier to understand. As we have pointed out, in the Biomedical Model, the causes and solutions to the disability are found in the individual, and generally the social solution and the built environment are ignored. In contrast, the Environmental and Functional models of disability posit that society can cause disabilities, exaggerate disabilities, and, in the words of some disability scholars, "make disabilities" (Higgins, 1992). Two examples illustrate these models. Itzak Perlman, the world-famous violinist and a survivor of polio, stated that people with disabilities experience two problems: (a) the physical inaccessibility of the environment and (b) the attitudes of the people without disabilities toward disability and people with disabilities (J. F. Smart, 2004). As difficult as these problems are, it can be seen that neither problem concerns the disability itself (or the individual with the disability). Indeed, one of the results of the ADA has been the increased public awareness that many of the problems and obstacles experienced by people with disabilities are due to their environments. Also, it can be seen that for Perlman's major professional function, playing the violin, his difficulty in walking is not a functional disability. The definition of disability varies with the roles expected of the individual. In addition, it can be seen that both of Perlman's difficulties can be ameliorated.

World War II and the resulting demands for a large number of military personnel changed both the functional and environmental definitions of disability. During World War I and World War II, many men who had been residents of institutions for the long-term care of individuals with mental retardation entered the U.S. military and fought in the wars' battles. Sobsey (1994) told of 13 men from such an institution in Connecticut who, in spite of being labeled as having mental retardation, enlisted to fight in World War II. Four of these men were promoted to higher ranks, and seven were wounded in action. In spite of their war records, most of these men returned to the institution after the war. Sobsey concluded, "wars and labor shortages have repeatedly redefined who has mental retardation" (p. 132). It can be seen that nothing in the disability or the individual changed, but rather changes in the environment occurred.

These two examples also illustrate the disabling effects of prejudice and discrimination, and therefore in both the Environmental and Functional models, the potential exists for incorporating some degree of societal prejudice and discrimination when attempting to render a rating of the severity of a disability. For example, a young African American man with schizophrenia would probably experience more prejudice and discrimination than a European American man who is blind. Medical ratings of the level of severity of these two disabilities might be relatively equal, but the difficulties experienced are probably much greater for the man with schizophrenia, mostly because of societal attitudes. Schizophrenia is a disability that is considered highly stigmatizing, and blindness is not. Furthermore, other perceived characteristics of the individual who "carries" the disability label (such as racial/cultural/ethnic identification, gender, sexual orientation, or age) intersect with the public perception of the disability.

There is a tendency to think that each individual's environment and functions are exclusively unique to that individual. However, broad, general changes in both environment and function can affect the daily life of an individual with a disability. For example, in a society based on physical labor such as farming or mining, a physical disability presents more difficulties than a cognitive disability, but in a service-, information-, and technology-based economy, a physical disability does not cause as many difficulties as does a cognitive disability. Liachowitz (1988) in her book, *Disability as a Social Construct: Legislative Roots,* made a compelling argument that literally overnight the federal government has the capability to define disability and, therefore, to determine who has a disability. Nazi Germany is an extreme but clear-cut illustration of the Environmental Model and its power to shape the response to disability. Because of the political–social environment (Nazism), "Aryan" Germans with disabilities were systematically mass murdered by their government (Friedlander, 1995; Gallagher, 1990).

The causal attributions of these two models are not as sharply defined and as easily understandable as those of the Biomedical Model; certainly, one of the strengths of the Biomedical Model is its strong explanatory power. Nonetheless, both the Functional Model and the Environmental Model possess strengths that the Biomedical Model does not. In addition, the bases of the Functional and Environmental models are more closely related to the theoretical assumption and practice orientations of most counselors.

Viewing the client as a complete person with skills, abilities, and demands and conceptualizing the client within a context allow the counselor to see the client as more than a disability. If the disability is not the only factor in the equation of disability, then the diagnoses and labels attached to the individual will not acquire as much power to define the individual to himself or herself and to others. It will be more difficult to dehumanize people with disabilities and to think of the person with a disability as "not one of us." Labels and diagnoses, and the professionals who render them, will not be as powerful as they once were.

In contrast to the Biomedical Model, the Environmental and Functional models deal more flexibly with psychiatric disabilities that are

> episodic, highly responsive to context and environment, and exist along a spectrum, which theoretically could be cause for hope—people with mental disabilities are frequently strong, talented, competent, and capable, and their environments can be structured in a way to support and increase their strengths, talents, competence, and capabilities. (Stefan, 2001, p. 10)

Because an individual's cultural identification defines his or her functions, roles, and environment to a great extent, the Functional and Environmental models provide a better basis from which to understand and respond to the disabilities experienced by individuals who are not White, middle-class, heterosexual, male, or European American (D. W. Smart & Smart, 1997b; J. F. Smart & Smart, 1997). The Functional and Environmental models are also more appropriate for chronic conditions, which most disabilities are. With chronic conditions, after medical stabilization, the treatment focus is on maintaining the highest quality of life, avoiding secondary disabilities and complications, supporting independence, acquiring the appropriate assistive technology, and assisting the individual in negotiating developmental tasks. It can be seen that most of these interventions require functional and environmental adaptations—rather than focusing solely on "rehabilitating" the individual.

In the Functional and Environmental models, it is more difficult to dehumanize individuals with disabilities because of the following factors: (a) categorization by disability type is less likely; (b) the power differential is reduced when the individual is viewed as a total person and not as a stigmatized, medicalized category; and (c) partial responsibility for the response to the disability devolves upon "society" to provide a physically accessible and nonprejudiced environment.

Perhaps most important, the discomfort, anxiety, defensiveness, and existential angst experienced because of the fear of acquiring a disability are decreased when individuals without disabilities take the opportunity to associate with friends, colleagues, and clients with disabilities. Thus, by viewing the individual as more than the disability and conceptualizing the environment and the functional requirements as major determinants of the difficulties experienced by people with disabilities, the fear of acquiring a disability will be greatly reduced.

THE SOCIOPOLITICAL MODEL

The Sociopolitical Model, also referred to as the Minority Model of Disability (Hahn, 1985, 1988, 1991, 1996, 1997; Kleinfield, 1979), is the most recently developed model and, more important, is a fundamental and radical change from the previous models. The Sociopolitical Model (in contrast to the Biomedical Model and the Environmental and Functional models) has the capability to explain and describe more of the day-to-day life of people with disabilities. Certainly, for most people with disabilities, the prejudice and discrimination found in the broader society are more of an obstacle than are medical impairments or functional limitations.

Madeline Will (cited in Weisgerber, 1991), former assistant secretary for education and head of the Office of Special Education and Rehabilitation Services underscored this:

> Most disabled people [*sic*] … will tell you that despite what everyone thinks, the disability itself if not what makes everything different. What causes the difficulties are the attitudes society has about being disabled, attitudes that make a disabled person embarrassed, insecure, uncomfortable, dependent. Of course, disabled people [*sic*] rarely talk about the quality of life. But it has precious little to do with deformity and a great deal to do with society's own defects. (p. 6)

In this model, people with disabilities view themselves as members of a U.S. minority group. Indeed, some disability rights advocates have described Americans with disabilities as "foreigners in their own country" (Higgins, 1992). The hallmarks of this model include self-definition, self-determination, the elimination (or reduction) of the prejudice and discrimination (sometimes referred to as "handicapism"), rejection of medical diagnoses and categories, and the drive to achieve full equality and civil rights under U.S. law.

The Sociopolitical Model refuses to accept the inferior, dependent, and stigmatizing definition of disability; furthermore, in this model, disability is defined as a social construction in that the limitations and disadvantages experienced by people with disabilities have nothing to do with the disability but are only social constructions and therefore unwarranted. If society constructs disability, society can also deconstruct disability. Stigmatization, prejudice, discrimination, inferiority, and handicapism are not inevitable, natural, or unavoidable consequences of disabilities. Inherent in this definition of disability are three aspects: (a) People with disabilities must define disability; (b) people with disabilities must refuse to allow "experts" or "professionals" to define the disability, determine the outcomes of their lives, or judge the quality of their lives; and (c) people with disabilities refuse the "disabled role" of deviance and pathology. While in the past, professionals defined disabilities and the experiences available to individuals with disabilities, disability rights advocates assert their rights to self-definition and self-determination. It can be seen that much of the Sociopolitical Model seeks to displace the "expert in control" basis of the Biomedical Model.

In the past, the disabled role was determined by people who did not have disabilities and therefore had no experience in managing a disability on a day-to-day basis. Individuals with disabilities were expected to learn the rules of this role; to live the rules; and, most important, to believe in the rules. The rules and expectations of this role, although unwritten, were strongly enforced, and individuals who did not comply with these expectations often experienced severe consequences, including the lack of services and social isolation. These rules included the following: always be cheerful; face the disability with courage, optimism, and motivations; manage the disability as well as possible (in the view of others); adhere to medical and rehabilitation regimens; request only those accommodations and assistance that others feel are necessary; make others comfortable with the disability; and keep all aspirations at a reasonable level, or stated differently, do not ask for much. Often, a person with a disability who is perceived to have adopted the disabled role is considered to be a "Tiny Tim" by disability rights advocates.

Adherents of the Sociopolitical Model resist medical categorization by diagnosis and, indeed, view this categorization to be a source of prejudice and discrimination (although they acknowledge that prejudice and discrimination were not the intention of the medical profession). According to the Sociopolitical Model, categorization has resulted in (a) teaching individuals who bear the diagnoses to accept the meanings of these labels as their self-identity, (b) allowing the general public to avoid focusing on the universal problems of people with all types of disabilities, (c) fragmenting the disability community so that it cannot form broad coalitions with which to effect sociopolitical changes, and (d) leading "society" to believe that disability is inferiority and that, therefore, the prejudice and discrimination toward people with disabilities are inevitable consequences of the inferiority.

Thus, the Sociopolitical Model minimizes dependence on an academic discipline or professional area of expertise, and it does not consider causal attribution to be a relevant concern. This model is considered to be an interactional model. Disability, in this model, is not viewed as a personal tragedy but as a public concern.

Many scholars and researchers state that the prejudice and discrimination directed toward people with disabilities have been more pervasive than the prejudice and discrimination directed toward any other group of people, and, further, much of this has been due to the Biomedical Model. In their book, Fleischer and Zames (as cited in McCarthy, 2003) pointed out the tendency to over look prejudice against persons with disabilities:

> In *The Anatomy of Prejudice* (1996), Elisabeth Young-Bruehl analyzes what she believes to be "the four prejudices that have dominated American life and reflection in the past half-century—anti-Semitism, racism, sexism, and homophobia." No reference is made to disability discrimination. Misrepresented as a health, economic, technical, or safety issue rather than discrimination, prejudice based on disability frequently remains unrecognized. (p. 210)

Albrecht (1992) summarized,

> More *recent* studies suggest that prejudice against impaired persons is more intense than that against other minorities. Bowe (1978) concludes that employer attitudes toward impaired workers are "less favorable than those toward elderly individuals, minority group members, ex-convicts, and student radicals," and Hahn (1983) finds

that handicapped persons are victims of great animosity and rejection than many other groups in society. (p. 245)

Proponents of the Sociopolitical Model assert that this prejudice and discrimination against individuals with disabilities is long-standing, systematic, and institutionalized in American life. The ADA (1990) states,

Individuals with disabilities are a discrete and insular minority who have been faced with restrictions and limitations, subjected to a history of purposeful unequal treatment, and relegated to a position of political powerlessness in our society, based on characteristics that are beyond the control of such individuals and resulting from stereotypical assumptions not truly indicative of the individual ability of such individuals to participate in and contribute to society. (Seventh Finding)

The ADA (1990) further asserts, "Unlike individuals who have experienced discrimination on the basis of race, color, sex, national origin, religion, or age, individuals who have experienced discrimination on the basis of disability have often had no legal recourse to redress such discrimination" (Fourth Finding). Moreover, it is the prejudices, stereotypes, and stigma, and not the disability itself, that are the true handicap and obstacle.

Much like other civil rights movements in the United States and, indeed, building on the history and the methods of the successes of African Americans and the women's movement, the disability rights advocates view the only commonality among people with disabilities as being the prejudice and discrimination they experience. If the occurrence of the disability appears to be unfair and unpredictable, then society's response to disability can nevertheless be equitable, moral, and predictable. A perfect world is not a world without disabilities but a world in which accommodations and services are provided to people with disabilities, and, more important, disability is not viewed as inferiority.

THE POWER OF MODELS

Lack of Interagency Collaboration

All four broad models answer the question, "What is a disability?" (Berkowitz, 1987). Because each model provides a different answer to this question, the needs of the individual with a disability are also determined differently in each of the models (Bickenbach, 1993). All four models contain a definition of disability that reduces it to a single dimension, thus ignoring and excluding other important aspects. Therefore, all of these models are considered to be reductionistic, unidimensional, and somewhat time bound and culture bound. As a result, these incomplete definitions of disability may impede the type of interagency collaboration that has the potential to provide a range of services to individuals with disabilities. In addition, funding policies (which pay for services) are often based on these unidimensional definitions. Occasionally, the meanings ascribed to the disability experience by professional service providers and funding agencies may remain invisible simply because these meanings are not questioned or challenged.

Despite these basic differences, three of the models of disability lump individuals into categories such as "the blind," "the mentally ill," or "quads" (M. G. Eisenberg, Griggins, & Duval, 1982; Wright, 1991). Furthermore, the simple act of "placing" or "assigning" people to categories robs them of their individuality; to counteract this, counselors can assist clients with disabilities in dealing with the effects of automatic categorization.

These definitions of disability vary with the purposes, values, and needs of the definers. Zola's (1993) chapter, "Disability Statistics, What We Count and What It Tells Us," provides an excellent introduction to the varying definitions of disability. Zola's title clearly communicates that definitions (and statistics) of disability are a reflection of the values and needs of the defining group, and because of this, none of the models can be entirely value free or morally neutral.

Blaming the Victim

Models ask the questions, "Who is responsible for the disability" and "Who is responsible for the solution?" (Berkowitz & Hill, 1986; Yelin, 1992). Again, each model answers these questions differently. Determining the onset or acquisition of the disability attempts to understand *how* the disability occurred, or more precisely stated, the etiology of the disability. Often, the search for the etiology or cause of the disability becomes distorted, resulting in implicit or explicit blame, fault, and moral accountability placed on the individual or his or her parents. Nonetheless, for purposes of calculating financial benefits and allocation of services, many disability programs require a clear-cut causal attribution. It is true that regardless of etiology or causal attribution, the treatment of a particular type and severity of disability is almost identical. However, the response of the general population, and hence the personal experience of the person with the disability, is a result of the public's assumptions of causal attribution. For example, an individual who is born with spina bifida is often considered a victim, whereas a person who acquires a spinal cord injury in combat is thought to be a hero, and a person who acquires a spinal cord injury while intoxicated and speeding on a motorcycle, without a helmet, is viewed as a culprit. The attribution of responsibility also determines which professions serve people with disabilities (Albrecht, 1981; Davis, 1997; Reno et al., 1997).

The history of these models can be easily traced simply by looking at the attributions of cause and responsibility in each model and the resulting formulation and implementation of policies and services. Furthermore, these attributions have had a profound effect on the lack of counseling services provided to people with disabilities, simply because the Biomedical Model of disability has dominated. Most important, attribution theory (Heider, 1958) has the power to individualize and privatize the experience of disability by looking for (and seemingly finding) both the cause and the solution for the disability wholly within the individual rather than within the social system. Attribution theories that privatize disability (rather than viewing disability as a public concern) often view the individual as a "patient" or as a "victim" or both.

The models described in this chapter place varying emphasis on the medical, functional, environmental, and sociopolitical needs and rights of the person with a disability. Three of the models emphasize definitions of disability rather than determining ways in which to intervene. In order for needs to be met, they must be clearly defined (Zola, 1989). For example, in the Biomedical Model, needs are considered to be solely medical; in the Environmental and Functional models, the needs are thought to be those of adapting the environment and functional requirements to fit the requirements of the individual with the disability; and in the Sociopolitical Model, the needs are considered to be full social integration and civil rights. The counseling interventions that flow from each model dictate different responses from the counselor. In order to be even minimally effective, counselors should understand the implications of each model for their manner of practice.

Shaping Self-Identities and Daily Lives

One model, the Biomedical Model, provides labels, diagnoses, categories, and theories of causation and responsibility that are derived from seemingly authoritative and prestigious sources. Diagnostic categories, however, can often be distorted to become stereotypes and uninformed assumptions (Clendinen & Nagourney, 1999). Moreover, these stereotypes are continually socially reinforced in the media and in the educational system, eventually becoming an accepted part of the social environment and, consequently, often remain unidentified and unquestioned (Stone, 1984). The individual with a disability may come to accept these diagnoses, and occasionally the stereotypes, as self-identifiers (Goffman, 1963). Often the individual with a disability is required to label himself or herself with a negative diagnosis or other label to be declared eligible for services and benefits. If disability is thought to be an unbearable personal tragedy, the individual (with a disability) is often effectively taught to be both inferior and dependent.

Despite the fact that these models are only representations of reality, and not reality itself, the assumptions, definitions, and history of each model are so persuasive and long-standing that they are often mistaken for fact (Hannah & Midlarsky, 1987). In addition, the personal daily functioning of the individual with a disability is determined, in large part, by assumptions derived from these models. Where the individual lives, how (and if) the individual is educated, the type and quality of professional services offered, and the degree of social integration afforded the individual are all influenced by the model of disability that is implemented.

Determining Which Academic Disciplines Teach About the Disability Experience

The disability experience, despite the large number of individuals with disabilities, remains invisible in most university curricula (Bauman & Drake, 1997; Hogben & Waterman, 1997). Students in counseling training programs, with the exception of rehabilitation counseling (Thomas, 2004), are typically not required to learn about people with disabilities. Simply because disability has been considered solely a biological and medical concern, only medical schools and the allied health professions have offered course work in disability issues. The "medicalization" of the disability experience has effectively kept the history and viewpoints of people with disabilities outside the realm of counseling education and professional training. Models of disability have provided the explanatory rationale for academic disciplines and therefore most graduates of counseling programs do not possess competencies to provide services to clients with disabilities. Olkin and Pledger (2003) reported that students are trained *not* to notice the absence of disability issues. In their view, the lack of disability information "in curricula, and among peers and professors—is a powerful statement about the marginalization of people with disabilities" (p. 297). Furthermore, research on disability and people with disabilities, including rigorously designed and executed studies, is often of questionable value because of negative and biased assumptions toward disability. Certainly, any disability-related research study is only as valid as the model of disability upon which it is based. Myerson (1988) provided the following summary:

> The number of investigations that are flawed from inception by prejudicial commonsense assumptions, by theoretical bias, or by methodological error remains high. … These errors are functions, in great part, not of [the researchers'] incompetence in the mechanics of research, but of asking the wrong questions, of incorrect notions of the meaning of disability to those who live with it, and of lack of understanding. … A particular source of error is the narrowly trained clinician who believes that clinical criteria are appropriate measures of problems that arise from systematic social injustice. (pp. 182–183)

Myerson concluded that "like others, to the extent that their thinking incorporates cultural myths, [researchers] become prisoners of plausible but erroneous hypotheses" (p. 183).

IMPLICATIONS FOR THE COUNSELING PROFESSION

Biology is still a factor in the equation of disability; however, biology does not matter as much as has been previously thought (J. F. Smart, 2005c). For counselors, this assumption has important implications because for the client with a disability, self-identity and the conceptualization of his or her life situation are derived from these basic concepts. In contrast, many professionals may, consciously or unconsciously, ascribe more importance to the biological and physical aspects of the disability than the client does. The individual with a disability certainly does not conceive of his or her life in these four neatly (and artificially) explained models. However, counselors can, albeit unintentionally, reinforce the status quo by unquestioningly accepting the assumptions, including expectations for the client's self-actualization, of these models and their labels and diagnoses. Clients with disabilities, on the other hand, may enter the counseling relationship with the expectation of receiving inaccurate (and often negative) diagnoses and inadequate services, often provided in offices that are inaccessible. Nevertheless, counselors are in a unique position to recognize the interplay of personal characteristics and environmental factors in a developmental context. Furthermore, counselors have long recognized the value of empowerment for all clients. The following is a listing of some implications for the counseling profession.

1. Counselors should engage in an ongoing examination of clients' feelings about the experience of disability and the resulting interaction of the counselor's own identity with that of the client. Taken to the extreme, the counselor may focus more on himself or herself if the disability of the client arouses feelings of existential angst, anxiety, and defensiveness, much of which is a result of the widely held view of the Biomedical Model of disability. If the counselor views disability as a tragic inferiority, then he or she will more likely experience a negative, emotional response to the client with a disability. Countertransference, and other emotional reactions to the disability of the client, may prevent the counselor from fully understanding the client and therefore negatively affect the counseling relationship.

2. Counselors should recognize that most individuals with disabilities do not accept the basic tenets of the Biomedical Model of disability. Rather, they may view the disability as a valued part of their identity; see positive aspects in having the disability; not view the disability as tragic or limiting or being an inferiority; and would not choose to eliminate the disability if they could. At times, it may be necessary to ask the client about his or her identity as a person with a disability. Counselors must recognize that clients with disabilities want respect and not sympathy (Harris, 1992). Indeed, sympathy and lowered expectations may be considered to be stigmatizing and prejudicial; sympathy and lowered expectations toward people with disabilities often result in withholding helpful and honest feedback, reduce the range of opportunities open to the individual, foster dependence, and subtly communicate the message to clients with a disability that standards will be lowered for them because they are not perceived (by the counselor) to be capable.

3. Counselors should recognize that the disability is simply one part of the individual's identity. As does everyone, the client with a disability has multiple identities and multiple roles. Disability is not the "master status." Furthermore, a deeper and more complete understanding of the client's varied identities, functions, and environments will facilitate the implementation of the Environmental and Functional models of disability in the counseling process. Disability identity also constantly shifts and develops, as do all identities.

4. Counselors know that empowerment refers to the processes and outcomes relating to issues of control, critical awareness, and participation (Perkins & Zimmerman, 1995). For clients with disabilities,

   empowerment values provide a belief system that governs how our clients and we as professionals can work together. Based on this paradigm shift, there are substantial changes to be made to our practice. ... Empowerment values include attention toward health, adaptation, and competence, and the enabling environment. As professionals, our goal is to promote our clients' full participation and integration into their communities. The collaboration ... is itself an empowering process. (Tate, 2001, p. 133)

5. As with any other client, the counselor may occasionally need to guard against imposing his or her values on the client with a disability (Norcross, 2002). Clients with disabilities have, at times, interpreted their counselors' guidance as a type of the "Try Harder Syndrome," or some individuals with disabilities have felt themselves to have been given the negative label by counselors of denying their disability. Often, clients with disabilities are not denying the presence, implications, or permanence of the disability, but rather they are denying the "disabled role" of pathology, inferiority, and deviance. Therefore, these clients may terminate counseling prematurely because they have felt misjudged.

6. The power differential between counselor and client with a disability should be addressed. Often, the power differential is increased when the client has a disability and the counselor does not. If the counselor subscribes to the Biomedical Model, with its strong normative emphasis, this increased power differential may impede the establishment of rapport and trust. Furthermore, this power imbalance in the therapeutic setting may simply reflect the broader world in which the client functions.

7. Counselors should listen to their clients and be willing to hear about experiences of prejudice and discrimination experienced by their clients with disabilities. Learning the basic tenets of the Sociopolitical Model of disability will provide counselors with some introductory understanding of this stigmatization and discrimination, and, accordingly, counselors will be able to set aside some of their preconceived notions concerning the experiences of their clients with disabilities. Counselors should recognize that many clients with disabilities may not seek services at counseling agencies because they understand that often the counselors at these agencies may reinforce the prejudice and discrimination of the broader culture. On the other hand, counselors need to avoid attributing all the client's issues and problems to prejudice and discrimination. Nonetheless, for most people with disabilities, self-identification as a person with a disability does not automatically translate into group consciousness or political action (Scotch, 1988).

8. Counselors should recognize that, for many of them, their professional training may be inadequate to prepare them with the skills and competencies to work with clients with disabilities. Also, some theoretical approaches and counseling practices have their basis in the Biomedical Model and therefore simply "adapting" these approaches and orientations for clients with disabilities may be at best ineffective and at worst harmful. Stated differently, the little professional training counselors have received may be faulty and ill conceived. Counselors who do not have adequate training must seek opportunities for additional education.

9. Counselors should examine their willingness to broaden their vision about the experience of disability. On one hand, counselors may have strong needs to be knowledgeable, skilled, and helpful, but on the other hand, counselors may view disability as

ambiguous and inferior. Students in counseling programs should seek out course work (such as is available in rehabilitation counseling programs) and other workshops that focus on disability issues. Certainly, information about a client's identity and feelings about his or her disability must come from that individual, but obtaining a broad knowledge of the topic of disability is imperative. It is not ethical or appropriate to expect clients with disabilities to teach counselors about the world of disability.

10. Both outreach efforts and collaborative learning among counseling professions can be achieved by learning which agencies people with disabilities typically go to for assistance (such as state vocational rehabilitation offices) and then establishing professional relationships with these agencies.

11. Professionals, in all aspects of counseling, should intervene at institutional and political levels when appropriate and possible. Although individual counseling and support for clients with disabilities can make a contribution to the larger society, advocating for changes in systems and policies, alerting the public to manifestations of prejudice and discrimination in the media, and advocating for environmental accessibility can also be valuable contributions. Counselors, both as individuals and as part of statewide, regional, or national professional organizations, can create change.

12. Counselors should recognize that it is necessary to clearly articulate the assumptions about models of disability that underlie research studies. Research can be more sharply focused if the basic assumptions and values about people with disabilities are made clear. Articulating these values as they relate to one or more of the four models of disability would help both researchers and consumers of research evaluate the research findings.

In order to provide ethical and effective services to clients with disabilities, counseling professionals in all aspects of the field will be required to examine the ways in which they conceptualize the experience of disability. For some counseling professionals, many of these ideas, derived from the models of disability, may be new and different ways of responding to people with disabilities. For others, these ideas will provide a useful adjunct to the counseling services or the counseling training and education they provide.

REFERENCES

Akabas, S. H. (2000). Practice in the world of work. In P. Allen-Meares & C. Garvin (Eds.), *The handbook of social work: Direct practice* (pp. 449–517). Thousand Oaks, CA: Sage.

Albrecht, G. L. (Ed.). (1981). *Cross national rehabilitation policies: A sociological perspective.* Beverly Hills, CA: Sage.

Albrecht, G. L. (1992). *The disability business: Rehabilitation in America.* Newbury Park, CA: Sage.

American Psychiatric Association. (2000). *Diagnostic and statistical manual of mental disorders* (4th ed., text rev.). Washington, DC: Author.

Americans with Disabilities Act of 1990, 42 U.S.C.A. § 12101.

Bauman, H. D. L., & Drake, J. (1997). Silence is not without voice: Including deaf culture within the multicultural curricula. In L. J. Davis (Ed.), *Disability studies reader* (pp. 307–314). New York: Routledge.

Berkowitz, M. (1987). *Disabled policy: America's programs for the handicapped.* London, England: Cambridge University Press.

Berkowitz, M., & Hill, M. A. (Eds.). (1986). *Disability and the labor market: Economic problems, policies, and programs.* Ithaca, NY: Cornell University Press.

Bickenbach, J. E. (1993). *Physical disability and social policy.* Toronto, Ontario, Canada: University of Toronto.

Bickenbach, J. E., Somnath, C., Badley, E. M., & Ustun, T. B. (1999). Models of disablement, universalism and the International Classification of Impairments, Disabilities and Handicaps. *Social Science & Medicine, 48,* 1173–1187.

Bowe, F. (1980). *Rehabilitation America: Toward independence for disabled and elderly people.* New York: Harper & Row.

Brant, E. N., & Pope, A. M. (Eds.). (1997). *Enabling America: Assessing the role of rehabilitation science and engineering.* Washington, DC: National Academy Press.

Byrom, B. (2004). A pupil and a patient: Hospital schools in progressive America. In S. Danforth & S. D. Taff (Eds.), *Crucial readings in special education* (pp. 25–37). Upper Saddle River, NJ: Pearson-Merrill, Prentice Hall.

Clendinen, D., & Nagourney, A. (1999). *Out for good: The struggle to build a gay rights movement in America.* New York: Simon & Schuster.

Conrad, P. (2004). The discovery of hyperkinesis: Notes on the medicalization of deviant behavior. In S. Danforth & S. D. Taff (Eds.), *Crucial readings in special education* (pp. 18–24). Upper Saddle River, NJ: Pearson-Merrill, Prentice Hall.

Davis, L. J. (1997). Constructing normalcy: The bell curve, the novel, and the invention of the disabled body in the nineteenth century. In L. J. Davis (Ed.), *Disability studies reader* (pp. 307–314). New York: Routledge.

Dembo, T. (1982). Some problems in rehabilitation as seen by a Lewinian. *Journal of Social Issues, 38,* 131–139.

Eisenberg, L. (1996). Foreword. In J. E. Mezzich, A. Kleinman, H. Fabrega Jr., & D. L. Parron (Eds.), *Culture and psychiatric diagnosis: ADSM-IV perspective* (pp. xiii–xv). Washington, DC: American Psychiatric Association.

Eisenberg, M. G., Griggins, C., & Duval, R. J. (Eds.). (1982). *Disabled people as second-class citizens.* New York: Springer.

Employment and Disability Institute. (1996). National health interview survey. Retrieved August 10, 2003, from www.disabilitystatistics.org

Friedlander, H. (1995). *The origins of Nazi genocide: From euthanasia to the final solution.* Chapel Hill: University of North Carolina Press.

Gallagher, H. G. (1990). *By trust betrayed: Patients, physicians, and the license to kill in the Third Reich.* New York: Holt.

Gill, C. J., Kewman, D. G., & Brannon, R. W. (2003). Transforming psychological practice and society: Policies that reflect the new paradigm. *American Psychologist, 58,* 305–312.

Goffman, E. (1963). *Stigma: Notes on the management of spoiled identity.* Englewood Cliffs, NJ: Prentice Hall.

Hahn, H. (1985). Toward a politics of disability: Definitions, disciplines, and policies. *Social Science Journal, 22,* 87–105.

Hahn, H. (1988). The politics of physical differences: Disability and discrimination. *Journal of Social Issues, 44,* 39–47.

Hahn, H. (1991). Alternative views of empowerment: Social services and civil rights. *Journal of Rehabilitation, 57,* 17–19.

Hahn, H. (1993). The political implications of disability definitions and data. *Journal of Disability Policy Studies, 4,* 41–52.

Hahn, H. (1996). Antidiscrimination laws and social research on disability: The minority group perspectives. *Behavioral Sciences and the Law, 14,* 41–59.

Hahn, H. (1997). Advertising the acceptable employment image: Disability and capitalism. In L. J. Davis (Ed.), *The disability studies reader* (pp. 172–186). New York: Routledge.

Hannah, M. E., & Midlarsky, E. (1987). Differential impact of labels and behavioral descriptions on attitudes toward people with disabilities. *Rehabilitation Psychology, 32,* 227–238.

Harris, R. (1992). Musing from 20 years of hard earned experience. *Rehabilitation Education, 6,* 207–212.

Hayes, P. A. (2001). *Addressing cultural complexities in practice: A framework for clinicians and counselors.* Washington, DC: American Psychological Association.

Heider, F. (1958). *The psychology of interpersonal relations.* New York: Wiley.

Higgins, P. C. (1992). *Making disability: Exploring the social transformation of human variation.* Springfield, IL: Thomas.

Hogben, M., & Waterman, C. K. (1997). Are all of your students represented in their textbooks? A content analysis of coverage of diversity issues in introductory psychology textbooks. *Teaching of Psychology, 24,* 95–100.

Hulnick, M. R., & Hulnick, H. R. (1989).Life's challenges: Curse or opportunity? Counseling families of persons with disabilities. *Journal of Counseling & Development, 68,* 166–170.

Humes, C. W., Szymanski, E. M., & Hohenshil, T. H. (1989). Roles of counseling in enabling persons with disabilities. *Journal of Counseling & Development, 68,* 145–150.

Kemp, N. T., & Mallinckrodt, B. (1996). Impact of professional training on case conceptualization of clients with a disability. *Professional Psychology: Research and Practice, 27,* 378–385.

Kiesler, D. J. (1999). *Beyond the disease model of mental disorders.* Westport, CT: Praeger.

Kirk, S. A., & Kutchins, H. (1992). *The selling of the DSM: The rhetoric of science in psychiatry*. New York: Aldine Degruyter.

Kleinfield, S. (1979). *The hidden minority: A profile of handicapped Americans*. Boston, MA: Atlantic Monthly Press.

Liachowitz, C. H. (1988). *Disability as a social construct: Legislative roots*. Philadelphia: University of Pennsylvania Press.

Longmore, P. K. (1995). Medical decision making and people with disabilities: A clash of cultures. *Journal of Law, Medicine and Ethics, 23*, 82-87.

McCarthy, H. (1993). Learning with Beatrice A. Wright: A breath of fresh air that uncovers the unique virtues and human flaws in us all. *Rehabilitation Education, 10*, 149-166.

McCarthy, H. (2003). The disability rights movement: Experiences and perspectives of selected leaders in the disability community. *Rehabilitation Counseling Bulletin, 46*, 209-223.

Melia, R. P., Pledger, C., & Wilson, R. (2003). Disability and rehabilitation research. *American Psychologist, 58*, 289-295.

Myerson, L. (1988). The social psychology of physical disability. *Journal of Social Issues, 44*, 173-188.

Nagi, S. Z. (1969). *Disability and rehabilitation: Legal, clinical, and self-concepts and measurements*. Columbus: Ohio State University Press.

Norcross, J. C. (Ed.). (2002). *Psychotherapy relationships that work: Therapist contributions and responsiveness to patient needs*. New York: Oxford University Press.

Olkin, R. (1999). *What psychotherapists should know about disability*. New York: Guilford.

Olkin, R., & Pledger, C. (2003).Can disability studies and psychology join hands? *American Psychologist, 58*, 296-298.

Perkins, D. D., & Zimmerman, M. A. (1995). Empowerment theory: Research and applications. *American Journal of Community Psychology, 23*, 569-579.

Peterson, D. B. (2002). *International Classification of Functioning, Disability, and Health (ICF): A primer for rehabilitation psychologists*. Unpublished manuscript, New York University.

Pledger, C. (2003). Discourse on disability and rehabilitation issues. *American Psychologist, 58*, 279-284.

Pope, A. M., & Tarlov, A. R. (1991). *Disability in America: Toward a national agenda for prevention*. Washington, DC: National Academies Press.

Reno, V. P., Mashaw, J. L., & Gradison, B. (Eds.). (1997). *Disability: Challenges for social insurance, health care financing, and labor market policy*. Washington, DC: National Academy of Social Insurance.

Schur, E. M. (1971). *Labeling deviant behavior: Its sociological implications*. New York: Harper & Row.

Scotch, R. K. (1988). Disability as a basis for a social movement: Advocacy and the politics of definition. *Journal of Social Issues, 44*, 159-172.

Singer, P. (2000). *Writings on an ethical life*. New York: Ecco.

Smart, D. W., & Smart, J. F. (1997a). *DSM-IV* and culturally sensitive diagnosis: Some observations for counselors. *Journal of Counseling & Development, 75*, 392-398.

Smart, D. W., & Smart, J. F. (1997b). The racial/ethnic demography of disability. *Journal of Rehabilitation, 63*, 9-15.

Smart, J. F. (2001). *Disability, society and the individual*. Austin, TX: Pro-Ed.

Smart, J. F. (2004). Models of disability: The juxtaposition of biology and social construction. In T. F. Riggar & D. R. Maki (Eds.), *Handbook of rehabilitation counseling* (pp. 25-49). New York: Springer.

Smart, J. F. (2005a). Challenges to the biomedical model of disability: Changes to the practice of rehabilitation counseling. *Directions in Rehabilitation Counseling, 16*, 33-43.

Smart, J. F. (2005b). The promise of the International Classification of Functioning, Disability, and Health (ICF). *Rehabilitation Education, 19*, 191-199.

Smart, J. F. (2005c). *Tracing the ascendant trajectory of models of disability: Confounding competition or a cross-model approach?* Unpublished manuscript, Utah State University, Logan.

Smart, J. F., & Smart, D. W. (1997). Culturally sensitive informed choice in rehabilitation counseling. *Journal of Applied Rehabilitation Counseling, 28*, 32-37.

Sobsey, D. (1994). *Violence and abuse in the lives of people with disabilities: The end of silent acceptance*. Baltimore: Brookes.

Stefan, S. (2001). *Unequal rights: Discrimination against people with mental disabilities and the Americans with Disabilities Act*. Washington, DC: American Psychiatric Association.

Stone, D. A. (1984). *The disabled state*. Philadelphia: Temple University Press.

Tanenbaum, S. J. (1986). *Engineering disability: Public policy and compensatory technology*. Philadelphia: Temple University Press.

Tate, D. G. (2001). Hospital to community: Changes in practice and outcomes. *Rehabilitation Psychology, 46*, 125-138.

Tate, D. G., & Pledger, C. (2003). An integrative conceptual framework of disability. *American Psychologist, 58*, 289-295.

Thomas, K. R. (2004). Old wine in a slightly cracked new bottle. *American Psychologist, 59,* 274–275.

Thomason, T., Burton, J. F., Jr., & Hyatt, D. R. (Eds.). (1998). *New approaches to disability in the workplace.* Madison: University of Wisconsin Press.

Trieschmann, R. (1987). *Aging with a disability.* New York: Demos.

U.S. Department of Education, Office of Special Education and Rehabilitation Services, National Institute on Disability and Rehabilitation Research. (2000). *Long-range plan 1999–2003.* Washington, DC: Author.

Weisgerber, R. S. (1991). *Quality of life for persons with disabilities.* Gaithersburg, MD: Aspen.

Wilson, J. (2003, October). *Johnny Lingo: Helping clients to fulfill their potential.* Speech given at the national training conference of the National Council on Rehabilitation Education/Rehabilitation Services Administration/Council of State Administrators of Vocational Rehabilitation, Arlington, VA.

Wolfensberger, W. (1972). *The principle of normalization in human services.* Toronto, Ontario, Canada: National Institute on Mental Retardation.

World Health Organization. (1980). *International Classification of Impairments, Disabilities, and Handicaps: A manual of classification relating to the consequences of disease.* Geneva, Switzerland: Author.

World Health Organization. (2001). *International Classification of Impairments, Disabilities, and Handicaps: A manual of classification relating to the consequences of disease.* Geneva, Switzerland: Author.

Wright, B. A. (1991). Labeling: The need for greater person-environment individuation. In C. R. Snyder & D. R. Forsythe (Eds.), *Handbook of social and clinical psychology* (pp. 469–487). Elmsford, NY: Pergamon.

Yelin, E. H. (1992). *Disability and the displaced worker.* New Brunswick, NJ: Rutgers University Press.

Zola, I. K. (1989). Toward a necessary universalizing of a disability policy. *Milbank Quarterly, 67,* 401–428.

Zola, I. K. (1993). Disability statistics, what we count and what it tells us. *Journal of Disability Policy Studies, 4,* 9–39.

6

Changes in Attitudes Toward People With Handicaps

BEATRICE A. WRIGHT

AFFIRMATION OF HUMAN RIGHTS

A most important document appeared in 1948 when the General Assembly of the United Nations adopted the Universal Declaration of Human Rights. That Declaration not only affirmed that it is possible for all of humanity to agree in general on what is important to every human being but, more than that, it also forthrightly stated that "every individual and every organ of society" has a responsibility to promote the matters contained in the Declaration.

Since then, in fact, different persons and organs of society have formulated principles to serve as guidelines for action to ensure the fuller realization of human dignity. In 1973, the American Hospital Association published a "Patient's Bill of Rights" consisting of 12 points. These rights are considered to be so fundamental that every patient in a hospital setting is to be informed of them. The rights include such items as the right of the patient to respectful care and to consideration of privacy, the right to receive information necessary to give informed consent to any procedure or treatment, and the right to be advised if the hospital proposes to engage in human experimentation affecting his or her care. The document concludes with this significant emphasis. "No catalog of rights can guarantee for the patient the kind of treatment he has a right to expect.... [For such treatment] must be conducted with an overriding concern for the patient, and, above all, the recognition of his dignity as a human being."[3]

In addition to the rights of patients in general, a formulation of the basic rights of the mentally ill and the mentally retarded was published in 1973.[8] These rights are articulated in three broad categories, namely, the right to treatment, the right to compensation for institution-maintaining labor, and the right to education. Prototype court cases are presented to show that litigation can be a valuable tool and catalyst in protecting the rights of the mentally handicapped.

A set of 18 value-laden beliefs and principles published in 1972 provides guidelines for rehabilitation of people with disabilities.[12] The general tenor of these principles may be conveyed by citing a few of them:

1. Every individual needs respect and encouragement; the presence of a handicap, no matter how severe, does not alter these fundamental rights.

From "Changes in attitudes toward people with handicaps," by B. Wright, 1973, *Rehabilitation Literature, 34,* 354–368. Copyright ©1973 by the National Easter Seal Society for Crippled Children and Adults. Reprinted by permission of the Editor. Also published in *The Psychological and Social Impact of Illness and Disability,* 1st Edition, 1977.

2. The assets of the person must receive considerable attention in the rehabilitation effort.
3. The active participation of the client in the planning and execution of his rehabilitation program is to be sought as fully as possible.
4. The severity of a handicap can be increased or diminished by environmental conditions.
5. Involvement of the client with the general life of the community is a fundamental principle guiding decisions concerning living arrangements and the use of resources.
6. All phases of rehabilitation have psychological aspects.
7. Self-help organizations are important allies in the rehabilitation effort.

For each of these principles, implications for action are elaborated. For example, principle 1 further asserts that "A person is entitled to the enrichment of his life and the development of his abilities whether these be great or small and whether he has a long or short time to live." "A Bill of Rights for the Disabled"[1] published in 1972, highlights 16 rights that apply to such areas as health, education, employment, housing, transportation, and civil rights. To take transportation as an example, it is resolved that programs and standards be established for the "modification of existing mass transportation systems and the development of new specially designed demand-schedule transportation facilities."

"A Bill of Rights for the Handicapped" was recently adopted by the United Cerebral Palsy Association (UCPA).[11] Among the 10 rights listed are the right to health and educational services, the right to work, the right to barrier-free public facilities, and the right to petition social institutions and the courts to gain such opportunities as may be enjoyed by others but denied the handicapped because of oversight, public apathy, or discrimination.

Also in accord with the stress on civil rights is the recent declaration of intent by the Canadian Rehabilitation Council for the Disabled, which delineates 14 areas to which these rights pertain. These areas include treatment, education, recreation, transportation, housing, spiritual development, legal rights, and economic security.

Accepting the handicapped person as a full human being means accepting him or her as having the full range of human needs, including those involving the sexual areas of life. The past few years have witnessed a much greater awareness of the importance of this matter. A brief summary of specialized studies and conferences in a number of countries was presented at the Twelfth World Congress of Rehabilitation International in 1972.[5] In this enlightening presentation, Chigier listed six rights with regard to sexual behavior of individuals in general and then traced the extent to which persons with disabilities are assisted or prevented from achieving these rights. Among the rights examined were the right to be informed about sexual matters, the right to sexual expression, the right to marry, and the right to become parents. While recognizing certain problems that come with greater freedom in these areas, the thrust of the analysis is directed toward constructive solutions that will enable severely disabled and mentally retarded persons to realize these rights more fully. Also in 1972, a beautiful article appeared on management of psychosexual readjustment in the spinal cord–injured male.[7] It deals specifically with the kinds of sexual activities open to the cord-injured person and how the possibilities for sexual fulfillment can be enhanced between two people who care for each other.

Legislation helps to give reality to principles of human rights by making provision for the financing and administration of relevant services. The First International Conference on Legislation Concerning the Disabled was held in 1971. The principles guiding the recommendations reflect changing attitudes toward people with handicaps. For example, it is pointed out that "the ultimate objective of all legislation for the disabled is complete integration of the disabled in the community and to enable the disabled person to lead as normal a life as possible regardless of productive capacity."[6] The conference further emphasized that real progress can be achieved only when legislation is designed to foster "respect for the personality and human rights of the individual."[6]

MANIFESTATIONS IN PRACTICE

Fortunately, the explicit expression of principles and ideals set forth in the aforementioned documents is increasingly becoming manifest in practice. Let us consider, as an example, the concept of integration, which has been regarded as a principle that can more fully ensure the realization of human rights for most people. What is necessary to appreciate is that, once integration becomes a guiding principle, certain matters were not at issue until they quickly assume vital importance. The location of institutions and the houses in which handicapped people can live becomes important because their location within communities enables participation of the handicapped in community offerings. Architectural barriers become an issue because their elimination enables people with a wide range of physical abilities to have access to events within buildings at large. The organization of services becomes a challenge because integration rather than segregation is fostered when special needs can be met within general community facilities, such as hospitals, comprehensive rehabilitation centers, schools, recreation areas, churches, and community centers. Transportation assumes special significance because integration requires that the person have a way to get to the integrated facilities that exist. And, when these issues receive sufficient attention, ways to improve the situation become apparent.

A case in point is the increasing accommodation of handicapped children within regular schools. Helping to make such integration a reality are special classes, resource teachers, and teacher aides. The following conclusion, based on a review of children with hearing impairments, is also applicable to children with other handicapping conditions: "Recent experience indicates that children can manage in the ordinary school with more severe hearing impairments than has been generally considered possible."[9] Lest there be a too-ready overgeneralization, however, I hasten to add that this conclusion does not obviate the need for special groupings of children in particular instances and for special purposes.

Integration is not an answer for all circumstances. It will ill serve handicapped children unless their special needs are met through necessary accommodations within the community setting that nurtures a climate of full respect for the dignity of each individual. Nor must integration imply that, where handicapped people are integrated within general community settings, there is no need for handicapped people to get together. Sharing and solving mutual problems, participating in specially designed activities together, and finding needed companionship are some of the rewards that can be provided by self-help, recreation, and other groups. This does not mean that people should be forced to join such groups, that the groups are appropriate for all people with handicaps, or that these groups should preempt association with people who are not handicapped. But it does mean that such groups should not be discredited as fostering segregation, as limiting adaptation to a nonhandicapped world, or as implying overconcern with personal problems. It does mean that groups like these should be valued for providing the opportunity for people to meet together, have fun together, and to affirm and assert themselves together.

A second example of change in practice is the greater involvement of people with handicaps in leadership positions in agencies working on their behalf. Agencies are increasingly recognizing that handicapped people themselves have special contributions to make in the development of services directed toward meeting the needs and enriching the lives of clients. The UCPA, for example, has enumerated the kinds of roles that adults with cerebral palsy are especially equipped to fill by virtue of their special vantage point.[10] It is explicitly pointed out that adults with cerebral palsy should serve on boards of directors and on *all* committees, that they can help with educating parents, that they can provide constructive role models and share personal experiences with young cerebral palsied children and teenagers, and that in-service training programs for such leadership roles are important just as are other in-service training efforts. A recent survey conducted by the UCPA of New York on "The Status of the Cerebral Palsied Adult as a Board, Committee, or Staff Member in UCPA Affiliates" revealed that one or more cerebral palsied adults were on the Board of Directors in 24% of the 227 local agencies who replied and served as staff members in 16%.[10] It was urged that these percentages be increased.

A third reflection in practice of the affirmation of human dignity is the enormously significant effort on the part of people with handicaps to speak out and act on their own behalf, an effort that so clearly parallels the efforts of other minority groups. Sometimes the effort has taken the form of individual action, as in the case of a blind woman who, in 1964, filed a complaint in criminal court against being refused restaurant service because she was accompanied by her seeing-eye dog. Sometimes the protest involved civil disobedience, as in 1967, when a group of seven persons were refused restaurant service because four of them were blind and had guide dogs. They refused to leave the premises until, after the owner contacted the Health Department, they were allowed to remain. Sometimes the effort involved street demonstrations, as in 1970, when a group of university paraplegic students undertook a 100-mile wheelchair trek to promote employment of the handicapped.

Sometimes the effort was extended beyond a single issue to include wide-ranging problems of concern to large numbers of people with handicaps. Thus, in 1970, after winning the case of a young woman confined to a wheelchair, who had been refused a teaching license, the law institute that was involved extended its services to all cases of infringement of civil rights of the handicapped. Among these new cases were a bedridden man who was refused an absentee ballot in a federal election and a blind man who was denied a teacher's license. Recently, a National Center for Law and the Handicapped was established. Sometimes the effort on the part of the handicapped solicited the support of an entire community as in the case of the Committee for the Architecturally Handicapped, organized by two University of Kansas students. Curb cuts in town and on campus, the remodeling of buildings, the revamping of architectural plans for new construction, and the appearance of the international symbol of access attest to the success of this effort.

Parent groups have had a long and impressive history of involvement on behalf of children with disabilities; currently, people with handicaps themselves are gaining the sense of strength and accomplishment that comes from actively participating in advancing their own cause. The number of self-help and mutual-aid groups keeps growing. There are publications by people with handicaps for people with handicaps, such as *Accent on Living*, *Rehabilitation Gazette* (formerly *Toomey j Gazette*), *Paraplegia News*, and *The Braille Technical Press. Stuttering*, published for specialists in the field of speech pathology, primarily consists of papers presented at an annual conference by speech pathologists who stutter. All of these efforts reflect a greater readiness on the part of people with handicaps to acknowledge their own handicaps and to become actively involved with improving their circumstances and increasing understanding of their problems.

PROSPECTS

Attitudes toward the handicapped have seen such marked change since World War II that I believe the reader will be able to guess whether the article from which the following is quoted was published before 1950 or after. It deals with the birth of a child with Down's syndrome (mongolian mental retardation):

> The problems presented by the arrival into a family of one of these accidents of development are many.... Because the mongolian is so incompetent in the ordinary technics of living, his mother soon becomes a complete slave to his dependency. As a result, she devotes all of her time to his necessary care, neglecting her other household duties, her other children..., and inevitably, her husband. The effect of all this is that all other satisfying areas of living are blotted out.... With the passing years,... [the mongol's] brothers and sisters refuse to bring other children into the house,... and are obsessed with a feeling of family shame no matter how unjustifiable it may be.... There is only one adequate way to lessen all this grief, fortunately a measure which most experienced physicians will agree to, and that is immediate commitment to an institution at the time of diagnosis.... When the diagnosis has been made in a newborn the mother is told that the baby is not strong enough to be brought to her at present.... Next, the father is asked to meet the physician immediately, bringing with him any close relatives...the nature of the problem is explained,...emphasizing its seriousness...and that immediate placement outside the family provides the only hope of preventing a long series of family difficulties.... [The mother] is asked, not to make the decision, but to accept the one which has already been made by the close relatives.... It means that the physician must take the lead in precipitating an immediate crisis in order to prevent much more serious difficulties later on. This is preventive medicine.[2]

The cues that one had in guessing correctly? There were many. In this article, the emphasis was on institutionalizing the child rather than on seeking ways to make it feasible for him to remain with his family, at least during his early years; the main responsibility for deciding the issue rested with the physician rather than with those directly concerned, that is, the family; gross devaluating generalizations were made concerning the devastating effects of having such a child; no consideration was given for the capacity of families, with the help of community resources, to be able to accept and adapt to new circumstances. It is not likely that the article in question could be published in a responsible professional journal today, an indication of how attitudes have changed in the past quarter of a century, even though, to be sure, there continue to be frequent breeches of the new directions in actual life settings.

We have seen how the ideals of human dignity and basic civil rights are being reflected in what is being said and done regarding people with handicaps. But how much can we count on continued progress? Not very much, I would argue. To assert otherwise would be to invite apathy. There is no guarantee that the right of each individual to respect and encouragement in the enrichment of his or her life will increasingly be honored, or that people with handicaps will increasingly have an important voice in influencing conditions that affect their lives. Although we can affirm that the changing attitudes described above are durable insofar as they are regarded as expressions of basic human rights, we must also recognize that they are fragile insofar as they are subject to the vicissitudes of broad-sweeping social and political circumstances. The lives of handicapped people are inextricably a part of a much wider socioeconomic political and ethical society affecting the lives of all people. It is therefore essential for all of us to remain vigilant to protect and extend the hard-won gains of recent decades and to be ready to counter undermining forces. Vigilance requires thoughtful action guided by continuing reevaluation of the effectiveness of present efforts and alertness to needs of changing conditions.

REFERENCES

1. Abramson, A. S., & Kutner, B. (1972). A bill of rights for the disabled. *Archives of Physical Medicine and Rehabilitation, 53*(3), 99–100.
2. Aldrich, C. A. (1947). Preventive medicine and mongolism. *American Journal of Mental Deficiency, 52*(2), 127–129.
3. American Hospital Association. (1973). *A Patient's Bill of Rights*. Chicago: Author. Also published as: *Statement on a Patient's Bill of Rights*; Affirmed by the Board of Trustees, Nov. 17, 1972. *Hospitals.* Feb. 16, 1973. 47 :4:41.
4. Canadian Council for Rehabilitation of the Disabled. (1973). A declaration of intent. *Rehabilitation Digest, 4*(4), 4–5.
5. Chigier, E. (1972). Sexual adjustment of the handicapped. In *Proceedings Preview: Twelfth World Congress of Rehabilitation International* (pp. 224–227, Vol. 1). Sydney, Australia.
6. First International Conference on Legislation Concerning the Disabled. (1972). *International Rehabilitation Review, Second Quarter, 23*(2), 18–19.
7. Hohmann, G. W. (1972). Considerations in management of psychosexual readjustment in the cord injured male. *Rehabilitation Psychology, 19*, 250–258.
8. Mental Health Law Project. (1973). *Basic rights of the mentally handicapped*. Washington, DC: Author (*1751 N St., N.W., 20036*).
9. Telford, C. W., & Sawrey, J. M. (1972). *The exceptional individual* (2nd Ed.). Englewood Cliffs, NJ: Prentice-Hall.
10. United Cerebral Palsy Associations. (1971). Survey shows few CP adults involved in UCP decision making. *Crusader, 6*, 2.
11. United Cerebral Palsy Associations. (1973). A Bill of Rights for the handicapped. *Crusader, 3*, 1–6. Also published separately.
12. Wright, B. A. (1972). Value-laden beliefs and principles for rehabilitation psychology. *Rehabilitation Psychology, 19*(1), 38–45.

I

Historical Perspectives on Illness and Disability: Conclusion

DISCUSSION QUESTIONS

1. Considering Darwinian eugenics, which groups of people (if you had to choose) would you consider to be the weaker species among us?
2. Why has there never been a consensus among humans regarding whether striving for the genetically perfect human being is a worthwhile scientific endeavor?
3. Considering the blatant prejudice and discrimination laws in the 1920s toward immigrants with perceived disabilities, do you think it is unthinkable that Americans would ever exterminate people with disabilities as the Nazis did?
4. Which of Livneh's origins of negative attitudes toward persons with disabilities do you believe to be the most influential in shaping people's opinions?
5. What do you believe are prevalent current societal attitudes toward people with disabilities and why?
6. What are some common misconceptions about individuals with a psychiatric disability or mental illness?
7. Why do you suppose there continues to be a stigma attached to persons with a psychiatric disability, and why do many of these people refrain from seeking counseling?
8. Why is the "minority group" model challenging the "functional limitations" model?
9. What are the differences between a sociopolitical perspective and the medical and/or economic definition of disability?
10. Which model of disability do you believe is the most empowering for persons with disabilities?
11. What strategies or methods need to be considered by rehabilitation professionals to help enhance more positive attitudes toward people with disabilities?

PERSONAL PERSPECTIVE

The meaning of these chapters in Part I take on an engaging implication with the Personal Statement of Dale Walsh, which is reprinted from the fifth edition. Personal statements show graphically and poignantly how the concepts presented in the literature assume a forceful meaning when they are "lived out" in daily life. Dr. Walsh, both a professional of mental health services and a consumer of these same services, discusses her own difficult recovery journey. She echoes the truth identified in several of the chapters that consumer empowerment is more than a vital component of recovery; it promotes an environment that really fosters recovery. In her statement of what stimulates coping with stigma and discrimination, associated with a severe mental health condition, she emphasizes the consumer's initiating behavior as it emerges from a participatory role in one's rehabilitation. This behavior of involvement is just one of many positive outcomes from the conceptual models of disability proposed in the chapters of Part I.

COPING WITH A JOURNEY TOWARD RECOVERY: FROM THE INSIDE OUT

DALE WALSH

I have worked in the field of mental health for about 30 years. I can talk about this part of my life easily. I have also been a survivor of a longterm psychiatric disability for most of my childhood and adult life, and I am a survivor of the mental health system, both public and private. This is the harder part of my life to talk about. I have walked on both sides of the fence, so to speak. I want to share with you my own personal path toward recovery and what I see as a consumer practitioner to be necessary to support the recovery process of people who use the mental health system.

First, a word about language. There is no clear consensus within either the professional mental health community or among the people who have actually experienced psychiatric treatment as to what we are to be called. In the 1970s, when people who were former "patients" started to come together and share their experiences, they called themselves just that—ex-patients or former patients. Later, as the movement developed and grew and people collectively began to express their anger, some people used the name "psychiatric inmate" to make clear their dissatisfaction with the prevailing power inequities of the medical model and with the way they were treated. In California, the term "client" came to be used, because it met the dual goals of neutrality and descriptiveness. And in the 1980s the term "consumer" began to be used, mostly by the mental health system and by family groups (usually groups of parents who had an adult child with a severe psychiatric disability) in an attempt to find a label that was nonstigmatizing, yet acceptable to them. Other people who have been through the mental health system and consider themselves in recovery may use the phrase "psychiatric survivors."

This debate over language is more than semantics. What people choose to call themselves is a key element in forming a group identity. It is also an indication of people's sense of empowerment and the place they feel they occupy within the hierarchy of the system of mental health care or services. It is important for the mental health system to be respectful and to take careful note of the names or phrases used to describe the people who use their services. Since I knew I was one, I have called myself a "survivor" or "person with a psychiatric disability." Recently I have been with some colleagues who prefer the phrase "person with a psychiatric label." I like that because the phrase speaks to the stigma carried and experienced by those of us who have been through psychiatric "treatment."

I have been dealing with the aftereffects, the stigma, and the shame of having a psychiatric disability for most of my life. As a child I was overly good. I was very anxious. I had multiple physical problems, nightmares, and trouble sleeping. As an adult, I have always been restricted in performing many of life's everyday functions—going to a shopping mall

Note: This chapter is based on a presentation at the Alliance for the Mentally Ill/Department of Mental Health Curriculum and Training Committee Annual Conference in Boston, MA April 19, 1996.

From *Psychiatric Rehabilitation Journal*, Fall 1996, 20(2), p. 859. Reprinted with permission. Reprinted from 5th Edition of *The Psychological and Social Impact of Disability*, 2007, Springer Publishing Company.

or to the bank, taking vacations or doing other leisure activities, going to social events like weddings, and working full time. Many times just leaving my house has been too anxiety provoking for me to handle. I have had many episodes of depression so severe that basic functioning has been difficult. Most of the time I live with some level of anxiety and a sense of terror and foreboding that come not from the present but from my past history of abuse. Feeling safe in the world is something I work on on a daily basis.

For many years I believed in a traditional medical model. I had a disease. I was sick. I was told I was mentally ill, that I should learn to cope with my anxiety, my depression, my pain, and my panic. I never told anyone about the voices, but they were there, too. I was told I should change my expectations of myself and realize I would always have to live a very restricted life.

After I was diagnosed, I was put in a box up on a shelf. Occasionally I was taken down and my medication was changed. But no one really talked to me. No one helped me figure out why I should be content to take my medication and be grateful things were not worse. After all, at least I did not have to live my life in the back wards of a state hospital.

Because of my history and because of the society in which I lived, I easily turned the notion of illness into thinking there was something wrong with me. I was the problem. I felt deformed, everything I did was wrong. I had no place in the world. I was a freak. I was deeply ashamed of who I was and I tried my best to cover up my abnormality. I learned from those around me that psychiatric disability and its aftereffects were something to hide. As a result I lived marginally. I worked in a constant state of terror and tried to look normal. For the most part I succeeded—but at a tremendous cost to myself in terms of my energy, my self-image, my fear, and my inferiority. There were times when the stresses got to be too much and I ended up hospitalized, defeated, and feeling a failure because I couldn't tolerate even the day-to-day problems of what seemed to be a fairly simple life.

I worked in the field of mental health and I was very careful not to let anyone know my shameful secret. I was constantly terrified someone would find me out. I kept myself in entry-level positions because I was having a hard enough time without the added stress of climbing up the ladder in my field. I went to therapy. I took my medication and waited to feel better. I waited and waited. . . .

I sometimes felt angry at my caregivers, but mostly I felt angry at myself. At times my symptoms were better but I wasn't. I felt powerless. I felt empty. I looked outside myself to the doctors and professionals to cure me, or at least take away some of my pain. But they didn't. Maybe I was one of those hopeless cases. I felt despair and deep loneliness.

This old patriarchal system of treatment and culture of disease is characterized by a hierarchical arrangement of power, a mechanistic view of the mind, causality due to organic forces outside the person's self, an emphasis on a person's deficits, and treatment administered by an expert—always at a professional distance. Did they think they might catch it? Why were they all so careful to maintain that professional distance? For years I felt trapped because I knew no other way to look at myself and my process.

Then about 8 years ago I read *The Courage to Heal.* I started talking to people—professionals and survivors who knew about the effects of trauma and psychiatric disability. I was lucky enough to stumble on a 12- step and other self-help groups. Finally my symptoms, my dreams, and my fears started making sense. I discovered the principles and the practices of recovery. I discovered hope. I had lived for years in despair because the pills and the therapy did not make me better. I began to see that if my life was to become better, I would have to do it myself. I saw that other people with histories similar to mine had been able to move beyond their symptoms. I started working with a therapist who was able to communicate to me that she trusted and believed in my own capacity to grow and move forward. She was willing to assist me but she respected my own pacing. I began to believe

I could actually participate in a healing process. As I looked within myself I discovered over the following years, slowly and sometimes painfully, that healing, making positive changes in my life, and feeling better were all possible. Especially helpful to this process were several self-help groups where I didn't have to hide, where people understood and were engaged in struggles similar to mine. I saw people who were further along in their recovery who served as role models. I also got to know people who were not so far along as I was whom I could mentor. Giving back and learning how to get out of myself and into someone else's frame of reference has been, and continues to be, an important step in my recovery.

What I found through my own experience is that in order to travel the path of true recovery I could not rely on externals, wait, hope to be rescued, or be made better because of someone or something outside me. Instead, I learned that both the power and the possibility of change reside within me. I could make decisions that would affect my life. But I found I could not do this alone. I needed a supportive community around me. Slowly and gradually I found people who understood. I found friends and support people who could help me hold the hope when I was going through tough times and when I reached what felt like an insurmountable obstacle. These people believed in my capacity to heal. As I learned to take risks, I found that I could actually set and accomplish goals very much like people who were chronically normal.

Recovery is not a return to a former level of functioning. I have heard so many people—professionals and survivors alike—say that mental illness is not curable. I agree that we can never go back to our "premorbid" selves. The experience of the disability, and the stigma attached to it, changes us forever. Instead, recovery is a deeply personal and unique process of changing one's attitudes, values, self-concept, and goals. It is finding ways to live a hopeful, satisfying, active, and contributing life. Everyone is changed by major happenings in their lives.We cannot return to the past. Recovery involves the development of a new meaning and purpose in one's life. It is looking realistically at both the limitations and the possibilities. It is much more than mere symptom relief.

As I continued on my path of recovery, I found I could handle responsible jobs. I am now slowly expanding my social network as I feel safer in the world and more comfortable with who I am. And, very importantly, I have come out of the closet and announced publicly, as a representative of those with psychiatric labels, who I am, where I have been, and where we as a community of oppressed people can go if we can find our voices, recapture our power, and exercise it to take charge of our lives and our journey toward wholeness. I am still in recovery, for it is a process not a sudden landing.

Discovering and participating in this culture of healing has given me the hope and courage to travel the path of recovery. This is a culture of inclusion, hope, caring, and cooperation; of empowerment, equality, and humor; of dignity, respect, and trust. Forming relationships and creating systems of mental health care based on these principles are vital to supporting the growth of people who are users of the system. Traditionally, people who have been labeled as mentally ill have been considered to have poor judgment. They need to be taken care of. They do not know what is best for them. They are told what is wrong with them, what they need, what their future is to be like, and what is in their best interest. The stigma and discrimination that those of us who are labeled as mentally ill have suffered steals our hope, isolates us, and is a barrier to our healing.

Part of healing and recovery is the ability to participate as full citizens in the life of the community. As psychiatric survivors begin to break their silence and advocate for their humanity, the call and demand for basic civil rights becomes increasingly stronger. People want to be able to make their own choices about their own lives. They want to be seen, heard, and taken seriously. They want to be part of the decision making that so deeply affects their everyday experiences. This taking back of power and being taken seriously are both necessary components of recovery.

The notion that there is a recovery process that goes on internally within each person with a psychiatric label, often very separate from the treatment the person receives, is a new and somewhat threatening concept of the psychiatric treatment community. As recovery begins to be talked about and recognized by psychiatric survivors, it offers a way of taking back dignity, self-responsibility, and a sense of hope for the future.

By taking back power from the system of care, a consumer/survivor acknowledges that the ability to cope and heal comes from within. No one else, including the best of service providers, can do anything but facilitate the healing process. However, this facilitation—if it takes the form of good attention, respect, validation, and genuine connection—is an essential part of recovery.

Empowerment is a vital component of our recovery. Allowing and supporting a change within a program, agency, or system requires trust among administrators, staff members, and the people served. This change requires a shift from power being retained exclusively by administrators to it being shared among all constituencies. It requires a willingness to take risks in not only allowing, but actively encouraging, people to work toward their own goals. It means that choice and self-determination are to be considered foremost when consumer/survivors and staff members are developing treatment and rehabilitation plans. When treatment or rehabilitation is seen as more than prescribing the right formula, and when the emphasis is placed on maintaining the functioning and identity of the person, an atmosphere that promotes recovery is created. We who use the mental health system need to play a significant role in the shaping of the services, policies, and research that affect us. We need to have a place at the table and become participants in a shared dialog.

When people assert control over their own lives and make their own decisions, they also take on responsibility for the consequences of their decisions. Often, as service providers, we want to protect people from failure. We know, or at least think we know, what is best. We do not like to see people fail, both because of the pain it may cause to the person, but also because of the pain and feelings of failure we may experience. Sometimes when psychiatric survivors decide to make changes in their lives, they may not succeed. And, like other people, they may or may not learn from their failures. Like other people, they have a right to take risks. And sometimes they succeed, surpassing all expectations.

How many of you have tried something new and found it did not work? An investment perhaps? Or maybe a new relationship, or a marriage? You were allowed to take these risks even if the money you put into the investment was money you could not afford to lose, even if the relationship was the same kind of destructive relationship you had been through in the past. Maybe you learned from these situations, but maybe you didn't. People with psychiatric labels have these same rights. Part of sharing power is nurturing, encouraging, and fostering these rights.

Decision making in an environment that fosters recovery involves more people and more time. It is much easier for an administrator to make a decision alone than to bring it to the community for discussion and input. Often, decision making has to be taught to people who have grown accustomed to having their decisions made for them, who have been told so many times that, because of their "illness," they are unable to make responsible choices, and that any preferences they do express should be discounted because they are sick and unstable.

It takes time, patience, and a lot of listening to teach people to take the major risk of making their own choices again. But this type of power sharing through conversation can provide for a climate of equality, which can ensure that all people can be free to express and reach for their own hopes and aspirations. Power sharing allows both staff members and clients alike to become much more involved in, and invested in, their own growth. In an environment that fosters recovery, the barriers of discrimination and stigma, which destroy self-esteem, perpetuate learned helplessness, and convince people they are incapable of self-determination, are broken down.

Many people who have been diagnosed as mentally ill hate labels and object strongly when people are called schizophrenic, bipolar, or borderline. After people are diagnosed, everything that happens to them is seen through the filter of their labels. A couple of years ago I was admitted to a hospital on an emergency basis. The next morning I called my office to say I wouldn't be in because I was in the hospital. At the time I worked in a very progressive agency with several people who themselves had psychiatric disabilities. My colleagues assumed I was in a psychiatric unit. These same colleagues called every psychiatric unit in the Boston area trying to find me. In reality, I had been admitted to the hospital because of a respiratory infection. They had assumed that if I was in the hospital on an emergency basis of course I was having a psychiatric emergency.

An environment that fosters recovery must be one in which hope is an essential component of each activity. Often people with psychiatric labels have lost hope. They see their disability as a death sentence. They think they can never get any better. When you are in the midst of despair it is almost impossible to see the other side. Too often providers echo these feelings and cement them into reality for those with whom they work. Have you ever found yourself angry at a person who has given up hope? I have.

During difficult times it can be easier to give up. Do we blame ourselves? Sometimes. This can serve to fuel our own despair. More often, though, I think professionals blame the people who are in despair. Despairing clients are seen as lazy, noncompliant, and manipulative, and they don't want to get better. They don't want help. They should be discharged from the program so they can hit bottom, then maybe they will appreciate how good they had it.

In a system where this continually happens, people within the system and the system itself can get caught up in the despair and become rigid, distancing, and lifeless. As an administrator, I try to use these times to take an honest look at the services my agency is providing: are they relevant to what people need and want? Are staff members burning out and in need of support from me or from each other? In these days of more work and fewer resources I often find that the issues, the traumas, and the life experiences of the people who use the mental health center trigger myself and my staff. We can only be with people in their pain to the extent we are willing to be with our own pain within our own life experiences. I model this with my staff by talking about the feelings the work evokes in me. And I invite others to share also. I have found that creating an environment of safety for staff members as well as for clients is necessary for this open sharing to go on. Safety to reveal one's own vulnerabilities without fear of sanctions is vital for an environment that fosters recovery. Confidentiality, respect, and sincere attempts to empathize and demonstrate understanding to others are components of such an environment. Well-developed interpersonal skills, on the part of both staff members and administrators, can serve to support the atmosphere of safety and compassion.

When I decided to return to school to get my doctorate, I did so for several reasons. First of all I wanted to learn more. Second, I thought that the title "doctor" before my name would help me feel validated, and that I had a place in the world. And third, because I wanted to give back some of what had been given to me by those who supported my recovery. As I looked at various programs I was disappointed at the values and the sterility of the various programs. Then I talked to someone at Boston University, where I had gotten my master's many years before. I liked the idea of rehabilitation with its emphasis on functioning rather than illness and limitations. It was suggested to me that I read some of Bill Anthony's work to see if the principles expressed resonated with my own. As I did, I found that both the principles and practices gave a context and a structure as well as a guide for helpers to foster recovery instead of encouraging passivity and compliance. In psychiatric rehabilitation the person and his or her preferences and thoughts are essential to the process. When I learned of the values of involvement, choice, comprehensiveness, support, and growth potential, I saw these were the same values that helped free me from feeling trapped in traditional treatment. I was excited at the possibility of learning how to put these values into practice with other survivors of the psychiatric system. I learned in the very best way possible—by teaching. I taught courses in rehabilitation counseling for 4 years. Over the past several years I have been using these principles to help mental health systems put a recovery paradigm into practice. I have seen, in myself and in the people with whom I work, that when these values form the basis of the structure and program-ming within a system, people learn to take responsibility for themselves and their actions. These principles provide the soil for people to choose to grow and change. I have come to think of psychiatric rehabilitation as providing an external structure, while recovery is the internal process.

Through recovery I have found myself capable of making changes toward more sat-isfaction and success in my life. The quality of my life has greatly improved. I still have my limitations—I am not a finished product. And from an acceptance of my limitations has come a belief in my own unique possibilities. I have the power to move toward wholeness.

PERSONAL PERSPECTIVE EXERCISE

1. Dr. Walsh, both a professional mental health service provider and consumer of mental health services, discusses her personal difficulty as a "person with a psychiatric dis-ability" or a "survivor." She indicates that there is no clear consensus among clients/consumers and professionals within the mental health community on "what we are to be called." Discuss how the language of disability can help or harm people with psychiatric disabilities and what life areas may be impacted by the language of stereotypes.

2. Dr. Walsh states, "After I was diagnosed, I was put in a box up on a shelf." What exactly did she mean by this statement? What was the significance and impact on her?

3. Dr. Walsh suggests that discovering and participating in a healing path provided her with hope and courage for recovery. What specific actions did Dr. Walsh take that empow-ered her with an increased self-concept and the ability to live her life in a more hopeful way?

4. Dr. Walsh mentions that when an individual asserts control over his or her life and makes his or her own decisions, he or she takes on responsibility for the consequences of the decisions. What does she mean when she states "asserting control" and "taking responsibility"?

5. Dr. Walsh makes several significant statements about mental health services in the United States. Discuss the following points: (a) How does the mental health system view people with psychiatric disabilities? (b) What support systems and resources are deficient and how does this affect the client/consumers' independence?

6. Dr. Walsh, at one point in her career, decided to return to school to work on a doctorate with a specialty in rehabilitation counseling and psychiatric rehabilitation. What reasons does she give for returning to school?

II

The Personal Impact of Disability: Introduction

*P*art II transitions nicely into the personal impact of illness and disability on the individual and uniquely blends the issues with theory and practice. Of the seven chapters, four have undergone significant updates since the last edition. Following Part I and the exploration of disability from a sociological perspective, Part II looks inward at the potential implications from the interrelationship between an individual and his or her environment when living with a disability. As such, relevant authors discuss various theories of adaptation to disability, gender differences regarding sexuality, multicultural perspectives, and quality of life. This section concludes with a personal perspective by the renowned Dr. Albert Ellis who himself lived with a number of disabling conditions.

Chapter 7 by Livneh and Antonak regarding the psychosocial adaptation to chronic illness and disability (CID) provides counselors with a primer that succinctly establishes the foundation for this section. The authors discuss some of the major reactions to congenital and adventitious disabilities including stress and threats to body image, grieving the loss, stages of adjustment, various coping mechanisms of adapting to disability, and intervention strategies. A brief discussion is also presented regarding common psychometric measures to help assess one's adaptation to CID.

Chapter 8 by Phemister and Crewe is unique in that it is the only chapter in any psychosocial textbook that explores the topic of objective self-awareness and stigma for persons with visible disabilities. In their discussion, the authors define the differences between subjective and objective self-awareness, and once again highlight the critical individual–environment interrelationship on one's self-concept that is based in part, on one's feedback and perception of how society or the outside world responds and views them. In this fascinating chapter, the authors discuss the potential psychosocial ramifications of stigma and provide guidance for counselors regarding the implications and working with persons with visible disabilities.

Chapter 9 by Nosek is an updated look at the psychosocial issues of women with disabilities. The authors have devoted much of their professional career to exploring women's issues and nicely delineate demographic and health statistics for women with physical disabilities and the potential subsequent psychological implications regarding stress, self-esteem, and connectedness in society. A brief discussion also ensues pertaining to the closeted but prevalent occurrence of physical and sexual abuse of this population.

Chapter 10 by Miller and Marini is also an updated chapter dealing with both male and female issues regarding sexuality and, specifically, spinal cord injury (SCI), as well as its implications and practical counseling strategies when working with this population. The significance of this chapter explores the definition of sexuality, common myths, and misconceptions regarding sexuality and disability; the medical and physiological impact of SCI for men and women; and basic sex counseling strategies conceptualized within a five-component framework (physical appearance, personality and behavioral traits, courtship factors, sexuality encounter, and long-term intimacy) adapted from Vash's original work on the topic.

Chapter 11 by Marini is also updated exploring the cross-cultural counseling issues of males who sustain a disability. Marini addresses ethnic and racial differences regarding worldview and specifically each group's perceptions and treatment of its members with a disability. Particular to men's issues, the author touches upon societal perceptions of masculine traits, perceptions of disability, and the impact a severe disability may have on a male's perceptions of himself. Three major models of adjustment or adaptation to disability are discussed and applied to tangible counseling strategies for working with this population.

Chapter 12 by North and Surís is also an updated chapter addressing the psychiatric and psychological issues that face survivors of major disasters. This poignantly revamped chapter expounds upon what has unfortunately continued to increase in the United States over the past decade, namely, an increase in natural disasters including more powerful hurricanes, fires, and tornadoes; an increase in terrorism; and an increase in technological accidents including infrastructure accidents (e.g., bridge collapses, natural gas explosions, and toxic chemical accidents). The authors focus predominantly, however, on the human condition impact of post-traumatic stress disorder (PTSD), other psychiatric disorders, and both pharmacological and nonpharmacological interventions for PTSD.

Chapter 13 by Bishop explores the theoretical and contextual definition of quality of life as it applies to adapting to CID. He describes the disability centrality model, noting the significance individual's place on various life domains, and the psychological impact a CID may have if important life domains are negatively affected. Bishop asserts that quality of life may be reduced if satisfaction and control of personally important domains cannot be achieved or regained. Clinical implications for counselors and counseling interventions are described through this model.

7

Psychological Adaptation to Chronic Illness and Disability: A Primer for Counselors

Hanoch Livneh and Richard F. Antonak

Chronic illnesses and disabling conditions are common occurrences in the lives of many individuals. It has been estimated that approximately 54 million Americans (about 1 in 5) have physical, sensory, psychiatric, or cognitive disabilities that interfere with their daily living (Bowe, 2000). Furthermore, (a) more than 9 million Americans with disabilities are unable to work or attend school; (b) costs of annual income support (e.g., supplemental security income and social security disability insurance) and medical care provided by the U.S. government to assist people with disabilities are about $60 billion; (c) disabilities are higher among older people, minorities, and lower socioeconomic groups; and (d) 8 of the 10 most common causes of death in the United States are associated with chronic illness (Eisenberg, Glueckauf, & Zaretsky, 1999; Stachnik, Stoffelmayr, & Hoppe, 1983).

Many disability- and nondisability-related factors interact to create a profound effect on the lives of individuals with chronic illness and disabilities (CID). Among these, the most commonly recognized factors include the degree of functional limitations, interference with the ability to perform daily activities and life roles, uncertain prognosis, the prolonged course of medical treatment and rehabilitation interventions, the psychosocial stress associated with the incurred trauma or disease process itself, the impact on family and friends, and the sustained financial losses (e.g., reduced income and increased medical bills).

The intent of this article is to provide the reader with an overview of (a) the dynamics (i.e., process) of psychosocial adaptation to CID, (b) methods commonly used to assess psychosocial adaptation to CID, and (c) intervention strategies applied to people with CID.

THE DYNAMICS OF PSYCHOSOCIAL ADAPTATION TO CID

The onset of CID is typically associated with a disease process (e.g., multiple sclerosis [MS] and cancer) or a traumatic injury (spinal cord injury and traumatic brain injury). CID is also dichotomized into congenital, or evident at birth (e.g., spina bifida and cerebral palsy), and adventitious, or acquired later in life (Parkinson's disease and amputation). In this chapter, we focus on psychosocial adaptation to acquired disabling conditions.

This overview of the literature on psychosocial adaptation to CID is grouped under three headings: basic concepts, CID-triggered reactions, and CID-related coping strategies.

From "Psychological adaptation to chronic illness and disability: A primer for counselors," by H. Livneh and R. Antonak, 2005, *Journal of Counseling & Development, 83,* 12–20. ACA. Reprinted with permission. No further reproduction authorized without written permission from the American Counseling Association.

BASIC CONCEPTS

Included here are the concepts of stress, crisis, loss and grief, body image, self-concept, stigma, uncertainty and unpredictability, and quality of life (QOL).

Stress

Individuals with CID normally face an increase in both the frequency and severity of stressful situations (Falvo, 1999; Horowitz, 1986). Increased stress is experienced because of the need to cope with daily threats that include, among others, threats to (a) one's life and well-being; (b) body integrity; (c) independence and autonomy; (d) fulfillment of familial, social, and vocational roles; (e) future goals and plans; and (f) economic stability (Falvo, 1999).

Crisis

The sudden onset of many medical impairments and disabilities (e.g., myocardial infarction, spinal cord injury, traumatic brain injury, and amputation) and that of life-threatening diagnoses or loss of valued functions (e.g., cancer and vision impairment) is highly traumatic. As such, these conditions constitute a psychosocial crisis in the life of the affected person (Livneh & Antonak, 1997; Moos & Schaefer, 1984). Although crisis, by definition, is time limited (e.g., Janosik, 1984), during its presence, life is affected by disturbed psychological, behavioral, and social equilibrium. The psychological consequences of crisis are, in contrast, long lasting and may even evolve into pathological conditions such as post-traumatic stress disorder (PTSD).

Loss and Grief

The crisis experienced following the onset of a traumatic or progressive CID triggers a mourning process for the lost body part or function. In a manner parallel to that evidenced following the loss of a loved one, the individual exhibits feelings of grief, bereavement, and despair (Parkes, 1975; Wright, 1983). The term *chronic sorrow* has often been used to depict the grief experienced by persons with CID (Burke, Hainsworth, Eakes, & Lindgren, 1992; Davis, 1987). Unlike grief associated with nonbodily losses, CID serves as a constant reminder of the permanency of the condition. Furthermore, daily triggering events act to remind the affected person of the permanent disparity between past and present or future situations (Teel, 1991).

Body Image

Body image has parsimoniously been defined as the unconscious mental representation or schema of one's own body (Schilder, 1950). It evolves gradually and reflects interactive forces exerted by sensory (e.g., visual, auditory, and kinesthetic), interpersonal (e.g., attitudinal), environmental (e.g., physical conditions), and temporal factors. CID, with its impact on physical appearance, functional capabilities, experience of pain, and social roles, is believed to alter, even distort, one's body image and self-concept (Bramble & Cukr, 1998; Falvo, 1999). Successful psychosocial adaptation to CID is said to reflect the integration of physical and sensory changes into a transformed body image and self-perception. Unsuccessful adaptation, in contrast, is evidenced by experiences of physical and psychiatric symptoms such as unmitigated feelings of anxiety and depression, psychogenic pain, chronic fatigue, social withdrawal, and cognitive distortions (Livneh & Antonak, 1997).

Self-Concept

One's self-concept and self-identity are linked to body image and are often seen as conscious, social derivatives of it (Bramble & Cukr, 1998; McDaniel, 1976). However, self-concept and self-identity may be discordant for many individuals with visible disabilities. The sense of self (i.e., self-identity), which is privately owned and outwardly presented, may be denied in social interactions with others who respond to the person as "disabled" first (i.e., focusing on appearance rather than identity), thereby losing sense of the person's real self (Kelly, 2001). The person's self-esteem, representing the evaluative component of the self-concept, gradually shows signs of erosion and negative self-perceptions following such encounters.

Stigma

The impact of stereotypes and prejudice acts to increase stigma toward people with CID (Corrigan, 2000; Falvo, 1999). Restrictions imposed by CID lead to deviations from several societal norms and expectations (e.g., utilization of health care services and occupational stability). They are, therefore, viewed negatively by society and result in stigmatizing perceptions and discriminatory practices. Moreover, when internalized by people with CID, these stigmatizing encounters with others result in increased life stress, reduced self-esteem, and withdrawal from social encounters, including treatment and rehabilitation environments (Falvo, 1999; Wright, 1983).

Uncertainty and Unpredictability

Although the course of some CIDs is rather stable or predictable (e.g., amputation and cerebral palsy), most conditions may be regarded as neither stable nor predictable (e.g., epilepsy, cancer, diabetes mellitus, and MS). Put differently, the insidious and variable course of these conditions is fraught with intermittent periods of exacerbation and remissions, unpredictable complications, experiences of pain and loss of consciousness, and alternating pace of gradual deterioration. Indeed, the concept of "perceived uncertainty in illness" was coined by Mishel (1981, p. 258) to depict how uncertainty, or the inability to structure personal meaning, results if the individual is unable to form a cognitive schema of illness-associated events. Medical conditions, such as cancer and MS, which are marked by heightened levels of perceived uncertainty regarding disease symptoms, diagnosis, treatment, prognosis, and relationships with family members, were found to be associated with decreased psychosocial adaptation (Mishel, 1981; Wineman, 1990).

Quality of Life

The ultimate psychosocial outcome in rehabilitation practice is believed to be that of post-CID QOL (Crewe, 1980; Roessler, 1990). As a global and multifaceted construct, QOL includes the following functional domains (Flanagan, 1982; Frisch, 1999): (a) intrapersonal (e.g., health, perceptions of life satisfaction, and feelings of well-being), (b) interpersonal (e.g., family life and social activities), and (c) extrapersonal (e.g., work activities and housing). In the context of adaptation to CID, for QOL, there are typically assumptions in two primary domains: successful restructuring of previously disrupted psychosocial homeostasis and attainment of an adaptive person-environment (reality) congruence. Furthermore, QOL is considered to be linked to a more positive self-concept and body image, as well as to an increased sense of control over CID, and QOL is negatively associated with perceived stress and feelings of loss and grief (Dijkers, 1997; Falvo, 1999).

CID-TRIGGERED RESPONSES

Clinical observations and empirical research on the psychosocial process of adaptation to CID have been marred by conflicting findings and heated debate. In this section, we focus on the most frequently experienced psychosocial reactions to CID as cited in the rehabilitation research and disability studies literatures.

Shock

This short-lived reaction marks the initial experience following the onset of a traumatic and sudden injury or the diagnosis of a life-threatening or chronic and debilitating disease. The reaction is characterized by psychic numbness, cognitive disorganization, and dramatically decreased or disrupted mobility and speech.

Anxiety

This reaction is characterized by a panic-like feature on initial sensing of the nature and magnitude of the traumatic event. Reflecting a state-like (i.e., situationally determined) response, it is accompanied by confused thinking, cognitive flooding, and a multitude of physiological symptoms including rapid heart rate, hyperventilation, excess perspiration, and irritable stomach.

Denial

This reaction, also regarded as a defense mechanism mobilized to ward off anxiety and other threatening emotions, involves the minimization and even complete negation of the chronicity, extent, and future implications associated with the condition. Denial involves selective attention to one's physical and psychological environments. It includes wishful thinking, unrealistic expectations of (full or immediate) recovery, and at times, blatant neglect of medical advice and therapeutic or rehabilitation recommendations. Although denial may successfully mitigate anxiety and depression when used selectively and during initial phases of adaptation, its long-term impact is often considered maladaptive and life threatening (Krantz & Deckel, 1983; Meyerowitz, 1983).

Depression

This reaction, commonly observed among people with CID, is considered to reflect the realization of the permanency, magnitude, and future implications associated with the loss of body integrity, chronicity of condition, or impending death. Feelings of despair, helplessness, hopelessness, isolation, and distress are frequently reported during this time. Although depression has been found to be a wide-spread reaction among persons with CID (e.g., Rodin, Craven, & Littlefield, 1991; Turner & Noh, 1988), it is still unclear if it is (as some theoreticians and clinicians argue) a pre-requisite to ultimate acceptance of the condition or attaining successful psychosocial adaptation (Wortman & Silver, 1989).

Anger/Hostility

There action of anger/hostility is frequently divided into internalize danger (i.e., self-directed feelings and behaviors of resentment, bitterness, guilt, and self-blame) and externalized hostility (i.e., other- or environment-directed retaliatory feelings and behaviors; Livneh & Antonak, 1997). When internally directed, self-attributions of responsibility for the condition onset or failure to achieve successful outcomes are evident. In contrast, externally oriented attributions of responsibility tend to place blame for the CID onset or unsuccessful treatment efforts on other people (e.g., medical staff and family members) or aspects of the external environment (e.g., inaccessible facilities and attitudinal barriers). Behaviors commonly observed during this time include aggressive acts, abusive accusations, antagonism, and passive-aggressive modes of obstructing treatment.

Adjustment

This reaction, also referred to in the literature as reorganization, reintegration, or reorientation, comprises several components: (a) an earlier cognitive reconciliation of the condition, its impact, and its chronic or permanent nature; (b) an affective acceptance, or internalization, of oneself as a person with CID, including a new or restored sense of self-concept, renewed life values, and a continued search for new meanings; and (c) an active (i.e., behavioral) pursuit of personal, social, and/or vocational goals, including successful negotiation of obstacles encountered during the pursuit of these goals.

CID-ASSOCIATED COPING STRATEGIES

The literature on CID-related coping strategies is vast (Moos, 1984; Zeidner & Endler, 1996). In this section, only a cursory overview of the most commonly reported strategies, directly related to coping with CID, is undertaken. First, however, the concept of coping is briefly discussed and its relevance to CID is illustrated.

Coping has been viewed as a psychological strategy mobilized to decrease, modify, or diffuse the impact of stress-generating life events (Billings & Moos, 1981; Lazarus & Folkman, 1984). Foremost, among the defining characteristics of coping are those of (a) including both stable (i.e., trait-like) and situationally determined (i.e., state-like) elements; (b) accessibility to conscious manipulation and control; (c) hierarchical organization that spans the range from macroanalytic, global styles of coping (e.g., locus of control and optimism), to micro-analytic, specific behavioral acts; and (d) being structurally multifaceted, including affective, cognitive, and behavioral aspects (Krohne, 1993; Zeidner & Endler, 1996). In addition, clinical and empirical studies of coping emphasize its (a) amenability to assessment by psychometric measures (there are currently over 20 psychological measures that purport to assess from 2 to almost 30 coping styles and strategies) and (b) divergent theoretical underpinnings (the nature of coping has been viewed differently by clinicians from various theoretical persuasions including psychodynamic, interpersonal, and cognitive behavioral).

Research on coping with CID has spanned a wide range of conditions such as cancer, heart disease, spinal cord injury, epilepsy, MS, amputation, rheumatoid arthritis, and diabetes, as well as the experience of pain. Commonly assumed in these research endeavors is the existence of two broad categories of coping strategies, namely, disengagement and engagement coping strategies.

Disengagement Coping Strategies

These strategies refer to coping efforts that seek to deal with stressful events through passive, indirect, even avoidance-oriented activities such as denial, wish-fulfilling fantasy, self- and other-blame, and resorting to substance abuse (Tobin, Holroyd, Reynolds, & Wigal, 1989). This group of coping strategies is often associated with higher levels of psychological distress (i.e., increased negative affectivity), difficulties in accepting one's condition, and generally poor adaptation to CID.

Engagement Coping Strategies

These strategies refer to coping efforts that defuse stressful situations through active, direct, and goal-oriented activities such as information seeking, problem solving, planning, and seeking social support (Tobin et al., 1989). This group of coping strategies is commonly linked to higher levels of well-being, acceptance of condition, and successful adaptation to CID.

During the chronic, but often remitting and exacerbating, course of medical conditions and physical disabilities, coping strategies are differentially adopted to meet the fluctuating demands necessitated by the changing physical, psychosocial, spiritual, economic, and environmental needs of the person. The rehabilitation and disability studies literature suggests that coping strategies could occupy several roles in their relationship to psychosocial adaptation to CID. These include (a) direct or causal, such that their use might differentially determine or influence psychosocial adaptation; (b) indirect or mediating, such that their use acts to mediate between certain demographic (e.g., age), disability-related (e.g., severity or duration of condition), or personality (e.g., level of perceived uncertainty) variables, and outcomes of adaptation to CID; and (c) outcome variables, such that the type and valence of coping strategies are an indicator of how successful psychosocial adaptation is.

ASSESSMENT OF PSYCHOSOCIAL ADAPTATION TO CID

Over the past half-century, a large number of measures of psychosocial adaptation to and coping with CID have been reported in the literature. In this section, only those psychometrically sound measures most frequently reported in the literature are reviewed. Readers may refer to the study by Livneh and Antonak (1997) for a comprehensive discussion of these and other measures.

GENERAL MEASURES OF ADAPTATION TO CID

Millon Behavioral Health Inventory

The Millon Behavioral Health Inventory (MBHI; Millon, Green, & Meagher, 1979) is a 150-item self-report questionnaire, organized into 20 clinical scales. The scales are classified into four domains that include (a) coping styles, (b) psychogenic attitudes, (c) psychosomatic complaints, and (d) a prognostic index. The MBHI seeks to (a) describe the psychological styles of medical service recipients, (b) examine the impact of emotional and motivational needs and coping strategies on disease course, and (c) suggest a comprehensive treatment plan to decrease the impact of deleterious psychological reactions. The strengths of the MBHI include its sound psychometric (i.e., reliability and validity) properties, clinical usefulness, and applicability to a wide range of medical and rehabilitation settings. Weaknesses include empirically unconfirmed domain structure and potential reactivity influences and response bias.

Psychosocial Adjustment to Illness Scale

The Psychosocial Adjustment to Illness Scale (PAIS; Derogatis, 1977; Derogatis & Lopez, 1983) is a 46-item instrument designed to measure psychosocial adaptation to medical illnesses and chronic diseases. The scale can be administered both as a semistructured psychiatric interview by a trained clinician and as a self-report measure (PAIS-SR). In addition to an overall adjustment score, seven subscales are provided. These include health care orientation, vocational environment, domestic environment, sexual relationships, extended family relationships, social environment, and psychological distress (i.e., indicating reactions of anxiety, depression, guilt, and hostility, as well as levels of self-esteem and body image). The strengths of the PAIS include the psychometric robustness of its scales, having both self-report and clinician interview forms, and the availability of norm scores for several medical conditions (e.g., cancer, MS, and renal failure). Weaknesses include lack of data on possible response bias influences.

Acceptance of Disability Scale

The Acceptance of Disability (AD; Linkowski, 1971) scale is a 50-item, 6-point, summated rating scale developed to measure the degree of acceptance of disability as theorized by

Dembo, Leviton, and Wright (1956). Items are summed to yield a single score representing changes in one's value system following the onset of physical disability.

Major strengths inherent in the AD scale include its theory-driven rationale, reliability, and use in a large number of English-speaking and non-English-speaking countries. Weaknesses are suggested by the lack of investigation of its factorial structure, its unidimensional approach to a complex construct, and lack of data on response bias influences.

Sickness Impact Profile

The Sickness Impact Profile (SIP; Bergner et al., 1976; Gilson et al., 1975) comprises 136 items that yield, in addition to scores on 12 subscales, a global scale score; three scales can be combined to create a physical dimension score (i.e., ambulation, mobility, and body care and movement), four scales can be combined and yield a psychosocial dimension score (i.e., social interaction, alertness behavior, emotional behavior, and communication), and the five remaining scales are viewed as independent categories and are typically scored separately (i.e., sleep and rest, eating, work, home management, and recreation and pastimes). Respondent-perceived impact of sickness is measured by directing the respondent to choose descriptors of currently experienced, sickness-related behavioral dysfunction.

The strengths of the SIP include its comprehensive and rigorous psychometric development and properties, extensive use with patients diagnosed with a variety of physical and health conditions, and the availability of a Spanish-language version. Weaknesses may be related to its yet-to-be tested factorial structure and susceptibility to defensiveness and response set.

Reactions to Impairment and Disability Inventory

The Reactions to Impairment and Disability Inventory (RIDI; Livneh & Antonak, 1990) is a 60-item, multidimensional, self-report summated rating scale. Its intended use is to investigate eight clinically reported classes of psychosocial reactions to the onset of CID. The eight psychosocial reaction scales include shock, anxiety, denial, depression, internalized anger, externalized hostility, acknowledgment, and adjustment. The strengths of the RIDI include its comprehensive psychometric development, scale reliability, and multidimensional perspective on adaptation to CID. Weaknesses are suggested by scant concurrent validity data, lack of normative data across disabling conditions, and potential confounding effects of response bias influences.

Handicap Problems Inventory

The Handicap Problems Inventory (HPI; Wright & Remmers, 1960) is a 280-item checklist of problems believed to be attributed to the presence of physical disability. Respondents are asked to mark those problems that are caused or exacerbated by the existence of the condition. Items on the inventory are grouped into four life domains that include personal, family, social, and vocational subscales. The strengths of the HPI include domain comprehensiveness, its documented internal reliability estimates, and available normative data. Weaknesses include lack of supportive data on its validity, possible response bias, and its inordinate length.

SPECIFIC MEASURES OF ADAPTATION TO CID

A sizeable number of measures related to psychosocial adaptation to specific CIDs have been reported in the rehabilitation and disability studies literatures. Because of space constraints, these measures will not be reviewed here. Interested readers may refer to the study by Livneh and Antonak (1997) for a comprehensive review of these scales. Readers may also wish to directly consult the following:

1. Measures of adaptation to cancer that include the Mental Adjustment to Cancer Scale (Watson et al., 1988).
2. Measures of adaptation to diabetes that include the Diabetic Adjustment Scale (Sullivan, 1979).
3. Measures on adaptation to epilepsy and seizure disorders that include the Washington Psychosocial Seizure Inventory (Dodrill, Batzel, Queisser, & Temkin, 1980).
4. Measures of adaptation to traumatic brain injury that include the Portland Adaptability Inventory (Lezak, 1987).
5. Measures of adaptation to rheumatoid arthritis that include the Arthritis Impact Measurement Scale (Meenan, 1982, 1986).
6. Measures of adaptation to spinal cord injuries that include the psychosocial questionnaire for spinal cord injured persons (Bodenhamer Achterberg-Lawlis, Kevorkian, Belanus, & Cofer, 1983).
7. Measures of adaptation to visual impairments that include the Nottingham Adjustment Scale (Dodds, Bailey, Pearson, & Yates, 1991).
8. Measures of adaptation to hearing impairments that include the social-emotional assessment inventory for deaf and hearing-impaired students (Meadow, Karchmer, Peterson, & Rudner, 1980).

Counselors and clinicians who consider adopting traditional psychological measures (e.g., the Minnesota Multiphasic Personality Inventory, Beck Depression Inventory, and Spielberger's State-Trait Anxiety Inventory) to address psychosocial adaptation to CID must be cognizant of the following two issues:

1. Physical and physiological symptoms (e.g., fatigue, weakness, and sleep problems) directly associated with a number of CIDs (e.g., spinal cord injury, MS, and Parkinson's disease) often mimic indicators of depression and anxiety among members of these populations. Counselors who work with people with CID should therefore (a) pay careful attention and differentiate, whenever possible, the more authentic indicators of depression and anxiety (typically cognitive and affective correlates) from those associated with the condition's physiological concomitants and (b) gain understanding of the literature that has examined the confounding effects of CID-triggered physiological symptoms on the scoring and interpretation of traditional psychological measures (e.g., Morrison, 1997; Pollak, Levy, & Breitholtz, 1999; Skuster, Digre, & Corbett, 1992).
2. Most traditional psychological and psychiatric measures lack scoring norms based on responses from populations of people with CID. This lack of normative data for people with CID renders these measures suspicious, even misleading, when their findings are interpreted indiscriminately. Counselors who adopt, or contemplate modifying, psychological tests for use with people with CID should carefully review the *Standards for Educational and Psychological Testing* (American Psychological Association, 1999) and Bolton (2001) for specific suggestions on this matter.

INTERVENTION STRATEGIES FOR PEOPLE WITH CID

Numerous theory-driven, reaction-specific, and clinically documented intervention strategies to assist people with CID successfully adapt to their conditions have been reported in the literature. In the following section, we review the major approaches to psychosocial interventions applied to people with CID.

Theory-Driven Interventions

These interventions focus on the clinical applications of widely recognized personality theories and therapeutic models to persons with CID and the perceived merits of their use with this population. Among the more commonly applied theories are psychoanalytic, individual (Adlerian), Gestalt (Perls), rational-emotive-behavioral (Ellis), cognitive (Beck), and behaviorist (Riggar, Maki, & Wolf, 1986; Thomas, Butler, & Parker, 1987).

When adopting theory-driven interventions, clinicians typically follow a three-step sequence. First, core concepts from a particular theory (e.g., defense mechanisms, feelings of inferiority, unfinished life situations, and irrational beliefs) are identified and examined. Second, the usefulness of these concepts, within the context of psychosocial adaptation to CID (e.g., understanding the process of grieving for loss of body parts or functions) is scrutinized. Third, the benefits derived from these concepts, for practical counseling interventions, for people with CID are assessed and, if deemed appropriate, are applied to their life situations. Readers may wish to refer to the study by Chan, Thomas, and Berven (2002), English (1971), Livneh and Antonak (1997), Livneh and Sherwood (1991), and Shontz (1978) for detailed reviews of these interventions.

Psychosocial Reaction-Specific Interventions

These eclectic interventions aim at offering a logical match between specific psychotherapeutic strategies and those reactions (or experiences) evoked during the process of adaptation to CID (e.g., anxiety, depression, denial, and anger). Worded differently, the counselor seeks to link specific counseling strategies with clinically observed, or client-reported, psychosocial reactions (Dunn, 1975; Livneh & Antonak, 1997; Livneh & Sherwood, 1991). It is generally argued that strategies regarded as supportive, affective-insightful, or psychodynamic in nature (e.g., person-centered therapy, Gestalt therapy, and Jungian therapy) may be more useful during earlier phases of the adaptation process. In contrast, strategies viewed as more active-directive, goal-oriented, or cognitive behavioral in nature (e.g., cognitive therapy, behavioral therapy, and coping skills training) may be more beneficial during the later stages (Dunn, 1975; Livneh & Antonak, 1997; Marshak & Seligman, 1993). To illustrate the above rationale, two examples are provided. First, disability or loss-triggered depression can be approached by encouraging the client to vent feelings associated with grief, isolation, guilt, shame, and mourning for the lost function (e.g., mobility, vision, and health). Protracted depression can be further managed by reinforcing social contacts and activities and by practicing self-assertiveness, self-determination, and independent living skills. Second, reactions (feelings and behaviors) of self-directed or other-directed anger may be dealt with by teaching and practicing anger expression in socially sanctioned forms, such as the pursuit of artistic endeavors and, if feasible, sports-related activities. Other strategies could include practicing behavior modification techniques to reduce physically and verbally aggressive acts.

Global Clinical Interventions

These comprehensive clinical interventions are geared toward assisting people with specific CIDs (e.g., cancer, heart disease, and spinal cord injury) in successfully adapting to their condition and its impact on their lives. More specifically, these interventions provide the client and his or her family and significant others with emotional, cognitive, and behavioral support. In addition, these interventions equip the client with adaptive coping skills that could be successfully adopted when facing stressful life events and crisis situations. Among the most commonly encountered global clinical interventions are the following:

1. *Assisting clients to explore the personal meaning of the CID.* These strategies rest heavily on psychodynamic principles and focus on issues of loss, grief, mourning, and suffering. Emphasis is also placed on encouraging clients to vent feelings leading to acceptance of condition permanency, altered body image, and realization of decreased functional capacity. A three-phase approach by Rodin et al. (1991) to treating depression in medically impaired individuals best illustrates this strategy (i.e., assisting clients in expressing grief and mourning, providing clients with opportunities to seek personal meaning of their CID, and training clients to attain a sense of mastery over their emotional experiences).

2. *Providing clients with relevant medical information.* These strategies emphasize imparting accurate information to clients on their medical condition, including its present status, prognosis, anticipated future functional limitations, and when applicable, vocational implications. These approaches are best suited for decreasing initial levels of heightened anxiety and depression, as well as the potentially damaging effects of unremitting denial (Ganz, 1988; Razin, 1982).

3. *Providing clients with supportive family and group experiences.* These strategies permit clients (usually with similar disabilities or common life experiences) and, if applicable, their family members or significant others to share common fears, concerns, needs, and wishes. These experiences also allow clients to acquire greater insight and to gain social support and approval from other group participants, family members, and professional helpers. Common group modalities include educational groups, psychotherapeutic groups, coping-skills training groups, and social support groups (Roback, 1984; Seligman, 1982; Telch & Telch, 1985). A group model by Subramanian and Ell (1989) for heart patients best exemplifies this approach because it incorporates (a) information on heart conditions and disability management, (b) coping-skills training to manage stressful life situations, and (c) cognitive skills teaching to manage maladaptive emotions.

4. *Teaching clients adaptive coping skills for successful community functioning.* These strategies, in a similar vein to those of group-based coping-skills training, focus on instilling in clients coping skills that will allow them to face a wide range of stressful conditions typically encountered by people with CID in physical, social, educational, and vocational settings. These skills include assertiveness, interpersonal relations, decision making, problem solving, stigma management, and time management skills. Craig and coauthors (Craig, Hancock, Chang, & Dickson, 1998; Craig, Hancock, Dickson, & Chang, 1997) have used a cognitive behavioral therapy coping program to train clients who have sustained spinal cord injury. The authors' multifaceted approach uses relaxation techniques, visualization techniques, cognitive restructuring, and social and self-assertiveness skills training to help participants cope with psychosocial difficulties encountered on release into the community.

SUMMARY

Approximately one in five Americans is currently diagnosed with CID. People with CID often encounter physical, psychological, social, educational, financial, and vocational barriers that greatly interfere with their QOL. In this chapter, we have attempted to provide counselors with the most useful and pragmatic concepts, processes, assessment tools, and intervention strategies related to psychosocial adaptation to CID.

When working with individuals who have sustained CID, counselors are commonly called to draw on their expertise in the areas of (a) stress, crisis, and coping with loss and grief; (b) the impact of traumatic events on self-concept, body image, and QOL; and (c) the effects of disability-linked factors (e.g., uncertainty and unpredictability) and societal reactions (e.g., stigma and prejudice) on psychosocial adaptation to CID.

Counselors must also be cognizant of, and demonstrate clinical acumen when observing, clients' psychosocial reactions to their conditions and the external environment. Several CID-triggered responses (at times described as phases) have been discussed. These include (a) reactions of shorter duration that are more commonly experienced earlier in the adaptation process (e.g., shock and anxiety); (b) reactions of longer duration that normally suggest distressed and unsuccessful coping efforts (e.g., depression and anger); and (c) reactions that signal successful adaptation to the condition and renewed life homeostasis (adjustment).

Of the many measures available for assessing psychosocial adaptation to CID, six have been reviewed in this chapter. They were selected because of their (a) applicability to a wide range of CIDs, (b) sound psychometric development and structure, (c) frequent citations in the rehabilitation and disability studies literatures, and (d) clinical and research potential.

Assessment of clients' levels of psychosocial adaptation to their condition should pave the way to appropriate selection of intervention strategies. To this end, the chapter concludes with an overview of four psychosocial strategies most commonly applied to counseling people with CID. Reviewed were interventions based on innovative applications of traditional personality and psychotherapeutic interventions. Next, interventions that seek to address reactions linked to the onset of CID (e.g., anxiety, depression, and anger) were highlighted. Finally, global, eclectic, clinical approaches that were typically developed for specific disabilities (e.g., cancer, heart conditions, and spinal cord injury) were illustrated. The last group of interventions offers the counselor fertile ground for applying comprehensive, multifaceted approaches geared to meet the wide range of psychological, social, and vocational needs of clients with CID.

REFERENCES

American Psychological Association. (1999). *Standards for educational and psychological testing* (4th ed.). Washington, DC: Author.

Bergner, M., Bobbitt, R. A., Kressel, S., Pollard, W. E., Gilson, B. S., & Morris, J. R. (1976). The sickness impact profile: Conceptual formulation and methodology for the development of a health status measure. *International Journal of Health Services, 6*, 393–415.

Billings, A. G., & Moos, R. H. (1981). The role of coping responses and social resources in attenuating the stress of life events. *Journal of Behavioral Medicine, 4*, 139–157.

Bodenhamer, E., Achterberg-Lawlis, J., Kevorkian, G., Belanus, A., & Cofer, J. (1983). Staff and patient perceptions of the psycho-social concerns of spinal cord injured persons. *American Journal of Physical Medicine, 62*, 182–193.

Bolton, B. (Ed.). (2001). *Handbook of measurement and evaluation in rehabilitation* (3rd ed.). Gaithersburg, MD: Aspen.

Bowe, F. (2000). *Physical, sensory, and health disabilities: An introduction.* Upper Saddle River, NJ: Merrill.

Bramble, K., & Cukr, P. (1998). Body image. In I. M. Lubkin (Ed.), *Chronic illness: Impact and interventions* (4th ed., pp. 283–298). Boston: Jones and Bartlett.

Burke, M. L., Hainsworth, M. A., Eakes, G. G., & Lindgren, C. L. (1992). Current knowledge and research on chronic sorrow: A foundation for inquiry. *Death Studies, 16*, 231–245.

Chan, F., Thomas, K. R., & Berven, N. L. (Eds.). (2002). *Counseling theories and techniques for rehabilitation health professionals.* New York: Springer.

Corrigan, P. W. (2000). Mental health stigma as social attribution: Implications for research methods and attitude change. *Clinical Psychology: Science and Practice, 7*, 48–67.

Craig, A., Hancock, K., Chang, E., & Dickson, H. (1998). The effectiveness of group psychological intervention in enhancing perceptions of control following spinal cord injury. *Australian and New Zealand Journal of Psychiatry, 32*, 112–118.

Craig, A., Hancock, K., Dickson, H., & Chang, E. (1997). Long-term psychological outcomes in spinal cord injured persons: Results of a controlled trial using cognitive behavior therapy. *Archives of Physical Medicine and Rehabilitation, 78*, 33–38.

Crewe, N. M. (1980). Quality of life: The ultimate goal in rehabilitation. *Minnesota Medicine, 63*, 586–589.

Davis, B. H. (1987). Disability and grief. *Social Casework, 68*, 352–357.

Dembo, T., Leviton, G. L., & Wright, B. A. (1956). Adjustment to misfortune—A problem of social-psychological rehabilitation. *Artificial Limbs, 3*(2), 4–62.

Derogatis, L. R. (1977). *Psychological adjustment to illness scale.* Baltimore: Clinical Psychometric Research.

Derogatis, L. R., & Lopez, M. (1983). *Psychosocial adjustment to illness scale (PAIS & PAIS-SR): Scoring, procedures and administration manual.* Baltimore: Clinical Psychometric Research.

Dijkers, M. (1997). Quality of life after spinal cord injury: A meta analysis of the effects of disablement components. *Spinal Cord, 35*, 829–840.

Dodds, A. G., Bailey, P., Pearson, A., & Yates, L. (1991). Psychological factors in acquired visual impairment: The development of a scale of adjustment. *Journal of Visual Impairment and Blindness, 85*, 306–310.

Dodrill, C. B., Batzel, L. W., Queisser, H. R., & Temkin, N. R. (1980). An objective method for the assessment of psychological and social problems among epileptics. *Epilepsia, 21*, 123–135.

Dunn, M. E. (1975). Psychological intervention in a spinal cord injury center: An introduction. *Rehabilitation Psychology, 22*, 165–178.

Eisenberg, M. G., Glueckauf, R. L., & Zaretsky, H. H. (Eds.). (1999). *Medical aspects of disability: A handbook for the rehabilitation professional.* New York: Springer.

English, R. W. (1971). The application of personality theory to explain psychological reactions to physical disability. *Rehabilitation Research and Practice Review, 3*, 35–47.

Falvo, D. (1999). *Medical and psychosocial aspects of chronic illness and disability* (2nd ed.). Gaithersburg, MD: Aspen.

Flanagan, J. C. (1982). Measurement of quality of life: Current state of the art. *Archives of Physical Medicine and Rehabilitation, 63*, 56–59.

Frisch, M. B. (1999). Quality of life assessment/intervention and the quality of life inventory. In M. E. Maruish (Ed.), *The use of psychological testing for treatment planning and outcome assessment* (pp. 1277–1331). Mahwah, NJ: Erlbaum.

Ganz, P. A. (1988). Patient education as a moderator of psychological distress. *Journal of Psychosocial Oncology, 6*, 181–197.

Gilson, B. S., Gilson, J. S., Bergner, M., Bobbitt, R. A., Kressel, S., Pollard, W. E., & Vesselago M. (1975). The Sickness Impact Profile: Development of an outcome measure of health care. *American Journal of Public Health, 65*, 1304–1310.

Horowitz, M. J. (1986). *Stress response syndromes* (2nd ed.). Northvale, NJ: Aronson.

Janosik, E. H. (1984). *Crisis counseling: A contemporary approach.* Belmont, CA: Wadsworth.

Kelly, M. P. (2001). Disability and community: A sociological approach. In G. L. Albrecht, K. D. Seelman, & M. Bury (Eds.), *Handbook of disability studies* (pp. 396–411). Thousand Oaks, CA: Sage.

Krantz, D. S., & Deckel, A. W. (1983). Coping with coronary heart disease and stroke. In T. G. Burish & L. A. Bradley (Eds.), *Coping with chronic disease: Research and applications* (pp. 85–112). New York: Academic Press.

Krohne, H. W. (Ed.). (1993). *Attention and avoidance.* Seattle, WA: Hugrefe & Huber.

Lazarus, R. S., & Folkman, S. (1984). *Stress, appraisal, and coping.* New York: Springer.

Lezak, M. D. (1987). Relationship between personality disorders, social disturbance, and physical disability following traumatic brain injury. *Journal of Head Trauma and Rehabilitation, 2*(1), 57–59.

Linkowski, D. C. (1971). A scale to measure acceptance of disability. *Rehabilitation Counseling Bulletin, 14*, 236–244.

Livneh, H., & Antonak, R. F. (1990). Reactions to disability: An empirical investigation of their nature and structure. *Journal of Applied Rehabilitation Counseling, 21*(4), 13–21.

Livneh, H., & Antonak, R. F. (1997). *Psychosocial adaptation to chronic illness and disability.* Gaithersburg, MD: Aspen.

Livneh, H., & Sherwood, A. (1991). Application of personality theories and counseling strategies to clients with physical disabilities. *Journal of Counseling & Development, 69*, 525–538.

Marshak, L. E., & Seligman, M. (1993). *Counseling persons with physical disabilities: Theoretical and clinical perspectives.* Austin, TX: Pro-Ed.

McDaniel, J. W. (1976). *Physical disability and human behavior* (2nd ed.). New York: Pergamon Press.

Meadow, K. P., Karchmer, M. A., Peterson, L. M., & Rudner, L. (1980). *Meadows/Kendall social-emotive assessment inventory for deaf students: Manual.* Washington, DC: Gallaudet College, Pre-College Programs.

Meenan, R. F. (1982). The AIMS approach to health status measurement: Conceptual background and measurement properties. *Journal of Rheumatology, 9*, 785–788.

Meenan, R. F. (1986). New approach to outcome assessment: The AIMS questionnaire for arthritis. *Advances in Internal Medicine, 31*, 167–185.

Meyerowitz, B. E. (1983). Postmastectomy coping strategies and quality of life. *Health Psychology, 2*, 117–132.

Millon, T., Green, C. J., & Meagher, R. B. (1979). The MBHI: A new inventory for the psycho-diagnostician in medical settings. *Professional Psychology, 10*, 529–539.

Mishel, M. (1981). The measurement of uncertainty in illness. *Nursing Research, 30*, 258–263.

Moos, R. H. (Ed.). (1984). *Coping with physical illness: New perspectives* (Vol. 2). New York: Plenum.

Moos, R. H., & Schaefer, J. A. (1984). The crisis of physical illness. In R. H. Moos (Ed.), *Coping with physical illness: New perspectives* (Vol. 2, pp. 3–31). New York: Plenum.

Morrison, J. (1997). *When psychological problems mask medical disorders: A guide for psychotherapists.* New York: Guilford.

Parkes, C. M. (1975). Psychosocial transitions: Comparison between reactions to loss of a limb and loss of a spouse. *British Journal of Psychiatry, 127*, 204–210.

Pollak, J., Levy, S., & Breitholtz, T. (1999). Screening for medical and neuro developmental disorders for the professional counselor. *Journal of Counseling & Development, 77*, 350–358.

Razin, A. M. (1982). Psychosocial intervention in coronary artery disease: A review. *Psychosomatic Medicine, 44*, 363–387.

Riggar, T. F., Maki, D. R., & Wolf, A. W. (Eds.). (1986). *Applied rehabilitation counseling.* New York: Springer.

Roback, H. B. (Ed.). (1984). *Helping patients and their families cope with medical problems.* San Francisco: Jossey-Bass.

Rodin, G., Craven, J., & Littlefield, C. (1991). *Depression in the medically ill: An integrated approach.* New York: Brunner/Mazel.

Roessler, R. T. (1990). A quality of life perspective on rehabilitation counseling. *Rehabilitation Counseling Bulletin, 34*, 82–91.

Schilder, P. (1950). *The image and appearance of the human body.* New York: Wiley.

Seligman, M. (1982). Introduction. In M. Seligman (Ed.), *Group psychotherapy and counseling with special populations* (pp. 1–26). Baltimore: University Park Press.

Shontz, F. C. (1978). Psychological adjustment to physical disability: Trends in theories. *Archives of Physical Medicine and Rehabilitation, 59*, 251–254.

Skuster, D. Z., Digre, K. B., & Corbett, J. J. (1992). Neurologic conditions presenting as psychiatric disorders. *Psychiatric Clinics of North America, 15*, 311–333.

Stachnik, T., Stoffelmayr, B., & Hoppe, R. B. (1983). Prevention, behavior change, and chronic disease. In T. G. Burish & L. A. Bradley (Eds.), *Coping with chronic disease: Research and applications* (pp. 447–473). New York: Academic Press.

Subramanian, K., & Ell, K. O. (1989). Coping with a first heart attack: A group treatment model for low-income Anglo, Black, and Hispanic patients. *Social Work in Groups, 11*, 99–117.

Sullivan, B. J. (1979). Adjustment in diabetic adolescent girls: I. Development of the Diabetic Adjustment Scale. *Psychosomatic Medicine, 41*, 119–126.

Teel, C. S. (1991). Chronic sorrow: Analysis of the concept. *Journal of Advanced Nursing, 16*, 1311–1319.

Telch, C. F., & Telch, M. J. (1985). Psychological approaches for enhancing coping among cancer patients: A review. *Clinical Psychology Review, 5*, 325–344.

Thomas, K., Butler, A., & Parker, R. M. (1987). Psychosocial counseling. In R. M. Parker (Ed.), *Rehabilitation counseling: Basics and beyond* (pp. 65–95). Austin, TX: Pro-Ed.

Tobin, D. L., Holroyd, K. A., Reynolds, R. V., & Wigal, J. K. (1989). The hierarchical factor structure of the coping strategies inventory. *Cognitive Therapy and Research, 13*, 343–361.

Turner, R. J., & Noh, S. (1988). Physical disability and depression: A longitudinal analysis. *Journal of Health and Social Behavior, 29*, 23–37.

Watson, M., Greer, S., Young, J., Inayat, Q., Burgess, C., & Robertson, B. (1988). Development of a questionnaire measure of adjustment to cancer: The MAC scale. *Psychological Medicine, 18*, 203–209.

Wineman, N. M. (1990). Adaptation to multiple sclerosis: The role of social support, functional disability, and perceived uncertainty. *Nursing Research, 39*, 294–299.

Wortman, C. B., & Silver, R. C. (1989). The myth of coping with loss. *Journal of Consulting and Clinical Psychology, 57*, 349–357.

Wright, B. A. (1983). *Physical disability—A psychosocial approach.* New York: Harper & Row.

Wright, G. N., & Remmers, H. H. (1960). *Manual for the handicap problems inventory.* Lafayette, IN: Purdue Research Foundation.

Zeidner, M., & Endler, N. S. (Eds.). (1996). *Handbook of coping: Theory, research, applications.* New York: Wiley.

8

Objective Self-Awareness and Stigma: Implications for Persons With Visible Disabilities

ANDREW A. PHEMISTER AND NANCY M. CREWE

*D*oes self-consciousness affect how a person thinks or behaves in different situations? Social scientists and psychologists have studied this question for over a century and many have said, "yes, it does" (Cooley, 1902; James, 1890; Mead, 1934). For instance, giving a presentation, interviewing for a job, and inviting someone on a date are all common situations that will likely cause a person to feel more self-aware and sometimes self-critical (cf. Silvia & Duval, 2001; Duval & Wicklund, 1972). After such an event, the person may feel quite negative about his or her appearance and performance. "I was terrible!" "Now they will never hire me!" and "I looked foolish!"

It has been exhaustively discussed among scholars that inherent to such self-conscious events lies a "fulcrum" of awareness that balances a person directly between the anxiety-provoking experience of self as *both* object and subject. May (1967) fittingly referred to this experience as the "human dilemma" and asserted that such dual awareness (of self as object and subject) is a necessary element to gratification in life. Perception of approval from others can lead to increased confidence and self-esteem, whereas perception of disdain or negative evaluation can produce the opposite results. People in general receive varying degrees of positive and negative appraisal, but does this dilemma of self-awareness impact a person differently when others can see that the person has a disability? From experiences, many people can probably relate to the above self-critical statements (e.g., "I looked foolish!"). However, on closer inspection, such statements imply a deeper issue regarding the proposed dilemma of self-awareness, especially when visible disability is a factor. It is well observed that persons with disabilities experience social stigma much more than the general population, and the enduring presence of stigma in our society suggests that the answer to the above question might also be "yes,"—that because of stigma, it is conceivable that the acute experience of self-awareness may affect persons with visible disabilities differently than able-bodied persons. Stigma affects people who are in some way different from majority expectations (Coleman, 1997) and, in fact, even *perceived* stigma was found to be an independent predictor of depression in persons with leg amputations (Rybarczyk, Nyenhuis, Nicholas, Cash, & Kaiser, 1995).

Stigma has been around for a long time, and social scientists have been studying it closely for perhaps just as long (e.g., Allport, 1954; Cooley, 1902; Fine & Asch, 1995; Heatherton, Kleck, Hebl, & Hull, 2000). In the early 1960s, Goffman (1963, p. 9) posed the

From "Objective self-awareness and stigma: Implications for persons with visible disabilities," by A. Phemister and N. Crewe, 2004, *Journal of Rehabilitation 70*, 33–37. Reprinted with permission of the National Rehabilitation Association.

question, "how does the stigmatized individual respond to his [sic] situation?". In response to his own question, Goffman asserted that for some stigmatized individuals, "it will be possible for him to make a direct attempt to correct what he sees as the *objective* basis of his failing," for instance, plastic surgery for certain deformities (emphasis added, see below).

In keeping with these observations, this chapter is concerned with the large number of persons with disabilities who may always be at risk of experiencing social stigma. The goal of this chapter is to employ a critical theory of self-awareness that offers much to the phenomenology of disability in a conceptual examination of the impact of stigma on persons with visible disabilities. Below is an introduction to the theory of *objective self-awareness* (OSA; Duval & Wicklund, 1972) and some recent developments. This is followed by a discussion of research on stigma, and the integration and implications of both OSA and stigma to disability studies and individual adjustment to disability.

OSA AND VISIBLE DISABILITY

In its original form, the theory of *objective self-awareness* was a comprehensive theory intended to explain why individuals conform their behaviors, appearance, and beliefs to those of others (Duval & Wicklund, 1972). Duval and Wicklund formulated their theory on the basis of a distinction between two forms of conscious attention. They postulated that individuals have one innate consciousness with directional properties; attention can be dually focused either *outward* toward the environment or *inward* toward oneself. However, it was emphasized that attention cannot be simultaneously focused outward and inward and that a person can only attend to one thing at a time. For instance, a person is unable to focus attention on a personal characteristic while driving a nail into wood. Duval and Wicklund identified outward attention as the state of *subjective* self-awareness and defined it as attention that is focused on environmental characteristics. In subjective self-awareness, the person is the "subject" who is observing and perceiving the various aspects of their environment. However, given this, it may seem more accurate to say that a subjectively self-aware individual is actually *environment* aware rather than *self*-aware, and as Duval and Wicklund explained, this is indeed accurate—at least in the "usual sense of the term" (p. 2). But, the person is self-aware in that he or she receives and perceives feedback from the environment regarding his or her behaviors, attitudes, and so on. Subjective self-awareness arises directly from the experience of oneself as the source of perception and action.

On the other hand, the theory asserted that when a person is *objectively* self-aware, then he or she has become *acutely* aware of those personal characteristics that most distinguish him or her from the majority. The occurrence of OSA can be understood in three ways. First, as indicated, the term "objective" specifies where attention is directed. That is, in a state of OSA, the person's attention is focused exclusively on the self; the person is the "object" of his or her own attention and is now seeing himself or herself as he or she thinks others do. It is this self-focused attention that induces an acute state of OSA. Second, induced OSA was theorized to automatically elicit comparisons between the self and perceived standards for social correctness in terms of specific behaviors, attitudes, traits, and so on. Such standards of correctness were said to determine who or what a "correct" person is. For instance, a t-shirt and cutoffs typically are not considered appropriate attire for a job interview, and the person wearing them will draw much attention. Finally, if discrepancies are detected between a person and one or more standards, then negative affect was theorized to surface, and in order to reduce the negative affect, the person would either conform as best he or she could or avoid the situation altogether. Another consequence of this is that the person may also avoid other similar situations in which they feel objectively self-aware (e.g., formal gatherings).

Additionally, whether a person is objectively or subjectively self-aware, OSA theory contends that whatever is the focus of attention in any given situation will draw causal attributions (i.e., responsibility). It has been demonstrated that objectively self-aware persons are more likely to attribute the source of an event to themselves (Duval, 1971; Duval & Lalwani, 1999; Lalwani & Duval, 2000). According to the theory, attributing cause to oneself will occur because the objectively self-aware person is experiencing him or herself as somehow different and exhibiting salient characteristics that distinguish them from the majority. What this implies is that when a person with a visible disability (e.g., using a wheelchair or a having facial deformity) enters into a situation where he or she is the only one with such a characteristic, then they will likely become objectively self-aware and focus attention on that characteristic. They will perceive themselves as they think others perceive them.

More recently, however, new research has initiated fundamental changes to Duval and Wicklund's theory. One major change relevant to persons with visible disabilities emerged from controlled experiments on an individual's perceived rate of progress relative to the perceived discrepancy size. Duval, Duval, and Mulilis (1992) conducted three experiments using male introduction to psychology students. At one point, the participants were asked to meet an experimental standard by determining which of five two-dimensional figures when folded would match a three-dimensional figure previously displayed. It was discovered that when the participants were high in OSA and perceived sufficient progress toward reducing the discrepancy (i.e., meeting the experimental standard), they maintained involvement and effort. However, when participants high in OSA perceived insufficient progress to reduce the discrepancy, then they would relax their efforts and avoid involvement.

This new finding for the theory of *objective self-awareness* is significant to an examination of stigma and visible disability because, generally, our society values good health, a particular physique, and the concept of "body beautiful" (Hahn, 1993; Wright, 1983). This is a social standard that, for many people with disabilities, simply cannot be met—a discrepancy that cannot be reduced—and, if that is the case, then what happens? Coleman (1997) stated that human differences are the basis for stigma and those individuals who have differences may feel *permanently* stigmatized in situations where their differences are pronounced (emphasis added). More importantly, Coleman further asserted that stigmas mirror our social and cultural beliefs, which, if so, and unless social attitudes change, could mean that the stigmatized individual will continually be struggling against the grain.

"NOTES ON STIGMA," OSA, AND VISIBLE DISABILITY

In his classic work, *Stigma: Notes on the Management of Spoiled Identity*, Goffman (1963) stated that stigma represents a special discrepancy between a person's "virtual social identity," which refers to what society assumes about a person, and his or her "actual social identity," which refers to those attributes that a person could in fact be proved to possess. Goffman went on to define stigma as a term that highlights a deeply discrediting personal attribute that leads to assumptions about the person's character and abilities and often results in various forms of discrimination.

In general, however, stigma is considered a social construction that is essentially based on individual or group differences and results in the devaluation of the persons who possess those differences (see Coleman, 1997; Dovidio, Major, & Crocker, 2000). Stigma dehumanizes and lessens the social value of an individual because he or she is appraised as being "marked," flawed, or otherwise less than average (Dovidio et al., 2000; cf. Goffman, 1963). Several researchers have categorized stigma in various ways that make it easier to comprehend. For instance, Goffman (1963) identified three types of stigma: "abominations of the body" (e.g., physical deformities), "blemishes of individual character" (e.g., mental disorders and unemployment), and "tribal stigma" or "tribal identities" (e.g., race, religion, etc.). Similarly, Jones et al. (1984) defined six dimensions of stigma: (1) concealability (i.e., visibility), (2) course (i.e., salience and prognosis), (3) disruptiveness (i.e., during interpersonal interactions), (4) aesthetics (i.e., attractiveness), (5) origin (i.e., congenital vs. acquired conditions and personal responsibility), and (6) peril (i.e., threat of contagion).

Recently, however, it was argued that one of the most important issues to consider about stigma is its *visibility* (Crocker, Major, & Steele, 1998). Crocker et al. asserted that the visibility of a particular stigmatizing attribute determines the schema through which an individual is understood or perhaps "defined" by society. This is significant to consider for persons with visible disabilities because if we apply this to a situation in which a person feels objectively self-aware, then, according to Duval and Wicklund's theory, it is plausible that the person may also feel highly self-critical as a direct result of OSA interacting with the stigmatizing attribute.

To elaborate, it has been argued that during any given situation where too much or too little attention is directed at one person (e.g., staring at or ignoring the person altogether), then that person's comfort and anxiety levels could be dramatically affected causing embarrassment and even shame (Buss, 1980; cf. Goffman, 1963). For a person with a visible disability, such attention may be a daily experience and a constant reminder that he or she "is" different (e.g., uses a wheelchair). Social Darwinism (Spencer, 1872) is implied in social appraisals like these because, invariably, when one person feels that he or she does not "fit in" (or must work harder in order to do so), then a social hierarchy is imposed. Social Darwinism is characterized by the phrase "survival of the fittest" and promotes the ideology that inferior races exist relative to superior races. For instance, in their controversial book, *The Bell Curve*, Herrnstein and Murray (1994) argued that social inferiority is a direct consequence of genetic inferiority. In other words, for whatever reason, some people are "naturally" meant to be inferior. Social Darwinism has received little support but is still reflected in the attitudes and behaviors of our society today (i.e., stigma, prejudice, and discrimination).

Several experiments have revealed that feeling self-focused and self-aware in the presence of others can greatly impact a person's sense of physical attractiveness and self-evaluations (Thornton & Moore, 1993), the expression of their personal beliefs (Scheier, 1980; Wicklund & Duval, 1971), their level of shyness and social dysfunction (Bruch, Hamer, & Heimberg, 1995), and their individuation and feeling uncomfortably distinct from others (Ickes, Layden, & Barnes, 1978). It is, therefore, conceivable that the social appraisals of a person's difference, vis-à-vis stigma, and causal attributions, could impact the adjustment process of an individual with a visible disability in ways we are not yet sure of, but are very important to understand.

In contrast, Buss (1980) argued that most people who experience increased self-awareness during social situations generally would not experience any ill effects (e.g., increased anxiety levels), presumably because they have not experienced the stigma that is often associated with having a visible disability (cf. Bruch et al., 1995). Yet, what seems pivotal is the extent to which the inducement of OSA may lead the individual to interpret the negative appraisals as being *realistically* based. In other words, can one's personal beliefs about oneself stand up against the perception that others believe differently—and for how long?

IMPLICATIONS FOR OSA AND STIGMA

In a discussion on stigma effects and self-esteem, Crocker and Quinn (2000) argued that feelings of self-worth, self-regard, and self-respect are not stable characteristics. Instead, they are constructed in situ as a function of the connotative meanings that a person attributes to a particular situation (cf. Heatherton & Polivy, 1991; Phemister, 2002; Sommers & Crocker, 1999). Crocker and Quinn asserted that what people bring to different situations are their sets of beliefs, attitudes, and values, and when something negative (or positive) occurs, then self-esteem is subsequently affected by the meaning that they attribute to those events. The presumption here is that OSA and personal meanings may be phenomenologically linked. To illustrate, being turned down for both a date and a job will likely hold different implications for a person depending on which meant more to them. That is, the more something is desired by a person (e.g., getting a job), then the more meaningful it may be. Likewise, the more meaningful something is, the more he or she may feel objectively self-aware about appearing and performing in such a way that the event has a satisfactory outcome (e.g., being nicely dressed and trying to conceal an attribute that is believed will hinder the chances of being hired). But, if the person is rejected, then corresponding with the greater meaning ascribed to the situation, he or she could also experience a more heartfelt disappointment. Thus, for example, the individual may find it easier to invite another person on a date than to interview for another job and, as a result, perhaps avoid further interviews.

Symbolic interactionists such as Cooley (1902) compared the phenomenon of social appraisals to a "looking glass" and argued that we are continually affected by what we see reflected in another's eye (cf. Hewitt, 2000). Using Duval and Wicklund's (1972) theory as a backdrop, how likely is it that a person with a visible disability would indeed avoid situations where he or she feels objectively self-aware and stigmatized? Moreover, what if these situations were vital to one's quality of life such as in the case of interviewing for a job? For adults who have already established and maintained a lasting identity (e.g., vocational, familial, educational, and financial stability), this may not pose such a problem. However, for younger individuals who are likely to still be forming their identities, it is reasonable to assume that a prolonged state of OSA may negatively affect the beliefs they have regarding their competencies, abilities, and self-esteem (cf. Duval, Duval, & Mulilis, 1992), especially it seems if the person also attributes responsibility to his or her stigmatizing differences.

It has long been argued that society's attitudes and behaviors can and do dramatically impact individuals well after any actual interaction has occurred (Goffman, 1963; Laing, 1965; Szasz, 1961). Ronald Laing and Thomas Szasz in particular are well known for their theories that mental illness emerges from untenable social interactions, such as in the family, or as a socially imposed "myth" that justifies the mistreatment of certain individuals. Likewise, the self-identification literature stresses that groups of people cue relevant information in a person's memory about himself or herself, the group, and the relationship between the person and the group (see Neisser & Jopling, 1997; Schlenker, 1986). Social appraisals can activate social roles, memories, present images, and conceivable goals for an individual in the present moment. Underscoring all of this is the minority group paradigm, which holds as a standard maxim that handicaps emerge from societally imposed barriers (Hahn, 1985). It is, therefore, conceivable that, if a person were to continually encounter stigmatizing situations, then he or she may begin to feel utterly unable to meet the standards set for those situations and, over time, form a new resolution about those situations and his or her assets in them (e.g., "Based on my experiences, I can see that I am not employable"). This resolution can be seen as reflecting the stigma and perhaps causal attributions that the person perceived others to have about him or her. Such a resolution may likely be a determining factor for the future choices a person makes regarding particular situations ("I will give up interviewing for jobs.") (cf. Magnusson, 1981; Pervin, 1981; Rommetveit, 1981). As a result, an individual may decide to engage primarily in situations that promote a desired identity and avoid situations that demote a desired identity. In effect, the person will "settle for less," which is clearly a significant barrier to the successful adaptation to life with a disability. This is significant because adaptation to disability connotes the restoration of a personal sense of wholeness, of bodily experience and integrity, and harmony, or *balance*, in life (see Charmaz, 1995; Trieschmann, 1988, Vash, 1981; Wright, 1983; Zola, 1991). That is, a person's life may feel "lopsided" if there are desired situations (e.g., finding employment) that are avoided because of the erroneous introjection of other's stigmatizing attitudes.

In conclusion, what we can glean from Duval and Wicklund's theory is that when a person with a visible disability is perpetually at risk of being objectively self-aware and stigmatized, then he or she could perhaps become more susceptible to such erroneous introjection—a "hypothesis" that appears reinforced by the continuing existence of social Darwinism and discrimination against persons with disabilities.

REFERENCES

Allport, G. (1954). *The nature of prejudice*. Reading, MA: Addison-Wesley.

Bruch, M., Hamer, R., & Heimber, R. (1995). Shyness and public self consciousness: Additive or interactive relation with social interaction. *Journal of Personality, 63*, 47–63.

Buss, A. (1980). *Self-consciousness and social anxiety*. San Francisco: W. H. Freeman and Company.

Charmaz, K. (1995). The body, identity, and self: Adapting to impairment. *The Sociological Quarterly, 36*, 657–680.

Coleman, L. (1997). Stigma: An enigma demystified. In L. Davis (Ed.), *The disability studies reader*. New York: Rutledge.

Cooley, C. H. (1902). *Human nature and the social order*. New York: Charles Scribner's Sons.

Crocker, J., Major, B., & Steele, C. (1998). Social stigma. In D. Gilbert, T. S. Fiske, & G. Lindzey (Eds.), *Handbook of social psychology* (4th ed., Vol. 2, pp. 504–553). Boston, MA: McGraw-Hill.

Crocker, J., & Quinn, D. (2000). Social stigma and self: Meanings, situations, and self-esteem. In T. Heatherton, R. Kleck, M. Hebl, & J. Hull (Eds.), *The social psychology of stigma* (pp. 153–183). New York: The Guilford Press.

Dovidio, J., Major, B., & Crocker, J. (2000). Stigma: Introduction and overview. In T. Heatherton, R. Kleck, M. Hebl, & J. Hull (Eds.), *The social psychology of stigma* (pp. 1–32). New York: The Guilford Press.

Duval, S. (1971). *Causal attribution as a function of focus of attention*. Unpublished manuscript. University of Texas.

Duval, S., & Wicklund, R. (1972). *A theory of objective self-awareness*. New York: Academic Press.

Duval, T. S., Duval, V. H., & Mulilis, J. P. (1992). Effects of self-focus, discrepancy between self and standard, and outcome expectancy favorability on the tendency to match self to standard or to withdraw. *Journal of Personality and Social Psychology, 62*, 340–348.

Duval, T. S., & Lalwani, N. (1999). Objective self-awareness and causal attributions for self-standard discrepancies: Changing self or changing standards of correctness. *Society for Personality and Social Psychology, 25*, 1220–1229.

Fine, M., & Asch, A. (1995). Disability beyond stigma: Social interaction, discrimination, and activism. In N. G. Rule, & J. B. Veroff (Eds.), *The culture and psychology reader* (pp. 536–558). New York: New York University Press.

Goffman, E. (1963). *Stigma: Notes on the management of spoiled identity*. New York: Simon and Schuster, Inc.

Hahn, H. (1985). Changing perception of disability and the future of rehabilitation. In L. G. Perlman, & G. F. Austin (Eds.), *Social influences in rehabilitation planning: A blueprint for the future*. A Report of the Ninth Mary Switzer Memorial Seminar, Alexandria. VA: National Rehabilitation Association.

Hahn, H. (1993). The politics of physical difference: Disability and discrimination. In M. Nagler (Ed.), *Perspectives on disability* (pp. 39–47). Palo Alto, CA: Health Markets Research.

Heatherton, T., Kleck, R., Hebl, M., & Hull, J. (2000). *The social psychology of stigma*. New York: Guilford Press.

Heatherton, T., & Polivy, J. (1991). Development and validation of a scale for measuring state self-esteem. *Journal of Personality and Social Psychology, 60,* 895–910.

Herrnstein, R., & Murray, C. (1994). *The bell curve: Intelligence and class structure in American life.* New York: Free Press.

Hewitt, J. P. (2000). *Self and society: A symbolic interactionist social psychology* (8th ed.). Boston: Allyn and Bacon.

Ickes, W., Layden, M., & Barnes, R. (1978). Objective self-awareness and individuation: An empirical link. *Journal of Personality, 46,* 146–161.

James, W. (1890). *The principles of psychology.* New York: Henry Holt and Company.

Jones, E., Farina, A., Hastorf, A., Markus, H., Miller, D., & Scott, R. (1984). *Social stigma: The psychology of marked relationships.* New York: Freeman.

Laing, R. D. (1965). *The divided self: An existential study in sanity and madness.* New York: Penguin Books.

Lalwani, N., & Duval, T. S. (2000). The moderating effects of cognitive appraisal processes on self-attribution of responsibility. *Journal of Applied Social Psychology, 30,* 2233–2245.

Magnusson, D. (Ed.). (1981). *Toward a psychology of situations.* Hillsdale, NJ: Lawrence Erlbaum Associates, Inc.

May, R. (1967). *Psychology and the human dilemma.* New York: W.W. Norton and Company.

Mead, G. H. (1934). *Mind, self, and society.* Chicago, IL: University of Chicago Press.

Neisser, U., & Jopling, A. (Eds.). (1997). *The conceptual self in context: Culture, experiences, and self-understanding.* Cambridge: Cambridge University Press.

Pervin, L. (1981). The relation of situations to behavior. In D. Magnusson (Ed.), *Toward a psychology of situations* (pp. 157–169). Hillsdale, NJ: Lawrence Erlbaum Associates, Inc.

Phemister, A. A. (2002). Investigating the effects of objective self-awareness on the meaning attributions and job-hunting behaviors of persons with visible disabilities (Doctoral dissertation, Michigan State University, 2002). *Dissertation Abstracts International, 63,* 4421.

Rommetveit, R. (1981). On meanings of situations and social control of such meaning in human communication. In D. Magnusson (Ed.), *Toward a psychology of situations* (pp. 99–128). Hillsdale, NJ: Lawrence Erlbaum Associates, Inc.

Rybarczyk, B., Nyenhuis, D., Nicholas, J., Cash, S., & Kaiser, J. (1995). Body image, perceived social stigma, and the prediction of psychosocial adjustment to leg amputation. *Rehabilitation Psychology, 40,* 95–109.

Scheier, M. (1980). Effects of public and private self-consciousness on the public expression of personal beliefs. *Journal of Personality and Social Psychology, 39,* 514–521.

Schlenker, B. (1986). Self-identification: Toward an integration of the public and private self. In R. Baumeister (Ed.), *Public and private self* (pp. 212–230). New York: Springer-Verlag.

Silvia, P., & Duval, T. S. (2001). Objective self-awareness theory: Recent progress and enduring problems. *Personality and Social Psychology Review, 5,* 230–241.

Sommers, S., & Crocker, J. (1999). *Hopes dashed and dreams fulfilled: contingencies and stability of self-esteem among graduate school applicants.* Chapter presented at the annual meeting of the Midwestern Psychological Association, Chicago.

Spencer, H. (1872). *Social statics; or, the conditions essential to human happiness specified, and the first of them developed.* New York: Appleton.

Szasz, T. (1961). *The myth of mental illness.* New York: Dell.

Thornton, B., & Moore, S. (1993). Physical attractiveness contrast effects: Implications for self-esteem and evaluations of the social self. *Personality and Social Psychology Bulletin, 19,* 474–480.

Trieschmann, R. (1988). *Spinal cord injuries: Psychological, social and vocational rehabilitation* (2nd ed.). New York: Demos.

Vash, C. L. (1981). *The psychology of disability.* New York: Springer Publishing Company.

Wicklund, R., & Duval, S. (1971). Opinion change and performance facilitation as a result of objective self-awareness. *Journal of Experimental Social Psychology, 7,* 319–342.

Wright, B. A. (1983). *Physical disability: A psychosocial approach* (2nd ed.). New York: Harper Collins.

Zola, I. (1991). Bringing our bodies and ourselves back in: Reflections on a past, present, and future "medical sociology." *Journal of Health and Social Behavior, 32,* 1–16.

9

Psychosocial Disparities Faced by Women
With Physical Disabilities

MARGARET A. NOSEK

*W*omen with disabilities constitute one of the largest and most disadvantaged populations in the United States. Despite the magnitude of the psychological, social, physical, and environmental challenges they face across the life span and the disproportional
share of health care costs they incur, only a small fraction of research on disability topics is
dedicated to their concerns. Women like me, who live with disabilities, are nevertheless in
every corner of the country, at every socioeconomic level, part of every minority, in every
type of relationship, and in every vocation, living as successfully as they can. A careful look
will place these women in one category or another, but most do not even identify as having a disability. It did not take me very long to realize I had a disability, but it took decades
before I understood what it meant to be a woman.

The major driving force in my career has been my desire to make that journey toward
successful living a little easier for my sisters in disability. As founder and executive director of the Center for Research on Women with Disabilities, I have had a hand in dozens
of research projects over the past 20 years, substantiating our many disadvantages with
population-based statistics, survey data, and interviews with hundreds of women with various types of disability. I have networked with and studied the research of others, looking
for theories and connections that might help us understand why we face such enormous
socioeconomic and health disparities. It is not enough to say it is due to our disability! If that
were so, why then are some women with relatively minor disabling conditions totally devastated by them in every aspect of their lives, yet other women with very severe limitations
are able to achieve their vocational and family goals and manifest fulfillment. Across almost
all of our studies, disability type, age at onset, and severity of limitations have consistently
failed to explain the difference in outcome variables. All that we have learned points to one
undeniable truth—disability is a complex phenomenon, but psychological and social factors make all the difference in the outcomes.

The purpose of this chapter is to help rehabilitation counselors understand the myriad factors that affect the psychological and social health of women with disabilities. After
giving some background on the historical roots of the rehabilitation response to women
and a description of the demographic and health characteristics of this population, I will
present a heuristic, holistic model for understanding the reality of our lives and strategies for helping us achieve optimal health. The pivotal construct of self-esteem will be
discussed first, followed by social connectedness, its polar opposite—abuse—and the

consequences of disparities—stress and depression. The chapter ends with recommenda-tions on strategies rehabilitation researchers and practitioners can use to include gender in their examination of individual and program outcomes and thereby advance the field.

HISTORY OF RESEARCH ON WOMEN WITH DISABILITIES

The study of disability and rehabilitation has made its most significant advances during and after periods of war and therefore has been primarily concerned with the health and vocational problems of men. Guidelines for clinical treatment and interventions for rein-tegration into society have been developed for the most part based on the needs of men with spinal cord injury, amputation, and other adventitious musculoskeletal problems. Any services rendered to women used male norms and approached the needs of women accord-ing to traditional social roles. For issues related to congenital disabling conditions, such as cerebral palsy, spina bifida, or neuromuscular disorders, and adult-onset chronic disabling conditions, such as joint and connective tissue disorders (arthritis, lupus) or multiple sclero-sis, gender has rarely been considered important in research or intervention development.

Interest in examining the needs of women with disabilities took an early focus on sexu-ality in response to the overwhelming preponderance of literature on the fertility and erectile dysfunction of spinal cord injured men (Charlifue, Gerhart, Menter, Whiteneck, & Manley, 1992; Griffith & Trieschmann, 1975). When the sexuality of women with disabilities was studied, it was often narrowly defined as fertility, pregnancy, labor, and delivery as demon-strated by the number of studies on menstruation, fertility, pregnancy, and childbirth (Axel, 1982; Carty & Conine, 1988; Comarr, 1976; Jackson & Varner, 1989; Jackson & Wadley, 1999; Leavesley & Porter, 1982; Verduyn, 1986) and women's self-reports that if their fertility was not compromised, they were made to feel as if no other aspects of sexuality should matter (Cole, 1975). In one of the few early studies dealing specifically with sexual issues of women with spinal cord injuries, Charlifue et al. (1992) discovered that 69% of 231 women surveyed were satisfied with their postinjury sexual experiences but were not content with sexual information provided during rehabilitation, feeling a need for more literature, counseling, and peer support. In another early study of gynecologic health care of women with disabili-ties, 91% had received breast and pelvic examinations and Papanicolaou smears, but only 19% had received counseling about sexuality; women with paralysis, impaired motor func-tion, or obvious physical deformity were rarely offered contraceptive information or methods (Beckmann, Gittler, Barzansky, & Beckmann, 1989). Only one-third believed their health care provider knew enough about their disability to provide adequate sexual information.

The study of health and wellness in the context of disability for women is a relatively new avenue of investigation, opened only after challenges to entrenched stereotypes that dis-ability is the opposite of health and that gender is far less important than the characteristics of the disability itself. Interest in research on women with disabilities followed a decade after the rise of interest in women's health and interest in wellness and the prevention of second-ary conditions in people with disabilities after the deficit in the literature was noted by sev-eral researchers and feminist disability rights activists (Altman, 1985; Barnartt, 1982; Deegan & Brooks, 1985; Fine & Asch, 1985). According to Altman (1996), before 1990, there was only one publication on demographics about women with disabilities using national population-based data and a few on access to benefits by women with disabilities. Although some infor-mation about women with disabilities could be found in publications about people with disabilities in general (LaPlante, 1991; McNeil, 1997), Altman (1996) was the first to examine statistical information about risks, causes, and consequences of disability among women at the national level. Aside from one very useful compilation of data from multiple national statistical data sources and individual research studies on the demographics, education, employment, and health status of girls and women with disabilities (Jans & Stoddard, 1999), there have been very few efforts to examine population-based data sets for statistics related to women with disabilities. Notable advances have been made in refining the wording of disability definitions in national surveys, and many analyses have been conducted to reveal the changing demographics of the disabled population (Brault, 2008; Waldrop & Stern, 2003), yet no detailed information has been published about gender differences in these statistics.

DEMOGRAPHIC AND HEALTH STATISTICS

There is a distinct lack of consistency in the few studies that have examined national data sets to describe the population of women with disabilities. Data from the 1994–1995 Survey of Income and Program Participation (Jans & Stoddard, 1999; McNeil, 1997) use a functional- and employment-based definition of disability and show that women with disabilities comprise 21% of the population of women in the United States, outnumbering men with disabilities (28.6 million vs. 25.3 million). Using the new set of definitions (hearing, visual, cognitive, ambulatory, self-care, and independent living disability), data from the 2008 American community survey show somewhat lower statistics, with 12.4% of all women in the United States (nearly 19 million) and 11.7% of all men (17.1 million) having some type of disability (Erickson, Lee, & von Schrader, 2009). Quite a different disability rate surfaces when the definition of physical functioning (in terms of nine daily activities) in the National Health Interview Survey data set is used. Seventeen percent of women (19.9 million) in 2006 had at least one physical difficulty compared with 12% of men (12.3 million), and more women than men had difficulty performing each of the nine physical activities. When results are considered by single race, sex, and ethnicity, non-Hispanic Black women were more likely to find at least one of the nine physical activities very difficult or impossible to do compared with the other single race-sex or single race-ethnicity groupings (Pleis & Lethbridge-Cejku, 2006, p. 9). People who have difficulty in physical function comprise only one subset of the disabled population; therefore, the actual number of women with any kind of disability-related limitation may be much greater than reported earlier.

According to the 1994 and 1995 National Health Interview Survey (Chevarley, Thierry, Gill, Ryerson, & Nosek, 2006), women with three or more functional limitations, compared to women in general, were less likely to be married (40% vs. 63%), more likely to be living alone (35% vs. 13%), more likely to have only a high school education or less (78% vs. 54%), less likely to be employed (14% vs. 63%), more likely to be living in households below the poverty level (23% vs. 10%), particularly in the 18 to 44 age group, and less likely to have private health insurance (55% vs. 74%). Other studies (Jans & Stoddard, 1999; McNeil, 1997) have shown that men earn substantially higher monthly incomes than women whether or not they have a disability ($2,190 vs. $1,470 for men vs. women without disabilities; $1,262 vs. $1,000 for men vs. women with severe disabilities). Men with work disabilities are more likely to receive benefits from Social Security (30.6% vs. 25.6%), but women with work disabilities are more likely to receive food stamps, Medicaid, and housing assistance.

In terms of health care needs, women with functional limitations, especially younger women, are more likely to see a specialist, delay getting care due to cost, and be unable to get care for general medical conditions or surgery, mental health needs, dental needs, prescription medicine, or eyeglasses. Although hypertension, depression, stress, smoking, and being overweight are concerns for women in general, these problems are significantly greater among women with functional limitations (Chevarley et al., 2006). Nearly a third of women with three or more functional limitations rate their overall health as poor compared to less than 1% of women with no limitations.

The prevalence of disability is highly correlated with age, with 40% of women 65 years and older having at least one functional limitation. The most prevalent disabling condition in women is back disorder (15.3%), followed by arthritis (13.3%), cardiovascular disease (9.7%), asthma (5.3%), orthopedic impairment of lower extremity (4.2%), mental disorders (3.3%), diabetes (3.3%), and learning disability and mental retardation (2.5%). Men are also most often disabled by back disorders (15.9%), but the list varies from there, with cardiovascular disease (11.4%), followed by orthopedic impairment of lower extremity (6.1%), arthritis (5.8%), asthma (5.4%), learning disability and mental retardation (5.0%), mental disorders (4.6%), and diabetes (2.9%) (LaPlante & Carlson, 1996). For disabilities resulting from trauma, such as spinal cord injury (DeVivo & Chen, 2011) and brain injury (TBI National Data and Statistics Center, 2010), men outnumber women, 4 to 1. Women, however, have a greater prevalence of many physically disabling health conditions compared to men, such as joint and connective tissue disorders (rheumatoid arthritis, fibromyalgia) (Lawrence et al., 2008), systemic lupus erythematosus (Bernatsky et al., 2009), osteoporosis (Johnell & Kanis, 2006), and multiple sclerosis (Noonan et al., 2010).

The most limiting characteristic shared by a high percentage of women with physical disabilities is that of low economic status. For women with disabilities aged 16 to 64 years, nearly two and one-half times as many live in poverty as do their counterparts with no disability (28.1% vs. 11.9%) (U.S. Census Bureau, 2006). Women with disabilities share the economic-related problems of women in general, including low wages and occupational segregation (Schaller & DeLaGarza, 1995). They may, however, also experience restricted career opportunities associated with the nature of their disabilities, gender plus disability socialization experiences, and a lack of role models or mentors (Patterson, DeLaGarza, & Schaller, 1998). Women with gradual-onset disabilities, such as arthritis, fibromyalgia, lupus, multiple sclerosis, and neuromuscular disorders, may live on the edge of poverty because they are unable to maintain their level of employment as symptoms increase. Reducing their hours or changing jobs usually means lower pay and no health insurance. Earning even a minimal salary makes them ineligible for government-funded health care (Medicaid, Medicare). Women with early-onset disabilities or traumatic injuries, who have no other means of support from spouse or family, often cannot afford to work. They must maintain a state of poverty in order to qualify for the government-funded medical, personal assistance, food, and housing benefits they need to survive. The health care that is available to them through Medicaid is the lowest tier in the dysfunctional health care system of this country (Nosek, 2010b). Those who have disabilities that are severe enough to make working unfeasible qualify for Social Security and Medicare and fair far better.

Despite an increasing number of publications purporting to characterize the population of people with disabilities, consistent and detailed reports of findings about the number of women with disabilities living in the United States and their specific demographic and health characteristics are not available. Despite a substantial amount of federal funding allocated to identifying and removing health disparities and developing health promotion interventions, women with disabilities have not garnered a position on the priority list. Indeed, they are not even considered a health disparities population (Nosek & Simmons, 2007).

The demographic characteristics of the population of women with disabilities will change substantially in the coming years due to the improved survival rate of low birthweight newborns, resulting in higher rates of children with activity limitation and permanent disability (National Center for Health Statistics, 2006), as well as the aging and functional decline of baby boomers. The combination of longer life expectancy and increased disability rates is expected to more than triple the number of persons over age 65 with severe or moderate disabilities in the next 50 years (Siegel, 1996). Our society does not seem prepared for the rapidly expanding population of women with disabilities across the life span who may face serious and worsening social disadvantages (Nosek, 2006).

To illustrate more specifically the need to examine the disability-related needs of women, we will now present evidence from the literature and our own studies about five major psychosocial problems that are disproportionately severe for women with disabilities compared to men with disabilities and women in general. The topics to be discussed are depression, stress, self-esteem, social connectedness, and abuse.

A MODEL FOR UNDERSTANDING HEALTH IN THE CONTEXT OF DISABILITY FOR WOMEN

There has been considerable discussion of the disability relevance of health and wellness models that include biological, psychological, social, and spiritual elements (Myers & Sweeney, 2004; Nosek, 2005; Roberts & Stuifbergen, 1998). After putting these together with what I have learned from many years of living and studying independent living (Nosek & Fuhrer, 1992) and feminism (Nosek, 2010a), I am convinced that there has not been enough attention placed on context, particularly for women. Context is not only the environment but the entirety of a woman's past experience and current living situation in our patriarchal society. As a longtime student of Eastern philosophy and religion, I have come to understand that spirituality is not just one part of the analytic model; it is the whole thing (Nosek, 1995; Nosek & Hughes, 2001; Nosek et al., 2004). I have now begun to teach this model by using a tetrahedron, a three-sided pyramid, as a visual aid. The visible faces represent in equal measure the biological, psychological, and social elements of being. Without any one of them, the integrity of the structure cannot be maintained. The part that is not visible is the base of the tetrahedron, which represents context. Without considering that element, it is impossible to understand why women with disabilities experience such extreme health disparities. The entire structure, including the base and all that surrounds it, is a manifestation of spirituality or, as some would prefer to phrase it, the feeling of essence or connection with a higher power (see Figure 9.1).

This heuristic allows for a holistic approach to health promotion. I describe the construct of context as including factors that are either internal to the individual or external in the environment and tend to not be easily changed, but some of them can be modified through management strategies (Nosek, 2005). These include health history, disability characteristics, demographics, relationships, values and beliefs, life experiences, and environmental resources. The category of environmental resources encompasses many aspects of

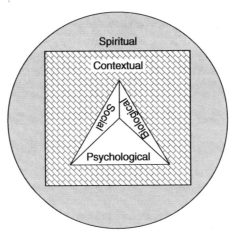

FIGURE 9.1

A contextual model of health.

the micro-, meso-, exo-, and macrosystems in which people with disabilities live, including access to financial resources, education level, the built and natural environment, technology, information from the print and broadcast media and the Internet, instrumental social support and services, and access to health care services. At the Center for Research on Women with Disabilities, we postulate that psychological factors, such as self-esteem and self-efficacy, together with social connectedness can mediate the effect of context on health behaviors and health outcomes (see Figure 9.2). By creating and testing health promotion interventions that offer information, goal setting and action planning, and opportunities for women with disabilities to connect with one another, women can be empowered to improve their health behaviors and health outcomes. To date, we have had success in using this approach to address general health promotion, aging and health promotion, self-esteem enhancement, stress reduction, and self-management of depression for women with physical disabilities. Attending face-to-face workshops, however, is difficult for some women who deal with significant mobility impairments, transportation and environmental barriers, lack of personal assistance, and interference in their daily lives from pain and fatigue. To circumvent these participation barriers, we have begun testing the effectiveness of offering our intervention programs using the Internet, both via interactive website and 3D immersive virtual environments, such as Second Life (Nosek et al., in press).

SELF-ESTEEM

Self-esteem and its related constructs appear to play a central role in the psychological well-being of persons with functional limitations (O'Leary, Shoor, Lorig, & Holman, 1988) including women with physical disabilities (Abraido-Lanza, Guier, & Colon, 1998). It can be threatened at times of declining health and increased functional limitation associated with the development of secondary health conditions such as pain, fatigue, and other new symptoms (Burckhardt, 1985; Mahat, 1997; Schlesinger, 1996; Taal, Rasker, & Wiegman, 1997). In the context of disability, self-worth may be compromised by internalizing the devaluation that society tends to assign physical impairment (Wright, 1960).

The literature offers convincing evidence that positive self-esteem is fundamental to psychological and social well-being. It has been defined as a comparison of accomplishment to hopes, and a personal awareness and recognition of all of one's being (James, 1890; May, 1953). The effect of interpersonal feedback and the environment is a link to a sense of belongingness, societal contribution, and gaining approval from significant others (Adler, Ansbacher, & Ansbacher, 1979). Our research suggests that this is particularly true for women with disabilities (Nosek, 1996; Nosek, Hughes, Swedlund, Taylor, & Swank, 2003).

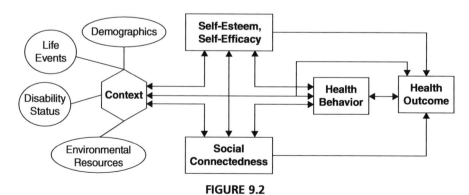

FIGURE 9.2

A health promotion model for women with physical disabilities.

Feminist theory posits that for women "the primary experience of self is relational, that is, the self is organized and developed in the context of important relationships" (Surrey, 1991, p. 51). Because of this relational context of sense of self, a woman's perception about how others view her disability may become internalized and incorporated into her definitions and evaluation of self, resulting in low self-esteem.

Disability is a stigmatizing phenomenon as shown by the lower levels of self-esteem observed among individuals with disabilities compared to those without disabilities (Craig, Hancock, & Chang, 1994; Felton, Revenson, & Hinrichsen, 1984; Magill-Evans & Restall, 1991; Walsh & Walsh, 1989). When combined with women's social devaluation, its effects on sense of self can be profound. The relevant literature portrays a woman who is challenged to accommodate increased needs for personal assistance; to grieve multiple losses, increased vulnerabilities, and externally imposed invisibility; to maintain self-efficacy for inclusion; to test self-evaluation against societal devaluation equating functional abilities with personal value; and to deal with environmental factors such as barriers to employment and health care, interpersonal violence, and inaccessibility. Yet, clinical experience suggests many women who acquire disability at birth or later develop and maintain positive self-worth. The literature on the self-esteem in the context of disability fails to explain these differences and the connections between self-esteem and health outcomes, particularly as related to gender. Our national study of women with physical disabilities revealed that this population experiences low self-esteem and the problems associated with it, such as depression, unemployment, social isolation, limited opportunities to establish satisfying relationships, and emotional, physical, and sexual abuse (Nosek, Howland, Rintala, Young, & Chanpong, 2001).

People with disabilities must continually cope with assaults to their self-esteem by negative societal attitudes, which would have us believe that individuals with disabilities are "ill, pitiful, asexual, and incapable of employment" (Perduta-Fulginiti, 1996, p. 298). Finally, the literature validates our clinical picture of women who—like those in our face-to-face group intervention studies—must mobilize fierce, personal efficacy for coping with and connecting to the contextual experience of disability. The link of self-esteem with health status is evidenced by decreased self-esteem related to symptom exacerbation, increased functional limitation, and/or the emergence of secondary health conditions (Gatten, Brookings, & Bolton, 1993; Maynard & Roller, 1991; Schlesinger, 1996).

Self-esteem in adulthood has been linked to childhood experiences. We explored relations among a set of precursor variables (age, education, severity of disability, and childhood experiences, including overprotection, familial affection, and school environment) and a set of adult outcome variables (intimacy, employment, and health maintenance behavior) (Nosek et al., 2003). We hypothesized that variables related to one's sense of self (self-cognition, social isolation, and self-esteem) would mediate the effects of the precursor variables on adult outcomes. The sample included 881 women, including 475 with physical disabilities and 406 without disabilities, aged 18 to 65 years who were Caucasian (82%), African American (9%) or other ethnic minority women (9%). Our findings indicated that the women with disabilities had significantly less education, were more overprotected during childhood, and had lower rates of salaried employment than the women without disabilities. Additionally, women with disabilities had significantly lower self-esteem and self-cognition and greater social isolation. The self variables did prove to mediate the effect of the precursors on the outcomes in a number of ways. Self-esteem, for example, mediated the impact of family affection and school environment on intimacy and mediated the impact of some of the precursor variables on employment and health maintenance.

Self-esteem appears to be a malleable factor in women with disabilities. We developed a psychoeducational, peer-led, self-esteem enhancement program for women with disabilities (Hughes, Taylor, Robinson-Whelen, Swedlund, & Nosek, 2004). In collaboration with five centers for independent living (CIL), we recruited 102 participants and randomly assigned them to either CIL services alone or CIL services plus the program on self-esteem. The results indicated that participants in the intervention showed significantly greater improvement on two measures of self-esteem, self-efficacy, and depression. The two groups did not differ significantly on social connectedness. We concluded that women with physical disabilities can benefit from peer-led self-esteem enhancement interventions and that such interventions should be incorporated into CIL services.

SOCIAL CONNECTEDNESS

Intimate relationships and other sources of connectedness and support may offer people with disabilities an important validation of self-worth (Crisp, 1996); however, social isolation has been strongly associated with health problems and mortality (Berkman & Syme, 1979). Relationships often provide positive social support that serves important functions for the well-being of people with physical disabilities (Patrick, Morgan, & Charlton, 1986). Social isolation is regarded by some as a very common secondary condition associated with any primary disability (Coyle, Santiago, Shank, Ma, & Boyd, 2000; Ravesloot, Seekins, & Walsh, 1997). Physical restrictions, such as fatigue and pain, may discourage people from making contact and connecting with others. Common knowledge and clinical experience suggest that the combination of multiple environmental barriers, negative societal messages, and diminished social opportunities may lead women with disabilities to become disconnected and isolated from sources of support and intimacy, employment opportunities, and health-promoting opportunities.

Part of the theoretical foundation for our intervention research is the importance of social connectedness and self-efficacy in relation to self-esteem and other outcomes. First, social connectedness serves as a foundation for self-esteem in women (Jordan, Kaplan, Miller, Stiver, & Surrey, 1991). Feminist theory postulates that women's groups may reduce social isolation by offering participants an opportunity to share common life experiences and connect more effectively with one another (Burden & Gottlieb, 1987; Jordan et al., 1991; McManus, Redford, & Hughes, 1997; Walker, Sechrist, & Pender, 1987) and address topics difficult to discuss in mixed-gender groups (Enns, 1992). In the context of disability, greater self-esteem has been associated with better integration in social networks (Crisp, 1996). Women with physically disabling and chronic health conditions appear to benefit from the presence of mutually supportive relationships with one another (Crigger, 1996; Fine & Asch, 1988; Hughes, Nosek, Howland, Groff, & Mullen, 2003; Hughes, Robinson-Whelen, Taylor, & Hall, 2006; Hughes et al., 2004; Reid-Cunningham, Snyder-Grant, Stein, Tyson, & Halen, 1999). In our group intervention studies, we have drawn successfully on the use of peer leaders, a practice grounded in the independent living movement with its emphasis on role modeling, consumer participation, and empowerment (Nosek & Fuhrer, 1992).

In our group intervention studies, women shared how they yearn for and benefit from opportunities to develop caring relationships with one another, to heal their shared multiple losses, and to strive for optimal wellness. Women with physically disabling conditions may clearly benefit from the resources of supportive relationships (Hughes, Swedlund, Petersen, & Nosek, 2001).

ABUSE

It took a long time for abuse against women with disabilities to surface in the research literature. For most of history, it was an accepted practice and sometimes even encouraged;

women with disabilities were safe targets because they were less able to fight back and less likely to be believed (Pelletier, 1989). Canadians were the first to take a serious look at the issue. Disabled Women's Network Canada/Réseau d'action des femmes handicapées du Canada (DAWN-RAFH) conducted a survey of the needs and concerns of women with disabilities in 1989 and analyzed responses from 245 women (Pelletier, 1989). They found that 40% had been raped, abused, or assaulted and 64% had been verbally abused; girls with disabilities had a less than equal chance of escaping violence; women with disabilities had little access to services for victims of violence; and women with multiple disabilities reported being multiply abused. They also asked about perpetrators, reporting of violence, and response to violence, as well as passing an organizational action agenda related to these findings. Sadly, abuse of women with disabilities is a little different in the United States 20 years later, but at least we can describe it more accurately.

While early research focused primarily on physical, sexual, and emotional violence against women with disabilities, additional forms of disability-specific violence have now been documented (Nosek, Foley, Hughes, & Howland, 2001; Powers, Hughes, & Lund, 2009). Examples include destruction of medical equipment and communication devices, withholding, stealing or overdosing of medications, physical neglect, and financial abuse (Curry, Powers, Oschwald, & Saxton, 2004; Gilson, DePoy, & Cramer, 2001; McFarlane et al., 2001; Nosek, Foley et al., 2001; Saxton et al., 2001). Rates of abuse vary considerably across studies depending on the definitions used and the types of disabilities represented in the sample. A comparison of the abuse experienced by a large sample of women with disabilities with their nondisabled women friends found comparable rates of abuse (Young, Nosek, Howland, Chanpong, & Rintala, 1997). Most studies, however, show significantly higher rates of violence among women with disabilities (Powers et al., 2009) and that they are more likely to experience physical and sexual violence (Brownridge, 2006; Martin et al., 2006; Powers et al., 2002; Smith, 2008), increased severity of violence (Brownridge, 2006; Nannini, 2006; Nosek, Howland, & Hughes, 2001), multiple forms of violence (Curry et al., 2004; Martin et al., 2006; Nosek, Foley et al., 2001), and longer duration of violence (Nosek, Howland, & Hughes, 2001). A consistent theme across the research is the complex intersections of disabled women's experience of impairment, poverty, isolation, reliance on others for support, discrimination, and other factors that may restrict women's violence awareness, safety-promoting behavior, and access to resources (Copel, 2006; Hassouneh-Phillips, McNeff, Powers, & Curry, 2005; Nosek, Hughes, Taylor, & Taylor, 2006).

Contrary to what some may believe, disability does not serve as a protective factor against abuse for women (Nosek, Foley et al., 2001). We strongly recommend that counselors use a very simple screening tool that we developed, the Abuse Assessment Screen—Disability (McFarlane et al., 2001), which includes four items assessing physical, sexual, and disability-related abuse in the past year. We found that women who were positive for abuse tended to be younger, had more education, had greater mobility impairments, were more socially isolated, and reported more symptoms of depression (Nosek et al., 2006). This important topic is discussed in greater detail in Chapter 23.

STRESS

Women in the general population have reported higher levels of perceived stress than their male counterparts (Cohen & Williamson, 1988). We also know that having a physical disability constitutes a chronic life strain (Turner & Wood, 1985). Thus, women with physical disabilities are at increased risk for experiencing stress and its negative health consequences as a result of being both female and having a disability (Coyle et al., 2000; Hughes, Taylor, Robinson-Whelen, & Nosek, 2005; Rintala, Hart, & Fuhrer, 1996). This was substantiated by an analysis of the National Health Interview Survey (Chevarley et al., 2006) that showed, after adjusting for age, women with three or more functional limitations are 10 times more likely to report having difficulty with day-to-day stress than women without limitations (21% vs. 2%). Hughes and colleagues (2005), who observed elevated levels of perceived stress in a sample of 415 women with physical disabilities, reported that greater perceived stress was linked with lower levels of social support, greater pain limitations, and recent experience with abuse. According to an analysis of data from the National Health Interview Survey, 1992 and 1994, women with disabilities (three or more functional limitations) are 10 times more likely to report having difficulty with day-to-day stress than women with no limitations (21% vs. 2%) when age was adjusted (Chevarley, Thierry, Gill, Reyerson, & Nosek, 2005).

Stress reflects the extent to which individuals perceive their lives to be unpredictable, uncontrollable, and overloading (Cohen & Williamson, 1988). Although everyone lives with some degree of stress, its impact on people with disabilities may be more severe due to the fact that they often have a more vulnerable physical and psychological health status (Turner & Noh, 1988) and fewer resources to buffer the effects of stress. Social support, which has been well studied as a stress buffer (Cohen & Wills, 1985), is often lacking or inadequate among women with disabilities (Crewe & Clarke, 1996; Rintala et al., 1996). Hughes and colleagues found that, after controlling for demographics and disability characteristics, perceived stress is greater for women with physical disabilities who have less social support, greater pain, and experience with abuse in the past year (Hughes, Robinson-Whelen, Taylor, Petersen, & Nosek, 2005).

Elevated blood pressure, chronic pain, and irritable bowel syndrome are generally acknowledged as being associated with high levels of stress, but less known is its effect on worsening disability symptoms. Stress has been associated with greater disability among those with arthritis (Weinberger, Tierney, Booher, & Hiner, 1990), elevated depressive symptomatology in spinal cord injury (Hughes et al., 2001; Rintala et al., 1996), greater symptom severity in systemic lupus erythematosus (Adams, Dammers, Saia, Brantley, & Gaydos, 1994), increased disease progression in multiple sclerosis (Schwartz et al., 1999), and exacerbations of disease activity in rheumatoid arthritis (Zautra et al., 1998).

A task force of the American Psychological Association asserted that women are likely to experience stress related to social isolation, poverty, violence, and other forms of victimization and chronic health problems (McGrath et al., 1990). Women with disabilities are often faced with the uncertainty of health problems; lack of physical fitness related to mobility limitations, pain, and illness; inadequate nutrition; abuse and violence; environmental barriers in health care settings and the workplace; and unemployment, lower wages, and poverty (Crewe & Clarke, 1996; Nosek, 2000). Other stressors related to a woman's disability include the need for personal assistance, changes in appearance, interruption of daily activities, and increased planning, time, and effort for activities of daily living (Crewe & Clarke, 1996).

Only one effort to date has been made to develop an intervention that helps women with disabilities manage stress. Hughes and colleagues together with women with disabilities modified the standard approach to stress management to include elements of feminist theory and peer role modeling from the independent living movement. This intervention offers information, opportunities to practice coping and management skills, goal setting and action planning to increase self-efficacy, social connectedness, and peer support. When the intervention was tested in a randomized clinical trial, the intervention group showed greater improvement on measures of stress, pain, and role limitations owing to physical health compared the wait-listed control group. Perceived stress was supported as a mediator of the effect of the intervention on mental health. There was also support for social connectedness and self-efficacy as mediators of the relation between the intervention and perceived stress (Hughes et al., 2006).

DEPRESSION

Depression is a complex phenomenon among women who live with the culturally devalued status of being female and having a disability (Fine & Asch, 1988; Gill, 1996; Nosek, Hughes, & Robinson-Whelen, 2008). As women, they are twice as likely to experience depression as men (Coyle & Roberge, 1992; Rintala et al., 1996; U.S. Department of Health and Human Services, 1999) primarily due to women's experience of being female in our culture (McGrath et al., 1990), including gender-based roles and socialization experiences (Fedele, 1994; Jordan et al., 1991; Miller, 1976). As women living with disabilities, they may experience disproportionately high rates of depressive symptomatology compared to other women, with estimates ranging from 30% (11) to 59% (Chevarley et al., 2006; Ferguson & Cotton, 1996; Hughes et al., 2001; U.S. Department of Health and Human Services, 2000; Ward et al., 1999). Younger women with three or more functional limitations are more frequently depressed (30%) than women without disabilities (4%) and are eight times more likely to report having experienced major depression in the past year (Chevarley et al., 2006).

Some of the somatic criteria for depression (e.g., fatigue, sleep disturbance) are also common disability-related symptoms that may lead to overestimating depression (Aikens et al., 1999). On the other hand, those same symptoms can mask psychological distress (Franklin, 2000) and leave depression in women with disabilities underdetected and undertreated. Depression has been associated with conditions that often accompany disability, such as cerebral involvement or medications for the underlying disease (Cameron, 1987), pain (Kraaimaat, Van Dam-Baggen, & Bijlsma, 1995; Tate, Forchheimer, Kirsch, Maynard, & Roller, 1993), and environmental factors (Turner & Noh, 1988), such as social isolation (Murphy, Dickens, Creed, & Bernstein, 1999).

Hughes and colleagues examined depression in a sample of 443 women with physical disabilities living in the community, the majority of whom had minority backgrounds and low income (Hughes, Robinson-Whelen et al., 2005). Using the self-report Beck Depression Inventory II (BDI-II) (Beck, Steer, & Brown, 1996) cutoff for significant depressive symptomatology (≥17), 51% of the respondents scored in the mildly depressed range or higher and 31% scored in the moderately or severely depressed range. Women classified as depressed compared to nondepressed women were significantly younger and had shorter duration of disability. Only 44% of the women classified as depressed on the BDI-II had received recent treatment for depression, and those identified as Hispanic being the least likely to have received treatment.

Rural women with physical disabilities may face even greater barriers to mental health than their urban counterparts due to greater social and geographical isolation, lack of access to health-related resources, transportation problems, and communication barriers (Levine, Lishner, Richardson, & Porter, 2001; Mulder et al., 2000). A study of 135 rural women with physical disabilities who exceeded the cutoff for depression on the BDI-II indicated that most of the women reported moderate to severe depression, and nearly one out of five reported thoughts of suicide (Hughes, Nosek, & Robinson-Whelen, 2007).

CONCLUSION

The life situation of women with disabilities is complex and permeated with attitudinal, social, and economic obstacles to psychosocial well-being. The evidence is irrefutable that women with disabilities are a substantial segment of the population and face more serious disadvantages than men with disabilities or women in general in achieving their life goals. Population-based research has documented very high rates of mental and physical health problems among women with disabilities, yet attention to these problems in the clinical research literature is minimal and far out of proportion to their magnitude.

The field of rehabilitation counseling has been slow to rouse regarding the importance of recognizing gender differences in the experience of disability and developing approaches that have proven to be effective in counseling women. The way of women is holistic with a very strong emphasis on mutual benefit and social connectedness. Since rehabilitation counseling as a profession has its roots in the wars of the 20th century, it is understandable that it grew out of a masculine, competitive base. To maintain its relevance for a future that is witnessing the rising status of women, rehabilitation research and counseling must develop and test new approaches that incorporate balance of biological, psychological, social, contextual, and spiritual elements.

We believe that rehabilitation researchers and practitioners are ready to take action to address the needs of women. We recommend that researchers

1) Remove unnecessary enrollment criteria that would exclude or tend to exclude women with disabling conditions, such as
   a) Limiting age to under 65, unless a working-age sample is essential to the design
   b) Conducting surveys or exams in inaccessible facilities
   c) Requiring telephonic response to questions
   d) Requiring attendance at a clinic or an event.

2) Eliminate procedures that require manual dexterity or mobility when these are not essential for the phenomenon under investigation (e.g., minimum competency screens, intelligence tests).

3) During recruitment, take special measures to ensure that announcements reach minority, low-income, low-education, and sensory-impaired women.

4) Set the parameters for your study carefully and state exclusion criteria in all publications of findings.

5) Always include gender as an independent variable in all data analyses. Do not simply control for gender because that, in effect, pretends that a woman is a man.

6) Advance the careers of students who are women with disabilities by offering scholarships, giving opportunities to make presentations to academic audiences, and introducing them to leaders in their field.

We recommend that rehabilitation counselors and administrators

1) Be aware of gender bias when developing rehabilitation plans for women consumers

2) Use only those assessment instruments and tools that have been validated for both genders

3) Consider, as appropriate, the woman's life situation and if abuse is suspected, refer her to community resources for battered women

4) Be vigilant for signs of stress and depression and, as appropriate, refer for psychological counseling

5) Encourage all consumers to become involved in the independent living movement or other peer support groups

6) Include gender as a variable in analyzing consumer and program outcomes

7) Ensure that advisory boards for rehabilitation services have equal representation of women and men with disabilities

It is not difficult to see that some of these recommendations cannot be implemented until more research has been conducted. When assessment techniques that are common in rehabilitation settings have been proven valid for women, when counselors have information and training about how disability can affect women differently than men, when success is defined by the same standards for both women and men, and when as many women as men have reached the highest levels of rehabilitation research, education, administration, and practice, then we will begin to see progress toward a truly inclusive society.

REFERENCES

Abraido-Lanza, A. F., Guier, C., & Colon, R. M. (1998). Psychological thriving among Latinas with chronic illness. *Journal of Social Issues, 54*, 405–424.

Adams, S. G., Dammers, P. M., Saia, T. L., Brantley, P. J., & Gaydos, G. R. (1994). Stress, depression, and anxiety predict average symptom severity and daily symptom fluctuation in systemic lupus erythematosus. *Journal of Behavioral Medicine, 17*, 459–477.

Adler, A., Ansbacher, H. L., & Ansbacher, R. R. (Eds.). (1979). *Superiority and social interest.* New York: Norton.

Aikens, J. E., Reinecke, M. A., Pliskin, N. H., Fischer, J. S., Wiebe, J. S., McCracken, L. M., et al. (1999). Assessing depressive symptoms in multiple sclerosis: Is it necessary to omit items from the original Beck Depression Inventory? *Journal of Behavioral Medicine, 22*(2), 127–142.

Altman, B. M. (1985). Disabled women in the social structure. In S. E. Browne, D. Conners, & N. Stern (Eds.), *With the power of each breath* (pp. 69–76). Pittsburgh, PA: Cleis Press.

Altman, B. M. (1996). Causes, risks, and consequences of disability among women. In D. M. Krotoski, M. A. Nosek, & M. A. Turk (Eds.), *Women with physical disabilities: Achieving and maintaining health and well-being* (Vol. 35–55). Baltimore: Paul H. Brookes.

Axel, S. (1982). Spinal cord injured women's concerns: Menstruation and pregnancy. *Rehabilitation Nursing, 10*, 10–15.

Barnartt, S. N. (1982). The socio-economic status of deaf women: Are they doubly disadvantaged? In J. Christiansen & K. Egelston-Dodd (Eds.), *Socioeconomic status of the deaf population* (pp. 1–31). Washington, DC: Gallaudet College.

Beck, A. T., Steer, R. A., & Brown, G. K. (1996). *Manual for Beck Depression Inventory-II.* San Antonio, TX: Psychological Corporation.

Beckmann, C. R. B., Gittler, M., Barzansky, B. M., & Beckmann, C. A. (1989). Gynecologic health care of women with disabilities. *Obstetrics and Gynecology, 74*, 75–79.

Berkman, L. F., & Syme, S. L. (1979). Social networks, host resistance, and mortality: A nine-year follow-up study of Alameda County residents. *American Journal of Epidemiology, 109*, 186–204.

Bernatsky, S., Joseph, L., Pineau, C. A., Belisle, P., Lix, L., Banerjee, D., et al. (2009). Polymyalgia rheumatica prevalence in a population-based sample. *Arthritis and Rheumatism, 61*(9), 1264–1267.

Brault, M. W. (2008). *Americans with disabilities: 2005.* Washington, DC: US Census Bureau.

Brownridge, D. A. (2006). Partner violence against women with disabilities: Prevalence, risk, and explanations. *Violence Against Women, 12*, 805–822.

Burckhardt, C. S. (1985). The impact of arthritis on quality of life. *Nursing Research, 34*, 11–16.

Burden, D. S., & Gottlieb, N. (1987). Women's socialization and feminist groups. In C. M. Brody (Ed.), *Women's therapy groups: Paradigms of feminist treatment* (pp. 24–39). New York: Springer.

Cameron, O. G. (1987). Some guidelines for a pragmatic approach to the patient with secondary depression. In O. G. Cameron (Ed.), *Presentations of depression: Depressive symptoms in medical and other psychiatric disorders* (pp. 417–423). New York: John Wiley and Sons.

Carty, E. A., & Conine, T. A. (1988). Disability and pregnancy: A double dose of disequilibrium. *Rehabilitation Nursing, 13*, 85–92.

Charlifue, S. W., Gerhart, K. A., Menter, R. R., Whiteneck, G. G., & Manley, M. S. (1992). Sexual issues of women with spinal cord injuries. *Paraplegia, 30*, 192–199.

Chevarley, F., Thierry, J. M., Gill, C. J., Ryerson, A. B., & Nosek, M. A. (2006). Health, preventive health care, and health care access among women with disabilities in the 1994–1995 National Health Interview Survey. *Women's Health Issues, 16*(6), 297–312.

Cohen, S., & Williamson, G. M. (1988). Perceived stress in a probability sample of the United States. In S. Spacapan & S. Oskamp (Eds.), *The social psychology of health: Claremont symposium on applied social psychology* (pp. 31–67). Newbury Park, CA: Sage.

Cohen, S., & Wills, T. A. (1985). Stress, social support, and the buffering hypothesis. *Psychological Bulletin, 98*, 310–357.

Cole, T. M. (1975). Spinal cord injured patients and sexual dysfunction. *Archives of Physical Medicine and Rehabilitation, 56*, 11–12.

Comarr, A. E. (1976). Sexual response of paraplegic women. *Medical Aspects of Human Sexuality, 10*, 124–128.

Copel, L. C. (2006). Partner abuse in physically disabled women: A proposed model for understanding intimate partner violence. *Perspectives in Psychiatric Care, 42*(2), 114–129.

Coyle, C. P., & Roberge, J. J. (1992). The psychometric properties of the Center for Epidemiological Studies-Depression Scale (CES-D) when used with adults with physical disabilities. *Psychology & Health, 7*, 69–81.

Coyle, C. P., Santiago, M. C., Shank, J. W., Ma, G. X., & Boyd, R. (2000). Secondary conditions and women with physical disabilities: A descriptive study. *Archives of Physical Medicine and Rehabilitation 81*(10), 1380–1387.

Craig, A. R., Hancock, K., & Chang, E. (1994). The influence of spinal cord injury on coping styles and self-perceptions two years after the injury. *Australian and New Zealand Journal of Psychiatry, 28*, 307–312.

Crewe, N. M., & Clarke, N. (1996). Stress and women with disabilities. In D. Krotoski, M. A. Nosek, & M. A. Turk (Eds.), *Women with physical disabilities: Achieving and maintaining health and well-being* (pp. 193–202). Baltimore: Paul H. Brookes.

Crigger, N. J. (1996). Testing an uncertainty model for women with multiple sclerosis. *Advances in Nursing Science, 18*, 37–47.

Crisp, R. (1996). Community integration, self-esteem, and vocational identity among persons with disabilities. *Australian Psychologist, 31*, 133–137.

Curry, M. A., Powers, L. E., Oschwald, M., & Saxton, M. (2004). Development and testing of an abuse screening tool for women with disabilities. *Journal of Aggression, Maltreatment and Trauma, 8*(4), 123–141.

Deegan, M. J., & Brooks, N. A. (Eds.). (1985). *Women and disability: The double handicap*. New Brunswick, NJ: Transaction Books, Rutgers University.

DeVivo, M. J., & Chen, Y. (2011). Trends in new injuries, prevalent cases, and aging with spinal cord injury. *Archives of Physical Medicine and Rehabilitation, 92*, 332–338.

Enns, C. Z. (1992). Self-esteem groups: A synthesis of conscious-raising and assertiveness training. *Journal of Counseling and Development, 71*, 7–13.

Erickson, W., Lee, C., & von Schrader, S. (2009). *2008 Disability Status Report: The United States*. Ithaca, NY: Cornell University Rehabilitation Research and Training Center on Disability Demographics and Statistics.

Fedele, N. (1994). *Relationships in groups: Connection, resonance, and paradox: Work in progress, No. 69*. Wellesley, MA: Stone Center Working Papers Series.

Felton, B. J., Revenson, T. A., & Hinrichsen, G. A. (1984). Stress and coping in the explanation of psychological adjustment among chronically ill adults. *Social Science and Medicine, 18*(10), 889–898.

Ferguson, S. J., & Cotton, S. (1996). Broken sleep, pain, disability, social activity, and depressive symptoms in rheumatoid arthritis. *Australian Journal of Psychology, 48*(1), 9–14.

Fine, M., & Asch, A. (1985). Disabled women: Sexism without the pedestal. In M. J. Deegan & N. A. Brooks (Eds.), *Women and disability: The double handicap* (pp. 6–22). New Brunswick, NJ: Transaction, Inc.

Fine, M., & Asch, A. (Eds.). (1988). *Women with disabilities: Essays in psychology, culture, and politics*. Philadelphia: Temple University Press.

Franklin, D. J. (2000). Depression: Information and treatment [Electronic Version]. *Psychology Information Online*.

Gatten, C. W., Brookings, J. B., & Bolton, B. (1993). Mood fluctuations in female multiple sclerosis patients. *Social Behavior and Personality, 21*, 103–106.

Gill, C. (1996). Becoming visible: Personal health experiences of women with disabilities. In D. M. Krotoski, M. A. Nosek, & M. A. Turk (Eds.), *Women with physical disabilities: Achieving and maintaining health and well-being* (pp. 5–15). Baltimore: Paul H. Brookes.

Gilson, S. F., DePoy, E., & Cramer, E. P. (2001). Linking the assessment of self-reported functional capacity with abuse experiences of women with disabilities. *Violence Against Women, 7*(4), 418–431.

Griffith, E. R., & Trieschmann, R. B. (1975). Sexual functioning in women with spinal cord injury. *Archives of Physical Medicine and Rehabilitation, 56*, 18–21.

Hassouneh-Phillips, D., McNeff, E., Powers, L. E., & Curry, M. (2005). Invalidation: A central process underlying maltreatment of women with disabilities. *Women and Health, 41*(1), 33–50.

Hughes, R. B., Nosek, M. A., Howland, C. A., Groff, J., & Mullen, P. D. (2003). Health promotion workshop for women with physical disabilities: A pilot study. *Rehabilitation Psychology, 48*, 182–188.

Hughes, R. B., Nosek, M. A., & Robinson-Whelen, S. (2007). Correlates of depression in rural women with physical disabilities. *Journal of Obstetric, Gynecologic, and Neonatal Nursing, 36*(1), 105–114.

Hughes, R. B., Robinson-Whelen, S., Taylor, H. B., & Hall, J. W. (2006). Stress self-management: An intervention for women with physical disabilities. *Women's Health Issues, 16*(6), 389–399.

Hughes, R. B., Robinson-Whelen, S., Taylor, H. B., Petersen, N., & Nosek, M. A. (2005). Characteristics of depressed and non-depressed women with physical disabilities. *Archives of Physical Medicine & Rehabilitation, 86*(3), 473–479.

Hughes, R. B., Swedlund, N., Petersen, N., & Nosek, M. A. (2001). Depression and women with spinal cord injury. *Topics in Spinal Cord Injury Rehabilitation, 7*(1), 16–24.

Hughes, R. B., Taylor, H. B., Robinson-Whelen, S., & Nosek, M. A. (2005). Perceived stress in women with physical disabilities: Identifying psychosocial correlates. *Womens Health Issues, 15*, 14–20.

Hughes, R. B., Taylor, H. B., Robinson-Whelen, S., Swedlund, N., & Nosek, M. A. (2004). Enhancing self-esteem in women with physical disabilities. *Rehabilitation Psychology, 19*(4), 295–302.

Jackson, A. B., & Varner, R. E. (1989). Gynecological problems encountered in women with acute and chronic spinal cord disabilities. *Abstracts Digest*, 111–112.

Jackson, A. B., & Wadley, V. (1999). A multicenter study of women's self-reported reproductive health after spinal cord injury. *Archives of Physical Medicine and Rehabilitation, 80*(11), 1420–1428.

James, W. (1890). *Principles of psychology.* New York: Dover.

Jans, L., & Stoddard, S. (1999). *Chartbook on women and disability in the United States: An InfoUse report.* Washington, DC: U.S. Department of Education, National Institute on Disability and Rehabilitation Research.

Johnell, O., & Kanis, J. A. (2006). An estimate of the worldwide prevalence and disability associated with osteoporotic fractures. *Osteoporosis International, 17*, 1726.

Jordan, J. V., Kaplan, A. G., Miller, J. B., Stiver, I. P., & Surrey, J. L. (1991). *Women's growth in connection.* New York: Guilford Press.

Kraaimaat, F. W., Van Dam-Baggen, C. M., & Bijlsma, J. W. (1995). Depression, anxiety and social support in rheumatoid arthritic women without and with a spouse. *Psychology and Health, 10*, 387–396.

LaPlante, M. P. (1991). *Disability risks of chronic illnesses and impairments.* Washington, DC: National Institute on Disability and Rehabilitation Research, U.S. Department of Education.

LaPlante, M. P., & Carlson, D. (1996). *Disability in the United States: Prevalence and causes, 1992: Disability Statistics Report: Report 7.* Washington, DC: National Institute on Disability and Rehabilitation Research, U.S. Department of Education.

Lawrence, R. C., Felson, D. T., Helmick, C. G., Arnold, L. M., Choi, H., Deyo, R. A., et al. (2008). Estimates of the prevalence of arthritis and other rheumatic conditions in the United States: Part II. *Arthritis & Rheumatism, 58*(1), 26–35.

Leavesley, G., & Porter, J. (1982). Sexuality, fertility and contraception in disability. *Contraception, 26*, 417–441.

Levine, P., Lishner, D., Richardson, M., & Porter, A. (2001). Face on the data: Access to health care for people with disabilities living in rural communities. In R. M. Moore III (Ed.), *The hidden America: Social problems in rural America for the twenty-first century* (pp. 179–196). Cranbury, NJ: Associated University Press.

Magill-Evans, J. E., & Restall, G. (1991). Self-esteem of persons with cerebral palsy: From adolescence to adulthood. *American Journal of Occupational Therapy, 45*, 819–825.

Mahat, G. (1997). Perceived stressors and coping strategies among individuals with rheumatoid arthritis. *Journal of Advanced Nursing, 25*, 1144–1150.

Martin, S. L., Ray, N., Sotres-Alvarez, D., Kupper, L. L., Moracco, K. E., Dickens, P. A., et al. (2006). Physical and sexual assault of women with disabilities. *Violence Against Women, 12*, 823–837.

May, R. (1953). *Man's search for himself.* New York: New American Library.

Maynard, F. M., & Roller, S. (1991). Recognizing typical coping styles of polio survivors can improve rehabilitation. *American Journal of Physical Medicine and Rehabilitation, 70*, 70–72.

McFarlane, J., Hughes, R. B., Nosek, M. A., Groff, J. Y., Swedlund, N., & Mullen, P. D. (2001). Abuse assessment screen-disability (AAS-D): Measuring frequency, type, and perpetrator of abuse towards women with physical disabilities. *Journal of Women's Health and Gender-Based Medicine, 10*(9), 861–866.

McGrath, E., Keita, G. P., Strickland, B. R., Russo, N. F., McGrath, E., Keita, G. P., et al. (1990). *Women and depression: Risk factors and treatment issues: Final report.* Washington, DC: American Psychological Association's National Task Force on Women and Depression.

McManus, P. W., Redford, J. L., & Hughes, R. B. (1997). Connecting to self and others: A structured group for women. *The Journal for Specialists in Group Work, 22*, 22–30.

McNeil, J. M. (1997). *Americans with disabilities 1994–1995.* Washington, DC: U.S. Census Bureau.

Miller, J. B. (1976). *Toward a new psychology of women.* Boston: Beacon Press.

Mulder, P. L., Shellenberger, S., Streiegel, R., Jumper-Thurman, P., Danda, C. E., Kenkel, M. B., et al. (2000). *The behavioral health care needs of rural women: An APA Report to Congress*: American Psychological Association.

Murphy, H., Dickens, C., Creed, F., & Bernstein, R. (1999). Depression, illness perception and coping in rheumatoid arthritis. *Journal of Psychosomatic Research, 46*, 155–164.

Myers, J. E., & Sweeney, T. J. (2004). The indivisible self: An evidence-based model of wellness. *Journal of Individual Psychology, 60*(3), 234–245.

Nannini, A. (2006). Sexual assault patterns among women with and without disabilities seeking survivor services. *Women's Health Issues, 16*(6), 372–379.

National Center for Health Statistics. (2006). *Health, United States, 2006, with chartbook on trends in the health of Americans*. Hyattsville, MD: National Center for Health Statistics.

Noonan, C. W., Williamson, D. M., Henry, J. P., Indian, R., Lynch, S. G., Neuberger, J. S., et al. (2010). The prevalence of multiple sclerosis in 3 US communities. *Preventing Chronic Disease [electronic resource], 7*(1), A12.

Nosek, M. A. (1995). The defining light of Vedanta: Personal reflections on spirituality and disability. *Rehabilitation Education, 9*(2–3), 171–182.

Nosek, M. A. (1996). Wellness among women with physical disabilities. *Sexuality and Disability, 14*(3), 165–182.

Nosek, M. A. (2000). The John Stanley Coulter lecture. Overcoming the odds: the health of women with physical disabilities in the United States. *Archives of Physical Medicine and Rehabilitation, 81*, 135–138.

Nosek, M. A. (2005). Wellness in the context of disability. In J. Myers & T. Sweeney (Eds.), *Wellness in counseling: Theory, research, and practice*. Alexandria, VA: American Counseling Association.

Nosek, M. A. (2006). The changing face of women with disabilities: Are we ready? *Journal of Women's Health and Gender-Based Medicine, 15*(9), 996–999.

Nosek, M. A. (2010a). Feminism and disability: Synchronous agendas in conflict. In H. Landrine & N. Russo (Eds.), *Handbook of diversity in feminist psychology* (pp. 501–533). New York: Springer Publishing Company.

Nosek, M. A. (2010b). Healthcare apartheid and quality of life for people with disabilities. *Quality of Life Research, 19*(4), 609–610

Nosek, M. A., Foley, C. C., Hughes, R. B., & Howland, C. A. (2001). Vulnerabilities for abuse among women with disabilities. *Sexuality and Disability, 19*(3), 177–190.

Nosek, M. A., & Fuhrer, M. J. (1992). Independence among people with disabilities: I. A heuristic model. *Rehabilitation Counseling Bulletin, 36*(1), 6–20.

Nosek, M. A., Howland, C., & Hughes, R. B. (2001). The investigation of abuse and women with disabilities: Going beyond assumptions. *Violence Against Women, 7*(4), 477–499.

Nosek, M. A., Howland, C. A., Rintala, D. H., Young, M. E., & Chanpong, G. F. (2001). National study of women with physical disabilities: Final report. *Sexuality and Disability, 19*(1), 5–39.

Nosek, M. A., & Hughes, R. B. (2001). Psychospiritual aspects of sense of self in women with physical disabilities. *Journal of Rehabilitation, 67*(1), 20–25.

Nosek, M. A., Hughes, R. B., Howland, C. A., Young, M. E., Mullen, P. D., & Shelton, M. (2004). The meaning of health for women with physical disabilities: A qualitative study. *Family & Community Health, 27*(1), 6–21.

Nosek, M. A., Hughes, R. B., & Robinson-Whelen, S. (2008). The complex array of antecedents of depression in women with physical disabilities: Implications for clinicians. *Disability and Rehabilitation, 30*(3), 174–183.

Nosek, M. A., Hughes, R. B., Swedlund, N., Taylor, H. B., & Swank, P. (2003). Self-esteem and women with disabilities. *Social Science and Medicine, 56*(8), 1737–1747.

Nosek, M. A., Hughes, R. B., Taylor, H. B., & Taylor, P. (2006). Disability, psychosocial, and demographic characteristics of abused women with physical disabilities. *Violence Against Women, 12*(9), 1–13.

Nosek, M. A., Robinson-Whelen, S., Hughes, R. B., Porcher, E., Davidson, G., & Nosek, T. M. (2011). Self-esteem in second life: An inworld group intervention for women with disabilities. *Journal of Virtual Worlds Research, 4(1)*. https://journals. toll. org/jvwr/article/view/3538/5545

Nosek, M. A., & Simmons, D. K. (2007). People with disabilities as a health disparities population: The case of sexual and reproductive health disparities. *California Journal of Health Promotion 5, Special Issue (Health Disparities & Social Justice)*, 68–81.

O'Leary, A., Shoor, S., Lorig, K., & Holman, H. R. (1988). A cognitive behavioral treatment for rheumatoid arthritis. *Health Psychology, 7*, 527–544.

Patrick, D. L., Morgan, M., & Charlton, R. H. (1986). Psychosocial support and change in the health status of physically disabled people. *Social Science and Medicine, 22*, 1347–1354.

Patterson, J. B., DeLaGarza, D., & Schaller, J. (1998). Rehabilitation counseling practice: Considerations and interventions. In R. M. P. E. M. Szymanski (Ed.), *Rehabilitation counseling: Basics and beyond* (3rd ed., pp. 269–302). Austin, TX: Pro-Ed.

Pelletier, J. (1989). Beating the odds: Violence and women with disabilities. Retrieved July 3, 2011, from http://www.dawncanada.net/ENG/Engodds.pdf

Perduta-Fulginiti, P. S. (1996). Impact of bladder and bowel dysfunction on sexuality and self-esteem. In D. M. Krotoski, M. A. Nosek, & M. A. Turk (Eds.), *Women with physical disabilities: Achieving and maintaining health and well-being* (pp. 287–298). Baltimore: Paul H. Brookes.

Pleis, J. R., & Lethbridge-Cejku, M. (2006). Summary health statistics for U.S. adults: National Health Interview Survey, 2005. National Center for Health Statistics. *Vital Health Statistics, 10*(232).

Powers, L. E., Curry, M. A., Oschwald, M., Maley, S., Eckels, K., & Saxton, M. (2002). Barriers and strategies in addressing abuse within personal assistance relationships: A survey of disabled women's experiences. *Journal of Rehabilitation, 68*(1), 4–13.

Powers, L. E., Hughes, R. B., & Lund, E. M. (2009). Interpersonal violence and women with disabilities: A research update. *Applied Research Forum, National Online Resource Center on Violence Against Women* Retrieved July 3, 2011, from http://www.vawnet.org/advanced-search/summary.php?doc_id=2077&find_type=web_desc_AR

Ravesloot, C., Seekins, T., & Walsh, J. (1997). A structural analysis of secondary conditions experienced by people with physical disabilities. *Rehabilitation Psychology, 42*(1), 3–16.

Reid-Cunningham, M., Snyder-Grant, D., Stein, K., Tyson, E., & Halen, B. (1999). *Work in progress: Women with chronic illness: Overcoming disconnection*. Wellesley, MA: The Stone Center.

Rintala, D. H., Hart, K. A., & Fuhrer, M. J. (1996). Perceived stress in individuals with spinal cord injury. In D. Krotoski, M. A. Nosek, & M. A. Turk (Eds.), *Women with physical disabilities: Achieving and maintaining health and well-being* (pp. 223–242). Baltimore: Paul H. Brookes.

Roberts, G., & Stuifbergen, A. K. (1998). Health appraisal models in multiple sclerosis. *Social Science & Medicine, 47*, 243–253.

Saxton, M., Curry, M. A., Powers, L. E., Maley, S., Eckels, K., & Gross, J. (2001). "Bring my scooter so I can leave you": A study of disabled women handling abuse by personal assistance providers. *Violence Against Women, 7*(4), 393–417.

Schaller, J., & DeLaGarza, D. (1995). Issues of gender in vocational testing and counseling. *Journal of Job Placement, 11*, 6–14.

Schlesinger, L. (1996). Chronic pain, intimacy, and sexuality: A qualitative study of women who live with pain. *Journal of Sex Research, 33*, 249–256.

Schwartz, C. E., Foley, F. W., Rao, S. M., Bernardin, L. J., Lee, H., & Genderson, M. W. (1999). Stress and course of disease in multiple sclerosis. *Behavioral Medicine, 25*, 110–116.

Siegel, J. (1996). *Aging into the 21st century*. Retrieved August 31, 2006, from www.aoa.gov/prof/Statistics/future_growth/aging21/health.asp#Disability

Smith, D. L. (2008). Disability, gender and intimate partner violence: Relationships from the behavioral risk factor surveillance system. *Sexuality and Disability 26*(1), 15–28.

Surrey, J. (1991). The self in relation: A theory of women's development. In J. V. Jordan, A. G. Kaplan, J. B. Miller, I. P. Stiver, & J. L. Surrey (Eds.), *Women's growth in connection: Writings from the stone center* (pp. 51–66). New York: Guilford.

Taal, E., Rasker, J. J., & Wiegman, O. (1997). Group education for rheumatoid arthritis patients. *Seminars in Arthritis and Rheumatism, 26*(6), 805–816.

Tate, D. G., Forchheimer, M., Kirsch, N., Maynard, F., & Roller, A. (1993). Prevalence and associated features of depression and psychological distress in polio survivors. *Archives of Physical Medicine and Rehabilitation, 74*, 1056–1060.

TBI National Data and Statistics Center. (2010). *The traumatic brain injury model systems of care*. TBI National Data and Statistics Center, Englewood, CO.

Turner, R. J., & Noh, S. (1988). Physical disability and depression: A longitudinal analysis. *Journal of Health and Social Behavior, 29*, 23–37.

Turner, R. J., & Wood, D. W. (1985). Depression and disability: The stress process in a chronically strained population. *Research in Community and Mental Health, 5*, 77–109.

U.S. Census Bureau. (2006). B18030. Disability status by sex by age by poverty status for the civilian non-institutionalized population 5 years and over—universe: civilian noninstitutionalized population 5 years and over for whom poverty status is determined. Retrieved July 3, 2011, from U.S. Census: http://factfinder.census.gov/servlet/DTTable?_bm=y&-state=dt&-ds_name=ACS_2006_EST_G00_&-mt_name=ACS_2006_EST_G2000_B18030&-redoLog=true&-_caller=geoselect&-geo_id=01000US&-geo_id=NBSP&-format=&-_lang=en

U.S. Department of Health and Human Services. (1999). Executive summary mental health: Culture, race, and ethnicity, a supplement to mental health: a report of the surgeon general. Retrieved November 21, 2006, from http://www.surgeongeneral.gov/library/mentalhealth/cre/execsummary-1.html

U.S. Department of Health and Human Services. (2000). Healthy people 2010: Understanding and improving health and objectives for improving health. Retrieved March 16, 2007 from http://www.healthy-people.gov/Document/HTML/Volume1/06Disability.htm#_Toc486927301.

Verduyn, W. H. (1986). Spinal cord injured women, pregnancy and delivery. *Paraplegia, 24*, 231–240.

Waldrop, J., & Stern, S. M. (2003). Disability Status: 2000. *Census 2000 Brief* Retrieved April 18, 2011, from http://www.census.gov/prod/2003pubs/c2kbr-17.pdf

Walker, S. N., Sechrist, K. R., & Pender, N. J. (1987). The health-promoting lifestyle profile: Development and psychometric characteristics. *Nursing Research, 36*(2), 76–81.

Walsh, A., & Walsh, P. A. (1989). Love, self-esteem, and multiple sclerosis. *Social Science & Medicine, 29*, 793.

Ward, M. M., Lotstein, D. S., Bush, T. M., Lambert, R. E., van Vollenhoven, R., & Neuwelt, C. M. (1999). Psychosocial correlates of morbidity in women with systemic lupus erythematosus. *The Journal of Rheumatology, 26*(10), 2153–2158.

Weinberger, M., Tierney, W. M., Booher, P., & Hiner, S. L. (1990). Social support, stress, and functional status in patients with osteoarthritis. *Social Science and Medicine, 30*, 503–508.

Wright, B. A. (1960). *Physical disability: A psychological approach*. New York: Harper and Row.

Young, M. E., Nosek, M. A., Howland, C. A., Chanpong, G., & Rintala, D. H. (1997). Prevalence of abuse of women with physical disabilities. *Archives of Physical Medicine and Rehabilitation, 78*(12, Suppl. 5), S34–S38.

Zautra, A. J., Hoffman, J. M., Matt, K. S., Yocum, D., Potter, P. T., Castro, W. L., et al. (1998). An examination of individual differences in the relationship between interpersonal stress and disease activity among women with rheumatoid arthritis. *Arthritis Care and Research, 11*(4), 271–279.

10

Sexuality and Spinal Cord Injury Counseling Implications

EVA MILLER AND IRMO MARINI

Sexual concerns are often paramount following spinal cord injury (SCI). However, despite the sexual revolution in the mid-1970s, which spurred research in the area of sexuality, most of what is known about SCI on sexual function pertains to males. This is due in part to the fact that the majority of individuals with SCI are males (4:1) and because it is easier to study sexual response in males because of their external genitalia (Mona et al., 2000). Most early research regarding the sexual activity of women with SCI has been pessimistic and narrow in focus (Sipski & Alexander, 1997). Sipski and Alexander noted that part of the problem with the lack of research relates to low survival rates from years ago. The authors further suggested that it is difficult for some counselors to be objective about discussing sexuality due to their own values, biases, and experiences. Hwang (1997) and Leibowitz (2005) found that females with disabilities rarely receive sex education. This is because many such classes are offered as part of gym class where they have likely been excused, and due to the belief that "no one is going to marry them anyway" (p. 119). Hwang also noted that in a society where women are judged on their beauty and desirability, many women with disabilities are excluded in matters involving sexual relationships. On the other hand, men with SCI often experience problems with erectile dysfunction (DeForge et al., 2006), concerns regarding sexual satisfaction and self-image (Kedde & van Berlo, 2006; Mendes, Cardoso, & Savall, 2008), and issues relating to their adjustment to changes in sexual functioning (Burns, Mahalik, Hough, & Greenwall, 2008).

The purpose of this chapter is to identify some of the myths associated with SCI regarding male and female sexuality, to briefly explore the physiological and psychosocial implications of male and female sexuality for persons with an SCI, to summarize current models used to successfully work with men and women with SCI, and to provide a framework for counselors in identifying and addressing sexuality concerns among men and women with SCI.

SEXUALITY DEFINED

Sexuality is often difficult to define because of its different and sometimes incomplete or conflicting definitions. According to Lemon (1993), sexuality involves body image, self-esteem, social reactions, myths, feelings, and interpersonal relationships. Lefebvre (1997)

From "Female sexuality and spinal cord injury: Counseling implications," by E. Miller and I. Marini, 2004, *Journal of Applied Rehabilitation Counseling, 35(4)*, 17–25. Reprinted with permission from *Journal of Applied Rehabilitation Counseling.*

defined sexuality as verbal, visual, tactual, and olfactory communication that expresses intimacy and love. Medlar (1998) views sexuality as a natural and healthy part of living that encompasses physical, spiritual, emotional, and psychological dimensions that include one's sense of worth, desirability, and ability to give and receive love and affection within personal relationships. Unfortunately, the belief that people with disabilities are sexual and have sexual feelings and drives is frequently overlooked or ignored. Instead, they are often stereotyped as being asexual; lacking the same desire for sexual relationships as able-bodied persons (Sipski & Alexander, 1997). Women with disabilities are especially at risk for negative biases by others about their sexuality, and rehabilitation counselors and other human service professionals are not necessarily exempt from these attitudes.

SEXUALITY AND WOMEN WITH SCI

Sexuality among women with SCI was essentially ignored until the 1990s, and what little research does exist has often been a reflection of societal bias and is frequently limited to reproductive issues instead of areas such as sexual response, activity, and satisfaction (Moin, Durdevany, & Mazor, 2009; Nosek & Hughes, 2003; Sipski & Alexander, 1995a). For example, according to Basson (1998), common beliefs in Western society about female sexuality and disability are that only independently functioning women can handle sexual relationships, women with physical disabilities who are single are celibate, all women with physical disabilities are heterosexual, and women with physical disabilities should be grateful for sexual relationships. This notion is well illustrated by the fact that women typically experience pressure to have the "perfect" body and to adhere to their gender role, which includes a traditional, heterosexual marriage complete with children and possibly a job (Hwang, 1997; Livneh, 1991). According to Chenoweth (1993), it is because of these types of beliefs and attitudes that women with disabilities experience a "double strike," that is, being a woman and being disabled.

Limited education on the topic and phallocentric thinking (i.e., attitudes that a woman's sexuality exists only in relationship to her ability to satisfy her husband's needs) have also contributed to the lack of research on female sexuality and SCI. For example, Nosek et al. (1995) maintain that many adult women with physical disabilities lack basic knowledge of their reproductive health. In addition, women with disabilities are given Pap smear tests less frequently than able-bodied women due in part to the inaccessibility of gynecologists' offices and due to the assumption that they are asexual (Chance, 2002). Charlifue, Gerhart, Menter, Whiteneck, and Manley (1992) found that women with disabilities were generally satisfied with their postinjury sexual activities but reported a greater need for peer support, information, and counseling. Moin et al. (2009) found that women with physical disabilities (e.g., SCI) had the same sexual needs and desires as able-bodied women, yet their body image and sexual self-esteem were significantly lower. It has also been noted that even though it is essential that rehabilitation counseling students and seasoned counselors receive adequate training on the impact of disability on sexuality issues, this is often a low priority and virtually no literature dealing with this topic is available (Boyle, 1994).

SEXUALITY AND MALES WITH SCI

According to the National Spinal Cord Injury Statistical Center (2011), the number of people in the United States with SCI has been estimated to be approximately 265,000 persons, with males comprising 81% of these individuals. Following SCI, men frequently experience significant changes in their sexual functioning and are at increased risk for adjustment difficulties. Male sexual potency emphasizes the importance of male sexuality as a major indicator of masculinity and, from an early age, boys typically learn that men initiate sexual activity. Accordingly, for some males living with SCI, sexual dysfunction is associated with feelings of despair (Burns et al., 2008). In addition, the degree to which men adhere to masculine norms emphasizing sexual prowess may contribute to their adjustment to changes in sexual functioning following SCI. For example, Burns, Hough, Boyd, and Hill (2009) found that men with SCI who endorsed high levels of sexual desire had high rates of depression when they strongly adhered to traditional masculine norms for sexual prowess. This suggests that despite their strong interest in sexual activity, the injury-related performance difficulties males experience may undermine their sense of themselves as being masculine, possibly precipitating depression.

Sexual well-being among men with SCI has also been associated with age of onset, relationship status, and care dependency (Kedde & van Berlo, 2006); psychoeducation regarding SCI (Hess, Hough, & Tammoro, 2007); the degree of physiological impairment (Hvarness, Jakobsen, & Biering-Sorensen, 2007); and counselor attitudes and training relating to SCI (Kendall, Booth, Fronek, Miller, & Geraghty, 2003). It is also important to note that not all males with SCI report dissatisfaction with their sexuality.

COMMON MYTHS

Despite medical advances and the feminist movement that has challenged stereotypical female roles, numerous myths regarding men and women with SCI and their sexuality are still in existence. According to Tepper, Whipple, Richards, and Komisaruk (2001), accepted myths of the medical literature are that female sexuality is passive, that it is easier for a woman with an SCI to adapt to sexual changes than it is for a male, and that a loss of sexual functioning is less threatening to a woman than it is to a male. Farrow (1990) noted that individuals with SCI are assumed to be incapable, uninterested, or inactive sexually. Olkin (1999) cited several myths, including the most common one that persons with disabilities are asexual or lacking in basic sex drive. Other myths she described involve persons with physical disabilities being functionally incapable of having intercourse and not possessing the social skills and judgment to behave in a sexually appropriate manner (attributed to what Olkin believes is the result of the "spread effect"). Still another myth is that no able-bodied person will find someone with a disability desirable as a sex partner and, if they do, it is because the able-bodied person is "settling" or there is something wrong with them (Olkin, 1999).

Other commonly held myths by persons with SCI as well as significant others and the general public are that sex means intercourse, that sexual performance equals love, that sexual activity is natural and spontaneous, and that masturbation is sinful (Lemon, 1993). In addition, although the need to address sex and sexuality as a component of a holistic approach to the total rehabilitation process for men and women with SCI has been identified for over decades, little has been done to formally educate rehabilitation counselors in these areas. Instead, counselors are often forced to learn about human sexuality and disability through vicarious experiences and may subsequently feel unprepared or uncomfortable in discussing the issue of sexuality with their clients. Burling, Tarvydas, and Maki (1994) noted that some of the most common fears and misconceptions among counselors are that they believe sexuality is beyond the purview of their care, sexuality is not an appropriate area of concern for clients, and that if clients were interested or concerned about their sexuality, they would ask questions. Parritt and O'Callaghan (2000) found that counselors reported feeling anxious about raising the issue of sexuality with clients with disabilities because they feared they might upset the clients, they felt a sense of unknowing embarrassment about what people with disabilities do sexually, and they felt a need for safety in the therapeutic relationship prior to talking about disability and sex.

PHYSIOLOGICAL EFFECTS OF SCI ON WOMEN AND SEXUALITY

The level and degree of injury must be known in order to understand the implications of SCI on a person's sexual functioning. Tetraplegia refers to partial or permanent paralysis and potential loss or partial sensation in all four limbs, whereas paraplegia is indicative of partial or permanent paralysis and probable loss or dull sensation in only the lower extremities. The specific level of injury is determined by motor strength and sensory function at specific points and is defined as the last "normal" neurologic level of both motor and sensory functions (Crewe & Krause, 2002). Injuries are also classified as complete or incomplete, depending on nerve fiber damage. The injury can also affect multiple organ systems, including diminished respiratory capacity, alterations in skin integrity, and bowel and bladder function (Sipski & Alexander, 1995a).

Genitalia are almost invariably affected by SCI. For some, sensation may be altered or limited while others may experience complete loss of sensation in that part of the body. Sipski and Alexander (1995a) reported that vaginal lubrication and the ability to achieve orgasm after SCI is maintained by many women, albeit with more difficulty and altered orgasmic quality for some women. Sipski and Alexander (1995b) also found that women with SCI had the capacity to achieve orgasm approximately 50% of the time, regardless of whether they had complete or incomplete SCI.

In addition, the authors found that females with SCI preferred some type of genital stimulation to achieve orgasm and those able to achieve orgasm scored higher on measures of sexual information and sexual drive than did female subjects who were aorgasmic. However, similar to men, women with SCI have reported decreased sexual satisfaction and decreased frequency of sexual activities following SCI (Leibowitz, 2005; Sipski, 1997).

One reason for women's dissatisfaction and reduced sexual activity is that although sexual intercourse is neither the only nor always the most satisfying sexual activity, it is the most common (Farrow, 1990). Other types of erotic stimulation that are preferred by many women following SCI have been reported to be hugging, kissing, and touching usually just above the level of injury (Farrow, 1990). Areas that may become highly sensitive to stimulation include the neck, ears, lips, breasts, and nipples. Cuddling and massaging can also be highly pleasurable for women with SCI. For those who do choose to engage in sexual intercourse, penile-vaginal penetration can be accomplished by people with SCI in a variety of positions limited only by an individual's abilities, muscle strength, and desire. The level and severity of the injury also affect sexual activities and women with paraplegia are usually able to engage in top, bottom, and side positions whereas women with tetraplegia will more than likely need to be supine with the partner on top (Farrow, 1990).

Another area of concern for women with SCI is the appropriate contraception method. Birth control pills are typically not recommended for women with SCI due to the danger of blood clots caused by the combination of estrogen and progesterone (Farrow, 1990). The use of a diaphragm may also present several problems for women with SCI, including the need for dexterity and the ability to grasp, which is needed for insertion. In addition, weakened pelvic muscles may not allow for the diaphragm to remain in place, and the diaphragm may become dislodged. An intrauterine device (IUD) that is inserted into the uterus by a physician has sometimes been thought to be the best contraception choice; however, complications include pelvic inflammation, the possibility of a tubal pregnancy, and the fact that the expulsion of an IUD can go undetected due to the loss of sensation in the pelvic area. Levonorgestrel implants that are surgically placed in the inner upper arm have been used as a long-term contraceptive method. Levonorgestrel is a medication that does not have estrogen and requires no hand manipulation, making it appropriate for some women with SCI (Sipski, 1997). The combination spermicidal foam and condoms is one alternative that has been shown to be highly effective for women with SCI as this method does not require manual dexterity but can be used successfully for women with tetraplegia if their partner is willing to insert the foam and apply the condom. Sterilization of the male (vasectomy) or the female (tubal ligation) eliminates all worry about contraception, but serious consideration regarding this method of birth control is highly recommended since both procedures are usually permanent and irreversible (Farrow, 1990).

Although many women with SCI stop menstruating for several months postinjury, most are able to conceive and give birth. Unfortunately, most health care professionals including nurses and mental health counselors are unaware of how pregnancy affects physical disabilities (Lipson & Rogers, 2000). For those women who do become pregnant, it is important that their obstetricians are aware of the potential complications associated with pregnancy. Some of the more prevalent complications include anemia, problems with transfers due to weight gain, urinary tract infections, pressure sores, and, more significantly, autonomic dysreflexia (an abnormal reflex), which frequently occurs during labor in women with injuries above the T6 vertebral level (Sipski, 1997). Pregnant women with SCI may also benefit from being hospitalized for a short time prior to their due date if they lack sensation in the abdominal or pelvic area.

PHYSIOLOGICAL EFFECTS OF SCI ON MEN

Hess et al. (2007) conducted a study among males with paraplegia between the ages of 35–55 to assess the degree to which they believed their knowledge deficits interfered with their sexual performance. Although none of the participants reported a lack of sexual knowledge at the onset of the study, all indicated they were dissatisfied with their sexual functioning. Fifty percent of the participants reported a moderate improvement in their sexual function when taking an oral prescription of sildenafil, underscoring the benefits of including medication to enhance sexual performance.

Alexander et al. (2007) identified two primary elements of sexual functioning in males with SCI: male sexual response and male reproductive function. In terms of sexual response, males typically have two types of erections: psychogenic erections and reflex erections. The brain is the source of psychogenic erections. The process begins with sexual thoughts or seeing or hearing something stimulating or arousing. Signals from the brain are then sent through the nerves of the spinal cord down to the T10-L2 levels. The signals are then relayed to the penis and trigger an erection. A reflex erection occurs with direct physical contact to the penis or other erotic areas such as the ears, nipples, or neck. A reflex erection is involuntary and can occur without sexually stimulating thoughts. The nerves that control a man's ability to have a reflex erection are located in the sacral nerves (S2-S4) of the spinal cord. For men with SCI, the ability to have a psychogenic erection depends on the level and extent (complete or incomplete) of injury. Generally, men with low-level incomplete injuries are more likely to have psychogenic erections than men with higher level incomplete injuries. Men with complete injuries are less likely to experience psychogenic erections. However, most men with SCI are able to have a reflex erection with physical stimulation regardless of the extent of the injury if the S2-S4 nerve pathways are not damaged. Because each SCI is different, the impact of injury on sexual function can also differ. As such, treatment methods for erectile dysfunction vary and include oral medications such as sildenafil, tadalafil, and vardenafil HCI. For males who do not benefit from oral medications, penile injection therapy can be used and involves injecting a single drug or a combination of drugs into the side of the penis. This produces a hard erection that can last for 1–2 hours.

The possibility for men to father children has changed drastically in the past 20 years (Alexander et al., 2007). According to the Spinal Cord Injury Information Network (SCIIN, 2007), ejaculation problems are the primary issues to be resolved for men who want to become fathers. Approximately 90% of men with SCI experience anejaculation, which is an inability of men to ejaculate on their own during intercourse. Another potential problem is retrograde ejaculation, which is a condition wherein semen is deposited in the bladder instead of exiting the body through the urethra. Poor semen quality can also make it very difficult for men with SCI to fertilize the egg. Men with SCI make normal numbers of sperm, but the average number of motile sperm in semen from men with SCI is 20% compared to 70% in men in the general population. It is unknown why there is abnormally low sperm motility, but it does not appear to be related to level of injury, age, years postinjury, or frequency of ejaculation.

Because of problems with ejaculation, most men with SCI must rely on alternative techniques to achieve parenthood. The SCIIN (2007) reports that penile vibratory stimulation (PVS) can be used to achieve an erection, but its main purpose is to produce an ejaculate for those who wish to become fathers. A variety of vibrators/massagers are also available for this purpose. Some of these devices are specifically designed with the output power required to induce ejaculation in men with SCI. Estimations are that 55% of all men with SCI can respond to a high-amplitude vibrator, and 80% will respond if their injuries are above T10. PVS is usually recommended as a first treatment option because of the low investment of time and money. Although research (SCIIN, 2007) suggests that the better quality semen is obtained with PVS, Rectal Probe Electroejaculation (RPE) is an option if PVS is not successful. In RPE, a doctor inserts an electrical stimulation probe into the rectum and the controlled electrical stimulation produces an ejaculation. When sperm cannot be retrieved using PVS or RPE, minor surgery can be performed to remove sperm from the testicle. Collected sperm are subsequently used in artificial insemination techniques.

PSYCHOSOCIAL ASPECTS OF SCI AND SEXUALITY

Body image is an important aspect of a person's overall self-concept and self-esteem, especially in America where the emphasis on a "beautiful body" is more apparent than in any other society (Livneh, 1991). The relationship between body satisfaction and self-satisfaction is particularly strong among females, because of the emphasis our society places on attractiveness as an indicator of female worth. For women with SCI, body image and understanding one's self may be significantly impacted by the SCI, either directly or indirectly. Despite the emphasis Western society places on physique, Wright (1983) noted how adjustment to disability may be enhanced when individuals subordinate or deemphasize their worth based on their physique and instead begin to measure self-worth more on other personal attributes such as ones personality, intellect, or skills.

Men and women with SCI may also experience a sense of dependence and vulnerability because of limited financial resources, limited vocational opportunities, lack of social supports, and an increased need for personal assistance (Tate & Forchheimer, 2001). Other secondary conditions that may affect women with SCI include mobility and accessibility concerns, pain, spasticity, fatigue, muscle atrophy and body weight issues, concerns about developing romantic relationships, isolation, and depression (Nosek, 2000; Nosek & Hughes,

2003). Nevertheless, why some persons adapt to their SCI with relative ease while others struggle in their ability to understand and adjust to SCI continues to interest researchers (Janoff-Bulman, 2004; Tedeschi and Calhoun, 1995). Wright (1983) believed that some persons with disabilities adapt better than others due to cognitive changes in their values. Specifically, persons who are able to minimize focusing on their losses or what they no longer can do and begin focusing on their remaining assets, goals, interests, and abilities (enlarging one's scope of values) will typically respond better to their disability. In addition, restructuring comparative status values into asset values (e.g., believing a wheelchair helps with mobility rather than it is not better than walking) also can assist in adjustment.

Mona et al. (2000) examined a number of cognitive variables relating to sexuality among men and women with SCIs who were at least 2 years postinjury with varying degrees of severity. The factors assessed included levels of optimism about themselves and their situation, locus of control, self-esteem, and their purpose and meaning in life. The authors found that in addition to lower severity of injury, sexual adjustment was positively correlated with an internal locus of control, an optimistic outlook, having found a sense of meaning in one's life, and high self-esteem. However, beyond the cognitive constructs identified above, sexual self-esteem was found to be the best predictor of sexual adjustment in both men and women with SCI. In another study designed to assess qualitative sexual experiences of women with complete SCIs between levels T6 and T12, Tepper et al. (2001) found a number of variables to be related to levels of sexual adjustment. For example, women who acquired their disability later in life reported lower sexual self-esteem than women who acquired their disability early in life or at birth. The authors also found that cognitive-genital dissociation or the "shutting down" of one's sexuality based on the assumption that sexual pleasure was no longer possible because of absence of sensation in the genitals was common among the women surveyed. Instead, women tended to focus their energy on physical and vocational rehabilitation, bowel and bladder management, and other activities of daily living, with sex being a relatively low priority during the first few months postinjury. A lack of or inadequate sexuality education and counseling as well as asexual attitudes toward people with disabilities, concerns about body image, and negative feedback regarding sexuality from health professionals left many women in the study feeling as if they were no longer sexually desirable. However, with time (several months to years) and experience (e.g., ability to communicate sexual needs and desires and an increasing sense of value as a human being), women became more comfortable with their sexuality and developed improved sexual self-esteem (Tepper et al., 2001).

Westgren and Levi (1999) found that preinjury sexual behavior, positive attitudes toward sexuality, good communication skills, and perceived locus of control were better predictors of sexual adaptation than were age, extent of injury, and time since injury. It has also been suggested that sexual attitudes of people with SCI are more liberal than those of the general public but that females with SCI are far less experimental than males when it comes to engaging in untraditional sexual techniques (Westgren & Levi, 1999). Some of the reasons for their reticence include feeling unattractive, inadequate, and undesirable; lack of knowledge about techniques that can be used to make sexual activity a satisfying experience; and inhibitions about initiating alternative sexual techniques.

Kedde and van Berlo (2006) examined sexual satisfaction and sexual self-image among persons with SCI and other physical disabilities and found that men with late-onset disabilities showed lower levels of sexual satisfaction and body esteem than those with congenital disabilities. Although dependency issues had only a minor effect on males, lack of psychological well-being and feelings of helplessness were significantly correlated with their sexual and body esteem. However, age of onset of disability had no significant effect on women, suggesting that men with late-onset SCI and other physical disabilities may experience more adjustment problems than women with similar disabilities. Interestingly, the severity of injury did not have a great effect on sexual satisfaction and sexual self-esteem in men.

As with women with SCI, whether a man is in a romantic relationship can also influence his adjustment to his disability. There is also some consistency across the literature which maintains that relationships that begin after a SCI are more stable than those that begin preinjury (Ostrander, 2009). Other issues which can positively influence males' adjustment to SCI and their sexuality include having an internal locus of control, feeling sexually fulfilled, a high level of education, and being gainfully employed (Ostrander). Additional barriers to being a male with SCI include a lack of adequate personal assistance, physical inaccessibility (e.g., lack of transportation), and, like women, the "body beautiful" doctrine is increasingly becoming an ordeal for men (Sakellariou, 2006).

TREATMENT

The Council on Rehabilitation Education curriculum guidelines do not require extensive training in sexuality issues; subsequently, few rehabilitation counselors are generally trained to address the "specific skills" area of sexuality among persons with disabilities. There is no reason, however, why counselors cannot be minimally prepared to grant permission to discuss and provide limited information about sexuality issues. When clients learn to trust their counselor and rapport has been developed, any question or topic may become open for discussion if the client or counselor feels comfortable and conveys this to each other.

There are a number of methods which have been successfully used to assist persons with disabilities in overcoming sexuality issues. It is important to plan and provide opportunities for clients with SCI to discuss their sexual concerns because some individuals may feel uncomfortable to request sexually-related information for fear of being rejected or embarrassed. Although treatment models for decreased sexual desires, arousal disorders, and the inability to have orgasms have not been standardized for persons with SCI, sex therapy techniques similar to those used in the nondisabled population may be appropriate for women with SCI (Sipski, 1997).

One model that is currently being used with people with SCI is the PLISSIT model of sex therapy (Lemon, 1993). This model allows professionals to participate in therapy according to their level of skill, knowledge, and comfort. The aim of this model is to give an individual the permission to discuss sexual issues through counselor body language and verbalizations (P); to provide limited information about anatomy and physiology, dispelling myths, and prevention of STDs (LI); to provide women with SCI with specific suggestions regarding sexual expression, functioning with the disability, relationships, and satisfying a partner (SS); and to provide intensive therapy (IT) including medical procedures, counseling, fertility, childbirth, and hormonal imbalances. For clients with SCI, considerations might include physical appearance (e.g., wheelchair color, clothing choices), catheterization, drinking habits, sensation level and pain, lubrication methods, transferring, sexual positioning, spasticity, and learning how to identify areas of the relationship that may affect one's sexuality (e.g., role reversal). Cognitive restructuring is also used to help clients identify and change maladaptive ways of viewing their disability and sexuality-related issues.

Sensate focus exercises can also be used by counselors to help individuals and their partners identify residual sexual functioning and enhance the couples' repertoire of sexual and sensual behaviors (Lemon, 1993). Sensate focus is based on cognitive-behavioral theory aimed at minimizing anxiety performance while increasing intimacy behaviors and is considered IT. After discussing specific sexual behaviors and cognitions couples are experiencing difficulties with (e.g., low sex desire), homework assignments designed to gradually heighten sensory or tactile awareness or foreplay as well as improved verbal and nonverbal communication techniques are practiced. When giving homework assignments, it is important for counselors to describe in detail the activity that is required, the rationale for the activity, and then to suggest problem-solving exploration to determine barriers they encounter in carrying out the assignment. For example, a woman with an SCI with little sensation in the genital area might be counseled with her partner to have him focus more on caressing and/or kissing her neck, ears, breasts, and other areas where she has more sensation.

Using sensate focus, couples are initially given a form that is used to record specific types of sexual activity and whether the activity was pleasant and arousing. Additional exercises include visual exploration in which clients are instructed to spend approximately 30 minutes looking at their bodies with and without clothing, exploring their bodies using tactile exploration exercises, full body caresses to be completed alone or with a partner, and eventually coital activity (Lemon, 1993). Couples are continually encouraged to discuss with each other and the counselor how they feel about their sexuality, to pinpoint areas where sensation might remain, and to explore ways to enhance verbal and nonverbal communication.

The lack of training and reported discomfort of health care and rehabilitation professionals in dealing with SCI and sexuality has made the use of sexually explicit videos another attractive teaching model (Gill, 1988). Gill found that although 79% of rehabilitation professionals reported sexual adjustment was important to clients in rehabilitation, only 9% of the staff indicted feeling comfortable and having the expertise to discuss sexual issues. The use of videos and other sexually explicit materials for follow-up discussions is to communicate information and to develop more accepting attitudes about sexuality-related issues. However, caution must be used with this type of teaching because of the potential for graphic sexual images that may shock, embarrass, disgust, upset, and even block learning (Tepper, 1997). In order to avoid negative repercussions, Tepper has suggested that the videos be shown in a carefully planned sequence with time for discussion that is led by a knowledgeable and skilled facilitator.

Finally, it must be recognized that people with disabilities often internalize prevalent societal stereotypes about the nature of sexuality and disabilities and it may be difficult for them to develop a positive sexual self-concept when surrounded by negative messages about sexuality and attractiveness (Chance, 2002). Counselors must also feel comfortable with their own sexuality and must be willing to explore their attitudes and beliefs about sexuality as they relate to persons with disabilities in order to better understand how they may actually discourage client disclosure involving sexual relationships because of some of their own "hang-ups" about the subject. For example, Parritt and O'Callaghan (2000) found that therapists working with clients with disabilities thought that male partners of women with disabilities were likely to seek sex outside the relationship, they saw clients as being dependent, and they perceived clients' sexuality as "different" from that of able-bodied people. It is these types of stereotypical beliefs and attitudes that often raise doubts among people with disabilities, leaving them to question their sexuality by asking themselves "Am I normal?" and "Will I ever be normal again?" These attitudes can also lead to the exclusion of any type of discussions on sexuality-related issues during the rehabilitation process. Northcott and Chard (2000) found that although 86% of the participants in their study said their disability affected their sexual functioning, only 29% of the participants had received any formal advice or sex education from health professionals such as nurses or psychologists.

A FRAMEWORK FOR IDENTIFYING AND TREATING
SEXUALITY ISSUES IN WOMEN WITH SCI

In assisting rehabilitation counselors in better understanding the dynamics of sexuality and disability, the following five-component framework adapted from Vash (1981) is offered to help delineate specific sexuality concerns of women with SCI. Examples are provided when necessary with counseling suggestions. The five areas described below are sequentially outlined; however, they often overlap when social interaction progresses to sexual intimacy on the first date or soon thereafter.

Physical Appearance

Unless first meeting over the Internet (which is gaining wider acceptance), an individual's personal appearance is the first aspect with which he or she is evaluated. Western society places a high value on physical attractiveness (Livneh, 1991; Marini, 1994; Roessler & Bolton, 1978), and women with SCI as well as other persons with disabilities are generally not perceived or portrayed by the public or media in this manner. These first impression interactions are solely based on appearance and often dictate whether a relationship will be established.

Aside from the customary beautification techniques women use to enhance appearance (e.g., hygiene, dress, make-up), women with SCI have additional factors to consider. Since a wheelchair is typically viewed as an accessory or extension of the individual, model and color become important considerations. Today, there are literally hundreds of wheelchair designs and colors to choose from. Women with SCI must consider functional use versus design. In addition, although a number of feminine colors exist today, how these colors coordinate or clash with most clothing colors should be considered. Finally, a number of manual and electric standing wheelchairs allow individuals with SCI to stand if they choose. Standing not only impacts the quality of social interactions, but also may have a positive psychological affect on one's self-esteem in avoiding instances of being looked down at.

A second consideration of physical appearance pertains to physique. In most instances, the passage of time generally atrophies legs and other paralyzed muscles in persons with SCI. Current technology involving functional electrical stimulation of the legs on stationary bikes has successfully demonstrated how muscle mass may be maintained. Conversely, the sedentary lifestyle makes weight gain more problematic; therefore, women with SCI can be encouraged to exercise whatever remaining muscle groups are left as well as adhere to a balanced diet approved by their physician and/or nutritionist. A number of exercise equipment options are available for persons with SCI including nautilus, hand cycles, and sports wheelchairs. Overall, the central question for counselors and clients in this area is "How can physical appearance be enhanced?"

Personality and Behavioral Traits

This component involves social skills such as being a good listener, appropriate eye contact, and personality traits. Counselors can assess these traits through direct observation or by utilizing psychometric tests measuring personality. For women with SCI and others with similar disabilities, it is important that they do not monopolize the conversation about their disability, how it occurred, or complications extending from it. Sagatun (1985) found, however, that when disabled and nondisabled viewers watched six different videotaped interactions between a person using a wheelchair and a person with no disability, viewers without a disability preferred the interaction where the wheelchair user acknowledged his or her disability after initiating first contact. Viewers with a disability, however, preferred the interaction where the nondisabled individual asked about the disability and initiated first contact. Although persons without disabilities liked the idea of the wheelchair user mentioning the disability to "get it out of the way," viewers with disabilities disliked this approach because they perceived that mentioning their disability did not seem to flow in the general conversation. This suggests that there is a happy medium whereby briefly acknowledging one's disability appears advantageous as it serves to place nondisabled persons at ease, but dwelling on the topic can backfire and lead to what Roessler and Bolton (1978) call "prejudice inviting behavior."

Yuker (1988) analyzed the results of 318 interactions from 274 studies on interaction effects and found that attitudes toward persons with disabilities were rated more positively when these individuals were perceived as being competent, possessing good social and communication skills, and were willing to discuss their disability unemotionally. Additional well documented personality traits such as a sense of humor, extraversion, and social poise also correlated highly with positive attitude change (Yuker, 1988).

Courtship Factors

What important factors need to be considered when women with SCI begin dating? Having similar interests is a concern for everyone; however, noting probable physical limitations often precludes women with SCI from engaging in certain recreational activities such as tennis, skiing, racquetball, jogging or walking, cycling, hiking, and other similar sports. Nonetheless, women with low-level paraplegia may still be able to participate to some degree in games such as tennis, skiing (with modifications), and racquetball. In addition, assistive technology over the past decade has changed the landscape toward much greater participation possibilities in sports or recreational activities for all persons with a SCI. Today, people with low-level cervical SCI and below, with and without modified equipment, can actively participate in scuba diving, basketball, skiing, ice hockey, weightlifting, hunting, swimming, cycling, fishing, boating, billiards, and other sports.

Aside from the more physically involved leisure activities, women with SCI have a variety of other dating alternatives available to them as well. Counselors should assist women with SCI to develop a list of potential activities that they can pursue with their partner. The less demanding ones may include going to a movie, attending theater productions or concerts, going out to dinner, visiting bookstores and coffee shops, attending social gatherings, playing board or card games, and taking a walk or wheel. These activities may be especially appropriate for women with high-level cervical SCI.

Available technology and legislation such as the Americans with Disabilities Act (ADA) allows persons with SCI to ski, skate, bowl, hand cycle (for low-level SCI and below, synonymous with bicycling), fish (likely offshore or on a pontoon boat), stand erect, enter or exit a swimming pool, transfer to or from a car or other vehicle, and play billiards. Titles II and III of the ADA have had a significant impact on removing barriers to socialization for persons with disabilities. Any public place, event or activity such as restaurants, theaters, parks, sporting facilities, hotels, transportation, and other publicly used facilities or services must be accessible to persons with disabilities. In short, there should be a number of options to choose from regarding possible dating ideas for women with all levels of SCI. Nevertheless, it is still a good idea to call ahead to verify accessibility since there continue to be certain businesses that have not complied with the ADA (Blackwell, Marini, & Chacon, 2001). In cases where two wheelchair users are dating, additional factors must be considered regarding transportation issues, transferring, seating arrangements in certain instances, and the need for personal assistance.

Finally, due to the recent proliferation of online dating services, chat rooms, and basic internet or e-mail capabilities, women with SCI and other disabilities can become better acquainted with a potential partner and strategically decide at what point and in what way to convey having a disability. Counselors can assist clients in determining possible ways to convey this information. Nevertheless, Internet relationships established online initially work to minimize the superficial aspects of physical appearance and allow for greater intellectual intimacy to occur beforehand.

Sexual Encounter

This component of the relationship may arguably be the most difficult to explore for women with SCI. Concerns relating to body image, physical positioning, sexual self-confidence or performance issues, sensation level, myths and misconceptions about sex, bladder and bowel function, and spontaneity should be discussed. Vash (1981) noted how a perceived or actual altered body image (e.g., atrophied legs) may lead the individual with a disability to fear possible rejection once a potential mate sees them unclothed. Societal pressures regarding the perfect body are perhaps nowhere more crucial than during sex (Livneh, 1991; Vash, 1981).

Physical positioning will generally not be problematic for women with low-level SCI (e.g., T4 and below) who will most likely be able to engage in most any position unless experiencing problems with excessive weight, pain, severe muscle spasms or strength limitations (Farrow, 1990). Those with cervical or high-level thoracic SCI, however, may be limited largely to the missionary position unless physically maneuvered by an able-bodied partner or personal attendant. Relatedly, although giving oral sex to an able-bodied partner might be accomplished fairly spontaneously depending on the circumstances, sexual intercourse itself will be less spontaneous in most instances and may negatively affect immediate gratification desires.

As previously noted, intercourse will, in most cases of higher level SCI, be less spontaneous when transfers are involved or if catheterization and/or ostomy devices must be removed (Sipski & Alexander, 1995a; Tepper et al., 2001). Again, some women with SCI may fear ultimate rejection and possibly prolong or put off sexual advances by a partner for this reason. Counselors should discuss the intricacies of such issues and brainstorm ideas with their client in addressing these concerns. In addition, dispelling the myths of Hollywood movie sex (e.g., simultaneous partner orgasm, multiple orgasms) becomes important to minimizing performance anxiety. When both partners are wheelchair users and if one or both partners have a cervical SCI, the need for a personal assistant(s) or a third-party to assist in transferring, undressing, and positioning will be necessary. Unless both partners have previously discussed this alternative and negotiated this desire with a personal assistant, the encounter will be awkward at best.

Intimacy

The longevity of any intimate relationship involves much more than sexual compatibility. Partners must be able to communicate with one another as well as emotionally support each other (Sipski & Alexander, 1997; Vash, 1981). Basic marital tips generally recommended to other couples also apply here. What becomes different when having a long-term relationship with someone with an SCI depends on the severity of the injury and the need for personal assistance to carry out activities of daily living. When a partner becomes a primary caregiver (often due to financial constraints), the couple must be aware of potential caregiver burnout and role conflict between being a partner or lover and being a caregiver (McNeff, 1997). McNeff further noted that couples should establish boundaries as to what kinds of caregiving will be provided by the partner versus what type of assistance might best be provided by a personal attendant (e.g., bowel and bladder care).

Crewe and Krause (1988) found that couples who married after the onset of disability reported greater satisfaction with their sex lives, living arrangements, social lives, and emotional adjustment; whereas those already married when SCI occurred reported greater stress primarily caused by resentment and resignation. Crewe (1993) discussed role reversal in able-disabled partner relationships. For women with SCI, the role of mother, nurturer, and homemaker, albeit a gender stereotype, may affect the capacity to fulfill these roles either in part or wholly. Being unable to perform one or more of these gender roles can also diminish a woman's sense of self-worth (Rolland, 1994).

Generally speaking, there may be numerous sexuality-related concerns for persons with SCI and other disabilities. For women with SCI, common concerns will include physical appearance, dating ideas, social interaction skills from a wheelchair, sexual intimacy, and long-term issues such as motherhood, employment, and caregiving. By utilizing the five-component framework, counselors can assess specific issues the clients are experiencing to assist them in areas such as attracting potential mates, dating, and establishing a long-term relationship.

SUMMARY AND CONCLUSIONS

Despite the fact that most research on sexuality and SCI has been narrow in focus and has traditionally focused on males, developing an understanding of some of the physical and psychosocial factors associated with female sexuality and SCI can have a tremendous impact on their ability to establish and maintain intimate relationships. Dispelling some of the common myths regarding SCI and female sexuality can also have a major impact on how women with SCI perceive themselves in terms of their attractiveness and desirability.

Treatment models that emphasize the importance of providing information to individuals with SCI about their sexuality and facilitating heightened sensory awareness and improved verbal and nonverbal communication among couples have been especially helpful for assisting females in understanding overcoming their sexual reservations. The five-step counseling framework has also been shown to be an effective guide for counselors to use for assessing and treating specific client concerns regarding a woman's ability to attract, date, and develop a meaningful, romantic relationship. However, it should be noted that one of the most important counseling implications in the area of female sexuality and SCI is the counselor's ability to address sexuality-related issues in a manner that conveys to the client a level of comfort conducive to promoting opportunities for discussing a wide range of sexual topics and potential outcomes.

REFERENCES

Alexander, M.S., Bodner, D., Brackett, N.L., Elliot, S., Jackson, A.B., & Sonksen, J. (2007). Development of international standards to document sexual and reproductive functions after spinal cord injury: Preliminary report. *Journal of Rehabilitation Research & Development, 44*(1), 83–90.

Basson, R. (1998). Sexual health of women with disabilities. *Canadian Medical Association, 159*(4), 359–362.

Blackwell, T. M., Marini, I., & Chacon, M. (2001). The impact of the Americans with Disabilities Act on independent living. *Rehabilitation Education, 15*(4), 395–408.

Boyle, P. S. (1994). Rehabilitation counselors as providers: The issue of sexuality. *Journal of Applied Rehabilitation Counseling, 25*(1), 6–9.

Burling, K., Tarvydas, V. M., & Maki, D. R. (1994). Human sexuality and disability: A holistic interpretation of rehabilitation counseling. *Journal of Applied Rehabilitation Counseling, 25*(1), 10–16.

Burns, S. M., Hough, S., Boyd, B. I., & Hill, J. (2009). Sexual desire and depression following spinal cord injury: Masculine sexual prowess as a moderator. *Sex Roles, 61,* 120–129.

Burns, S. M., Mahalik, J. R., Hough, S., & Greenwall, A. N. (2008). Adjustment to changes in sexual functioning following spinal cord injury: The contribution of men's adherence to scripts for sexual potency. *Sexuality and Disability, 26,* 197–205.

Chance, R. S. (2002). To love and be loved: Sexuality and people with physical disabilities. *Journal of Psychology and Theology, 30*(3), 195–208.

Charlifue, S. W., Gerhart, K. A., Menter, R. R., Whiteneck, G. G., & Manley, M. S. (1992). Sexual issues of women with spinal cord injuries. *Paraplegia, 30,* 192–199.

Chenoweth, L. (1993). Invisible acts: Violence against women with disabilities. *Australian Disability Review, 2,* 22–28.

Crewe, N. M. (1993). Spousal relationships and disability. In F. P. Haseltine, S. S. Cole, & D. B. Gray (Eds.), *Reproductive issues for persons with physical disabilities.* Baltimore: Paul H. Brookes.

Crewe, N. M., & Krause, J. S. (1988). Marital relationships and spinal cord injury. *Archives of Physical Medicine and Rehabilitation, 69,* 435–438.

Crewe, N. M., & Krause, J. S. (2002). Spinal cord injuries. In M. G. Brodwin, F. Tellez, & S. K. Brodwin (Eds.), *Medical, psychosocial, and vocational aspects of disability* (pp. 279–291). Athens, GA: Elliott & Fitzpatrick, Inc.

DeForge, D., Blackmer, J., Garritty, C., Yazdi, F., Cronin, V., Barrowman, N., et.al. (2006). Male erectile dysfunction following spinal cord injury: A systematic review. *Spinal Cord, 44,* 465–473.

Farrow, J. (1990). Sexuality counseling with clients who have spinal cord injuries. *Rehabilitation Counseling Bulletin, 33*(3), 251–260.

Gill, K. M. (1988). Staff needs assessment data. Unpublished.

Hess, M. J., Hough, S., & Tammaro, E. (2007). The experience of four individuals with paraplegia enrolled in an outpatient interdisciplinary sexuality program. *Sexuality and Disability, 25,* 189–195.

Hvarness, H., Jakobsen, H., & Biering-Sorensen, F. (2007). Men with spinal cord injury have a smaller prostate than men without. *Scandinavian Journal of Urology and Nephrology, 41,* 120–123.

Hwang, K. (1997). Living with a disability: A woman's perspective. In M. L. Sispki & C. J. Alexander (Ed.), *Sexual function and people with disability and chronic illness: A health professionals guide* (pp. 3–12). Gaithersburg, MD: Aspen.

Janoff-Bulman, R. (2004). Posttraumatic growth: Three explanatory models. *Psychological Inquiry, 15*(1), 30–34.

Kedde, H., & van Berlo, W. (2006) Sexual satisfaction and sexual self-images of people with physical disabilities in the Netherlands. *Sexuality and Disability, 24*(1), 53–68.

Kendall, M., Booth, S., Fronek, P., Miller, D., & Geraghty, T. (2003). The development of a scale to assess the training needs of professionals in providing sexuality rehabilitation following spinal cord injury. *Sexuality and Disability, 21*(1), 49–64.

Lefebvre, K. A. (1997). Performing a sexual evaluation on the person with disability or illness. In M. L. Sipski & C. J. Alexander (Eds.), *Sexual function in people with disability and chronic illness* (pp. 19–45). Gaithersburg, MD: Aspen.

Leibowitz, R. Q. (2005). Sexual rehabilitation services after spinal cord injury: What do women want? *Sexuality and Disability, 23*(2), 81–107.

Lemon, M. A. (1993). Sexual counseling and spinal cord injury. *Sexuality and Disability, 11*(1), 73–97.

Lipson, J. G., & Rogers, J. G. (2000). Pregnancy, birth, and disability: Women's healthcare experiences. *Health Care for Women International, 21*(1), 1–11.

Livneh, H. (1991). On the origins of negative attitudes toward people with disabilities. In R. P. Marinelli, & A. E. Dell Orto (Eds.), *The psychological and social impact of disability* (3rd ed., pp. 181–196). New York: Springer.

Marini, I. (1994). Attitudes toward disability and the psychosocial implications for persons with SCI. *SCI Process 7*(4), 147–152.

McNeff, E. (1997). Issues for the partner of the person with disability. In M. L. Sipski & C. J. Alexander (Eds.), *Sexual function in people with disability and chronic illness* (pp. 19–45). Gaithersburg, MD: Aspen.

Medlar, T. (1998). The manual of policies and procedures of the SHIP sexuality education programme. *Sexuality and Disability, 16*(1), 21–42.

Mendes, A. K., Cardoso, F. L., & Savall, A. C. R. (2008). Sexual satisfaction in people with spinal cord injury. *Sexuality and Disability, 26,* 137–147.

Moin, V., Duvdevany, I., & Mazor, D. (2009). Sexual identity, body image, and life satisfaction among women with and without physical disability. *Sexuality and Disability, 27,* 83–95.

Mona, L. R., Krause, J. S., Norris, F. H., Cameron, R. P., Kalichrnan, S. C., & Lesondak, L. M. (2000). Sexual expression following spinal cord injury. *NeuroRehabilitation, 15,* 121–131.

National Spinal Cord Injury Statistical Center. (2011). Spinal cord injury facts and figures at a glance. Retrieved 24 April, 2011, from https://www.nscisc.uab.edu/public_content/pdf/Facts%202011%20 Feb%20Final.pdf (2011).

Northcott, R., & Chard, G. (2000). Sexual aspects of rehabilitation: The client's perspective. *British Journal of Occupational Therapy, 63*(9), 2-8.

Nosek, M. A. (2000). Overcoming the odds: The health of women with physical disabilities in the United States. *Archives of Physical Medicine and Rehabilitation, 81,* 135-138.

Nosek, M. A., & Hughes, R. B. (2003). Psychosocial issues of women with physical disabilities: The continuing gender debate. *Rehabilitation Counseling Bulletin, 46*(4), 224-233.

Nosek, M. A., Rintala, D. H., Young, M. E., Howland, C. A., Foley, C. D., & Chanpong, G. (1995). Sexual functioning among women with physical disabilities. *Archives of Physical Medicine and Rehabilitation, 7*(2), 107-115.

Olkin, R. (1999). *What psychotherapists should know about disability.* New York: Guilford Press.

Ostrander, N. (2009). Sexual pursuits of pleasure among men and women with spinal cord injuries. *Sexuality and Disability, 27,* 11-19.

Parritt, S., & O'Callaghan, J. (2000). Splitting the difference: An exploratory study of therapists' work with sexuality, relationships and disability. *Sexual Relationship Therapy, 15*(2), 151-169.

Roessler, R., & Bolton, B. (1978). *Psychosocial adjustment to disability.* Baltimore: University Park Press.

Rolland, J. (1994). In sickness and in health: The impact of illness on couples' relationships. *Journal of Marital and Family Therapy, 4*(20), 327-347.

Sagatun, I. J. (1985). The effects of acknowledging a disability and initiating contact on interaction between disabled and nondisabled persons. *The Social Science Journal, 22*(4), 33-43.

Sakellariou, D.(2006). If not disability, then what? Barriers to reclaiming sexuality following spinal cord injury. *Sexuality and Disability, 24,* 101-111.

Sipski, M. L. (1997). Sexuality and spinal cord injury: Where we are and where we are going. *American Rehabilitation, 23*(1), 26-29.

Sipski, M. L., & Alexander, C. J. (1995a). Spinal cord injury and female sexuality. *Annual Review of Sex Research, 6,* 224-244.

Sipski, M. L., & Alexander C. J. (1995b). Physiology parameters associated with psychogenic sexual arousal in women with complete spinal cord injuries. *Archives of Physical Medicine and Rehabilitation, 76,* 811-818.

Sipski, M. L., & Alexander, C. J. (1997). Impact of disability or chronic illness on sexual function. In M. L. Sispki & C. J. Alexander (Eds.), *Sexual function and people with disability and chronic illness: A health professionals guide* (pp. 3-12). Gaithersburg, MD: Aspen.

Spinal Cord Injury Information Network: Sexual function for men with spinal cord injury. Retrieved 16 June, 2011, from http://www.spinalcord.uab.edu/show.asp?durki=22405&print=yes (2007)

Tate, D. G., & Forchheimer, M. (2001). Health-related quality of life and life satisfaction for women with spinal cord injury. *Top Spinal Cord Injury Rehabilitation, 7*(1), 1-15.

Tedeschi, R. G., & Calhoun, L. G. (1995). *Trauma and transformation: Growing in the aftermath of suffering.* Thousand Oaks, CA: Sage.

Tepper, M. S. (1997). Use of sexually explicit films in the spinal cord injury rehabilitation process. *Sexuality and Disability, 15*(3), 167-181.

Tepper, M. S., Whipple, B., Richards, E., & Komisaruk, B. R. (2001). Women with complete spinal cord injury: A phenomenological study of sexual experiences. *Journal of Sex & Marital Therapy, 27,* 615-623.

Vash, C. L. (1981). *The psychology of disability.* New York: Springer.

Westgren, N., & Levi, R. (1999). Sexuality after injury: Interviews with women after traumatic spinal cord injury. *Sexuality and Disability, 17*(4), 309-319.

Wright, B. A. (1983). *Physical disability: A psychosocial approach.* New York: Harper & Row.

Yuker, H. E. (1988). *Attitudes toward persons with disabilities.* New York: Springer.

11

Cross-Cultural Counseling Issues of Males Who Sustain a Disability

IRMO MARINI

*T*he impact of a sudden traumatic disability to any individual can have profound implications in relation to his or her socialization, employment outlook, and basic independent functioning. Research pertaining to the psychosocial adjustment and reaction of persons who sustain an adventitious disability, such as spinal cord injury, often describe the individual as either going through certain stages of adjustment (Livneh, 1991; Shontz, 1975) or experiencing a continuous adaptation to the altered lifestyle (Kendall & Buys, 1998; Olkin, 1999).

For males from different ethnic and cultural backgrounds, the ramifications of their disability beliefs or schema, along with cultural beliefs regarding disability can significantly affect how they deal with their situations. Vash (1981) outlined the complexity of factors relating to one's reaction to disability. She identified four broad factors pertaining to *disability, person, culture, and environment*. Determiners relating to the *disability* include time of onset (acquired vs. congenital), type of onset (accident or self-inflicted), functions impaired, severity, visibility and stability of the disability, as well as the presence of pain. *Person* factors include gender, activities affected, interests/values/goals affected, remaining coping resources, personality variables, and spiritual beliefs. Factors relating to *culture* include community support, societal attitudes, social-political environment supporting disability issues and family dynamics. Finally, the factors relating to the *environment* pertain to physical barriers (curb cuts), accessible transportation, availability and cooperation from relevant support agencies.

Statistically, persons with disabilities remain the most disenfranchised population in virtually every society, no matter what their ethnicity. Over one-third of adults with disabilities in America have an annual income of $15,000 or less (Sue & Sue, 2003). Relatedly, the unemployment rate for persons with disabilities in the United States is estimated to be 65% (National Organization on Disability, 2004). Minorities with disabilities represent the least educated and the most poverty stricken and unemployed populous in most societies. Of the approximate 50 million persons with disabilities in the United States, over five million have no health insurance coverage (Olkin, 1999; Rubin & Roessler, 2008).

The focus of this chapter is to first provide a brief overview of key cultural differences among European Americans, Asian Americans, Latino or Hispanics, African Americans, and Native Americans. Next, the perceived masculinity of males is explored based on societal or cultural expectations. Third, an exploration of societal views toward disability is discussed,

From "Cross-cultural counseling issues of males who sustain a disability," by I. Marini, 2001, *Journal of Applied Rehabilitation Counseling,* 32, 36–44. Reprinted with permission of The National Rehabilitation Counseling Association.

noting cultural variations. Finally, implications for counselors who work with males with adventitious disabling injuries are outlined, focusing on specific counseling recommendations and talking points during sessions.

OVERVIEW OF CULTURAL DIFFERENCES AMONG ETHNIC GROUPS

A summary of fundamental cultural values and beliefs is presented to help distinguish perceptions toward disability in various cultures. Key characteristics of European American, Latino/Hispanic, Asian American, African American and Native American cultures are discussed. It cannot be overstated; however, that although this chapter discusses many commonalities between racial/ethnic groups, there are a multitude of specific individual differences (e.g., socioeconomic status, personality, upbringing) within groups, to where counselors should never assume that all persons of a particular group share similar cultural views as described here.

Latino/Hispanic perceptions of males or masculine traits somewhat overlap with those of Western society. In fact, the Latino/Hispanic family is somewhat more patriarchal with the wife deferring to the husband as the head of the household in first-generation homes. It is common in first-generation Latino/Hispanic families for the father to work while the mother remains home with the children (Locke, 1992; Garzon & Tan, 1992). The concept of "machismo" or male pride is prevalent among Latino/Hispanic males and unfortunately widely misunderstood (Anzaldua, 1987; Gonzalez, 1997 in Sue p. 294). Specifically, although machismo is generally misperceived as the tough, authoritarian, sometimes criminal type male, it actually describes a good-bad dichotomy of men. The good side of machismo is the proud, bread-winning, respectful, dignified, and family-responsible male who treats his family and the community with the utmost love and dedication (Anzaldua, 1987). Latino/Hispanic males who sustain a catastrophic disability are generally devastated if their ability to earn is compromised. Many continue to work if possible until they physically can no longer do so. Conversely, some Latino/Hispanic males view disability as a punishment from God, and believe that they must accept their fate in life, thus resigning themselves from participation in rehabilitation or attempts to alter their perceived fate (Rubin, Chung & Huang, 1998). Latinao belief in the supernatural and alternative medicine is also prominent. Puerto Ricans believe in espiritismo, Cubans in santiera, and Mexican Americans believe in curanderismo (Harris, Velasquez, White, & Renteria, 2004). Curanderismo is most widely believed since approximately 60% of this population living in the United States are of Mexican dissent. These healers or shamons are believed to have supernatural powers that include atonement, restoring balance, absolution for sinning, harmony through self-control, and spiritual healing. Spiritual healing can involve touching of the hands, prayer, massage and tea, especially, in treating emotional problems from supernatural causes such as fear and anxiety (susto), hexes (mal puesto), the evil eye (mal de ojo), and extreme jealousy (envidia) (Alegria, Guerra, Martinez, & Meyer, 1977).

Latino/Hispanic male role conflicts may occur if the male becomes disabled. Specifically, due to the expected role of being perceived as strong, feelings of isolation and depression may occur because many males perceive they cannot share their worries/anxieties with others, for fear of this being viewed as an additional sign of weakness. Role conflict will also likely occur if the male is unable to work and the wife has to become employed (Avila & Avila, 1995). In addition, regardless if a disability occurs in the family, the eldest daughter is expected to care for her siblings and/or ailing parents.

Asian Americans, similar to Latino/Hispanics, Native Americans, and African Americans are family oriented (collectivism), and view the needs of the family as more important than the needs of the individual (Rubin, Chung, & Huang, 1998). In the United States, there are 28 nationalities represented in the Asian American community, the largest of which includes Chinese, Filipinos, Japanese, Koreans, Asian Indians, and Vietnamese (U.S. Census Bureau, 1993). Traditional Chinese values embrace harmony with nature and society. This harmony constitutes a balance between the yin and yang; the two opposing forces in nature. Becoming sick or disabled is said to occur due to an imbalance between the yin and yang, often believed to be caused by God as punishment for having sinned (Lassiter, 1995). Family problems such as disability are viewed as having shamed or failed one's family, and all family members must bare the shame (Uba, 1994; Wong & Chan, 1994). Asian families tend to be secretive of family problems and often do not want to divulge the family shame. Asians also place a priority upon achievement; therefore, a disability which impedes one's ability to contribute to the family is again viewed as a devastating failure. Asian males are viewed as the head of the family power hierarchy, and the spouse is expected to take care of him, the children and the household. Asian males are the breadwinners and head of the household in Asian culture, commanding unquestionable loyalty and devotion from family members. This hierarchy follows the five Cardinal Relations rules of Confucianism (Chan, 1992). Overall, the fact that many Asian families believe disability is punishment for having sinned as well as the social stigma of failure, often leads the Asian family to keep the disability secret, and thus not actively seek out counseling (Sue & Sue, 1987). Asian, Latino/Hispanic, Native and African American family members also generally take care of all the disabled family member's needs, often creating unnecessary dependence and possibly learned helplessness.

Like all the other minority groups in the United States, Asian Americans have historically also been subjected to discrimination and anti-Asian sentiments (Chan, 1991; Choudhuri, 2009). As such, due to stories passed down from one generation to the other, distrust of Caucasian counselors or psychotherapists is not uncommon (Horsman, Rodriguez, & Marini, 2009). Asian Americans will often report physical symptoms of headaches or stomach problems in an effort to mask psychosomatic worries. Santos (2006) notes acculturative stress is especially exacerbated by post-traumatic stress for the Asian community who have left their country as refugees. Stories from Vietnamese, Cambodians, and Indochinese include imprisonment, physical and sexual assault, and death of family members (Mollica, Henderson, & Tor, 2002).

Among African Americans, religion is a highly valued priority. Research has indicated that for many African Americans, all people are believed to be God's children, including persons with disabilities. Studies indicate that the attitudes among African Americans toward persons with disabilities tend to be more positive than European Americans (Pickett, Vraniak, Cook, & Cohler, 1993; Rogers-Dulan & Blacker, 1995). Unlike Latino/Hispanic views, most African American men agree that a wife should work according to her desires (Smith, 1981). Alston, McCowen, and Turner (1994) note that it is this role flexibility in addition to access to extended family members (e.g., grandparents) in the African American household that allows for more successful adjustment when a disability occurs. This interdependence on one another, family role flexibility, and deep religious faith facilitate giving the family strength to adapt (Lee, Blando, Mizelle, & Orozco, 2007). It is not uncommon in African American culture for a family unit to be living with extended family, and, as with other minority groups, family comes first before individual desires.

Although many acculturated African Americans view all persons to be children of God, Jamaican culture generally sees disability as punishment for having sinned. Similarly, some Haitians view disability as personal failure bringing shame to oneself and one's family, and often ostracization by society. Some Haitians are afraid of persons with disabilities and believe they have been cursed by supernatural forces (Millington, 2011). Such beliefs can also lead to fears of contagion.

Some African Americans are also wary of Caucasian authority figures, partially stemming back to slavery, oppression, discrimination, and transgressions by the majority dating back to the eighteenth century (Horsman, Rodriguez, & Marini, 2009; Reid, 2009). Despite the relative success of the 1964 Civil Rights Act, African Americans continue to lag behind Whites in terms of employment, health coverage, education, and socio-economic status (Reid). African American males under age 24 also have the highest death and disability rates due to violent causes as well.

Native Americans also have large within-group and between-group differences. Over 60% of American Indians are of mixed heritage and differ in their level of acculturation (Trimble, Fleming, Beauvais, & Jumper-Thurman, 1996). Many Indians often view themselves as extensions of their tribe, which provides them with a sense of security and belonging. Personal accomplishments are acknowledged and honored if they somehow serve to benefit the whole tribe. For some Native Americans who leave the reservation, a sense of loss of self is experienced due to the detachment or loss of tribal identity (Anderson & Ellis, 1995). Women traditionally have a strong role in the family, and it is common for the extended family to include aunts, uncles, and grandparents who take part in raising the children. Since the extended family assists in child rearing and elders are held in high esteem in the family, Native males do not hold as strong a role as breadwinner or head of the household as do Latino/Hispanic and Asian husbands.

The poverty rate among Native Americans is high, with approximately one in four living in poverty. High unemployment rates exist on the reservation as well as problems with substance abuse (Swinomish Tribal Mental Health Project, 1991). Various studies on Native American issues indicate that although there are sometimes diverse within-group differences, common issues include a basic mistrust of European Americans, strong bonds to one's tribe, consideration of family and community needs before one's needs, low levels of success with acculturation off the reservation and cultural identity conflicts leading to substance abuse, suicide and low self-esteem (Sue & Sue, 1990). Native Americans do not view disability as a punishment for having sinned, and overall tend to treat their members with a disability as they would anyone else, without judging or stigmatizing a member with a disability. Native males with disabilities on the reserve continue to contribute what they can, and regardless of their contributions, are regarded with dignity and respect (Joe & Miller, 1987).

Finally, for European Americans, autonomy and independence are highly valued as signs of achievement (Fernandez & Marini, 1995). With European Americans being the majority in North America, the media often mirrors their views/values and beliefs. As such, television commercials and movies portray successful, physically attractive and independent people as top values to aspire toward (Livneh, 1991). Both husbands and wives often work and are approximately equally represented in the labor force (Szymanski, Ryan, Merz, Trevino, & Johnson-Rodriguez, 1996). In striving to be successful and independent, European Americans often leave home for college or work at an early age, and family cohesiveness is not as prevalent as it is with other minority groups (Sue & Sue, 2003). For a European American male to become disabled, the results can be devastating. Autonomy and independence become jeopardized, as does one's ability to become employed and perceived as successful. Indeed, as is next further outlined, a male's sense of self often becomes seriously compromised by a sudden catastrophic disability.

SOCIETAL PERCEPTIONS OF MASCULINE TRAITS

The concept of masculinity and masculine traits is well documented in various cultures (Bern, 1974, 1993; Brannon, 1976; Gerschick & Miller, 1995, 1997; Herek, 1986; Sprecher

& Sedikider, 1993; Tepper, 1997; Zilbergeld, 1992). Zilbergeld (1992) states that most lessons about male roles have been learned by age seven. He and other researchers have defined masculinity and masculine behavior as reflecting a cluster of male competency traits, including strength, self-reliance, success, sexual interest and prowess, active, independent, tough, no behaving like a "sissy," aggressive, dominant, stoic, never gives up, self-confident, athletic, assertive, and does not express emotions or becomes upset (Herek, 1986; Spence, Helmreich, & Stapp, 1974). In the United States, movie actors who traditionally depict the societal expected behavior of the perceived "real man" have included John Wayne, Clint Eastwood, Richard Roundtree, Bruce Lee, Geronimo, and Kirk Douglas to name a few.

Gender polarized traits become ingrained in us from various societal influences as projected by our culture, the media, family influences and religion. Little boys are brought up playing with toy soldiers, toy guns and contact sports; whereas, little girls are raised with dolls, toy kitchens and doll houses. Further, North American culture embraces the "body beautiful" concept which focuses on youth, health, physical/personal appearance, athletic prowess, and wholeness (Livneh, 1991; Roessler & Rubin, 1982; Wright, 1983; Zilbergeld, 1992).

Several empirical studies support the concept of masculine traits. Sprecher and Sedikider (1993) found that men express less emotion than women in close relationships, attributed to male social role expectations of self-control, toughness, and autonomy. Other findings indicate that men have problems asking for support and responding to such questions as "How do you feel?". Relatedly, Belle (1987) found that men tend to provide and receive less social support than women and are also less likely to seek social support to deal with problems. Other researchers have noted that many males do not seek social support because it signifies weakness and dependence, or have found self-disclosure to be inversely related to trait masculinity (Buda, Giordano, & Neren, 1985; Winstead, Derlega, & Wong, 1984). Subsequently, when a male incurs a severe disabling injury, his identity is compromised due to perceived loss of all his masculine traits.

Overall, the masculine traits described here are somewhat similarly shared across the five ethnic groups being discussed. Where there are subtle ethnic differences generally pertains to the European American traits of independence and assertiveness. In this regard, it has typically been found that being assertive or to question authority for Asians and Latino/Hispanics is generally considered rude and/or disrespectful (Rubin, Chung, & Huang, 1998). Also, although independence and autonomy are highly valued among European Americans, the other minority groups discussed here place a higher value on the needs of the family before the needs of the individual (Fernandez & Marini, 1995).

SOCIETAL ATTITUDES TOWARD DISABILITY

Having reviewed the masculine traits typically perceived to describe "real" men, we turn now to a brief literature review of societal views toward persons with disabilities. There exists a plethora of empirical and theoretical studies relating to the investigation of attitudes toward persons with disabilities (Anthony, 1972; Belgrave, 1984; Belgrave & Mills, 1981; Comer & Piliavin, 1975; Donaldson, 1980; English, 1971; Evans, 1976; Marini, 1992; Yuker, 1988). A critical review of the literature regarding attitudes and disability by Chubon (1982), however, found about 60% of the over 100 studies reviewed were empirical in nature. The remaining studies were conceptual or anecdotal, having little or no empirical basis.

The most compelling attitudes of able-bodied European Americans concerning their views of persons with disabilities indicate that persons with disabilities are generally thought of as objects of pity and/or admiration and perceived to be fundamentally different from nondisabled persons (Harris, 1991). Lyons (1991) adds that, in Western society, European Americans perceive persons with disabilities as helpless, incapable, and inferior. Although African and Native Americans may not share these perceptions, Asian and Latino/Hispanic cultures do have similar perceptions and often become overprotective of the disabled member, thus diminishing chances of the member becoming independent (Uba, 1994; Pickett et al., 1993). Aside from overprotection, Asian culture views the disability as a failure (Wong & Chan, 1994). Gething (1991) notes that societal attitudes can impact how people react toward a perceived minority. Subsequently, societal expectations can impact quality of life, job opportunities, and overall socialization as a stigmatized minority. Havranek (1991) states that the attitudes of others are often the most significant barriers that persons with disabilities encounter.

Livneh (1991) classified the origins of negative attitudes toward disability into 13 categories. Two of the categories are relevant to this discussion; psychodynamic mechanisms and the spread phenomena.

"Psychodynamic mechanisms" pertaining to societal beliefs suggest that if a person does not feel bad about the disability, he or she must be in denial (Dembo, Leviton & Wright, 1975). This expectation of having to mourn the loss poses a problem for males who typically attempt to hide or not show their emotions (Bem, 1993). As Olkin (1999) cities in referring to Wright's concept of the requirement of mourning, this reflects society's need for members to follow proper codes of conduct regarding how one ought to act and feel. It follows then that if an individual has a disability and does not feel sad about it, this disrupts the social order of conduct. A related mechanism, the "spread phenomena," refers to society's belief that a disability affecting one aspect of an individual (e.g., paralysis) affects all other aspects such as mental abilities and emotional stability. Thus, someone with paraplegia might also be perceived as having a developmental disability as well. This also becomes problematic for males who want to return to work and are perceived by employers as incapable, both mentally and physically, of performing the job despite the fact they have a physical disability.

DISABILITY IMPACT ON MASCULINITY

The trauma of a physical disability upon a man's sense of masculinity compromises virtually all of the traits ascribed by most societies for males. Men struggle with two sets of social dynamics. On the one hand, they attempt to live up to the pressures of being masculine (e.g., independent, healthy, autonomous, etc.), while, on the other hand, trying to disprove society's perception of them as passive, dependent, pitiful, sick, and incapable (Gerschick & Miller, 1995, 1997).

From her interviews of men with chronic disabilities, Charmaz (1995) found that males attempt to preserve aspects of their predisability self by maintaining qualities or attributes that *previously* defined their self-concept. As they adapt to their disability, males "preserve self" by limiting the impact of the disability in their daily lives and developing strategies to minimize the limiting aspects of their impairment.

Charmaz (1995) also noted that some males attempted to "recapture" all aspects of their past selves by ignoring their limitations. Wright (1983) defines this behavior as "as if" behavior, whereby an individual denies his or her limitations by acting as if he or she does not have a disability. When these men realized that it was not possible to ignore their disabilities, they became despondent and depressed. The despondence is described by Wright as having "succumb" to the limitations of the disability rather than more appropriately coping with it.

In other studies, Gerschick and Miller (1995) conducted 10 in-depth interviews with men who sustained either a paraplegia or tetraplegia by using an analytic induction approach. They noted three patterns of coping that interviewees used in dealing with the dominant masculinity standards. The first pattern, "reformulation," characterized males who redefined *idealial* masculine traits to conform to their new abilities. Males who needed a personal attendant to assist in performing activities of daily living (e.g., grooming, dressing) continued to view themselves as independent because they "controlled" the actions of the personal attendant. They also defined the term self-reliant to mean earning capacity and the ability to work and support oneself.

The second pattern of coping, defined as "reliance," characterized those males who relied heavily on the masculine ideals of strength, independence and sexual prowess. These males were troubled by the fact that they could not live up to these ideals. Some attempted to function independently even when they needed assistance. These men refused to ask for help and, instead, struggled to complete the task. Some men played wheelchair sports to remain competitive, while others viewed wheelchair sports as not being the "real" thing and therefore did not participate. Others became involved in risk-taking behavior.

The third pattern of coping described by Gerschick and Miller (1995, 1997) was "rejection" of the masculine ideals. This group of men with disabilities rejected the traditional notion of what made the "real" man. They created an alternate masculine identity by identifying themselves as "persons" and believed that mental ability was superior to physical strength. It appears that males with disabilities either attempt to adjust their perceptions of what it meant to be a man, denied their limitations by acting as if they were able-bodied, reluctantly succumbed to their fate, or redefined themselves as a person with a disability.

Males without disabilities likely share some of these same beliefs and reformulate the definition of masculine. For some, this may mean purchasing masculine-oriented material goods such as a speedboat, half-ton truck, or masculine clothing. For others, it may include maladaptive means of portraying masculinity such as gang activity, spousal and/or child abuse.

COUNSELING CONSIDERATIONS WHEN WORKING WITH MALES WITH DISABILITIES

The issues men from various cultures face in general after sustaining a debilitating permanent physical disability challenge the very essence of their male identity, often creating an identity crisis. Since role expectations for males restrict or prohibit their expressing emotions, many men maintain an image of toughness, while inwardly struggling with numerous unresolved issues. Such observations are sometimes construed by counselors as client's denial of disability. It is not only difficult for a male to disclose his problems for fear of being further perceived as weak, but it is also difficult to get many ethnic groups to agree to go for counseling (Sue & Sue, 1990). Sue and Sue note that approximately 50% of ethnic groups do not return for a second counseling session when the counselor is European American. African and Native Americans tend not to trust European American counselors based, in part, on past transgressions (White, 1994). Many Asians do not even make it to counseling, attempting instead to handle the disability within the family, due in part to the embarrassment the disability brings to the family (Wong & Chan, 1994). Many Latino/Hispanics, like

Asians, also believe that disability is punishment for having sinned and the impairment should be accepted as one's lot in life without seeking correction. Any conscious attempt to improve one's situation may be perceived as going against God's wishes (Smart & Smart, 1991).

It is beyond the scope of this chapter to outline counseling strategies specific to each ethnic group discussed here, however, the reader is referred to Sue and Sue (2003) for more detailed information on the "sensitivity" and awareness of counseling culturally diverse populations. The strategies discussed below relate to overlapping counseling issues of males with disabilities from various cultures.

There are at least seven clustered major schools of thought regarding how one adjusts or adapts to a traumatic disability, but only three are discussed here, and the reader is referred elsewhere for further information on the others (Marini, 2011). The first is Livneh's (1991) stage model of adjustment to loss. The *initial impact* is marked by shock and anxiety; *defense mobilization* identified by denial and bargaining with God or some higher power to live and/or be cured; *initial relaxation* marked by mourning the loss (and perhaps clinical depression) as well as internalized anger or self blame; *retaliation* observed as in directing anger outwardly at others; and, *acceptance* signified by an emotional and cognitive coming to terms with one's new disability identity. One generally transitions through these stages over time; however, may get stuck in a stage, regress back to a stage, or alternate/overlap between stages.

The recurrent model of adjustment (Davis, 1987; Kendall & Buys, 1998) similarly views the initial onset of a disability as overwhelming for the individual, analogous to a wildly swinging pendulum that gradually slows and steadies at center over time. As people adapt, they can develop new *cognitive schema*, defined as a new and more positive world view regarding how they see themselves as well as how others view them (however, new schema can be negative and self-defeating). Some individuals get stuck using old preinjury schema that no longer work. Wright (1983) describes this as "as if" behavior, as individual's attempt to function as if they did not have a disability. In order for the individual to successfully adapt to their disability, they must positively and cognitively reframe the meaning of their disability, gain control or master their environment, and preserve and enhance their new disability identity.

The third relevant model considers the intricate and complex interaction of an individual in his or her environment, otherwise known as the ecological and similar somatopsychology models (Marini, 2011; Vash & Crewe, 2004; Wright, 1983). Essentially, who we are and who we see ourselves to be is based not only on our perceived self-concept and self-esteem, but also mirrored or echoed by how we are treated by significant others and the community at large. Although individuals may have a positive view of themselves, if they are constantly devalued, discriminated against and otherwise ignored by others, it often becomes just a matter of time before one's self-concept and self-esteem are diminished (Hopps, Pepin, Arsenau, Frechette, & Begin, 2001; Li & Moore, 1998). Li and Moore (1998), for example, found that persons with disabilities generally were less accepting of their disability when responded to negatively by others, while Hopps et al. (2001) found that people with disabilities treated poorly by others reported feelings of loneliness and having poorer social skills.

There are typically several areas of worry/concern for males with disabilities. These can include how to financially support one's family; lack of job alternatives; perceived employer discrimination; perceived loss of sexuality and performance ability, as well as the ability to attract a mate; and, perceived social status as a poor, unemployed person with a disability. In many cases of having once been perceived as strong and independent, many males struggle with child-like feelings of dependency from the need to ask for assistance to complete the simplest of tasks. Such issues contradict the male identity of self-reliance, success and independence, as well as the ability to contribute and care for the family. Other issues pertain to loss of control of bodily functions and the fear of becoming a burden to the family with related frustrations of having to relearn basic human functions we generally acquire by age four. This dependency is often perceived as embarrassing and shameful by many injured males.

It should be noted that although the stage and recurrent models of adjustment to disability are commonly discussed in the literature, there is scant empirical information available which suggests that racial members of underrepresented groups experience either ways of adjusting. Conversely, there is little empirical-based evidence to suggest that ethnic members adjust to disability any differently than do European Americans. Cultural values and beliefs do, however, provide some insight as to what some of the concerns may be for ethnic males.

BASIC COUNSELING STRATEGIES FOR ETHNIC GROUPS

Sue and Sue (2003) recommend a number of basic counseling strategies for working with each ethnic group. For African American male clients, asking if they are uncomfortable working with a counselor from a different ethnic background (if relevant) is recommended. Exploring what their worldviews are and how they view their problem and possible solutions is also advised. It is also important to discuss how the African American male has responded to discrimination, be it due to race or disability. In addition, assessing the relative importance of the family, community and church provides clues as to how involved the family should be. Finally, note that, in general, a problem-solving time-limited approach works best for this population.

In counseling Asian American males, basic strategies include using restraint in gathering information due to the norm of keeping family matters private. Assess tangible issues such as financial or assistive device needs, and as with other ethnic groups, use a more direct problem-solving approach, making sure the client generates the solutions, rather than counselor imposed values to solving client problems. Again, being aware of the client's worldviews and focusing on concrete solutions to the presenting and/or future problems become important (Sue & Sue, 2003).

Basic counseling strategies for working with Native American males include exploring their values. Those on the reservation tend to hold more traditional values than those in the mainstream. Sue and Sue (2003) also recommend that the combination of client-centered and behavioral counseling approaches may work best with Native American clients. Exploring issues of acculturation and potential conflicts for the male client and his family is important as well as determining the strength of the family and extended family unit. Finally, remembering not to confront or stare at Native American clients (considered rude) and allowing the client to take his time in finishing his thoughts are key intrapersonal behaviors.

Finally, in counseling Latino/Hispanic males, counselors must be aware of the traditional male role and determine the level of acculturation. Assess whether there is an impact of racism or poverty in relation to the stated presenting problem. Discuss the desire or need for family involvement and what the impact of the client achieving his goals will have on the family. Note that Latino/Hispanic clients are generally respectful of authority, and once a strong rapport is developed, may develop a close personal bond with the counselor (Sue & Sue, 2003). With these basic ethnic group counseling strategies in mind, techniques for working with persons with acquired disabilities follow.

COGNITIVE REFRAMING RE SOCIETAL VIEWS OF DISABILITY

Recommendations for therapists begin with first having a thorough understanding of culture specific societal views of masculinity and disability. Many clients will harbor unresolved conflicts due to the extreme social role expectation contradictions between masculinity and disability. As noted in the recurrent model of adjustment, many males will initially strive to hold on to their preinjury schema as if they do not have a disability (Kendall & Buys, 1998; Wright, 1983). As injured individuals continue to realize these old schemas no longer work, they may experience anxiety, depression, and helplessness. Counselors should assist clients to reframe old schemas and build new schemas to function in the environment with the disability around the three themes noted earlier (Kendall & Buys, 1998). Counselors should be aware however, that some ethnic clients may not want to strive for independence or mastery of their environment. These values must be explored with minority clients and their families. For injured individuals and families who wish to see the disabled loved one become more independent, focusing on the client's remaining strengths while offering practical concrete suggestions to make positive changes becomes important (Kendall & Buys, 1998). Concrete strategies may include purchasing adaptive equipment, hiring personal attendants and furthering one's education to enhance employment marketability.

Another aspect to cognitive reframing relates to Albert Ellis's (1973) Rational Emotive Therapy (RET) and challenging client irrational beliefs about the presumed finality of their future. Clients who are not clinically depressed, but rather despondent and feeling hopeless/helpless about their situation could be questioned about what they believe their future holds. Those who feel their life is over should be tactfully challenged about what proof they have regarding their assertion. Counselors should be prepared to offer examples of persons with the same disabilities who have adjusted well.

SELF-INITIATING TALKING POINTS WITH CLIENTS

A second suggestion relates to the strategy that therapists will likely have to self-initiate discussions regarding the issues noted earlier. For the resistant client who continues to assert everything is "fine" and attempts to hide behind the stoic, strong male image, counselors must be able to differentiate denial versus masking what one really feels. Knowing the potential issues that males with disabilities may have, counselors may begin to initiate talking points with the client. Counselors can openly address the notion of clients not wanting to burden others with their problems so as to grant clients permission to talk about their pent-up fears. Counselors should also consider touching upon client issues such as sex, abandonment, health, career, finances, and so forth, then decide whether to move on or not to other issues, based on client response and nonverbal behavior. By letting clients know the counselor already understands and empathizes with the fear and anxiety clients must be feeling over these issues, clients may begin to open up and discuss their worries as well as perhaps experiencing their first catharsis, which they may have privately concealed or masked for so long.

ADDRESSING INAPPROPRIATE COPING MECHANISM ISSUES

The third issue to discuss pertains to inappropriate versus appropriate ways of dealing with stress such as alcohol/substance abuse, avoidance and reckless behavior. Statistics regarding persons with physical disabilities indicates that as many as 68% of them who sustain traumatic injuries have been under the influence of substances. Postinjury in many cases, substance abuse often continues among European Americans, not only because of preinjury use, but also to mask the pain experienced from the disability (Heinemann, 1993). In extreme cases of addiction, referral to a substance abuse program will be warranted. Ironically, drinking tolerance may be considered as masculine behavior for some males and thus perceived as a way to "hang on" to some of their masculinity.

Avoidance and isolating oneself from others may be another type of inappropriate response observed, particularly for minority clients. Again, cognitions of being embarrassed and perceived as a failure can lead clients into avoiding significant others who can bring meaning back to their life. Client's fears in this area should be explored and challenged regarding the differences between a person's physical appearance versus who he or she is as an individual.

A third area to observe and discuss is a client's mental status, especially pertaining to suicidal ideation. Suicide among European American males with spinal cord injury is about twice as high as the general population (Geisler, Jousse, Wynne-Jones, & Breithaupt, 1983). Persons of minority less frequently attempt suicide than European Americans, however, their rates are also higher than average. Death from unintentional injury and suicide are the leading causes of death among persons with spinal injury six months postinjury (Brown, 1998). As such, reckless behavior or suicidal ideation is another area which needs to be explored, especially during acute care rehabilitation.

UNDERSTANDING OF DISABILITY-SPECIFIC PHYSIOLOGY

A fourth suggestion is to become thoroughly familiar with the physiological changes of specific disability populations with which one is working. Aside from reading about the limitations, talk to treating therapists and physicians about an individual's functional limitations. From this, educate clients regarding sexual myths and functioning, health and wellness practices regarding taking care of oneself (e.g., managing stress, nutrition, drug/alcohol use, exercise, etc.), and the use of assistive devices for greater independence.

INTRODUCE CLIENTS TO ROLE MODELS WITH DISABILITIES

Finally, despite a non-disabled counselor's best efforts, nothing compares to recruiting successfully adjusted persons with the same disability as your clients to interact with, and see first-hand that a quality life can still be pursued and enjoyed. This can be accomplished individually or quite effectively in group counseling. Therapists should be cautious, however, to always first ask clients if they would like to meet and talk to someone who has lived with the disability. Most newly injured persons will have a certain period (usually right after injury), where their denial of the long-term prognosis is so great, they will resent and be unwilling to meet another person with a disability. Therapists should be prepared to broach the topic occasionally until the client is finally ready to meet the individual.

Today, persons with severe physical disabilities are living longer and healthier thanks to advances in medicine, assistive technology, pharmacological developments, and in some countries, empowering legislation. As such, the quality of life for this population continues to improve, with exciting new advances on the way. Physical barriers in the community and with transportation continue to be eliminated, opening the once closed doors of engaging in social activities that give us pleasure. Indeed, it may well be that the major issues that many males with disabilities face in industrialized countries, are not so much a lack of physical access, but rather dealing with the sometime negative attitudes and societal expectations of male roles.

REFERENCES

Alegria, D., Guerra, E., Martinez, C., & Meyer, G. G. (1977). El hospital invisible: A study of curanderismo. *Archives of General Psychiatry, 34,* 1354–1357.

Alston, R., McCowan, C. J., & Turner, W. L. (1994). Family functioning as a correlate of disability, adjustment for African Americans. *Rehabilitation Counseling Bulletin, 37,* 277–289.

Anderson, M. J., & Ellis, R. (1995). On the reservation. In N. A. Vacc, S. B. DeVaney, & J. Wittmer (Eds.), *Experiencing and counseling multicultural and diverse populations* (3rd ed., pp. 179–198). Bristol, PA: Accelerated Development.

Anthony, W. A. (1972). Societal rehabilitation: Changing society's attitudes toward the physically and mentally disabled. *Rehabilitation Psychology, 9*(3), 93–203.

Avila, D. L., & Avila, A. L. (1995). Mexican Americans. In N. A. Vacc, S. B. DeVaney, & J. Wittmer (Eds.), *Experiencing and counseling multicultural and diverse populations* (pp. 119–146). Bristol, PA: Accelerated Development.

Belgrave, F. Z. (1984). The effectiveness of strategies for increasing social interaction with a physically disabled person. *Journal of Applied Social Psychology, 14*(2), 147–161.

Belgrave, F. Z., & Mills, J. (1981). Effects upon desire for social interaction with a physically disabled person after mentioning the disability in different contexts. *Journal of Applied Social Psychology, 11,* 44–57.

Belle, D. (1987). Gender differences in the social moderators of stress. In R. C. Barnett, L. Biener, & G. K. Baruch (Eds.), *Gender and stress* (pp. 257–277). New York: Free Press.

Bern, S. L. (1974). The measurement of psychological androgyny. *Journal of Consulting and Clinical Psychology, 42*(2), 155–162.

Bem, S. L. (1993). *The lenses of gender: Transforming the debate on sexual inegality.* New Haven, CT: Yale University press.

Brannon, R. (1976). The male sex role: Our culture's blueprint of manhood, and what it's done for us lately. In D. David & R. Brannon (Eds.), *The forty-nine percent majority* (pp. 1–45). Reading, MA: Addison-Wesley.

Brown, W. J. (1998). Current psychopharmacologic issues in the management of major depression and generalized anxiety disorder in chronic spinal cord injury. *SCI: Psychosocial Process, 11*(3), 37–45.

Chan, S. (1991). *Asian-Americans: An interpretive history.* Boston: Twayne.

Chan, S (1992). Families with Asian roots. In E. W. Lynch & M. J. Hansen (Eds.), *Developing cross cultural competence: A guide for working with young children and their families* (pp. 181–257). Baltimore: Brookes.

Charmaz, K. (1995). Identity dilemmas of chronically ill men. In D. Sabo & D. Gordon (Eds.), *Men's health and illness: Gender, power and the body* (pp. 266–291). Thousand Oaks, CA: Sage.

Chouduri, D. D. (2009). Multicultural issues in counseling Asian-Americans. In I. Marini and M. Stebnicki (Eds.), *The professional counselor's desk reference* (pp. 219–229). New York: Springer.

Chubon, R.A. (1982). An analysis of research dealing with the attitudes of professionals toward disability. *Journal of Rehabilitation, Winter, 16,* 25–30.

Corner, R. C., & Piliavin, J. A. (1975). As others see us: Attitudes of physically handicapped and normals toward own and other groups. *Rehabilitation Literature, 36*(7), 206–221.

Davis, B. H. (1987). Disability and grief. *The Journal of Contemporary Social Work, 68,* 352–357.

Dembo, T., Leviton, G., & Wright, B. (1975). Adjustment to misfortune: A problem of social psychological rehabilitation. *Rehabilitation Psychology, 22,* 1–10.

Donaldson, J. (1980). Changing attitudes toward handicapped persons: A review and analysis of research. *Exceptional Children, 46,* 504–514.

Ellis, A. (1973). *Humanistic psychotherapy: The rational-emotive approach.* New York: Julian Press.

English, R. W. (1971). Correlates of stigma toward physically disabled persons. In R. P. Marinelli, & A. E. Dell Orto (Eds.), *The psychological & social impact of physical disability* (pp. 162–182). New York: Springer.

Evans, J. H. (1976). Changing attitudes toward disabled persons: An experimental study. *Rehabilitation Counseling Bulletin, 19,* 572–579.

Fernandez, M. S., & Marini, I. (1995). Cultural values orientation in counseling persons with spinal cord injury. *SCI Psychology Process, 8*(4), 150–155.

Gallagher, H. G. (1994). *FDR's splendid deception.* Arlington: Vandamere.

Garzon, F., & Tan, S. Y. (1992). Counseling Hispanics: Cross-cultural and Christian perspectives. *Journal of Psychology and Christianity, 11,* 378–390.

Geisler, W O., Jousse, A.T., Wynne-Jones, M., & Breithaupt, D. (1983). Survival in traumatic spinal cord injury. *Paraplegia, 21*(6), 364–373.

Gerschick, T. J., & Miller, A. S. (1995). Coining to terms: Masculinity and physical disability. In D. Sabo & D. Gordon (Eds.), *Men's health and illness: Gender, power, and the body* (pp. 183–204). Thousand Oaks, CA: Sage.

Gerschick, T. J., & Miller, A. S. (1997). Gender identities at the crossroads of masculinity and physical disability. In M. Gergen & S. Davis (Eds.), *Toward a new psychology of gender* (pp. 455–475). New York: Routledge.

Gething, L. (1991). Generality vs. specificity of attitudes towards people with disabilities. *British Journal of Medical Psychology, 64,* 55–64.

Gonzalez, G. M. (1997). The emergence of Chicanos in the twenty-first century: Implications for counseling, research, and policy. *Journal of Multicultural and Development, 25,* 94–106.

Harris, L. (1991). *Public attitudes towards people with disabilities.* New York: Louis Harris and Associates.

Harris, M., Velasquez, R. J., White, J., & Renteria, T. (2004). Folk healing and curanderismo within the contemporary Chicanao community. Current status. In R. J. Velasquez, L. M. Arellano, & B. W. McNeill (Eds.), *The handbook of chicana/o psychology and mental health* (pp. 111–126). Mahwah, NJ: Lawrence Erlbaum Associates.

Havranek, J. E. (1991). The social and individual costs of negative attitudes toward persons with physical disabilities. *Journal of Applied Rehabilitation Counseling, 22*(1), 15–21.

Heinemann, A. W. (1993). An introduction to substance abuse and physical disability. In A. W. Heinemann (Ed.), *Substance abuse and physical disability* (pp. 3–10). Binghamton, NY: Haworth Press.

Herek, G. M. (1986). On heterosexual masculinity. *American Behavioral Scientist, 29*(5), 563–577.

Hohmann, G. W. (1975). Psychological aspects of treatment and rehabilitation of the spinal cord injured person. *Clinical Orthopedics, 112,* 81–88.

Hopps, S., Pepin, M., Arseneau, I., Frechette, M., & Begin, G. (2001). Disability related variables associated with loneliness among people with disabilities. *Journal of Rehabilitation, 67*(3), 42–48.

Horsman, E. N., Rodriguez, V. J., & Marini, I. (2009). In I. Marini, & M. Stebnicki (Eds.), *The professional counselor's desk reference* (pp. 185–198). New York: Springer.

Joe, R.E., & Miller, D. (Eds.) (1987). *American Indian cultural perspectives on disability* (pp. 3–23). Tucson, AZ: University of Arizona, Native American Research and Training Center.

Kendall, E., & Buys, N. (1998). An integrated model of psychosocial adjustment following acquired disability. *Journal of Rehabilitation, 64,* 16–20.

Lassiter, S. M. (1995). *Multicultural clients: A professional handbook for health care providers and social workers.* Westport, CT: Greenwood.

Lee, W. M. L., Blando, J. A., Mizelle, N. D., & Orozco, G. L. (Eds.). (2007). *Introduction to multicultural counseling for helping professionals,* (2nd ed.). New York: Routledge.

Li, L., & Moore, D. (1998). Acceptance of disability and its correlates. *Journal of Social Psychology, 138*(1), 13–25.

Livneh, H. (1991). On the origins of negative attitudes toward people with disabilities. In R. P. Marinelli, & A. E. Dell Orto, *The psychological and social impact of disability* (3rd ed., pp. 181–196). New York: Springer.

Livneh, H. (1991). A unified approach to existing models of adaptation to disability: A model of adaptation. In R. P. Marinelli, & A. E. Dell Orto (3rd ed.), *The psychological and social impact of disability* (pp. 111–138). Springer: New York

Locke, D. C. (1992). *Increasing multicultural understanding: A comprehensive model.* Newbury Park, CA: Sage.

Lyons, M. (1991). Enabling or disabling? Students' attitudes toward persons with disabilities. *The American Journal of Occupational Therapy, 45*(4), 311–316.

Marini, I. (1992). The use of humor in counseling as a social skill for disabled clients. *Journal of Applied Rehabilitation Counseling, 23*(3), 30–36.

Marini, I. (2011). Theories of adjustment to disability by the individual. In I. Marini, N. M. Glover-Graf, & M. J. Millington (Eds.), *Psychosocial aspects of disability: insider perspectives and counseling strategies* (pp. 131–168). New York: Springer.

Millington, M. J. (2011). Culturally different issues and attitudes toward disability. In I. Marini, N. M. Glover-Graf, & M. J. Millington (Eds.), *Psychosocial aspects of disability: Insider perspectives and counseling strategies* (pp. 61–96). New York: Springer.

Mollica, R. F., Henderson, D. C., & Tor, S. (2002). Psychiatric effects of traumatic brain injury events in Cambodian survivors of mass violence. *British Journal of Psychiatry, 181*(4), 339–347.

National Organization on Disability. (2004) *The 2004 N.O.D./Harris survey of Americans with disabilities.* Washington, DC: Author.

Olkin, R. (1999). *What psychotherapists should know about disability.* New York: Guilford Press.

Pickett, S. A., Vraniale, D. A., Cook, J. A., & Cohler, B. J. (1993). Strength in adversity: Blacks bear burden better than Whites. *Professionals Psychology: Research and Practice, 24,* 460–467.

Reid, C. (2009). Multicultural issues in counseling African-Americans. In I. Marini & M. Stebnicki (Eds.), *The professional counselor's desk reference* (pp. 185–198). New York: Springer.

Roessler, R., & Rubin, S. E. (1982). *Case management and rehabilitation counseling.* Austin, TX: PRO ED.

Rogers-Dulan, J., & Blacker, J. (1995). African American families, religion, and disability: A conceptual framework. *Mental Retardation, 33,* 226–238.

Rubin, S. E., Chung, W., & Huang, W. (1998). Multicultural considerations in the rehabilitation counseling process. In R. T. Roessler & S. E. Rubin, *Case management and rehabilitation counseling* (3rd ed., pp. 185–230). Austin, DC: PRO ED.

Rubin, S. E., & Roessler, R. (2008). Philosophical and economic considerations in regard to disability rights and support for rehabilitation programs. In S. E. Rubin & R. Roessler (Eds.), *Foundations of the vocational rehabilitation process* (6th ed., pp. 143–166). Austin, TX: PRO ED.

Shontz, F. C. (1975). *The psychological aspects of physical illness and disability.* New York Macmillan.

Smart, J. F., & Smart, D. W. (1991). Acceptance of disability and the Mexican American culture. *Rehabilitation Counseling Bulletin, 34,* 357–367.

Smith, E. (1981). Cultural and historical perspectives in counseling Blacks. In D. Sue (Ed.), *Counseling the culturally different: Theory and practice* (pp. 141–185). New York: Wiley.

Spence, J. T., Helinreich. R. L., & Stapp, J. (1974). The personal attributes questionnaire: A measure of sex-role stereotypes and masculinity-femininity. *JSAS Catalog of Selected Documents in Psychology, 4,* 127.

Sprecher, S., & Sedikides, C. (1993). Gender differences in perceptions of emotionality: The case of close, heterosexual relationships. *Sex Roles, 28*(9/10), 511–530.

Sue, D., & Sue, S. (1987). Cultural factors in the clinical assessment of Asian Americans. *Journal of Counseling and Clinical Psychology, 55,* 479–487.

Sue, D. W., & Sue, D. (1990). *Counseling the culturally different: Theory and practice.* New York: John Wiley & Sons.

Sue, D. W., & Sue, D. (2003). *Counseling the culturally different: Theory and practice.* Hoboken, NJ: John Wiley & Sons.

Swinomish Tribal Mental Health Project (1991). *A gathering of wisdoms.* LaConner, WA: Swinomish Tribal Community.

Szymanski, E. M., Ryan, C., Merz, M. A., Trevino, B., & Johnson-Rodriguez, S. (1996). Psychosocial and economic aspects of work: Implications for people with disability. In E. M. Szymanski & R. M. Parker (Eds.), *Work and disability: Issues and strategies in career development and job placement* (pp. 9–38). Austin, TX: PRO ED.

Tepper, M. S. (1997). Living with a disability: A man's perspective. In M. Sipski, & C. Alexander (Eds.), *Sexual function in people with disability and chronic illness* (pp. 131–146). Gaithersburg, MD: Aspen.

Trimble, J. E., Fleming, C. M., Beauvais, F., & Jumper-Thurman, P. (1996). Essential cultural and social strategies for counseling Native American Indians. In P. B. Pedersen, J. G. Draguns, W. J. Lonner, & J. E. Trimble (Eds.), *Counseling across cultures* (4th ed., pp. 177–209). Thousand Oaks, CA: Sage Publications.

Uba, L. (1994). *Asian Americans.* New York: Guilford.

U.S. Bureau of the Census. (1995). *Population profile of the United States.* Washington, DC: U.S. Government Printing Office.

Vash, C. L. (1981). *The psychology of disability.* New York: Springer.

Vash, C. L., & Crewe, N. M. (2004). *Psychology of disability.* New York: Springer Publishing Co.

Winstead, B. A., Derlega, V. J., & Wong, P. T. P. (1984). Effect of sex-role orientation on behavioral self-disclosure. *Journal of Research in Personality, 18,* 541–553.

Wong, D., & Chan, C. (1994). Advocacy on self-help for patients with chronic illness: The Hong Kong experience. *Prevention in human services, 11*(1), 117–139.

Wright, B. A. (1983). *Physical disability: A psychosocial approach* (2nd ed.). New York: Harper & Row.

Yuker, H. E. (1988). *Attitudes toward persons with disabilities.* New York: Springer.

12

Psychiatric and Psychological Issues in Survivors of Major Disasters

CAROL S. NORTH AND ALINA M. SURÍS

LEARNING OBJECTIVE

Clinicians will become more skilled in recognizing symptoms of post-traumatic stress disorder (PTSD) and acute stress syndromes in patients who have survived various catastrophic experiences and will be offered guidelines for the psychosocial and psychopharmacological management of such conditions.

In this chapter, Drs. North and Surís defines three main types of disasters: natural ones, such as earthquakes; technological ones, such as accidental explosions; and attacks generated willfully by humans. Disaster survivors represent a population different from victims of individual calamities, such as automobile accidents and assaults. Personal trauma in general is associated with characteristics such as lower socioeconomic status, previous psychiatric illness, substance abuse, and novelty seeking, risk-taking personality traits—all of which tend to predict a poorer outcome following the traumatic event.

After reviewing the diagnostic criteria for PTSD, Drs. North and Surís point out that the most robust and reliable predictors of PTSD following disasters are female gender and predisaster psychopathology. After disasters, PTSD usually develops quickly; the delayed PTSD described in adult survivors of childhood sexual abuse and combat veterans is not typical of postdisaster experience. After considering issues such as chronicity and comorbidity, they go on to review psychosocial interventions and psychotherapeutic and pharmacologic treatments. Cognitive behavioral therapies (CBTs) have been shown to be effective in treating PTSD, while antidepressants are the mainstay of pharmacotherapy for PTSD.

The September 11 terrorist attacks brought the subject of disasters into sharp new focus in our nation's attention. Concerns about the specter of massive terrorism now lurk much larger than the usual transportation accidents, natural disasters, and other devastating catastrophes that had come to be almost routine in the news media.

In the wake of the September 11 attacks, recognition of the potential for serious and widespread mental health consequences of disasters and terrorism has spurred professionals in the field to respond to the resultant mental health needs associated with major disasters and prepare for the future. It is prudent for mental health professionals to keep abreast of current knowledge about mental health issues after disasters and be prepared to respond if they are needed to help.

This chapter will review the field of disaster mental health knowledge and examine the likelihood of postdisaster psychiatric disorders and predictors of individual outcomes. It will

From "Psychiatric and psychosocial issues in survivors of major disasters," by C. North, 2002, *Directions in Rehabilitation Counseling, 3(9)*, 105–114. The Hatherleigh Company, Ltd.

draw from empirical evidence gathered from actual studies of disasters. This knowledge will then be applied in a coherent framework of practical recommendations for the mental health field in disaster response, based closely on the findings of empirical research.

DISASTER TYPOLOGY

Three main types of disasters are recognized: (1) *natural disasters*, such as earthquakes, floods, tornadoes, and volcanoes, sometimes referred to as "acts of God"; (2) *technological accidents*, such as airplane crashes, structural collapses, and major explosions, involving human error rather than intent; and (3) intentionally generated human acts of mass trauma, including *terrorism*, such as the September 11 attacks. It is generally assumed that of all types of disasters, terrorism evokes the most severe mental health effects on its victims because of the heinous, intentional nature of the event. Data collected from the New York City area and nationally after the September 11 attacks suggested that the psychological effects were far-reaching, affecting not only those directly exposed but also people throughout the New York City and Washington, DC area, and people throughout the United States.[1-6]

Although psychological effects of major terrorist events may reverberate throughout an entire nation, it is important to recognize that PTSD by definition occurs only among those who are directly exposed to a traumatic event or indirectly exposed through the direct experience of loved ones. Other affected individuals and population groups can be expected to experience various levels of emotional distress.[7]

It may be difficult, if not impossible, to know whether these aspects of terrorism are directly linked to the mental health effects that follow or whether it is the wide scope and intensity of terrorist attacks, such as the bombing of the Murrah Federal Building in Oklahoma City and the September 11 attacks, that have historically marked such events and driven the mental health effects. It may never be possible to determine empirically whether this is actually the case, however, because it would require the study of a large number of disasters of different types and with varied scope and magnitude, using consistent methodology across all of the studies—a scientific feat that would be highly unlikely to occur. The utility of disaster typology in determining mental health effects of catastrophic events is further hampered because most disasters have at least some degree of overlap in typology based on the many elements involved.[8] For example, after the Great Midwestern Floods of 1993, when the Mississippi and Missouri Rivers overflowed their banks, many people blamed the Army Corps of Engineers for allowing water to flood certain areas. After a 1999 commercial airplane crash-landed in a severe storm in Little Rock, Arkansas, litigants sued the airline, claiming that the pilot's decision to land the airplane in such adverse weather conditions was an error in judgment.

Disaster survivors are a population different from victims of individual calamities such as motor-vehicle accidents, assaults, and work-related injuries. Research has identified personal risk factors that increase the likelihood of finding oneself in harm's way,[9] defining a population preselected for exposure to trauma based on preexisting characteristics, such as low socioeconomic status, previous psychiatric illness, substance abuse, and novelty-seeking and risk-taking personality traits. *These characteristics are many of the same ones that predict poor outcomes for individuals after traumatic events.* Therefore, it can be difficult to determine the degree to which post-trauma difficulties represent aspects of preexisting characteristics leading to trauma exposure or new behaviors in response the trauma.

Disasters, on the other hand, often select somewhat random cross-sections of the population on a more "equal opportunity" basis (with the major exception of floods, which may select victims of lower socioeconomic status, who have chosen to live on a flood plain where land is less expensive). Research studies of human response to stress resulting from disaster may provide the most representative data on adults coping with extreme stress.

DIAGNOSING PTSD AND ACUTE STRESS DISORDER

Much of what is known about human response to traumatic experiences has emerged from research on combat-veteran populations.[10] The most widely discussed psychiatric disorder that appears after traumatic events is PTSD.[11] This diagnosis first appeared in American Psychiatric Association diagnostic nomenclature in the *Diagnostic and Statistical Manual of Mental Disorders, Third Edition* in 1980,[12] largely in response to the need for a diagnosis to reflect the Vietnam experience, although the syndrome had been described in various forms during previous wars.

The first requirement for diagnosing PTSD is that it must occur in response to personal experience of a traumatic event that represents a threat to life or limb, either through direct personal contact or direct eyewitness of such an event, or vicariously through the sudden and unexpected experience of a loved one in such an event. To diagnose PTSD, one must identify in association with a qualifying event an illness that causes a great deal of distress or significant problems functioning, in conjunction with the presence of three types of symptoms that are new after the event. The symptoms are grouped as (1) intrusive recollection, which involves symptoms such as flashbacks, nightmares of the event, and unwanted, vivid images of the event; (2) avoidance and numbing symptoms in individuals who are so overwhelmed by the experience that they avoid anything that would remind them of it; their emotions may be numbed, and they may be isolated and distant from others; and (3) hyperarousal symptoms such as showing excessive vigilance against another encounter with danger, being keyed up and on edge (being jumpy and easily startled), and having difficulty sleeping and concentrating. Table 13.1 shows the complete symptom list. Meeting diagnostic criteria requires the presence of one new intrusive recollection symptom, three new avoidance and numbing symptoms, and two new hyperarousal symptoms. In addition, the symptoms must persist for at least 1 month for the diagnosis to be made.

Chronic PTSD is defined as lasting for more than 3 months, and delayed PTSD starts 6 months or more after the event. For those who do not qualify for a diagnosis of PTSD but are symptomatic during the passage of the requisite month of symptoms required for making the diagnosis, a new diagnosis of *acute stress disorder* was added to the *Diagnostic and Statistical Manual of Mental Disorders, Fourth Edition,* in 1994,[13] describing a similar condition that can be diagnosed in as early as 2 days. Once 4 weeks have passed, however, the diagnosis passes from acute stress disorder to PTSD in those who are still sufficiently

TABLE 12.1 PTSD Symptoms

Reexperiencing	Avoidance and Numbing	Hyperarousal
Intrusive Memories	Avoids Thoughts/Feelings	Insomnia
Nightmares	Avoids Reminders	Irritability/Anger
Flashbacks	Event Amnesia	Difficulty Concentrating
Upset by Reminders	Loss of Interest	Hypervigilance
Physiologic Reactivity Reminders	Detachment/Estrangement	Jumpy/Easily Startled
	Restricted Range of Affection	Sense of Foreshortened Future

symptomatic. Acute stress disorder also includes many of the same symptoms of all three PTSD symptom groups required for acute stress disorder plus dissociative symptoms. Although the diagnosis of acute stress disorder is so new that little is known about its course or outcome,[14] research indicates that the kinds of symptoms seen in acute stress disorder may predict later development of PTSD and other psychopathology.[15-17]

RISK FACTORS FOR PTSD

Research has identified predictors of risk for PTSD. One predictor that we might expect is *severity of the disaster* itself and the *degree of individual exposure to it.* Degree of exposure to the disaster agent has been found to be associated with incidence of PTSD. People who lived closest to Mt. St. Helens volcano at the time of its eruption had higher rates of PTSD than those lived farther away.[18,19] After an earthquake, severity of PTSD was found to decrease as the distance from the earthquake's epicenter increased.[20] After the Oklahoma City bombing, the level of injury predicted development of PTSD.[21] Exposure variables are not as routinely and robustly predictive of PTSD as one might intuitively expect, however.[22] Other aspects of the disaster exposure that may be associated with the mental health consequences may include elements of terror (fear for one's life), horror (contact with the grotesque), and loss of loved ones in the event.

Mental health consequences of disasters vary in different parts of the population affected. The effects of a disaster spread outward like concentric circles; the greatest impact is at the bulls-eye or the epicenter, targeting the victims directly in the path of the disaster agent, some of whom are injured and others who flee for their lives. As the impact of the disaster spreads outward in waves, the ripples affect others with decreasing intensity as they reach the periphery. Others strongly affected are those who lose close family members or friends in the disaster and eyewitnesses from a safe but close distance or late arrivals on the scene. Rescue workers may also be affected by exposure to gruesome aspects of body recovery and handling, danger and injury to themselves, and bereavement of colleagues or direct victims they know. Moving further outward in the concentric circle model, we encounter people affected indirectly through disruption of the usual conduct of their businesses (and business income) due to the disaster, people who lose jobs, large numbers of people whose lives may be disrupted by loss of electricity and other utilities, and people (such as commuters) who are more distant and are delayed by detours and damaged roads. More widespread economic consequences of far-reaching disasters may be followed by significant mental health consequences in the population.[23-27]

At the furthest extreme are those who are so far removed (e.g., people halfway across the country who only hear about the event indirectly or watch news coverage of it on television). These individuals may feel very upset by the news but are not candidates for PTSD based on just hearing or seeing news about the event. One must be directly present, an eyewitness, or a loved one of a direct victim of a disaster to develop PTSD.

The most robust and reliable predictors of PTSD after disasters have been found to be *female sex*[28-32] and *predisaster psychopathology.*[31,33,34] It should be no surprise that women have a higher prevalence of PTSD than men after disasters, given that PTSD is classified as an anxiety disorder; in the general population that is not affected by traumatic events, anxiety and depressive disorders are more prevalent among women than among men.[35] It is well established that preexisting psychopathology is a powerful predictor of PTSD after traumatic events.[31,36-40] However, prior psychiatric illness is neither necessary nor sufficient to develop PTSD after such an event. People with no prior psychiatric difficulties regularly develop PTSD after disasters, and many people with previous psychiatric illness do not have a recurrence afterward.[21,37,38] Among people exposed to mild events or with minimal exposure to more severe events, previous psychiatric history is a particularly important predictor of PTSD. With more severe events and greater exposure, psychiatric history is less important as more and more individuals without preexisting mental health difficulties succumb to PTSD.[41] Personality is an overlooked aspect of predisposing psychopathology. Research has shown that preexisting personality disorders predict postdisaster psychopathology.[42] A caveat is that experience of extreme events may alter people's patterns of interacting with others and the world in a way that may mimic personality disorder in the short term. In making a determination of whether the behaviors represent preexisting personality disorder, the key is to examine lifelong patterns of behavior that began long before the disaster and span the majority of the individual's life.

Other variables such as increased age, lack of education, and lower socioeconomic status have been identified as predictors of PTSD, but observations on these factors have been less uniform.[43] The apparent associations of these variables with psychopathology may lie with their confounding with significantly associated variables. For example, in two studies, lack of education was associated with PTSD only because it was a characteristic of women, who had a significantly higher incidence of PTSD than men.[21,38] An early indicator of PTSD may be available in the form of avoidance and numbing symptoms, which in two studies have been found to serve as powerful markers of the disorder.[21,44] After the Oklahoma City bombing,[21] those fulfilling PTSD's group C avoidance and numbing criteria (i.e., demonstrating three or more symptoms of this category) had 94% specificity and 100% sensitivity for PTSD. In other words, 94% of the people who met group C criteria also had full PTSD. Because the diagnostic criteria for PTSD require fulfillment of group C criteria, 100% of people with PTSD met group C criteria. In addition to predicting PTSD, the avoidance and numbing symptom group was also associated with preexisting psychopathology, difficulties functioning, treatment-seeking, diagnostic comorbidity, and use of alcohol or drugs to cope with the disaster.

PTSD INCIDENCE AND COURSE

The incidence of PTSD varies considerably after different disasters. Low rates (2%–8%) were identified in studies of a volcano,[44] after torrential rain and mudslides,[45] and after flooding and exposure to dioxin contamination.[46] Rates of more than 50% have been recorded in association with an airplane crash-landing[45] and with a dam break and flood.[47]

After disasters, PTSD begins quickly. After the Oklahoma City bombing, of those who developed PTSD, 76% reported onset of symptoms the day of the bombing, 94% within the first week, and 98% within the first month.[21] Delayed PTSD (beginning more than 6 months after the incident) was not observed after the Oklahoma City bombing[21] or after a mass-murder episode in Killeen, Texas.[38] The delayed PTSD that has been described after other kinds of trauma, such as in adult survivors of childhood sexual abuse[48] and combat veterans,[49] is not typical of postdisaster experience.

The course of PTSD tends toward chronicity. In a general population study of PTSD, more than one-half of all cases of PTSD continued unabated for more than 1 year.[50] Predictors of chronicity regardless of treatment included greater severity of PTSD, psychiatric comorbidity, interpersonal numbing, emotional reactivity, female sex, and family history of antisocial behavior. In the community, the duration of PTSD averages 3 years.

One-third of PTSD cases last 10 years or more.[51] Cases in women last on average four times as long as those in men. Few studies have followed the course of PTSD longitudinally after disasters. Approximately one-half of PTSD cases had recovered 1 year after a mass-murder episode, but few predictors of chronicity versus recovery from PTSD could be identified.[38]

OTHER PSYCHIATRIC DISORDERS

Psychiatric comorbidity is important in the diagnosis and management of post-traumatic psychopathology because of its prevalence and its potential to complicate the course and treatment of PTSD and its association with functional disability.[21] It is all too easy to stop searching for psychopathology once a diagnosis of PTSD is identified, despite experience that after disasters, PTSD may occur more frequently accompanied by another diagnosis than solo.[21,37] The most prevalent comorbid disorder is major depression, followed by alcohol-use disorder,[21,37,38] although among some populations, such as rescue workers, alcohol-use disorder may be more prevalent than major depression or PTSD, and in those groups it is almost always preexisting.[52,53]

After disasters, the alcohol- and drug-use disorders identified in survivors represent disorders that are almost always present before the event[54] Very few cases of alcohol or drug abuse arise anew in the postdisaster setting,[21] although substance abuse is quite prevalent among survivors of community traumas, and substance use is assumed to represent self-medication or efforts to cope with the traumatic event.[55-57] Anecdotal impressions that substance abuse surfaces after disasters may stem from people being flushed out of their private dwellings into public settings, such as on sandbagging brigades during impending floods and in shelters housing those whose homes were destroyed. If their usual behaviors include heavy drinking in the privacy of their own homes, persistence of these behaviors in public settings during and after the disaster can expose problems not seen before that may be misinterpreted as newly developed.

RESILIENCE

In the rush to identify psychiatric cases needing intervention after disasters, the resilience of the human spirit and the recognition that the majority of people do not become psychiatrically ill after disasters often go underappreciated. In that rush, those who do not meet diagnostic criteria for any psychiatric disorder, but who are clearly distressed by the event, may be overlooked or discounted. Strong feelings and emotional reactions a re nearly universal experiences after disasters. After the Oklahoma City bombing, for example, 96% of the survivors, even those without PTSD, reported having one or more PTSD symptoms.[21] Shortly after the September 11 terrorist attacks, a Pew poll of the general public[58] found that 7 out of 10 people acknowledged feeling depressed, nearly 1 in 2 reported trouble concentrating, and 1 in 3 had trouble sleeping. These experiences can hardly be considered pathological, given that they are the norm, reported by the majority after such extreme events. Some describe these responses as "normal responses to abnormal events." These highly prevalent symptoms tend to consist of PTSD group B (intrusive recall) and group D (hyperarousal) items that do not correspond to comorbidity or problems functioning.[21] Studies have shown that with time these symptoms generally diminish on their own as the process of healing proceeds.

Other findings that may also be easily neglected in considering mental health consequences of disasters represent positive outcomes, benefit, or growth after experiencing such a cataclysmic event. Despite the massive harm disasters bring to people and communities, some people do well or find positive elements in themselves or others that they would never have discovered otherwise.[59,60] A study of three different disaster sites found that 35%–95% of individuals interviewed reported such positive effects.[59]

MENTAL HEALTH INTERVENTION AFTER DISASTERS

Management of postdisaster mental health problems begins by identifying individuals at highest risk for PTSD and other psychopathology through early screening. Special attention should be paid to individuals with known risk factors: greater exposure to more severe disaster events, women, and individuals with previous psychopathology.[61] Because symptoms start early, efforts to identify people at risk for psychiatric disorders may also start early, even in the first few days when a diagnosis of PTSD cannot yet be made. Although delayed-onset PTSD is generally not seen after disasters, delay in seeking treatment and failure to seek treatment are common.[62] Therefore, along with screening cases, a goal of intervention outreaches to the affected population that typically is reluctant to venture outside its community or to accept help from strangers.[63,64] The main key to management of mental health effects after disasters is to subdivide the affected population into those who are psychiatrically ill versus those who are not psychiatrically ill but are subdiagnostically distressed. Because these two subpopulations are likely to require different treatment, they need triage for interventions tailored to their situation. Therefore, no one treatment approach is right for everyone. Treatment needs to be individualized.

PHARMACOTHERAPY FOR PTSD

A number of pharmacotherapeutic options are available for treatment of postdisaster psychopathology.[65] Because PTSD can cause considerable functional disability and pharmacotherapy reduces symptoms and improves comfort and functioning, use of medication in the treatment of this disorder is as vital as it is to the treatment of major depression. Antidepressant medications are the mainstay of pharmacotherapy for PTSD. Although tricyclic antidepressant and monoamine oxidase inhibitor agents have been documented to be efficacious in PTSD, the selective-serotonin reuptake inhibitors (SSRIs) are more widely used and studied currently, in large part because of their less toxic and more tolerable side effect profiles. Other agents, such as benzodiazepines, sedative hypnotics, and mood stabilizers, are not first-line agents of pharmacotherapy for PTSD.[66] Currently, only two antidepressant agents have been indicated by the Food and Drug Administration (FDA) for the treatment of PTSD, and only recently. Sertraline (Zoloft) was approved for treatment of PTSD in 1999,[67] but only for women because the supporting studies failed to demonstrate convincing benefit in male populations. Paroxetine subsequently received FDA approval for the treatment of PTSD. Many of the studies assessing these agents have failed to include instruments measuring hyperarousal, making it difficult to determine effectiveness of the medications with this symptom group.[66] Studies have shown that the therapeutic effects of these agents in the treatment of PTSD are independent of antidepressant properties.[68]

The antidepressant agents used to treat PTSD are also effective for the conditions that most often are comorbid with PTSD, and this is an important benefit. Not only do SSRIs benefit PTSD, but they are also mainstays of treatment for major depression, panic disorder, generalized anxiety disorder, and other anxiety disorders. Thus, the patient with comorbid PTSD may benefit in multiple ways from the same pharmacologic intervention. It is important to search for other disorders besides PTSD because they tend to be very treatable as well.

Effective pharmacotherapy in the treatment of PTSD is best provided in conjunction with supportive and cognitive behavioral psychotherapy.[69]

NONPHARMACOLOGIC INTERVENTIONS FOR PTSD
AND POSTDISASTER DISTRESS

It is critical to resist the temptation to pathologize normal distress following trauma. Normative distress can be difficult to differentiate from PTSD symptoms after a traumatic exposure. It has been shown that the majority of trauma survivors recover naturally from their symptoms within the 3 months following the incident.[70]

Different approaches are needed for those who are distressed but do not fulfill the criteria for PTSD after disasters. While it would be a disservice to these individuals to pathologize them by diagnosing them with a psychiatric disorder based on behaviors that are normative in the context of a highly unusual event and fail to meet diagnostic criteria, *their distress should not be discounted,* and some intervention may be appropriate. Distressed individuals not meeting the criteria for a psychiatric diagnosis sometimes contact mental health professionals seeking information and reassurance about what their symptoms mean and requesting assistance with short-term symptom management.

Psychoeducation approaches help provide the information and reassurance these people seek. These individuals can be reassured that their troublesome symptoms and unpleasant reactions do not necessarily mean that they are becoming psychologically unraveled or mentally ill. They can be told that, for most people, these experiences tend to lose intensity and fade away with the natural process of healing and the passage of time. Most survivors of disasters tend to cope by turning to their trusted loved ones for sharing, support, and starting the process of trying to make meaning of their experience and gain some perspective on it. This "natural talk" may help reduce discomfort and speed healing, although there is no evidence for its effects on preventing or ameliorating psychiatric illness after disasters.

For those who desire to share and begin to process their experience cognitively with other survivors of the disaster, *group formats* may be helpful. Some of these groups meet fairly spontaneously in loosely structured memorial services and workplace meetings after disasters.

A form of talking through an experience is a more organized activity termed "debriefing," which is widely used in many contexts from spontaneously informing someone about something that happened to a highly formalized and structured psychological debriefing format called "critical incident stress debriefing," developed by Mitchell.[71] This debriefing can take on elements of narrative revisitation of an experience, crisis intervention (critical incident stress debriefing), education or psychoeducation, prevention, stress management, and psychotherapy.[72]

Debriefing has been widely applied far beyond its original intended goals[73] to apply to diverse life experiences and provide a "magic bullet" of preventive intervention.[72]

Debriefing may not be for everyone. It must also be tailored to an individual's needs and to the setting and the time frame.[72] If debriefing is not suited to the individuals and the setting, prolongation or intensification of distress may occur. The rising popularity of debriefing has elicited messages of caution by professionals[74] against engaging in blanket application of this kind of intervention without a number of preliminary considerations. Despite a number of published articles claiming effectiveness of debriefing, methodological and conceptual difficulties have seriously limited the comparison to the extent that no database systematically evaluates the acute and long-term effectiveness of debriefing in randomized controlled trials.[74,75] At present, debriefing procedures have not been shown to prevent or reduce PTSD.

Before commencing psychotherapy for PTSD, careful evaluation of the patient is needed to determine the psychiatric diagnosis/diagnoses, identify the most distressing problem (which is not necessarily the trauma-related symptoms), evaluate the patient's resources, and, importantly, assess the patient's motivation and ability to commit to the selected treatment.[76]

Additionally, assessment of the presence of current suicidality and comorbid psychiatric illness such as depressive and substance-use disorders will aid the determination of the best timing and choice of treatment. Because avoidance is a hallmark symptom of PTSD, conducting a comprehensive informed consent procedure will help promote successful engagement in trauma-focused therapy for patients suffering from this disorder.

A number of psychotherapies are used to treat trauma-related psychological problems. CBT for PTSD is widely used and endorsed and has considerable evidence of efficacy.[77-79] CBTs include several components such as psychoeducation, anxiety management, exposure, and cognitive restructuring; exposure and cognitive restructuring are considered the most effective components.[80] The most widely studied CBTs are cognitive processing therapy and exposure therapy. Both are trauma-focused therapies based on the emotional processing model of PTSD that theorizes the emergence of PTSD as part of development of a fear network in memory that elicits escape and avoidance behaviors.[81] The goal of trauma-focused therapies is to act on these processes in the fear network, through imaginal and *in vivo* exercises in exposure therapy and through classic cognitive restructuring techniques in CBT. These treatments are structured interventions that require specialized training and commitment of both patients and therapists to complete a series of structured therapy sessions that include homework assignments.[82] It is unknown how much the research evidence established for these therapies in other types of trauma will apply to survivors of disaster because of limited evidence specific to disaster survivors including only one randomized controlled study in this population.[83]

BIOTERRORISM

Terrorism involving biological and chemical agents—bioterrorism—occupies a class by itself due to unique elements that are not shared by other disasters. An inherent aspect of bioterrorism that heightens fear and panic is that people cannot appraise their level of exposure because the effects may be delayed and the direct exposure may leave no acutely observable stigmata. The disaster agent in bioterrorism may go undetected for some time after the exposure, with the emotionally traumatic aspect occurring only when it comes to light that the individual may have been exposed. It is difficult for individuals to assess their own risk when they do not even know the status or the extent of their exposure to a hazardous agent. In bioterrorism, inability to appraise one's exposure to the agent leaves estimation of illness or damage to the imagination easily influenced by the level of fear in the individual potentially exposed. The psychiatric effects of bioterrorism thus become disconnected ("disarticulated") from the level of exposure.[84]

When people learn that they were possibly exposed to a biohazard, there is potential for many to be fearful and turn to the health system for protection. Large numbers seeking vaccines, antidotes, and treatments for symptoms, as well as reassurance of their worries about future illness, may overwhelm emergency rooms and other portals of care.

The second pattern involves responses more distant in time to the exposure. Models involving toxic chemical spills and contamination accidents may be relevant to these kinds of events. Previous studies of chemical spills and attacks have suggested that post-traumatic, anxiety, mood, and somatization symptoms may follow, as well as long-term concerns and fears about risk for cancer as a result of the exposure.[29,85-87] When managing psychological threats arising from bioterrorism and toxic contamination incidents, it is important to provide practical, accurate, and reassuring information and useful direction to avoid contributing to excessive fears among the public[88-90] Good risk communication and provision of such information may actually reduce the impact of bioterrorism by directing the public away from fears that produce counterproductive and unsafe behaviors and moving people toward accurately informed problem solving.[31,91,92]

REFERENCES

1. Galea S, Ahern J, Resnick H, et al. Psychological sequelae of the Sept 11 terrorist attacks in New York City. *New Engl J Med.* 2002;346:982-987.
2. Galea S, Resnick H, Ahern J, et al. PTSD in Manhattan, New York City, after the September 11th terrorist attacks. *J Urban Health.* 2002;79:340-353.
3. Galea S, Vlahov, D, Resnick H et al. Trends of probable PTSD in New York City after the September 11 terrorist attacks. *Am J Epidemiol.* 2003;158:514-524.
4. Schlenger WE, Caddell JM, Ebert L, et al. Psychological reactions to terrorist attacks: Findings from the national study of Americans' reactions to Sept 11. *JAMA.* 2002;288:581-588.
5. Schuster MA, Bradley DS, Lisa, HJ, et al. A national survey of stress reactions after the Sept 11, 2001, terrorist attacks. *New Engl J Med.* 2001;345:1507-1512.
6. Silver RC, Holman A, McIntosh, DN, Poulin, M, Gil-Rivas, V. Nationwide longitudinal study of psychological responses to Sept 11. JAMA. 2002;288:1235-1244.
7. North CS, Surís AM, Davis M, Smith RP. Toward validation of the diagnosis of posttraumatic stress disorder. *Am J Psychiatry.* 2009;166(1):1-8.
8. World Health Organization. *Psychosocial Guidelines for Preparedness and Intervention in Disaster.* MNH/PSF/91.3. Geneva: World Health Organization; 1991.
9. Breslau N, Kessler RC, Chilcoat HD, et al. Trauma and posttraumatic stress disorder in the community. *Arch Gen Psychiatry.* 1998;55:626-632.
10. Brewin CR, Andrews B, Valentine JD. Meta-analysis of risk factors for posttraumatic stress disorder in trauma-exposed adults. *J Consult Clin Psychiatry.* 2000;68:748-766.
11. Norris FH, Friedman MJ, Watson PJ, Byrne CM, Diaz E, Kaniasty K. 60,000 disaster victims speak: Part I. An empirical review of the empirical literature, 1981-2001. *Psychiatry.* 2002;65:207-239.
12. Robins LN, Helzer JE, Croughan J, Williams JBW, Spitzer RL. *NIMH Diagnostic Interview Schedule. Version 3.* Bethesda MD: National Institute of Mental Health; 1981.
13. Robins LN, Cottler L, Bucholz K, Compton W., North CS, Rourke KM. *Diagnostic Interview Schedule for DSMIV.* St. Louis, MO. Washington University; 1999.
14. Solomon Z, Mikulincer M. Combat stress reactions, posttraumatic stress disorder, and social adjustment: A study of Israeli veterans. *J Nerv Ment Dis.* 1987;175:277-285.
15. Solomon Z, Mikulincer M, Kotler M. A two year follow-up of somatic complaints among Israeli combat stress reaction casualties. *J Psychosomatic Res.* 1987;31:463-469.
16. Cardena E, Spiegel, D. Dissociative reactions to the San Francisco Bay area earthquake of 1989. *Am J Psychiatry.* 1993;150:474-478.
17. Weisæth L. The stressors and the post-traumatic stress syndrome after an industrial disaster. *Acta Psychiatr Scand.* 1989;80:25-37.
18. Shore JH, Vollmer WM, Tatum EL. Community patterns of posttraumatic stress disorders. *J Nerv Ment Disord.* 1989;177:681-685.
19. Shore JH, Tatum EL, Vollmer WM. Psychiatric reactions to disaster: The Mount St Helens experience. *Am J Psychiatry.* 1986;143:590-595.
20. Abdo T, al-Dorzi H, Itani AR, Jabr F, Zaghloul N. Earthquakes: Health outcomes and implications in Lebanon. *J Med Liban.* 1997;45:197-200.
21. North CS, Nixon SJ, Shariat S, et al. Psychiatric disorders among survivors of the Oklahoma City bombing. *JAMA.* 1999;282:755-762.
22. Sungur M, Kaya B. The onset and longitudinal course of a man-made post-traumatic morbidity: Survivors of the Sivas disaster. *Int J Psychiatry Clin Pract.* 2001;5:195-202.
23. Nandi A, Tracy M, Beard JR, Vlahov D, Galea S. Patterns and predictors of trajectories of depression after an urban disaster. *Ann Epidemiol.* 2009;19(11):761-770.
24. Norris FH, VanLandingham MJ, Vu L. PTSD in Vietnamese Americans following Hurricane Katrina: Prevalence, patterns, and predictors. *J Trauma Stress.* 2009;22:91-101.
25. Sastry N, VanLandingham M. One year later: Mental illness prevalence and disparities among New Orleans residents displaced by Hurricane Katrina. *Am J Public Health.* 2009;99(Suppl 3):S725-S731.
26. North CS, King RV, Fowler RL, et al Psychiatric disorders among transported hurricane evacuees: Acute-phase findings in a large receiving shelter site. *Psychiatri Ann.* 2008;38(2):104-113.

27. Bland RC. Psychiatry and the burden of mental illness. *Can J Psychiatry*. 1998;43:801–810.

28. Moore HE, Friedsam HJ. Reported emotional stress following a disaster. *Soc Forces*. 1959;38:135–138.

29. Lopez-Ibor JJ, Jr., Canas SF, Rodriguez-Gamazo M. Psychological aspects of the toxic oil syndrome catastrophe. *Br J Psychiatry*. 1985;147:352–365.

30. Steinglass P, Gerrity E. Natural disasters and posttraumatic stress disorder: Short-term vs. long-term recovery in two disaster-affected communities. *J Appl Soc Psychol*. 1990;20:1746–1765.

31. Weisæth L. Post-traumatic stress disorder after an industrial disaster. In: Pichot P, Berner P,Wolf R, Thau K, eds. *Psychiatry--The State of the Art*. New York: Plenum Press; 1985:299–307.

32. Kasl SV, Chisholm RE, Eskenazi B. The impact of the accident at Three Mile Island on the behavior and well-being of nuclear workers. *Am J Public Health*. 1981;71:472–495.

33. Steinglass P, Weisstub E, De-Nour AK. Perceived personal networks as mediators of stress reactions. *Am J Psychiatry*. 1988;145:1259–1264.

34. Feinstein A, Dolan R. Predictors of post-traumatic stress disorder following physical trauma: An examination of the stressor criterion. *Psychol Med*. 1991;21:85–91.

35. Blazer DG, Hughes D, George LK, Swartz M, Boyer R. Generalized anxiety disorder. In: Robins LN, Regier DA, eds. *Psychiatric Disorders in America: The Epidemiologic Catchment Area Study*. New York: The Free Press; 1991:180–203.

36. Bromet EJ, Parkinson DK, Schulberg HC. Mental health of residents near the Three Mile Island reactor: A comparative study of selected groups. *J Prev Psychiatry*. 1982;1:225–276.

37. Smith EM, North CS, McCool RE, Shea JM. Acute postdisaster psychiatric disorders: Identification of persons at risk. *Am J Psychiatry*. 1990;147:202–206.

38. North CS, Smith EM, Spitznagel EL. Posttraumatic stress disorder in survivors of a mass shooting. *Am J Psychiatry*. 1994;151:82–88.

39. Ramsay R. Post-traumatic stress disorder: A new clinical entity? *J Psychosomatic Res*. 1990;34:355–365.

40. McFarlane AC. The aetiology of post-traumatic morbidity: Predisposing, precipitating and perpetuating factors. *Br J Psychiatry*. 1989;154:221–228.

41. Hocking F. Psychiatric aspects of extreme environmental stress. *Dis Nerv Syst*. 1970;31:542–545.

42. Southwick SM, Yehuda R, Giller EL. Personality disorders in treatment-seeking combat veterans with posttraumatic stress disorder. *Am J Psychiatry*. 1993;150:1020–1023.

43. North CS. Human response to violent trauma. *Balliére's Clin Psychiatry*. 1995;1:225–245.

44. McMillen JC, North CS, Smith EM. What parts of PTSD are normal: Intrusion, avoidance, or arousal? Data from the Northridge, California earthquake. *J Traum Stress*. 2000;13:57–75.

45. Canino G, Bravo M, Rubio-Stipec M, Woodbury M. The impact of disaster on mental health: Prospective and retrospective analyses. *Int J Ment Health*. 1990;19:51–69.

46. Smith EM, Robins LN, Przybeck TR, Goldring E, Solomon SD. Psychosocial consequences of a disaster. In: Shore JH, ed. *Disaster Stress Studies: New Methods and North Findings*. Washington, DC: American Psychiatric Association; 1986:49–76.

47. Green BL, Lindy JD, Grace MC, et al. Buffalo Creek survivors in the second decade: Stability of stress symptoms. *Am J Orthopsychiat*. 1990;60:43–54.

48. McNally RJ, Clancy SA, Schacter DL, Pitman RK. Cognitive processing of trauma cues in adults reporting repressed, recovered, or continuous memories of childhood sexual abuse. *J Abnorm Psychol*. 2000;109:355–359.

49. Prigerson HG, Maciejewski PK, Rosenheck RA. Combat trauma: Trauma with highest risk of delayed onset and unresolved posttraumatic stress disorder symptoms, unemployment, and abuse among men. *J Nerv Ment Dis*. 2001;189:99–108.

50. Breslau N, Davis GC. Posttraumatic stress disorder in an urban population of young adults: Risk factors for chronicity. *Am J Psychiatry*. 1992;149:671–675.

51. Kessler RC, Sonnega A, Bromet E, Hughes M, Nelson CB. Posttraumatic stress disorder in the National Comorbidity Survey. *Arch Gen Psychiatry*. 1995;52:1048–1060.

52. North CS, Tivis L, McMillen JC, et al. Psychiatric disorders in rescue workers of the Oklahoma City bombing. *Am J Psychiatry*. 2002;159:857–859.

53. Boxer PA, Wild D. Psychological distress and alcohol use among fire fighters. *Scand J Work Environ Health*. 1993;19:121–125.

54. North CS, Ringwalt CL, Downs DL, Derzon J, Galvin D. The post-disaster course of alcohol use disorders in systematically studied survivors of ten disasters. *Arch Gen Psychiatry*. 2010; ePub Oct 4.

55. Zatzick DF, Roy-Byrne P, Russo JE, et al. Collaborative interventions for physically injured trauma survivors: A pilot randomized effectiveness trial. *Gen Hosp Psychiatry*. 2001;23:114–123.

56. Jacobsen LK, Southwick SM, Kosten TR. Substance use disorders in patients with posttraumatic stress disorder: A review of the literature. *Am J Psychiatry*. 2001;158: 1184–1190.

57. Saxon AJ, Davis TM, Sloan KL, et al. Trauma, symptoms of posttraumatic stress disorder, and associated problems among incarcerated veterans. *Psychiatr Serv*. 2001;52:959–964.

58. Associated Press. Poll: Americans depressed, sleepless. MSNBC. 9-19-2001. Washington, DC.
59. McMillen JC, Smith EM, Fisher RH. Perceived benefit and mental health after three types of disaster. *J Consult Clin Psychiatry.* 1997;6:733-739.
60. McMillen JC. Better for it: How people benefit from adversity. *Soc Work.* 1999;44:455-468.
61. Smith EM, North CS, Spitznagel EL. Post-traumatic stress in survivors of three disasters. *J Soc Behav Pers.* 1993;8:353-368.
62. Weisæth L. Acute posttraumatic stress: Nonacceptance of early intervention. *J Clin Psychiatry.* 2001;62:35-40.
63. North CS, Hong BA. Project C.R.E.S.T.: A new model for mental health intervention after a community disaster. *Am J Public Health.* 2000;90:1-2.
64. Lindy JD, Grace MC, Green BL. Survivors: Outreach to a reluctant population. *Am J Orthopsychiatry.* 1981;51:468-478.
65. Davidson JR. Pharmacotherapy of posttraumatic stress disorder: Treatment options, long-term follow-up, and predictors of outcome. *J Clin Psychiatry.* 2000;61(Suppl):52-59.
66. Cyr M, Farr MK. Treatment for posttraumatic stress disorder. *Ann Pharmacother.* 2000;34:366-376.
67. Schatzberg AF. New indications for antidepressants. *J Clin Psychiatry.* 2000;61(Suppl):9-17.
68. Davidson JRT, Rothbaum BO, van der Kolk BA, Sikes CR, Farfel GM. Multicenter, double-blind comparison of sertraline and placebo in the treatment of posttraumatic stress disorder. *Arch Gen Psychiatry.* 2001;58:485-492.
69. Southwick SM, Yehuda R. The interaction between pharmacotherapy and psychotherapy in the treatment of posttraumatic stress disorder. *Am J Psychother.* 1993;47: 404-410.
70. Foa EB, Cahill SP. Specialized treatment for PTSD: Matching survivors to the appropriate modality. In: Yehuda R, ed. *Treating Trauma Survivors with PTSD.* Washington DC: American Psychiatric Publishing; 2002.
71. Mitchell JT, Everly GS. *Critical Incident Stress Debriefing (CISD).* Ellicott City, MD: Chevron Publishing; 1995.
72. Raphael B, Wilson JP. Introduction and overview: Key issues in the conceptualization of debriefing. In: Raphael B, Wilson JP, eds. *Psychological Debriefing: Theory, Practice and Evidence.* Cambridge: Cambridge University Press; 2000:1-14.
73. Pitman RK, Altman B, Greenwald E, et al. Psychiatric complications during flooding therapy for posttraumatic stress disorder. *J Clin Psychiatry.* 1991;52:17-20.
74. Ursano RJ, Fullerton CS, Vance K, Wang L. Debriefing: Its role in the spectrum of prevention and acute management of psychological trauma. In: Raphael B, Wilson J, eds. *Psychological Debriefing: Theory, Practice and Evidence.* Cambridge: Cambridge University Press; 2000.
75. Raphael B, Meldrum L, McFarlane AC. Does debriefing after psychological trauma work? *BMJ.* 1995;310:1479-1480.
76. Shalev AY, Friedman MJ, Foa, EB, Keane TM. Integration and summary. In Foa EB, Keane TM, Friedman, MJ, eds. *Effective Treatments for* PTSD. New York: The Guilford Press; 2000: 361-362.
77. Institute of Medicine. *Treatment of Posttraumatic Stress Disorder: An Assessment of the Evidence.* Washington, DC: The National Academies Press; 2008.
78. Nemeroff CB, Bremner JD, Foa EB, Mayberg HS, North CS, Stein MB. Posttraumatic stress disorder: A state-of-the-science review. *J Psychiatr Res.* 2006;40(1):1-21.
79. Ponniah K, Hollon SD. Empirically supported psychological treatments for adult acute stress disorder and posttraumatic stress disorder: A review. *Depress Anxiety.* 2009;26(12):1086-1109.
80. http://www.ptsd.va.gov/professional/pages/overview-treatment-research.asp
81. Foa EB, Steketee GS, Rothbaum BO. Behavioral/cognitive conceptualizations of posttraumatic stress disorder. *Behav Ther.* 1989;20:155-176.
82. Cahill SP, Foa EB, Hembree EA, Marshall RD, Nacash N. Dissemination of exposure therapy in the treatment of posttraumatic stress disorder. *J Trauma Stress.* 2006;19(5):597-610.
83. Basoglu M, Salcioglu E, Livanou M, Kalender D, Acar G. Single-session behavioral treatment of earthquake-related posttraumatic stress disorder: A randomized waiting list controlled trial. *J Traum Stress.* 2005;18(1):1-11.
84. North CS, Pfefferbaum B, Vythilingam M, et al. Exposure to bioterrorism and mental health response among staff on Capitol Hill. *Biosecur Bioterror.* 2009;7(4):379-388.
85. Bowler RM, Mergler D, Huel G, Cone JE. Psychological, psychosocial, and psychophysiological sequelae in a community affected by a railroad chemical disaster. *J Traum Stress.* 1994;7:601-624.
86. Arata CM, Picou JS, Johnson GD, McNally TS. Coping with technological disaster: An application of the conservation of resources model to the Exxon Valdez oil spill. *J Traum Stress.* 2000;13:23-39.
87. Bowler RM, Mergler D, Huel G, Cone JE. Aftermath of a chemical spill: Psychological and physiological sequelae. *Neurotoxicology.* 1994;15:723-729.
88. North CS, Pollio DE, Pfefferbaum B, et al. Concerns of Capitol Hill staff workers after bioterrorism: Focus group discussions of authorities' response. J Nerv Ment Dis. 2005;193(8):523-527.

89. Moscrop A. Mass hysteria is seen as main threat from bioweapons. *BMJ.* 2001;323:1023.
90. Marks TA. Birth defects, cancer, chemical, and public hysteria. *Regul Toxicol Pharmacol.* 1993;2(Pt 1):44.
91. Covello CT, Peters RG, Wojteki JG, Hyde RC. Risk communication, the West Nile virus, and bioterrorism: Responding to the challenges posed by the intentional or unintentional release of a pathogen in an urban setting. *J Urban Health.* 2001;87:382–391.
92. National Research Council. *Chemical and Biological Terrorism: Research and Development to Improve Civilian Medical Response.* Washington, DC: National Academy Press; 1999.

13

Quality of Life and Psychosocial Adaptation to Chronic Illness and Acquired Disability: A Conceptual and Theoretical Synthesis

MALACHY BISHOP

*I*n contrast to persons with congenital disabilities, for whom research suggests that the process of body image and identity development is likely to be similar to that of children without disabilities (Grzesiak &Hicok, 1994; Livneh & Antonak, 1997; Wright, 1983), people who experience later-onset chronic illness or acquired disability (CIAD) may find their sense of self suddenly and dramatically challenged or altered. These persons may be faced with significant changes in their social and familial relationships and life roles while deal-ing concurrently with psychological distress, physical pain, prolonged medical treatment, and gradually increasing interference in or restriction of the performance of daily activities (Charmaz, 1983; Livneh & Antonak, 1997). Understanding how people navigate this process of adapting to CIAD-related changes and applying this understanding in the form of effec-tive clinical interventions has been an important focus of rehabilitation research for several decades (Elliott, 1994; Wright & Kirby, 1999).

Yet, despite the decades of research committed to understanding the dynamics of psychosocial adaptation, a review of the rehabilitation literature suggests a surprising lack of conceptual clarity and limited consensus about such fundamental questions as the nature of the process of adaptation and the appropriate conceptualization of outcome (Frank & Elliott, 2000; Livneh, 1988; Livneh & Antonak, 1997; Smart, 2001; Wright & Kirby, 1999). Further, in terms of the ultimate goal of this theoretical development, the translation of theory into practice, there is little evidence that adaptation theory has effectively translated into clinical intervention (Parker, Schaller, & Hansmann, 2003).

It has been suggested, for example, that few rehabilitation counselors either utilize the various existing measures of adjustment or adaptation in the counseling process, or assess the client's adaptation in terms of any extant theory (Bishop, 2001; Kendall & Buys, 1998). Rather, outside of the research context, measures specifically designed to assess adapta-tion rarely play a significant role in rehabilitation assessment, counseling, or planning. The failure of rehabilitation counselors to evaluate and address psychosocial adaptation in the counseling relationship likely results from a number of factors, including (a) the failure to understand the potential influence of adaptation on rehabilitation outcome, (b) the failure to see the clinical utility of extant theories of adaptation in the rehabilitation relationship, and (c) a lack of familiarity with, or confusion over, the many and frequently contradictory

From "Quality of life and psychosocial adaptation to chronic illness and acquired disability: A Con-ceptual and theoretical synthesis," by M. Bishop, 2005, *Journal of Rehabilitation, 71,* 5–13. Printed with permission from *Journal of Rehabilitation.*

theories or models of adaptation found in the rehabilitation counseling literature. The present chapter presents a model of adaptation to CIAD that may address some of these problems.

In the course of the decades, long exploration of the adaptation to disability process theories from fields of study outside of rehabilitation counseling have frequently contributed to both rehabilitation counseling practice and theoretical understanding. Such applications include, for example, that of Lewin's field theory (Lewin, 1951), operant learning principles (Elliott, 1994), and research from the medical sociology literature concerning the implications of chronic illness for the sense of self (Charmaz, 1983). Consistent with this approach, over the last two decades, rehabilitation researchers have suggested with increasing frequency that concepts from quality of life (QOL) research may provide an appropriate framework to understand the adaptation process (Crewe, 1980; Livneh, 1988, 2001; Livneh, Martz, & Wilson, 2001; Viney & Westbrook, 1982; Wright, 1983).

The twofold purpose of this chapter is (a) to explore this frequently proposed but underdeveloped relationship between adaptation to disability and QOL and (b) to propose a QOL-based model of adaptation to CIAD that has significant potential for enhancing both theoretical understanding and clinical application. This chapter begins with a review of those theoretical approaches to adaptation that have been prevalent in the rehabilitation counseling literature and the theoretical and clinical limitations associated with them. It is then proposed that a QOL perspective on adaptation may be seen to both encompass the important features of these extant approaches and address many of the limitations. Following this, a specific QOL-based model of adaptation, termed "disability centrality," is proposed. This model integrates concepts drawn from the QOL literature with existing models of adaptation from the rehabilitation literature. Because the proposed model relies on specific and contextual definitions of both QOL and adaptation, the definitions that are used in the proposed model are presented. Finally, the clinical implications of the proposed model are discussed.

DEFINING PSYCHOSOCIAL ADAPTATION

Although considerable disagreement exists concerning the specific nature of psychosocial adaptation (Livneh, 2001; Livneh & Antonak, 1997; Wright & Kirby, 1999), at a fundamental-level adaptation may be conceived as a process of responding to the functional, psychological, and social changes that occur with the onset and experience of living with a disability, chronic illness, or associated treatments. This process has been characterized in terms of movement toward some variously described outcome. Researchers have conceived both the process and the outcome in a great variety of ways (e.g., DeLoach & Greer, 1981; Kendall & Buys, 1998; Linkowski, 1971; Livneh & Antonak, 1997; Wright, 1983; Wright & Kirby, 1999).

In order to suggest that QOL represents an appropriate framework for defining and understanding the adaptation process, it is first necessary to understand how adaptation has been conceptualized to date. The following discussion reviews the current and historical approaches prominent in the rehabilitation literature, the limitations that have been associated with these approaches, and some points of theoretical consensus.

Current and Historical Approaches and Their Limitations

Early approaches to understanding the process of psychosocial adjustment to CIAD were based on a medical or psychopathological model and on the idea that "specific types of disabilities brought about specific types of personality characteristics or psychological problems" (Shontz, 2003, p. 178). It was believed that there existed "a direct relationship between the condition and psychosocial impairment" (Elliott, 1994, p. 231). Such theories failed, however, to reflect either the individuality or the complexity of the process of adaptation. Further, these early models neglected to consider the interaction between the individual and his or her social and physical environments. Over time, as it was increasingly observed that neither diagnosis nor degree of impairment, irrespective of other factors, served as important predictors of an individual's overall adaptation (Williamson, Schulz, Bridges, & Behan, 1994), such theories were increasingly recognized as incomplete and lacking empirical support or clinical utility.

Sequential or stage theories, in which adaptation is described in terms of movement through a predictable and terminal series of stages of adjustment, gained increasing acceptance in the 1970s and 1980s. The premise of such theories has been questioned in recent years. For example, the concept of a final stage of adjustment has repeatedly been rejected as un-realistic (Kendall & Buys, 1998; Parker, Schaller, & Hansmann, 2003). In addition, Kendall and Buys suggested that counselors working from this perspective may come to expect and identify as normal such reactions as depression and denial, and withhold or delay services until the client exhibits these responses according to the counselor's expectations. Stage theories have also been criticized as lacking both empirical validity (Elliott, 1994; Parker et al., 2003) and sufficient complexity to accurately represent the adaptation process, particularly in terms of progressive conditions (Kendall & Buys, 1998; Wortman & Silver, 1989).

More recent conceptualizations represent a more complex and comprehensive approach in which emphasis is placed on the interaction between the individual and the environments in which he or she lives. The conceptual framework of adaptation proposed by Livneh and Antonak (1997) and Livneh (2001) has been described as illustrative of the differences between early and modern approaches (Shontz, 2003). Livneh and Antonak proposed that four groups of variables influence adaptation outcomes, including social-demographic variables, disability-related variables, personality attributes, and physical/social environment. The comprehensive nature of such ecological or interactive models is more congruent with the observation that psychosocial adaptation is a highly complex and individual process. However, as has been suggested about stage or phase models (Kendall & Buys, 1998), ecological models are primarily descriptive rather than predictive. Because they fail to identify the motivating force behind the generally recognized movement toward adaptation (Kendall & Buys, 1998; Linkowski, 1971), such models have limited utility in terms of informing counseling intervention.

In terms of psychometric approaches to defining and measuring adaptation outcome, the measures most commonly used in research have been criticized for their unidimensional and atheoretical nature and their conceptual vagueness (Livneh & Antonak, 1997; Wright & Kirby, 1999). In the most frequently used measures, adaptation is operationalized as a unidimensional construct, measured as, for example: (1) pathological dimensions of personality (primarily the presence of depression or anxiety), (2) physical or behavioral complaints, (3) changes in productivity or reduction in performance, or (4) degree of disability acceptance (Livneh & Antonak, 1997). These unidimensional approaches to defining adaptation fail to encompass the complex and multidimensional nature of an individual's experience.

Other criticisms of existing theories of adaptation include their relative silence with regard to the individual differences that may be associated with gender and culture. Extant measures of adaptation have also been criticized for having a negatively skewed perspective (Smart, 2001; Wright & Kirby, 1999). That is, although individuals frequently report psychologically positive aspects of living with a disability (e.g., Smart, 2001; Wright, 1983; Wright & Kirby, 1999), unidimensional and deficit-oriented measures of adaptation are unable to register this aspect of experience.

Theoretical Consensus

Despite the ongoing debate about the adaptation process and appropriate conceptualization of outcome, two points of general consensus have consistently emerged across theories. The first is that the process of adaptation to the onset of disability involves a multidimensional response. The second is that this process is highly individual and unique.

Adaptation as a Multidimensional Construct

Because the onset of chronic illness and disability may potentially affect a range of psychological, physical, environmental, and social domains, rehabilitation researchers have consistently suggested that adaptation to chronic illness be measured multidimensionally (e.g., Jacobson et al., 1990; Livneh & Antonak, 1997; Shontz, 1965). For example, Jacobson et al. described adaptation to chronic illness in terms of self-esteem, psychological symptoms, behavioral problems, demonstrated skills in educational and social situations, and attitudes regarding the condition. Livneh and Antonak described adaptation as "(1) active participation in social, vocational, and avocational pursuits; (2) successful negotiation of the physical environment; and (3) awareness of remaining strengths and assets as well as existing functional limitations" (p. 8).

Adaptation as a Subjective Process

Research has also consistently indicated that significant variation exists within and across individuals in the adaptation process (Kendall & Buys, 1998). Inherent in more recent approaches to understanding the adaptation process is the subjective and phenomenological nature of the individual's response. That is, just as the condition itself fails to act as a predictor of adaptation, neither can the individual's response be predicted based on an objected analysis of specific features of either the person or the environment. Rather, the individual's personal and subjective analysis of his or her total situation appears to be the most important factor in guiding his or her response.

Adaptation Defined

Based on these points of current consensus, for the purpose of this chapter, adaptation to CIAD is defined as the individual's personal and highly individual response to disability-or illness-related disruptions across a wide range of life domains. These disruptions may be experienced, for example, in interpersonal relationships, in interaction with the physical environment, and as changes in psychological or emotional health and function.

Because adaptation is both multidimensional and subjective, it is suggested that an appropriate measure of adaptation to CIAD is necessarily on that (a) is sufficiently broad to assess change across a range of life domains and (b) is able to portray the individual's subjective experience of changes within those domains. For the purpose of this chapter it is suggested that QOL, appropriately defined, represents such a measure.

QUALITY OF LIFE DEFINED

Because QOL has been defined in numerous ways and applied in a variety of contexts, it is incumbent on researchers to identify the specific definition for their purpose. QOL has been defined in terms of both subjective and objective indices. Traditionally, researchers have focused on the objected indicators. These include externally manifested and measurable indices such as employment status, income, socioeconomic status, and size of support network (Bishop & Feist-Price, 2001). However, focusing solely on objective indicators has been found to account for only a small amount of the variance in overall QOL ratings (Diener, Suh, Lucas, & Smith, 1999), and there appears to be little correlation between objective indicators and subjective measures of overall well-being, QOL, life satisfaction, or personal happiness (Michalos, 1991; Myers & Diener, 1995).

Such findings have lead to the suggestion that overall QOL is largely regulated by internal mechanisms (Gilman, Easterbrooks, & Frey, 2004), and researchers have increasingly focused on more subjective components of QOL, for example, self-reported attitudes, perceptions, and aspirations (Gilman et al., 2004). This focus is increasingly prevalent in the rehabilitation counseling literature (Frank-Stromberg, 1988; Noreau & Sheppard, 1995; Rubin, Chan, & Thomas, 2003).

Based on the above noted consensus that adaptation to disability represents a subjective and multidimensional process, for the present purpose, QOL is defined in terms of the same characteristics. Specifically, QOL is defined as the subjective and personally derived assessment of overall well-being that results from evaluation of satisfaction across an aggregate of personally or clinically important domains. This specific definition of the broader QOL construct has alternately been referred to as subjective QOL (Frisch, 1999; Michalos, 1991) and subjective well-being (Ormel, Lindenberg, Steverink, & Verbrugge, 1999).

Inherent in this definition is the assumption that overall QOL is associated with satisfaction across a finite number of domains, or areas of life. Research on the QOL construct increasingly supports this assumption (Bowling, 1995; Cummins, 1997; Felce & Perry, 1995; Frisch, 1999). Over the last two decades, researchers in different fields of human study, and using different methodological approaches, have identified a fairly consistent set of core domains as important determinants of QOL (Bishop & Allen, 2003). Although the number of domains varies somewhat, those typically identified include (a) psychological well-being (defined in such terms as life satisfaction and freedom from depression or anxiety), (b) physical well-being, (c) social and interpersonal well-being, (d) financial and material well-being, (e) employment or productivity, and (f) functional ability (Bishop & Allen, 2003; Felce & Perry, 1995; George & Bearon, 1980; Jalowiec, 1990).

THE DISABILITY CENTRALITY MODEL

It is clear that, while not synonymous, subjective QOL and psychosocial adaptation may be said to share a number of conceptual similarities, including their multidimensional and subjective characteristics. Based on a linking of these similar constructs and the inclusion of additional concepts drawn from the QOL literature, the disability centrality model for measuring and understanding the impact of CIAD is proposed. The model's underlying conceptual tenets are listed below. This is followed by a brief discussion of the rationale for each tenet. Because the proposed model represents, to a great extent, an integration of existing theories, these underlying theories are described in the course of this discussion.

Conceptual Tenets

1 First it is proposed that an individual's overall QOL represents a summative evaluation of satisfaction or well-being in a number of life domains and particularly those that are of greater personal importance (or are more highly central) to the individual.

2 Through mechanisms originally identified by Devins et al. (1983), the onset of CIAD is proposed to result in a change in overall QOL. (Although this effect may typically be experienced as a reduction, this is not universally the case.) A reduction in overall QOL occurs to the extent that the disability, illness, or associated treatments act to reduce satisfaction in centrally important domains either by reducing the ability to participate in valued activities, roles, or relationships or by reducing perceived control over valued outcomes.

3 People seek (and actively work) to achieve and maintain a maximal level of overall QOL, in terms of an internal and personally derived set-point. This is achieved by working to close perceived gaps between the present and the desired level of QOL.

4 As a result of this homeostatic mechanism, when an individual experiences significant negative impact from the onset of a CIAD, three potential responses or outcomes may result: (a) importance change—People experience a shift in the importance of domains so that previously central but highly affected domains become less central to overall QOL, and peripheral but less affected domains, in which more satisfaction may be realized, become more central; (b) control change—Through processes that increase perceived control, such as self-management, treatment, or environmental accommodation, the negative impact in important domains is reduced and these domains remain central; or (c) neither change situation occurs, and the person continues to experience a reduced overall QOL.

QOL and Centrality

The first tenet simply summarizes the above discussion of the definition of QOL as a subjective and multidimensional construct. There is, however, an additional idea that is critical to the proposed model and concerns the concept of importance or centrality. In the QOL literature this concept has been referred to as domain importance.

Although there is growing consensus that people equate overall QOL with satisfaction within a limited set of life domains, it stands to reason that individuals will differ with regard to which domains are more personally meaningful or important. An individual may report a high overall level of QOL or life satisfaction despite being dissatisfied with some specific life domains. For this reason, many researchers have suggested that a single rating of overall QOL has limited practical and clinical utility (Cummins, 1996). Rather, QOL researchers have suggested that satisfaction in more highly valued areas of life will "have a greater influence on evaluations of overall [QOL] than areas of equal satisfaction but lesser importance" (Frisch, 1999, p. 56). A critical assumption underlying this perspective is that satisfaction in more important domains may mitigate, or compensate for, dissatisfaction in other areas (Campbell, Converse, & Rogers, 1976; Gladis, Gosch, Dishuk, & Crits-Christoph, 1999).

The concept of domain importance provides rationale for the use of the term "centrality" in the proposed model. This term has been used in the social psychology, sociology, and rehabilitation literature to refer to the importance that a person attributes to a role or life domain (Quantanilla, 1991; Rosenberg, 1979; Wheaton, 1990). For example, work centrality has been defined as "the degree of general importance that working has in the life of an individual at any given point in time" (Quantanilla, p. 85). In the proposed model, the term centrality refers to the importance an individual attributes to an area of life that is altered by the onset of CIAD.

The Impact of CIAD on QOL

Among the theories in which the impact of CIAD is described in terms of QOL, Devins's theory of illness intrusiveness is perhaps the best established and the most comprehensively researched in the rehabilitation literature. In essence, Devins has posited that chronic illness acts to disrupt an individual's life, and that this disruption may be interpreted in terms of its impact on well-being, or QOL (Devins et al., 1983). Specifically, chronic illness-induced lifestyle disruptions are proposed to compromise psychosocial well-being by reducing (a) positively reinforcing outcomes of participating in meaningful and valued activities, and (b) feelings of personal control, by limiting the ability to obtain positive outcomes or avoid negative ones (Devins et al., 1983; Devins & Shnek, 2001). Devins has further suggested that this impact can be assessed in terms of QOL domains. To assess this dynamic, Devins developed the Illness Intrusiveness Ratings Scale (Devins, et al., 1983), a self-report instrument that obtains ratings of the degree to which an illness or its treatment interferes with each of the 13 life domains that were identified by Flanagan (1978) as being important to QOL. Significant empirical support for this theory has been established by Devins and other researchers over the last two decades (Devins, 1994; Devins et al., 1983; Mullins et al., 2001).

Extension of the Illness Intrusiveness Model

The present model begins with Devins' fundamental assumption that QOL domains represent an appropriate format for assessing the impact of CIAD. However, based on current research in the QOL literature suggesting the importance of weighting more personally important domains, an extension of Devins's approach is proposed. Specifically, in addition to assessing the impact of CIAD in terms of QOL domains, it is also critical to understand the relative importance of each domain to the individual.

Because individuals differ in the value they place on various areas of their life, simply assessing the extent of CIAD-related disruption across a range of domains fails to take into account the differential importance of domains, and therefore provides an incomplete picture of the individual's experience. Rather, in order to effectively help an individual adapt to these changes, it is critical to understand the extent to which central versus peripheral aspects of one's QOL, and one's identity, are affected (Ryff & Essex, 1992). To a great extent the concept of domain importance, of centrality, explains why two individuals who appear objectively similar may express very different responses to the same condition.

Domain Control

Devins has suggested that the impact of CIAD on QOL occurs through two mechanisms; by reducing satisfaction and by reducing control. Related to this latter mechanism, Devins further suggested that interventions that increase the individual's control over the CIAD or its treatment will act to ameliorate this impact (Devins, 1994; Devins & Shnek, 2001). This second value also has significant implications for clinical intervention.

The onset of CIAD and its associated treatments can affect personal control in myriad ways. Treatment schedules, functional limitations, changes in cognitive function and mood, and other CIAD-associated changes can lead to limitations and restrictions that reduce opportunities to engage in valued activities or achieve desired outcomes (Sidell, 2001). Conversely, research among persons with chronic illnesses suggests that interventions that increase perceived control are associated with increased psychological and behavioral well-being (Endler, Kocovski, & Macrodimitris, 2001).

With regard to such interventions, a clinically useful distinction has been suggested between primary and secondary controls (Heckhausen & Schulz, 1995). Primary control refers to behaviors or cognitions that are aimed at altering the external environment and efforts taken to change the environment to meet the changing needs of the individual. Secondary control refers to changes in internal cognitive or psychological processes. These changes act to reduce the impact of uncontrollable and aversive realities through mechanisms such as altering expectations, disengaging from or changing unachievable goals, or reframing a negative experience in a positive way (Misajon, 2002). Rehabilitation counseling interventions aimed at assisting the client to increase control may be directed at both the external environment through, for example, environmental modification and accommodations and the internal environment through cognitive counseling techniques that enhance the individual's sense of control. Specific interventions in both areas are further discussed below.

Potential Response to the Impact of CIAD on QOL

Thus far it has been suggested that CIAD-related changes frequently lead to reduced overall QOL by reducing satisfaction and control in personally important domains. The final component of the disability centrality model proposes the mechanisms by which people adapt to this reduction in QOL. Specifically, based on research suggesting that a positive level of QOL is not only normative but also adaptive, it is proposed that people respond to this reduction in QOL by making adaptive changes in either domain importance or domain control.

QOL research with adults suggests that maintaining a positive level of QOL may be vital to adaptation. For example, Diener and Diener (1995) argued that a positive subjective QOL baseline is necessary from an evolutionary perspective in that it allows for greater opportunities for social and personal advancement, exploratory behavior, and reliable coping resources. The idea that people naturally seek to improve their perceived position with regard to their goals and aspirations is suggested generally in the work of many personality theorists, including, for example, Alfred Adler (in Ansbacher & Ansbacher, 1956). Carl Rogers (1963), and Abraham Maslow (1964), all of whom described people as inherently seeking to overcome perceived personal and situational deficits. Because people seek to maintain a relatively high level of QOL, when CIAD impacts QOL an adaptive response is to be expected. In the present model it is proposed that an individual's response takes the form of one of three processes or, more likely, some combination thereof.

Importance Change

When significant negative change is experienced in centrally important domains, the person may engage in or experience an adaptive shift, in which the central domain becomes less valued and previously peripheral but less affected domains gain more importance, or become more central. This form of value change was originally suggested in the acceptance of loss theory, initially described by Dembo, Leviton, and Wright (1956) and later further explicated by Wright (1960, 1983). This value change "represents an awakening interest in satisfactions that are accessible, and facilitates coming to terms with what has been lost" (Wright, 1983, p. 163).

This phenomenon of an adaptive shift has also received attention in the QOL literature, and has alternately been referred to as "preference drift" (Groot & Van Den Brink, 2000), "domain compensation" (Misajon, 2002), and most frequently, "response shift" (Schwartz & Sprangers, 1999, 2000). Similar to the concept of value change, response shift represents a change in an individual's evaluation of his or her QOL resulting from either (1) a change in the individual's internal standards of measurement, (2) a change in the individual's values (i.e., in the important domains constituting QOL), or (3) a redefinition of life quality (Schwartz & Sprangers, 1999). There is a growing body of literature and increasing empirical support associated with the response shift concept in the QOL literature (e.g., Andrykowski, Brady, & Hunt, 1993; Bach & Tilton, 1994).

Control Change

These potential responses are referred to as control change. In this case, through various processes that increase personal control, the impact in central domains is reduced and these domains remain important. Whereas the loss of perceived control is associated with decreased QOL, "feelings of vulnerability and helplessness can be offset by generating a sense of personal control over the illness" or disability (Misajon, 2002, p. 48). Both of these potential responses, importance change and control change, have important clinical implications which are further discussed below.

No Change

The third potential outcome is that despite a reduced level of satisfaction, no change occurs in either domain importance or sense of control and the individual continues to experience a reduction in his or her overall QOL. In this situation the individual may become involved in a cycle of increasing loss of control, decreased satisfaction, and decreasing QOL. Because the process of adapting to CIAD, as to other changes, is a continuously evolving and cyclic (Kendall & Buys, 1998; Livneh, 2001), it is likely that all people experience a phase of inertia for some duration before the types of changes described above occur.

CLINICAL IMPLICATIONS

Abraham Maslow (1966) once quipped that when the only tool one owns is a hammer, every problem begins to resemble a nail. The rehabilitation counselor's perspective on the process of psychosocial adaptation plays a significant role in guiding both service delivery and outcome expectations. The models and theories of adaptation prevalent in the rehabilitation literature (i.e., the counselor's tools) have frequently been criticized for engendering potentially limiting or, otherwise, problematic counseling approaches. The following discussion describes how, as a means of assisting counselors to understand and explore adaptation with their clients, the QOL perspective in general, and the disability centrality model in particular, offers a number of important advantages.

Advantages of a QOL Approach

As opposed to traditional unidimensional measures of adaptation, the multidimensional QOL framework offers counselors and their clients the opportunity to view the client's life holistically and understand the impact of CIAD in the context of the complex interactions of personal, social, and environmental domains. This approach also has significant potential for furthering understanding of individual differences in the response to disability. For example, analyzing the impact of CIAD on QOL in terms of the unique values that may emerge from gender differences, cultural background differences, and different disability or illness types may lead to the development of more effective interventions based on these differences.

Finally, assessing adaptation across QOL domains may help counselors distinguish between positive and negative experiences in response to disability, addressing the previously identified limitation of measures that focus on and are capable of assessing only the negative aspects of disability. Thus, it may be seen that as a general framework for assessing and understanding the impact of disability, QOL assessment has the potential to offer a more realistic, comprehensive, and informative approach.

Advantages of the Disability Centrality Approach

In addition to these general advantages, the disability centrality model offers counselors a specific approach to understanding and developing individually based counseling interventions. Essentially, the disability centrality model suggests that in order to comprehensively assess the impact of and response to disability, it is important to understand not only the level of impact experienced in different areas of life but also the importance placed upon these areas by the individual.

Rehabilitation counselors should explore the client's experience in the domains of mental health, physical health, family relations, social relations, relationships with partner or spouse, economic situation, leisure activity, and the religious or spiritual domain. Although information about the client's experiences in each of these domains is frequently discussed as a part of the intake interview, the present model offers a means of organizing this information in a way that allows for the prioritizing of interventions. For example, if work is discovered to be highly central for a client, and is also highly affected by the disability or illness, counselors may prioritize addressing work-related problems over concerns in less central areas. If, however, family relations are of primary importance, and are currently being significantly impacted, it is important that this area receives counseling attention. Indeed, until these more important issues are addressed, it is less likely that vocational planning will be successful.

Counseling Interventions

The proposed model suggests that counselors can assist clients in the adaptation process by (1) helping clients to experience increased control and (2) by exploring avenues for increasing satisfaction in currently peripheral domains. A number of interventions may be identified to enhance personal control over the illness or disability, the associated treatments, and the impact of the condition in important areas of a person's life. For example, Devins (1994), Devins and Shnek (2000), and others have suggested the importance of self-management or actively taking responsibility and informed control over managing one's disability or illness. Corbin and Strauss (1988) suggested that in order to effectively manage a CIAD, one must become knowledgeable about and a participant in one's own care. Self-management means that the client is an active and informed participant in the relationship with health care providers, adheres to and understands treatment regimens, and communicates adverse effects and questions. From the counselor's perspective, this involves helping the client (a) to actively monitor and evaluate physical and psychological well-being and (b) to be knowledgeable about his or her condition and the treatment.

Counselors may also increase the client's sense of control by helping the client to first clarify and then reach domain-specific goals. For example, if the client reports experiencing little control in the dimension of social relationships, the counselor may employ social skills training to increase the client's confidence and competence in social skills. Simultaneously, the counselor can help the client identify opportunities for social interaction. This process of enhancing the sense of personal control involves promoting success by initially developing measurable and achievable subgoals and encouraging the client for successful efforts. Finally, identifying functional and environmental accommodations at work or at home also represents a way to help the client experience increased control and mastery.

Counselors can also play a role in assisting clients in the process of adaptation by helping them to reevaluate the range and form of their participation in life domains. That is, by assisting the client to develop new interests, new social outlets, and new ways of engaging life, counselors may enable clients to increase the importance of or satisfaction within previously peripheral domains.

CONCLUSION

The importance of addressing the individual's adaptation to the onset of chronic illness and disability has consistently been highlighted as an essential component in the rehabilitation process. Dell Orto (1991) underscored the importance of addressing adaptation in the clinical relationship when he suggested that the enormity of chronic illness and disability "is so pervasive, powerful, and all-encompassing that coping with, challenging, and overcoming it cannot be left to chance" (p. 333).

This chapter provides a practical QOL-based framework for assessing adaptation in the counseling process. This framework also provides rehabilitation counselors specific interventions for enhancing clients' control over the impact of CIAD. Although the model presented in this article is not meant to represent a finished product, this synthesis of constructs is seen as a potentially useful beginning. Research specifically aimed at assessing the validity and utility of the combined model is currently under-way and further refinement of these ideas will be an important next step.

REFERENCES

Andrykowski, M. A., Brady, M. J., & Hunt, J. W. (1993). Positive psychosocial adjustment in potential bone marrow transplant recipients: Cancer as a psychosocial adjustment. *Psycho-Oncology, 2*, 261–276.

Ansbacher, H. L., & Ansbacher, R. R. (1956). *The individual psychology of Alfred Adler.* New York: Basic Books.

Bach, J. R., & Tilton, M. C. (1994). Life satisfaction and well-being measures in ventilator assisted individuals with traumatic tetraplegia. *Archives of Physical Medicine and Rehabilitation, 75*, 626–632.

Bishop, M. (2001). The recovery process and chronic illness and disability: Applications and implications. *Journal of Vocational Rehabilitation, 16*, 47–52.

Bishop, M., & Allen, C. A. (2003). Epilepsy's impact on quality of life: A qualitative analysis. *Epilepsy & Behavior, 4*, 226–233.

Bishop, M., & Feist-Price, S. (2001). Quality of life in rehabilitation counseling: Making the philosophical practical. *Rehabilitation Education, 15*(3), 201–212.

Bowling, A. (1995). What things are important in people's lives? A survey of the public' judgment to inform scales of health related to quality of life. *Social Science and Medicine, 41*, 1447–1462.

Campbell, A., Converse, P. E., & Rogers, W. L. (1976). *The quality of American life: Perceptions, evaluations, and satisfaction.* New York: Russell Sage.

Charmaz, K. (1983). Loss of self: A fundamental form of suffering in the chronically ill. *Sociology of Health and Illness, 5*, 168–195.

Corbin, J., & Strauss, A. (1988). *Unending work and care: Managing chronic illness.* San Francisco: Jossey-Bass.

Crewe, N. M. (1980). Quality of life: The ultimate goal in rehabilitation. *Minnesota Medicine, 63*, 586–589.

Cummins, R. A. (1996). The domains of life satisfaction: An attempt to order chaos. *Social Indicators Research, 38*, 303–328.

Cummins, R. A. (1997). *Comprehensive quality of life scale-Adult* (5th ed., ComQol-A-5). Melbourne: Deakin University School of Psychology.

Dell Orto, A. E. (1991). Coping with the enormity of illness and disability. In R. P. Marinelli & A. E. Dell Orto (Eds.), *The psychological and social impact of disability* (3rd ed., pp. 333–335). New York: Springer Publishing Co.

DeLoach, C., & Greer, B. G. (1981). *Adjustment to severe physical disability: A metamorphosis.* New York: McGraw-Hill.

Dembo, T., Leviton, G. L., & Wright, B. A. (1956). Adjustment to misfortune: A problem of social-psychological rehabilitation. *Artificial Limbs, 3*(2), 4–62.

Devins, G. M. (1994). Illness intrusiveness and the psychosocial impact of lifestyle disruptions in chronic life-threatening disease. *Advances in Renal Replacement Therapy, 1*, 125–263.

Devins, G. M., Blinik, Y. M., Hutchinson, T. A., Hollomby, D. J., Barre, P. E., & Guttmann, R. D. (1983). The emotional impact of end-stage renal disease: Importance of patients' perceptions of intrusiveness and control. *International Journal of Psychiatry in Medicine, 13*, 327–343.

Devins, G. M., & Shnek, Z. M. (2001). Multiple Sclerosis. In R. G. Frank & T. R. Elliott (Eds.), *Hand book of rehabilitation psychology* (pp.163–184). Washington, DC: American Psychological Association.

Diener, E., & Diener, C. (1995). Most people are happy. *Psychological Science, 7*, 181–185.

Diener, E., Suh. E. M., Lucas, R. E., & Smith, H. L. (1999). Subjective well-being: Three decades of progress. *Psychological Bulletin, 125*, 276–302.

Elliott, T. R. (1994). A place for theory in the study of psychological adjustment among persons with neuromuscular disorders: A reply to Livneh and Antonak. *Journal of Social Behavior and Personality, 9*, 231–236.

Endler, N. S., Kocovsky, N. L., & Macrodimitris, S. D. (2001). Coping, efficacy, and perceived control in acute versus chronic illness. *Personal and Individual Differences, 30,* 617–625.

Flanagan, J. C. (1978). A research approach to improving our quality of life. *American Psychologist, 33,* 138–147.

Frank, R. G., & Elliott, T. R. (2000). Rehabilitation psychology: Hope for a psychology of chronic conditions. In R. G. Frank & T. R. Elliott (Eds.), *Handbook of rehabilitation psychology* (pp. 3–8). Washington, DC: American Psychological Association.

Frank-Stromberg, M. (1988). *Instruments for clinical nursing research.* Norwalk, CT: Appleton & Lange.

Frisch, M. B. (1999). Quality of life assessment/intervention and the Quality of Life Inventory (QOLI). In M. R. Maruish (Ed.), *The use of psychological testing for treatment planning and outcome assessment* (2nd ed., pp. 1227–1331). Hillsdale, NJ: Lawrence-Erlbaum.

George, L., & Bearon, L. (1980). *Quality of life in older persons.* New York: Human Sciences Press.

Gilman, R., Easterbrooks, S., & Frey, M. (2004). A preliminary study of multidimensional life satisfaction among deaf/hard of hearing youth across environmental settings. *Social Indicators Research, 66,* 143–166.

Gladis, M. M., Gosch, E. A., Dishuk, N. M., & Crits-Christoph, P. (1999). Quality of life: Expanding the scope of clinical significance. *Journal of Consulting and Clinical Psychology, 67,* 320–331.

Groot, W., & Van Den Brink, H. M. (2000). Life satisfaction and preference drift. *Social Indicators Research, 50,* 315–328.

Grzesiak, R. C., & Hicok, D. A. (1994). A brief history of psychotherapy and disability. *American Journal of Psychotherapy, 48,* 240–250.

Heckhausen, J., & Schulz, R. (1995). A life-span theory of control. *Psychological Science, 102*(2), 284–304.

Jacobson, A. M., Hauser, S. T., Lavori, P., Woldsdorf, J. I., Herskowitz, R. D., Milley, J. E., et al. (1990). "Adherence among children and adolescents with insulin-dependent diabetes mellitus over a four-year longitudinal follow-up" 1. The influence of patient coping and adjustment. *Journal of Pediatric Psychology, 15,* 511–526.

Jalowiec, A. (1990). Issues in using multiple measures of quality of life. *Seminars in Oncology Nursing, 6,* 271–277.

Kendall, E., & Buys, N. (1998). An integrated model of psychosocial adjustment following acquired disability. *Journal of Rehabilitation, 64*(3), 16–20.

Lewin, K. (1951). *Field theory in social science: Selected theoretical papers.* New York: Harper & Row.

Linkowski, D. C. (1971). A scale to measure acceptance of disability. *Rehabilitation Counseling Bulletin, 14,* 236–244.

Livneh, H. (1988). Rehabilitation goals: Their hierarchical and multifaceted nature. *Journal of Applied Rehabilitation Counseling, 19*(3), 12–18.

Livneh, H. (2001). Psychosocial adaptation to chronic illness and disability: A conceptual framework. *Rehabilitation Counseling Bulletin, 44*(3), 151–160.

Livneh, H. & Antonak, R. F. (1997). *Psychosocial adaptation to chronic illness and disability.* Gaithersburg, MD: Aspen.

Livneh, H., Martz, E., & Wilson, L. M. (2001). Denial and perceived visibility as predictors of adaptation to disability among college students. *Journal of Vocational Rehabilitation, 16,* 227–2234.

Maslow, A. H. (1966). *The psychology of science: A reconnaissance.* New York: Harper and Row.

Maslow, A. H. (1964). The superior person. *Transaction, 1,* 17–26.

Michalos, A. C. (1991). *Global report on student well-being: Volume 1, Life satisfaction and happiness.* New York: Springer-Verlag.

Misajon, R. A. (2002). *The homeostatic mechanism: Subjective quality of life and chronic pain.* Unpublished doctoral dissertation, Deakin University, Australia.

Mullins, L. L., Cote, M. P., Fuemmeler, B. F., Jean, V. M., Beatty, W. W., & Paul, R. H. (2001). Illness intrusiveness, uncertainty, and distress in individuals with multiple sclerosis. *Rehabilitation Psychology, 46,* 139–153.

Myers, D. G., & Diener, E. (1995). Who is happy? *Psychological Science, 6,* 10–19.

Noreau, L., & Sheppard, R. J. (1995). Spinal cord injury, exercise and quality of life. *Sports Medicine, 20,* 225, 250.

Ormel, J., Lindenberg, S., Steverink, N., & Verbrugge, L. M. (1999). Subjective well-being and social production functions. *Social Indicators Research, 46,* 61–90.

Parker, R. M., Schaller, J., & Hansmann, S. (2003). Catastrophe, chaos, and complexity models and psychosocial adjustment to disability. *Rehabilitation Counseling Bulletin, 46,* 234–241.

Rogers, C. R. (1963). The concept of the fully functional person. *Psychotherapy: Theory, Research, and Practice, 1,* 17–26.

Rosenberg, M. (1979). *Conceiving the self.* New York: Basic Books Inc.

Rubin, S. E., Chan, F., & Thomas, D. L. (2003). Assessing changes in life skills and quality of life resulting from rehabilitation services. *Journal of Rehabilitation, 69*(3), 4–9.

Ryff, C. D., & Essex, M. J. (1992). The interpretation of life experiences and well-being: The sample case of relocation. *Psychology and Aging, 7*, 507–517.

Schwartz, C. E., & Sprangers, M. A. G. (1999). The challenge of response shift for quality of life based clinical oncology research. *Annals of Oncology, 10*, 747–749.

Schwartz, C. E., & Springers, M. A. G. (2000). *Adaptation to changing health: Response shift in quality of life research*. Washington, DC: American Psychological Association.

Shontz, F. C. (1965). Reaction to crisis. *Volta Review, 67*, 364–370.

Shontz, F. C. (2003). Rehabilitation psychology, then and now. *Rehabilitation Counseling Bulletin, 46*, 176–181.

Sidell, J. (2001). Adult adjustment to chronic illness: A review of the literature. *Health and Social Work, 22*(1), 5–12.

Smart, J. (2001). *Disability, society, and the individual*. Gaithersburg, MD: Aspen.

Viney, L. L., & Westbrook, M. T. (1982). Patients' psychological reactions to chronic illness: Are they associated with rehabilitation? *Journal of Applied Rehabilitation Counseling, 13*(2), 38–44.

Wheaton, B. (1990). Life transitions, role histories, and mental health. *American Sociological Review, 55*, 209–223.

Williamson, G. M., Schulz, R., Bridges, M. W., & Behan, A. M. (1994). Social and psychological factors in adjustment to limb amputation. *Journal of Social Behvaior and Personality, 9*, 249–268.

Wright, B. A. (1960). *Physical disability: A psychological approach*. New York: Harper & Row.

Wright, B. A. (1983). *Physical disability: A psychological approach*. New York: Harper & Row.

Wright, S. J., & Kirby, A. (1999). Deconstructing conceptualizations of "adjustment" to chronic illness: A proposed integrative framework. *Journal of Health Psychology, 4*, 259–272.

II

The Personal Impact of Disability: Conclusion

DISCUSSION QUESTIONS

1. When an individual sustains an adventitious or traumatic physical disability, do you believe they will transition through various stages of adjustment, or do people react in differing, random ways depending on their circumstances?
2. Does "how" an individual sustains a disability (e.g., having a leg amputated versus contracting multiple sclerosis) affect how that person will react or adjust to their disability?
3. What gender issues do women with disabilities face that males with disabilities may not?
4. What are societal expectations of males and females in America, and how are those expectations affected when a male or female has a physical disability?
5. Could you be attracted to, potentially date, and eventually marry a wheelchair user with a spinal cord injury? If not, what would be your major concerns given the individual was attractive, intelligent, and had a good personality.
6. If a client with a spinal cord injury approached you for advice on finding a partner, how would you approach the topic and/or what would be your anxiety in discussing sexuality issues?
7. What do you believe is a specific aspect of one's culture that can be a strong influence on a person's emotional reaction to a physical disability?
8. How might religious beliefs help and/or inhibit one's psychosocial adaptation or adjustment to disability?
9. Which ethnic/racial group(s) may be more resilient to adapting to a family member with the disability?
10. How can a disability impact or alter coping mechanisms?
11. What is of primary concern, and how would counselors best work with individuals who are survivors of major disasters?

PERSONAL PERSPECTIVE

One of the most well-known counseling therapists in the world speaks of his own life living with and in spite of illness and disabilities and how he coped with the physical and mental implications of his experiences. His process of adaptation is a fascinating journey. Of interest, Dr. Ellis's own physical disabilities add to his effectiveness as a therapist. He explains those behavioral strategies that emerge from his disability, such as self-disclosure and combating irrational thoughts, and how they can be included in intervention strategies. Dr. Ellis provides another thought provoking perspective on the realities of psychosocial adaptation. This was reprinted from the fifth edition.

USING RATIONAL EMOTIVE BEHAVIOR THERAPY TECHNIQUES TO COPE WITH DISABILITY

ALBERT ELLIS

I have had multiple disabilities for many years and have always used Rational Emotive Behavior Therapy (REBT) to help me cope with these disabilities. That is one of the saving graces of having a serious disability—if you really accept it, and stop whining about having it, you can turn some of its lemons into quite tasty lemonade.

I started using REBT with my first major disability soon after I became a practicing psychologist in 1943, at the age of 30. At age 19 I began to have trouble reading and was fitted for glasses, which worked well enough for sight purposes but left me with easily tired eyes. After I read or even looked steadily at people for no more than 20 minutes, my eyes began to feel quite fatigued, and often as if they had sand in them. Why? Probably because of my prediabetic condition of renal glycosuria.

Anyway, from 19 years onward I was clearly handicapped by my chronically tired eyes and could find no steady release from it. Today, over a half-century later, it is still with me, sometimes a little better, sometimes a little worse, but generally unrelieved. So I stoically accepted my tired eyes and still live with them. And what an annoyance it is! I rarely read, especially scientific material, for more than 20 minutes at a time, and I almost always keep my eyes closed when I am not reading, working, or otherwise so active that it would be unwise for me to shut them.

My main sight limitation is during my work as a therapist in the world. At our clinic at the Institute for Rational Emotive Behavior Therapy in New York, I usually see individual and group clients from 9:30 a.m. to 11:00 p.m., with a couple of half-hour breaks for meals, and mostly for half-hour sessions with my individual clients. So during each week I may easily see over 80 individual and 40 group clients.

Do I get tired during these long days of working? Strangely enough, I rarely do. I was fortunate enough to pick high-energy parents and other ancestors. My mother and father were both exceptionally active, on-the-go, people, until a short time before my mother died of a stroke at the age of 93 and my father died, also of a stroke, at the age of 80.

Anyway, for more than a half-century I have conducted many more sessions with my eyes almost completely shut than I have with them open. This includes thousands of sessions I have done on the phone without ever seeing my clients. In doing so, I have experienced some real limitations but also several useful advantages. Advantages? Yes, such as these:

1. With my eyes shut, I can focus unusually well on what my clients are telling me and can listen nicely to their tones of voice, speech hesitations and speed-ups, and other aspects of their verbal communications.

2. With my eyes closed, I can focus better, I think, on what my clients are telling themselves to make themselves disturbed: on their basic irrational meanings and philosophies that are crucial to most of their symptoms.

From *Professional Psychology: Research and Practice,* 1997, 28(1), pp. 17–22. Reprinted with permission. Included in the 5th Edition of *The Psychological and Social Impact of Disability,* Springer Publishing, 2007.

3. When I am not looking at my clients I am quite relaxed and can easily avoid bothering myself about how well I am doing. I avoid rating myself and producing ego problems about what a great therapist and noble person I am—or am not!

4. My closed eyes and relaxed attitude seem to help a number of my clients relax during the session themselves, to open up, concentrating on and revealing their worst problems.

5. Some of my clients recognize my personal disabilities: They see that I refuse to whine about my adversities, work my ass off in spite of them, and have the courage to accept what I cannot change. They therefore often use me as a healthy model and see that they, too, can happily work and live in spite of their misfortunes.

Do not think, now, that I am recommending that all therapists, including those who have no ocular problems, should often shut their eyes during their individual therapy sessions. No. But some might experiment in this respect to see what advantages closing their eyes may have, especially at certain times.

Despite the fact that I could only read for about 20 minutes at a time, I started graduate school in clinical psychology in 1942, when I was 28, finished with honors, and have now been at the same delightful stand for well over a half-century—still with my eyes often shut and my ears wide open. I am handicapped and partially disabled, yes—but never whining and screaming about my disabilities, and always forging on in spite of them.

In my late 60s my hearing began to deteriorate; and in my mid-70s I got two hearing aids. Even when working in good order, they have their distinct limitations and have to be adjusted for various conditions, and even for the voice loudness and quality of the voices of the people I am listening to. So I use them regularly, especially with my clients, but I am still forced to ask people to repeat themselves or to make themselves clearer.

So I put up with all these limitations and use rational emotive behavior therapy to convince myself that they are not awful, horrible, and terrible but only a pain in the ass. Once in a while I get overly irritated about my hearing problem—which my audiologist, incidentally, tells me will definitely get a little worse as each year goes by. But usually I live very well with my poor auditory reception and even manage to do my usual large number of public talks and workshops every year, in the course of which I have some trouble in hearing questions and comments from my audiences but still manage to get by. Too bad that I have much more difficulty than I had in my younger years.

I was diagnosed as having full-blown diabetes at the age of 40, so that has added to my disabilities. Diabetes, of course, does not cause much direct pain and anguish, but it certainly does lead to severe restrictions. I was quickly put on insulin injections twice a day and on a seriously restricted diet. I, who used to take four spoons of sugar in my coffee in my prediabetic days, plus half cream, was suddenly deprived of both. Moreover, when I stuck with my insulin injections and dietary restrictions, I at first kept my blood sugar regularly low but actually lost 10 pounds off my usually all-too-thin body. After my first year of insulin taking, I became a near-skeleton!

I soon figured out that by eating 12 small meals a day, literally around the clock, I could keep my blood sugar low, ward off insulin shock reactions, and maintain a healthy weight. So for over 40 years I have been doing this and managing to survive pretty well. But what a bother! I am continually, day and night, making myself peanut butter sandwiches, pricking my fingers for blood samples, using my blood metering machines, carefully watching my diet, exercising regularly, and doing many other things that insulin-dependent diabetics have to do to keep their bodies and minds in good order.

When I fail to follow this annoying regimen, which I rarely do, I naturally suffer. Over the many years that I have been diabetic, I have ended up with a number of hypoglycemic reactions, including being carried off three times in an ambulance to hospital emergency wards. And, in spite of me keeping my blood sugar and my blood pressure healthfully low over these many years, I have suffered from various sequelae of diabetes and have to keep regularly checking with my physicians to make sure that they do not get worse or that new complications do not develop. So, although I manage to keep my health rather good, I have several physicians who I regularly see, including a diabetologist; an internist; an ear, nose, and throat specialist; a urologist; an orthopedist; and a dermatologist. Who knows what will be next? Oh, yes: Because diabetes affects the mouth and the feet, my visits to the dentist and podiatrist every year are a hell of a lot more often than I enjoy making them. But, whether I like it or not, I go.

Finally, as a result of my advancing age, perhaps my diabetic condition, and who knows what else, I have suffered for the last few years from a bladder that is easily filled and slow to empty. So I run to the toilet more than I used to, which I do not particularly mind. But I do mind the fact that it often takes me much longer to urinate than it did in my youth and early adulthood. That is really annoying!

Why? Because for as long as I can remember, I have been something of a time watcher. I figured out, I think when I was still in my teens and was writing away like a demon, even though I had a full schedule of courses and other events at college, that the most important thing in my life, and perhaps in almost everyone else's life, is time. Money, of course, has its distinct value; so does love. But if you lose money or get rejected in your sex/love affairs, you always have other chances to make up for your losses, as long as you are alive and energetic. If you are poor, you can focus on getting a better income; if you are unloved and unmated, you can theoretically get a new partner up until your dying day. Not so, exactly, with time. Once you lose a few seconds, hours, or years, there is no manner in which you can get them back. Once gone, you can in no way retrieve them. Tempus fugit—and time lost, wasted, or ignored is distinctly irretrievable.

Ever since my teens, then, I have made myself allergic to procrastination and to hundreds of other ways of wasting time, and of letting it idly and unthinkingly go by. I assume that my days on earth are numbered and that I will not live a second more than I actually do live. So, unless I am really sick or otherwise out of commission, I do my best to make the most of my 16 daily hours; and I frequently manage to accomplish this by doing two or more things at a time. For example, I very frequently listen to music while reading and have an interesting conversation with people while preparing a meal or eating.

This is all to the good, and I am delighted to be able to do two things at once, to stop my procrastinating and my occasional day dreaming and, instead, to do something that I would much rather get done in the limited time that I have to be active each day and the all too few years I will have in my entire lifetime. Consequently, when I was afflicted by the problem of slow urination in my late seventies, I distinctly regretted the 5 to 15 minutes of extra time it began to take me to go to the toilet several times each day and night. What a waste! What could I effectively do about saving this time?

Well, I soon worked out that problem. Instead of standing up to urinate as I had normally done for all my earlier life, I deliberately arranged for most of the times I went to the john to do so sitting down. While doing so, I first settled on doing some interesting reading for the several minutes that it took me to finish urinating. But then I soon figured out that I could do other kinds of things as well to use this time.

For example, when I am alone in the apartment that I share with my mate, Janet Wolfe, I usually take a few minutes to heat up my regular hot meal in our microwave oven. While it is cooking, I often prepare my next hot meal as well as put it in a microwave dish in the refrigerator, so that when I come up from my office to our apartment again, I will have it quickly ready to put in the oven again. I therefore am usually cooking and preparing two meals at a time. As the old saying goes, two meals for the price of one!

Once the microwave oven rings its bell and tells me that my cooked meal is finished, I take it out of the oven, and instead of putting it on our kitchen table to eat, I take it into the bathroom and put it on a shelf by the side of the toilet, together with my eating utensils. Then, while I spend the next 5 or 10 minutes urinating, I simultaneously eat my meal out of the microwave dish that it is in and thereby accomplish my eating and urinating at the same time. Now some of you may think that this is inelegant or even boorish. My main goal is to get two important things—eating and urinating—promptly done, to polish them off as it were, and then to get back to the rest of my interesting life. As you may well imagine, I am delighted with this efficient arrangement and am highly pleased with having efficiently worked it out!

Sometimes I actually can arrange to do tasks while I am also doing therapy. My clients, for example, know that I am diabetic and that I have to eat regularly, especially when my blood sugar is low. So, with their permission, I actually eat my peanut butter and sugarless jelly sandwiches while I am conducting my individual and group sessions, and everyone seems to be happy.

However, I still have to spend a considerable amount of time taking care of my physical needs and dealing with my diabetes and other disabilities. I hate doing this, but I accept the fact that I have little other choice. So I use rational emotive behavior therapy (REBT) to overcome my tendencies toward low frustration tolerance that I may still have. I tell myself whenever I feel that I am getting impatient or angry about my various limitations:

> Too damned bad! I really do not like taking all this time and effort to deal with my impairments and wish to hell that I didn't have to do so. But alas, I do. It is hard doing so many things to keep myself in a relatively healthy condition, but it is much harder, and in the long run much more painful and deadly, if I do not keep doing this. There is no reason whatsoever why I absolutely must have it easier than I do. Yes, it is unfair for me to be more afflicted than many other people are. But, damn it, I should be just as afflicted as I am! Unfairness should exist in the world—to me, and to whomever else it does exist—because it does exist! Too bad that it does—but it DOES! (Ellis, 1979, 1980)

So, using my REBT training, I work on my low frustration tolerance and accept—yes, really accept—what I cannot change. And, of course, barring a medical miracle, I cannot right now change any of my major disabilities. I can live with them, and I do. I can even reduce them to some extent, and I do. But I still cannot get rid of them. Tough! But it is not awful. REBT, as you may or may not know, posits that there are two main instigators of human neurosis: First, low frustration tolerance (e.g., I absolutely must have what I want when I want it and must never, never be deprived of anything that I really, really desire). Second, self-denigration (e.g., when I do not perform well and win others' approval, as at all times I should, ought, and must, I am an inadequate person, a retard, a nogoodnik!).

Many disabled people in our culture, in addition to suffering from the first of these disturbances, suffer even more seriously from the second. People with serious disabilities often have more performance limitations in many areas (e.g., at school, at work, and at sports) than those who have no disabilities. To make matters worse, they are frequently criticized, scorned, and put down by others for having their deficiencies. From early childhood to old age, they may be ridiculed and reviled, shown that they really are not as capable and as "good" as are others. So not only do they suffer from decreased competence in various areas but also from much less approval than more proficient members of our society often receive. For both these reasons, because they notice their own ineptness and because many of their relatives and associates ignore or condemn them for it, they falsely tend to conclude, "My deficiencies make me a deficient, inadequate individual."

I largely taught myself to forgo this kind of self-deprecation long before I developed most of my present disabilities. From my early interest in philosophy during my teens, I saw that I did not have to rate myself as a person when I rated my efficacy and my lovability. I began to teach myself, before I reached my mid-20s, that I could give up most of my feelings of shame and could unconditionally accept myself as a human even when I did poorly, especially at sports. As I grew older, I increasingly worked at accepting myself unconditionally. So when I started to practice REBT in 1955, I made the concept of unconditional self-acceptance (USA) one of its key elements (Baiter, 1995; Dryden, 1995; Ellis, 1973, 1988, 1991, 1994, 1996; Hauck, 1991).

As you can imagine by what I stated previously in this chapter, I use my REBT-oriented high frustration tolerance to stop myself from whining about disabilities and rarely inwardly or outwardly complain about this. But I also use my self-accepting philosophy to refrain from ever putting myself down about these handicaps. For in REBT one of the most important things we do is teach most of our clients to rate or evaluate only their thoughts, feelings, and actions and not rate their self, essence, or being. So for many years I have followed this principle and fully acknowledged that many of my behaviors are unfortunate, bad, and inadequate, because they do not fulfill my goals and desires. But I strongly philosophize, of course, that I am not a bad or inadequate person for having these flaws and failings.

I must admit that I really hate growing old. Because, in addition to my diabetes, my easily tired eyes, and my poor hearing, old age definitely increases my list of disabilities. Every year that goes by I creak more in my joints, have extra physical pains to deal with, slow down in my pace, and otherwise am able to do somewhat less than previously. So old age is hardly a blessing!

However, as I approach the age of 82, I am damned glad to be alive and to be quite active, productive, and enjoying life. My brother and sister, who were a few years younger than I, both died almost a decade ago, and just about all my close relatives are also fairly long gone. A great many of my psychological friends and associates, most of who were younger than me unfortunately have died, too. I grieve for some of them, especially for my brother, Paul, who was my best friend. But I also remind myself that it is great that I am still very much alive, as is my beloved mate, Janet, after more than 30 years of our living together. So, really, I am very lucky!

Do my own physical disabilities actually add to my therapeutic effectiveness? I would say, yes—definitely. In fact, they do in several ways, including the following.

1. With my regular clients, most of whom have only minor disabilities or none at all, I often use myself as a model and show them that, in spite of my 82 years and my physical problems, I fully accept myself with these impediments and give myself the same unconditional self-acceptance that I try to help these clients achieve. I also often show them, directly and indirectly, that I rarely whine about my physical defects but have taught myself to have high frustration tolerance (HFT) about them. This kind of modeling helps teach many of my clients that they, too, can face real adversities and achieve USA and HFT.

2. I particularly work at teaching my disabled clients to have unconditional self-acceptance by fully acknowledging that their deficiencies are unfortunate, bad, and sometimes very noxious but that they are never, except by their own self-sabotaging definition, shameful, disgraceful, or contemptible. Yes, other people may often view them as horrid, hateful people, because our culture and many other cultures often encourage such unfair prejudice. But I show my clients that they never have to agree with this kind of bigotry and can actively fight against it in their own lives as well as help other people with disabilities to be fully self-accepting.

I often get this point across to my own clients by using self-disclosure and other kinds of modeling. Thus, I saw a 45-year-old brittle, diabetic man, Michael, who had great trouble maintaining a healthy blood sugar level, as his own diabetic brother and sister were able to do. He incessantly put himself down for his inability to work steadily, to maintain a firm erection, to participate in sports, and to achieve a good relationship with an attractive woman who would mate with him in spite of his severe disabilities.

When I revealed to Michael several of my own physical defects and limitations, such as those I mentioned previously in this chapter, and when I showed him how I felt sad and disappointed about them but stubbornly refused to feel at all ashamed or embarrassed for having these difficulties, he strongly worked at full self-acceptance, stopped denigrating himself for his inefficacies, shamelessly informed prospective partners about his disabilities, and was able to mate with a woman who cared for him deeply in spite of them.

In this case, I also used REBT skill training. As almost everyone, I hope, knows by now, REBT is unusually multimodal. It shows people with physical problems how to stop needlessly upsetting themselves about their drawbacks. But it also teaches them various social, professional, and other skills to help them minimize and compensate for their hindrances (Ellis, 1957/1975, 1988, 1996; Gandy, 1995). In Michael's case, in addition to teaching him unconditional self-acceptance, I showed him how to socialize more effectively; how to satisfy female partners without having perfect erections; and how to participate in some sports, such as swimming, despite his physical limitations. So he was able, although still disabled, to feel better and to perform better as a result of his REBT sessions. This is the two-sided or duplex kind of therapy that I try to arrange with many of my clients with disabilities.

3. Partly as a result of my own physical restrictions, I am also able to help clients, whether or not they have disabilities, with their low frustration tolerance (LFT). As I noted earlier, people with physical restrictions and pains usually are more frustrated than those without such impediments. Consequently, they may well develop a high degree of LFT. Consider Denise, for example. A psychologist, she became insulin dependent at the age of 30 and felt horrified about her newly acquired restrictions. According to her physicians, she now had to take two injections of insulin and several blood tests every day, give up most of her favorite fat-loaded and salt-saturated foods, spend a half-hour a day exercising, and take several other health-related precautions. She viewed all of these chores and limitations as "revolting and horrible," and became phobic about regularly carrying them out. She especially kept up her life-long gourmet diet and gained 20 extra pounds within a year of becoming diabetic. Her doctors' and her husband's severe criticism helped her feel guilty, but it hardly stopped her in her foolish self-indulgence.

I first worked with Denise on the LFT and did my best to convince her, as REBT practitioners often do, that she did not need the eating and other pleasures that she wanted. It was indeed hard for her to impose the restrictions her physical condition now required, but it was much harder, I pointed out, if she did not follow them. Her increased limitations were indeed unfortunate, but they were hardly revolting and horrible; I insisted that she could stand them, though never necessarily like them.

I at first had little success in helping Denise to raise her LFT because, as a bright psychologist, she irrationally but quite cleverly parried my rational arguments. However, using my own case for an example, I was able to show her how, at my older age and with my disabilities greater than hers, I had little choice but to give up my former indulgences or die. So, rather than die, I gave up putting four spoons of sugar and half cream in my coffee, threw away my salt shaker, stopped frying my vegetables in sugar and butter, surrendered my allergy to exercise, and started tapping my fingers seven or eight times a day for blood tests. When Denise heard how I forced my frustration tolerance up as my pancreatic secretion of insulin went down, and how for over 40 years I have thereby staved off the serious complications of diabetes that probably would have followed from my previous habits, and from her present ones, she worked on her own LFT and considerably reduced it.

Simultaneously, I also helped Denise with her secondary symptoms of neurosis. As a bright person and as a psychologist who often helped her clients with their self-sabotaging thoughts, feelings, and behaviors, she knew how destructive her own indulgences were, and she self-lambasted and made herself feel very ashamed of them, thereby creating a symptom about a symptom: self-downing about her LFT. So I used general REBT with her to help her give herself unconditional self-acceptance in spite of her indulging in her LFT. I also specifically showed her how, when I personally slip back to my pre-disability ways and fail to continue my antidiabetic exercise and other prophylactic routines, I only castigate my behavior and not my self or personhood. I therefore see myself as a goodnik who can change my no-goodnik actions, and this USA attitude helps me correct those actions. By forcefully showing this to Denise, and using myself and my handling of my disabilities as notable examples, I was able to help her give up her secondary symptoms—self-deprecation—and go back to working more effectively to decrease her primary symptom—low frustration tolerance.

I have mainly tried to show in this chapter how I have personally coped with some of my major disabilities for over 60 years. But let me say that I have found it relatively easy to do so because, first, I seem to be a natural-born survivor and coper, which many disabled (and nondisabled) people are not. This may well be my innate predisposition but also may have been aided by my having to cope with nephritis from my 5th to my 8th years and my consequent training myself to live with physical adversity. Second, as noted earlier, I derived an epicurean and stoic philosophy from reading and reasoning about many philosophers' and writers' views from my 16th year onward. Third, I originated REBT in January 1955 and have spent the great majority of my waking life teaching it to clients, therapists, and members of the public for over 40 years.

For these and other reasons, I fairly easily and naturally use REBT methods in my own life and am not the kind of difficult customer that I often find my clients to be. With difficult customers who have disabilities and who keep complaining about them and not working too hard to overcome and cope with them, I often use a number of cognitive, emotive, and behavioral techniques for which REBT is famous and which I have described in my book, *How to Cope With a Fatal Illness* (Ellis & Abrams, 1994) and in many of my other writings (Ellis, 1957/1975, 1985, 1988, 1994, 1996).

Several other writers also have applied REBT and cognitive behavior therapy (CBT) to people with disabilities, including Rochelle Balter (1995), Warren Johnson (1981), Rose Oliver and Fran Bock (1987), and J. Sweetland (1991). Louis Calabro (1991) has written a particularly helpful chapter showing how the anti-awfulizing philosophy of REBT can be used with individuals suffering from severe disabilities, such as those following a stroke, and Gerald Gandy (1995) has published an unusual book, *Mental Health Rehabilitation: Disputing Irrational Beliefs*.

The aforementioned writings include a great many cognitive, emotive, and behavioral therapy techniques that are particularly useful with people who have disabilities. Because, as REBT theorizes, human thinking, feeling, and acting significantly interact with each other, and because emotional disturbance affects one's body as well as one's physical condition and affects one's kind of and degree of disturbance, people who are upset about their disabilities often require a multifaceted therapy to deal with their upset state. REBT, like Arnold Lazarus's (1989) multimodal therapy, provides this kind of approach and therefore often is helpful to people with disability-related problems.

Let me briefly describe a few of the cognitive REBT methods that I frequently use with my clients who have disabilities and who are quite anxious, depressed, and self-pitying about having these handicaps. I bring out and help them dispute their irrational beliefs. Thus, I show these clients that there is no reason why they must not be disabled, although that would be distinctly desirable. No matter how ineffectual some of their behaviors are, they are never inadequate persons for having a disability. They can always accept themselves while acknowledging and deploring some of their physical and mental deficiencies. When other people treat them unkindly and unfairly because of their disabilities, they can deplore this unfairness but not damn their detractors. When the conditions under which they live are unfortunate and unfair, they can acknowledge this unfairness while not unduly focusing on and indulging in self-pity and horror about it.

Preferably, I try to show my disabled clients how to make a profound philosophical change and thereby not only minimize their anxiety, depression, rage, and self-pity for being disadvantaged but to become considerably less disturbable about future adversities. I try to teach them that they have the ability to consistently and strongly convince themselves that nothing is absolutely awful, that no human is worthless, and that they can practically always find some real enjoyment in living (Ellis, 1994, 1996; Ellis & Abrams, 1994). I also try to help them accept the challenge of being productive, self-actualizing, and happy in spite of the unusual handicaps with which they may unfortunately be innately endowed or may have acquired during their lifetime. Also, I point out the desirability of their creating for themselves a vital absorbing interest, that is, a long-range devotion to some cause, project, or other interest that will give them a real meaning and purpose in life, distract them from their disability, and give them ongoing value and pleasure (Ellis, 1994, 1996; Ellis & Harper, 1975).

To aid these goals of REBT, I use a number of other cognitive methods as well as many emotive and behavioral methods with my disabled clients. I have described these in many chapters and books, so I shall not repeat them here. Details can be found in *How to Cope With a Fatal Illness* (Ellis & Abrams, 1994).

Do I use myself and my own ways of coping with my handicaps to help my clients cope with them? I often do. I first show them that I can unconditionally accept them with their disabilities, even when they have partly caused these handicaps themselves. I accept them with their self-imposed emphysema from smoking or with their 100 extra pounds of fat from indulging in ice cream and candy. I show them how I bear up quite well with my various physical difficulties and still manage to be energetic and relatively healthy. I reveal some of my time-saving, self-management, and other discipline methods that I frequently use in my own life. I indicate that I have not only devised some sensible philosophies for people with disabilities but that I actually apply them in my own work and play, and I show them how. I have survived my handicaps for many years and damned well intend to keep doing so for perhaps a good number of years to come.

CONCLUSION

I might never have been that much interested in rational or sensible ways of coping with emotional problems had I not had to cope with a number of fairly serious physical problems from the age of 5 years onward. But rather than plague myself about my physical restrictions, I devoted myself to the philosophy of remaining happy in spite of my disabilities, and out of this philosophy I ultimately originated REBT in January 1955 (Ellis, 1962, 1994; Wiener, 1988; Yankura & Dryden, 1994). As I was developing REBT, I used some of its main principles on myself, and I have often used them with other people with disabilities. When

I and these others have worked to acquire an anti-awfulizing, unconditional self-accepting philosophy, we have often been able to lead considerably happier and more productive lives than many other handicapped individuals lead. This hardly proves that REBT is a panacea for all physical and mental ills. It is not. But it is a form of psychotherapy and self-therapy especially designed for people who suffer from uncommon adversities. It points out to clients in general and to physically disadvantaged ones in particular that however much they dislike the harsh realities of their lives, they can manage to make themselves feel the healthy negative emotions of sorrow, regret, frustration, and grief while stubbornly refusing to create and dwell on the unhealthy emotions of panic, depression, despair, rage, self-pity, and personal worthlessness. To help in this respect, it uses a number of cognitive, emotive-evocative, and behavioral methods. Its results with disabled individuals have not yet been well researched with controlled studies. Having used it successfully on myself and with many other individuals, I am of course prejudiced in its favor. But controlled investigations of its effectiveness are an important next step.

REFERENCES

Balter, R. (1995, Spring). Disabilities update: What role can REBT play? IRETletter, 1–4.
Calabro, L. E. (1991). *Living with disability*. New York: Institute for Rational Emotive Therapy.
Dryden, W. (1995). *Brief rational emotive behavior therapy*. London: Wiley.
Ellis, A. (1962). *Reason and emotion in psychotherapy*. Secaucus, NJ: Citadel.
Ellis, A. (1973). *Humanistic psychotherapy: The rational emotive approach*. New York: McGraw-Hill.
Ellis, A. (1975). *How to live with a neurotic: At home and at work* (Rev. Ed.). Hollywood, CA: Wilshire Books. (Original work published 1957.)
Ellis, A. (1979). Discomfort anxiety: A new cognitive behavioral construct. Part 1. *Rational Living*, 14(2), 3–8.
Ellis, A. (1980). Discomfort anxiety: A new cognitive behavioral construct. Part 2. *Rational Living*, 15(1), 25–30.
Ellis, A. (1985). *Overcoming resistance: Rational emotive therapy with difficult clients*. New York: Springer.
Ellis, A. (1988). *How to stubbornly refuse to make yourself miserable about anything—yes, anything!* Secaucus, NJ: Lyle Stuart.
Ellis, A. (1991). Using RET effectively: Reflections and interview. In M.D. Bernard (Ed.), *Using rational emotive therapy effectively* (pp. 1–33). New York: Plenum Press.
Ellis, A. (1994). *Reason and emotion in psychotherapy* (revised and updated). New York: Birch Lane Press.
Ellis, A. (1996). *Better, deeper and more enduring brief therapy*. New York: Brunner/Mazel.
Ellis, A., & Abrams, M. (1994). *How to cope with a fatal illness*. New York: Barricade Books.
Ellis, A., & Harper, R. A. (1975). *A new guide to rational living*. Hollywood, CA: Wilshire Books.
Gandy, G. L. (1995). *Mental health rehabilitation: Disputing irrational beliefs*. Springfield, IL: Thomas.
Hauck, P. A. (1991). *Overcoming the rating game: Beyond self-love—beyond self-esteem*. Louisville, KY: Westminster/John Knox.
Johnson, W. R. (1981). *So desperate the fight*. New York: Institute for Rational Emotive Therapy.
Lazarus, A. A. (1989). *The practice of multimodal therapy*. Baltimore, MD: Johns Hopkins University Press.
Oliver, R., & Bock, F. A. (1987). *Coping with Alzheimer's*. Hollywood, CA: Melvin Powers.
Sweetland, J. (1991). *Cognitive behavior therapy and physical disability*. Point Lookout, NY: Author.
Wiener, D. (1988). *Albert Ellis: Passionate skeptic*. New York: Praeger.
Yankura, J., & Dryden, W (1994). *Albert Ellis*. Thousand Oaks, CA: Sage.

PERSONAL PERSPECTIVE EXERCISE

1. What techniques or strategies did Albert Ellis use to adapt to his own multiple disabilities?

2. What would be some of the advantages and disadvantages to having a gradual-onset disabling condition, as he did, rather than a sudden-onset disability in terms of adaptation or adjustment?

3. How important do you believe having a sense of humor about one's limitations is to effectively dealing with one's disability?

4. As a world-renowned psychotherapist, educator, and book author, what cognitive, behavioral, and emotional traits do individuals like Ellis seem to possess that help them excel in life and be successful despite having a disability?

5. What information might you take from this remarkable personal story and perhaps integrate into your counseling practice with clients?

III

Family Issues in Illness and Disability: Introduction

*I*n Chapter 14 of this section, Prilleltensky draws on her research related to motherhood and parenting with a physical disability. This study further looks at the relationship between the child and mother and the child's well-being. The literature in this area continues to be sparse. Most of what is found focuses on the relationship between parents with a disability and how it relates to the psychosocial needs of their children's well-being. The unique aspect of this particular chapter explores the author's personal experiences of being a mother with muscular dystrophy and issues related to parenting. This is a very qualitative-oriented study, which interestingly finds that parents who have disabilities are quite independent within their families. There were no indications that the children and adolescents in this study had to act as the caregiver; rather, this relationship is typically found in more adult roles. In fact, some of the highest risk factors in parenting appear to be associated with high rates of poverty, single parenting with very little support system, and society's attitudinal barriers associated with women with physical disabilities. Prilleltensky's research concludes that the children within the families were not expected to carry out tasks that were inappropriate, burdensome, and restricting to their overall well-being; in fact, these children were quite well adjusted.

In keeping with the theme of parenting with a disability, the Case-Smith chapter also takes a qualitative approach to demonstrate the cultural differences, demands, and responsibilities in families that have children with disabilities. There is no doubt that parenting with a disability or being a parent of a child with a disability can be a stressful experience; however, the overall impact is not necessarily negative. Using a family systems model, Case-Smith's chapter examines ethnographic data, care-giving roles, social occupations, and self-identities of families with preschool-age children who have chronic medical conditions and disabilities. The Case-Smith study takes on the challenge of explaining to the reader the complex interplay of variables of parenting children with disabilities. These families ultimately have unique cultural differences that are separate from those families who parent children without disabilities. However, the strength of this qualitative study offers guidelines for rehabilitation practitioners on how to cultivate coping and resiliency strategies for families that have such challenges.

The chapter by Buki, Uman, Kogan, and Keen provides insight into one heterosexual, HIV-serodiscordant (i.e., one HIV-positive and one HIV-negative partner) couple's experience with AIDS. Through a series of interviews, the experience of a husband in the advanced stages of AIDS is described, as well as the experience of his wife who is his primary caregiver. A thematic analysis of these experiences reveals the emotional impact of the HIV diagnosis, the significant psychosocial changes in the couple's daily lives, their needs for social support, and their spiritual journeys. The chapter closes with several recommendations for counselors working with persons with AIDS and their heterosexual partners.

This is not your typical chapter on HIV/AIDS education, prevention, and treatment. Rather, because of its qualitative nature, the critical incidents provided in this study challenge not only the reader's intellect but the emotions in dealing with the psychosocial nature of persons who have such life-threatening disabilities.

The chapter by Pedersen and Revenson on parental illness, family functioning, and adolescent well-being demonstrates the psychosocial challenges of adolescents who live with parents who have a chronic illness. Most empirical studies discuss stress within the family dynamics and tend to focus on a parent with a chronic illness to try and establish the association between the severity of the illness and his or her adjustment. However, the unique contribution by these authors focuses on the developmental stage of adolescence by describing the unique psychosocial adjustment adolescents must go through in terms of coping tasks, role redistribution, and the long-term implications within the family. By discussing specific types of illnesses such as parents who have HIV/AIDS, breast cancer, diabetes, and other chronic illness, the reader can draw on specific research that discusses the qualitative nature of such illnesses. Rehabilitation professionals may utilize this material for generalization to practice settings. To better demonstrate and illustrate the critical psychosocial reactions of chronic illness within the family dynamics, and particularly adolescents, the authors offer a family ecological framework. This framework considers four basic principles: (a) social context, (b) interdependence within multiple systems, (c) reciprocal and interactive relationships between individuals and social systems, and (d) the multiple other variables that interact with the psychosocial adaptation of adolescents growing up in families that deal with chronic illnesses. Additionally, the authors offer to the reader a plethora of research within health psychology, early childhood development, and family medicine that reports on the interrelationships among parental illness, family functioning, and adolescent well-being.

Despite the limited research in this area, many studies support the hypothesis that parental illness negatively impacts some aspects of adolescent well-being, placing adolescents at greater risk for anxiety, depression, low self-esteem, and other maladaptive behavioral problems. Pedersen and Revenson conclude this chapter with a "blueprint" for future research on adaptation to parental illness, which should be valuable to practitioners to conceptualize programs and services for families and especially adolescents growing up in homes where there is a parent with a chronic illness.

Finally, Winske in Chapter 18 describes his personal experience living with muscular dystrophy and provides some empirical support regarding this neuromuscular disorder, while Lingerman provides a personal perspective on living with a child who has spina bifida. The authors talk about the devastating effects of family secrets and how the absence of communication between family members can cause difficulties in psychosocial adjustment and response to disability. Despite an account of life-changing events, these authors show how serious disruptions and crises within their families lead from just survival to spiritual growth and overall psychosocial well-being.

14

My Child Is Not My Carer: Mothers With Physical Disabilities and the Well-Being of Children

ORA PRILLELTENSKY

*T*his chapter is based on a study that explored the intersection of motherhood and physical disability. My own experience as a mother with muscular dystrophy has provided the impetus for this research. Elsewhere (Prilleltensky, 2003), I depict the pregnancy and early parenting experiences of mothers with disabilities, and their access (or lack thereof) to formal and informal supports. In this chapter, I focus on the relationship between disabled mothers and their children, and on the efforts of the former to enhance the well-being of the latter.

My use of the term *disability* is consistent with its reframing by disability scholars as a socially constructed disadvantage (Gill, Kewman, & Brannon, 2003). There are some substantive variations between the British social model of disability and the minority group model in the United States and it is beyond the scope of this chapter to explain them. Nonetheless, both models highlight issues of power, oppression, and civil rights, and share the premise that many of the barriers associated with disability are socially constructed and thus preventable. The impact of structural and attitudinal barriers on the lives of people with disabilities is manifested in the realm of parenting. Kirshbaum and Olkin (2002) refer to parenting as the "last frontier," where discrimination due to impairment is enacted. As a group, parents with disabilities and particularly mothers with disabilities have encountered others' skepticism regarding their capacity to function as parents. Prejudicial assumptions about their ability to provide care and about the psychological well-being of their children often underpin the resistance that many encounter (Campion, 1995; Kocher, 1994; Wates, 1997; Wates & Jade, 1999).

People with learning difficulties are particularly vulnerable to societal misconceptions that the mere presence of such impairments is inevitably counterindicated with the ability to parent. Work by Booth and Booth (1994) and others (Tymchuk, 1992, cited in Campion, 1995) has emphasized the need to deconstruct such assumptions, rather than hold them as truisms. Whereas individuals with intellectual and physical impairments share some common experiences of discrimination, this should not obscure important distinctions that may be of relevance to policy and practice. This chapter specifically explores the intersection of motherhood and physical disabilities and reviews literature that is specific to physical impairment. Whereas it cannot automatically be extrapolated to parents with other types of disabilities (e.g., intellectual and emotional), some of its implications and

From "My child is not my carer: Mothers with physical disabilities and the well being of children," by
O. Prilleltensky, 2004, *Disability and Society, 19,* 209–223. Reprinted with permission of Taylor
& Francis, Ltd.

conclusions may be of relevance and can thus advance work in these fields. Of course, the category of physical disabilities is not a uniform one and encompasses a wide range of conditions varying in severity, stability, and health status.

Despite the growing numbers of disabled adults who are having children, parents with disabilities continue to be primarily ignored by research and social policy (Meadow-Orlans, 2002; Olkin, 1999). The sparse literature that can be found on the topic typically focuses on the relationship between parental disability and children's well-being. In some cases, a negative impact is hypothesized, studied, and "verified" (Peters & Esses, 1985); in other cases, the correlation between indices of dysfunction in children and parental disability is explored (LeClere & Kowalewski, 1994); in others yet, the negative impact on children and the need to counsel them is taken as a given topic (Kennedy & Bush, 1979). Much of this literature has been critiqued on various grounds including unexamined assumptions, methodological flaws, and lack of differentiation between disability situations (Kelley, Sikka, & Venkatesan, 1997; Kirshbaum & Olkin, 2002; Meadow-Orlans, 2002; Prilleltensky, in press).

In the past decade, a body of literature on children who provide care to ill and disabled relatives (dubbed young carers) has gained prominence. One study emphasized the negative impact of such caring, referring to it as "a curse on children" (Sidall, 1994, p. 15). This issue has received increased attention not only from the popular media but also from researchers and policy analysts, most notably in Britain. Based on research carried out by Aldridge and Becker (1993) and others, arguments have been made regarding societal neglect of young carers, and their social, economic and educational disadvantage. A host of recommendations for respite services, drop-in centers and emotional support to these youngsters have emanated from this research (Aldridge & Becker, 1996).

The focus on young carers has been critiqued on a number of fronts. Olsen (1996) has drawn attention the artificial divide between this body of literature and one that explores the lives of parents with disabilities. He argues that researchers who have focused on young carers have neglected to emphasize the inadequacy of funded supports to meet the needs of their parents. He further objects to the unchallenged assumption that caring on the part of children is unquestionably associated with negative outcomes. Keith and Morris (1996) point to poverty, insensitive attitudes, and inadequate services as impediments to parental access to resources. Parents with disabilities are often reluctant to disclose their needs for services due to fear that their parental competence will be questioned (Keith & Morris, 1996; Thomas, 1997; Thorne, 1991).

Keith and Morris (1996) contend that the very terminology of young carers connotes taking charge of the individual requiring assistance. In other words, the child is assumed to be taking responsibility for the parent or even to be in the reversed role of parenting the parent. Not only is this association between the provision of assistance and role reversal harmful to children and parents alike, it is also an inaccurate description of the relationship dynamic in many such families. The misguided perception where disability is inevitably associated with dependency tends to undermine the parenting role of people with disabilities. Thus, parents who are unable to independently fulfill all of the physical tasks of child rearing may encounter skepticism regarding their ability to function as parents. Those requiring assistance with personal care are even more vulnerable to this kind of criticism (Keith, 1992; Keith and Morris, 1996; Lloyd, 2001; Morris, 2001; Olsen, 1996).

Those who have voiced concerns with some of the research and policy development on young carers also point to the danger of institutionalizing this phenomenon as an acceptable practice. After all, it is much cheaper to provide respite services and emotional support to young carers than to ensure that the entire family is properly serviced (Olsen and Parker, 1997). Indeed, a recent report on young carers in Australia (2002) contends that they need to be acknowledged and supported, given that there will never be sufficient resources to meet the needs of those who require care. Arguments of this nature, coupled with instances where services are withdrawn based on the availability of a young carer, are cautious reminders of the potentially disablist policies that may ensue from this discourse. The reader is referred to Aldridge and Becker (1996) and Olsen and Parker (1997) for a thorough understanding of the controversy that surrounds this issue.

Researchers who align themselves with disabled parents emphasize the importance of the overall family constellation, as well as sources of risks and protective factors external to the parental disability. The family's level of isolation versus support, the impact of poverty and disincentives for gainful employment, and inaccessible environments faced by many parents with disabilities are being raised as important contributing factors that should be considered in research (Blackford, 1999; Kelley et al., 1997; Kirshbaum & Olkin, 2002). Furthermore, some studies have found positive psychological adjustment among parents with cerebral palsy (Greer, 1985); lack of adverse effects of paternal disability (spinal cord injury) on the well-being of children (Buck & Hohmann, 1981, 1982); and similar interaction patterns between disabled and nondisabled mothers and their daughters (Crist, 1993).

What helps some families cope well despite the presence of risk factors, and what can be learned from their success in the presence of illness and disability? What supports do parents require that will assist them in caring for their children? These are some of the questions that warrant researchers' attention. Indeed, some studies have been instrumental in highlighting factors associated with positive functioning. For example, one study found that the family's ability to reflect on its performance and make adjustments in the face of illness was associated with a positive outcome (Hough, Lewis, & Woods, 1991; Lewis, Woods, Hough, & Bensley, 1989). Another study of parents with multiple sclerosis identified specific coping mechanisms that were utilized by well adjusted versus poorly adjusted families (Power, 1985).

An encouraging trend among some researchers and service providers is one of approaching these families with the purpose of identifying strengths. One such example is *Talking it Out in the Family*, a video portraying real-life situations of parental disability where the actors are the people living the experience (Blackford, 1990). Work conducted at Through the Looking Glass in California also operates from a strength-based orientation. Some examples are research that explores the impact of assistive technology on the transition to parenthood, an in-depth study of families that have positive parenting experiences and an investigation of factors that promote positive child outcomes, as well as those that increase risk (Kirshbaum, 1996; Kirshbaum & Olkin, 2002).

These types of studies can advance knowledge about specific coping strategies associated with positive outcome. They have clear implications for practice that can be used by professionals, parents with disabilities and those who are considering parenthood. Rather than minimizing difficulties or potentially problematic family situations, work of this nature attempts to identify and reduce socially created constraints to optimal functioning. Furthermore, as more research that explicitly sets out to "document the spectrum of capability in parents with disabilities" (Kirshbaum & Olkin, 2002, p. 70) is amassed, professional and public perceptions will continue to shift in a more favorable direction.

STUDY DESCRIPTION

This chapter draws on a larger study that focused on the intersection of motherhood and physical disability, and included women with disabilities with and without children (Prilleltensky, 2003). The main objective was to explore the meaning of motherhood for this group of women and their mothering experiences, issues, and priorities. For the purpose of the present chapter, I focus on mothers with disabilities.

I conducted two focus groups for mothers at a symposium on mothering with a disability. One group was for mothers of young children (under eight) and one for mothers of older children. Most of the women in the latter group had teenagers at home, while two had adult children. I also held 16 in-depth interviews with eight mothers, some of whom also participated in the focus groups. All mothers had a physical impairment and most were wheelchair users. All but one interview took place in participants' homes. Participants were well educated as a group, with approximately two-thirds of those interviewed holding a post-secondary degree. Some of the focus group participants, but none of the interviewees, belonged to a visible minority group.

Informed by a literature and by a pilot study, I constructed an interview guide that was used loosely and flexibly during the first interview. The interviews were approximately 90 minutes in length, and were audiotaped, transcribed, and sent to participants for review along with a 3- to 5-page summary. This served as the basis for the second interview. My approach to data analysis was informed by the work of Glesne and Peshkin (1992), Merriam (1988), and Seidman (1991), and consisted primarily of thematic organization of the data. Each transcript was carefully reviewed, excerpts were labeled according to categories, and categories were clustered into broader themes.

FINDINGS

Promoting Growth and Enhancing Well-Being in Children

Parenting is largely about the creation of a nurturing and caring atmosphere where children's physical and emotional growth can take place. This entails facilitating the expression of feelings, maintaining open lines of communication, and ensuring that children feel loved and protected. It also involves meeting children's physical and emotional needs, and making sure that the challenges they face are appropriate to their developmental phase.

Promoting their children's growth and enhancing their well-being was a central theme in most of the parent interviews and focus groups. At the most basic level, this includes measures to ensure that children are safe and out of harm. For one mother, given the nature of her impairment, this meant that she was never alone with her children for more than a few minutes when they were infants. Once they were old enough to sit on the footrest of her wheelchair and could respond to verbal instructions, she greatly enjoyed taking them for short outings on her own. As the children were maturing, she increasingly relied on verbal instructions to keep them safe:

> From a young age I taught them that if they listen to me I can keep them safe...like if a fire alarm goes, if they just listen to what I tell them they'll be safe you know, they're not going to burn to death. I think it's very important for children to feel safe. I don't want them to feel anxious like if they're home alone with me that there's more of a threat to their security than if they're home alone with their dad. Because even though there are things that I can't do, they still see that I get it done somehow. Like I know who to call or what to do or I can teach them to do things themselves.

Another mother of now-adult children had a number of surgeries when they were young. She knew that her then husband who was not involved in the children's care could not be trusted to look after them in her absence. Having no reliable co-parent, and devoid of other formal and informal supports, this mother had to make a very difficult decision:

I couldn't leave them with him...God knows what would have happened to them. So when I had to go into the hospital I had to make a big decision. I called Children's Aide.... I called them and they took the children into care while I was in the hospital because I was there sometimes 6 to 8 months [at a time]. My kids spend practically their whole childhood going in and out of Children's Aide.

The ramifications of these children being in and out of fostercare will be discussed later; relevant to the present discussion is this participant's belief that she had to temporarily relinquish her mothering role in order to ensure her children's safety and physical well-being.

Other participants noted their use of formal and informal supports as a way of ensuring that children's needs are always met, even if they are at times unable to fulfill those needs themselves. One single mother, whose health precludes her from being consistently available, assertively advocated for and was finally granted funded assistance. This assured her that "no matter how bad I feel I manage to come through or have someone else who is always there for the children."

A related theme that ran across a number of interviews and focus group discussions is the attempt to shield children from any burden related to maternal disability. A number of participants emphasized that they do not want their disability to become a source of hardship for their children. One mother noted that, although she encourages her children to help out, she doesn't want them to feel that they need to look after her:

They are developing skills to be a little more independent. But I don't want them to be adultified children. I don't want my children to take care of mommy. To be kind and respectful and to listen and to be responsible for their actions and to do simple things sometimes—that's great. To me, that's teaching morals and values of life. But for my children to take care of me I think is wrong. I think children should not be taking care of their parents.

Another mother expressed very similar sentiments:

I don't want my children to take on or have a sense that they have to take care of me. I am their parent. I think that a child has to be able to feel that they can be kids. And I guess you need to be able to say to yourself I'm going to take care of myself if it means getting the resources out there to help me take care of myself but to set a limit on what you expect of your children.

A third woman who utilizes attendant services for personal care emphasized the importance for her of having this service performed by a paid assistant. She expressed a concern that attendant services that are now publicly funded may be targeted for cuts in the future. She noted that her 7-year-old daughter helps out with the laundry. However, this was instituted with the goal of promoting the youngster's independence and sense of self-efficacy rather than as a necessity related to the mother's disability.

A related topic that came up in one of the focus groups is the attempt to protect children from the burden of worry. Interestingly, several women noted that the "super mom" role model that their own mothers provided as they were growing up made it difficult for them as mothers with disabilities:

When I was growing up the image that my mother portrayed is that you have to let your kids think that everything is fine...to constantly portray the image that everything is okay even though you feel like shit.... That was the image that I grew up with and that was the image I also felt I had to continue with my own kids and I think that caused a really severe depression because I couldn't do it...I couldn't be that super mom.

In response, another participant made eloquent connections between women's reflections on how they were parented and their similar attempts as mothers to shield their children from burden:

> We talk about our parents who looked as if they are so strong and everything is just fine and then behind it we realize that we try to do that too sometimes with our own kids simply because we don't want to burden them with the worry. We're there to make their life better.

THE CHALLENGE OF SETTING BOUNDARIES AND MANAGING CHILDREN'S BEHAVIOR

Nurturing a caring relationship goes hand in hand with managing behavior in a constructive way. Discipline and control are not ends in themselves; they are part of fostering congenial and harmonious relationships with youngsters. Parenting in the context of a physical disability may have specific implications for discipline and behavior management. Some parents with disabilities may not be able to catch a toddler who is trying to get away or pick up a child in the midst of a temper tantrum. Furthermore, the ongoing demands of parenting that are energy taxing for most parents, may be especially challenging for those whose energy is already in short supply.

Some participants discussed the disciplinary challenges they have come across, as well as strategies and techniques to overcome them. One mother found the toddler stage particularly taxing until she and her husband took a parenting course and came up with a consistent approach:

> We needed to come to some kind of a compromise and some consistency ... because how he dealt with it had implications for how I could deal with it.

They subsequently implemented a system of contracts and consequences giving as many choices as possible in accordance with the children's stage of development and maturation.

Another participant who has some funded assistance occasionally uses this support to implement consequences such as taking a young child to her room for "time-out". This would all be discussed ahead of time to ensure that the support person is indeed prepared to follow through on the mother's decision. As much as possible, this mother deals with misbehavior on a verbal level: "...I'm much more of an explainer and I try to reason with them even when they're quite little. I always wanted them to be able to deal with me on that verbal level." Now that the children are older it is increasingly easier to rely on verbal explanations and logical consequences as demonstrated by the following scenario at a public swimming pool:

> Can you imagine talking a kid out of a pool in July? Like the last thing they want to do is leave the water. But you know, they do, because the first time one of them wouldn't come when I called, then the next day it's like "I'm not taking you swimming today and this is why." I have to be [consistent]. It's the kiss of death if I'm not. And they go "Oh, we'll be good today, we'll get out" and I say "no, that's what you said yesterday so today you won't go swimming. Tomorrow I'll give you another chance."

This participant gave various other examples that attest not only to her consistent parenting style but also to her attempts to accentuate the positive and reinforce desirable behavior whenever possible. Her strong parenting skills notwithstanding, she jokingly indicated, "believe me, I don't do it as perfectly as it might sound that I do ... [sometimes] it just all falls apart and I scream at them."

Another participant who also relies on verbal communication and logical consequences encourages her young children to solve problems with words:

It's a totally nonviolent atmosphere that I have here. You have an anger problem, let's sit down and talk about it. I'll actually get them together and I'll say: "okay, you sit here and you sit there and I'll sit here. Now what is it that you're upset about? How can we make this better?" ... The other day, the seven year old says, "mom, you sound like a judge."

In addition to her solid parenting skills, this mother's ability to deal with conflicts and misbehavior in an effective manner is likely enhanced by the funded assistance she was able to secure as a single disabled mother. She conserves her energy by having someone else carry out household tasks, as well as provide direct care when she is in need of rest. Being able to get the rest she requires to replenish her strength allows her to be a more effective and compassionate parent. This point was further accentuated in a focus group by a participant who reflected on the years that she raised her son as a single mother:

Around the discipline issue, there are two things. One is the energy level, again depending on what your situation is. I couldn't be consistent to follow through on stuff because I was just wipedout. I felt that if I asked for help around that stuff I was giving up my child and in fact on one occasion someone did suggest the Children's Aide. I had wonderful help but not enough of it. Part of it was that it's not out there automatically and part of it was that I was afraid to disclose the need.

In the same group, a mother to teenagers shared the significant behavioral challenges she experienced when her daughter was a preschooler:

She'd come home at lunch and she'd walk through the door and start screaming...just screaming about stuff...it got to the point where I didn't talk to her hardly because it didn't matter what I said, it made her mad....I can remember thinking: "I'm not surprised some children get the shit kicked out of them by their parents," you know, because I can think of two or three times where I was just ready to strangle her.

Most parents who are honest with themselves can relate to this candid description of a highly intense situation where emotions run amok. Such scenarios are by no means unique to families of disabled parents, nor can they be said to characterize them. Nonetheless, it is perhaps significant that this mother experienced frequent change of homemakers when her children were very young and had little involvement in the day to day running of the house.

The mother whose children were in care during her hospitalizations experienced major disciplinary challenges. I asked her what it was like when her children returned home from care:

It was very hard when they came back. Of course, whoever they were staying with had rules and regulations, and things that they did and then I would have to try to get them to do what I wanted. It was really difficult. Then you had a man there that did a lot of yelling and spanking.

This mother spoke about the negative impact of frequent changes, an unstable family environment, and harsh and inconsistent disciplinary measures by the children's father. Consequently, she felt that her children were often out of control as adolescents.

The combined experience of study participants suggests that having access to appropriate resources and supports can have a facilitative impact on discipline and behavior management. Mothers who are inadequately supported are more likely to experience challenges while those who have access to formal and informal supports are better equipped to set boundaries, follow through and promote cooperative behavior.

RELATIONSHIP WITH CHILDREN

The preceding sections on enhancing children's well-being and providing structure and behavioral boundaries provide a backdrop for the types of relationships that study participants have with their children. The participant who successfully lobbied for funded assistance noted that it enabled her to play a more significant role in her children's life. She further commented on the diverse ways of carrying out parenting activities:

> My kids at a very young age, if they wanted me to read to them they knew they could either sit on my lap or beside me on the bed or if it was a heavy book they knew they'd have to help me hold it up. And they just did that quite spontaneously.

Now that her children are older and the relationship is based less and less on the provision of physical care, this mother feels that she can play an even greater role in the children's lives. She jokingly referred to this period in their lives as the "golden years" when they are no longer toddlers and have yet to enter the potentially rocky adolescent phase. In the focus group for mothers of older children, participants emphasized the more difficult and challenging adolescent years and made humorous references to "raging hormone syndrome" and "wonderful adolescent roller coaster ride."

For a number of participants, the fulfillment derived from motherhood is particularly magnified given the barriers that may have prevented them from experiencing it. Having been told early in life that she would not become a mother, one woman reflected on the joy of motherhood:

> I really treasure it when my eight-year-old still, you know, when I'm sitting on the couch, will curl up on my lap and put his head on my shoulder. Or my eleven-year-old when we're walking down the street, will put his arm around me. I think I'm so lucky to be where I am at this date and time because I may not have ever had the opportunity to enjoy this.

Another woman, who resisted pressures to undergo an abortion, gave a number of examples of the strong bond and intimacy that she has with her baby and the sense of "oneness" that new mothers often describe:

> I always think that it's too good to be true. I love him so much . . . and I feel so protective of him. I know what he needs. I know when he's complaining. I always know what he wants. I know exactly what he wants.

Recognizing the dynamic nature of a mother-child relationship, she reflected on what it may be like years from now when her infants grow up:

> You know what I think? I wonder if his friends will make fun of me. I wonder about that and I wonder if it'll be hard for him having a mom who is in a wheelchair. I wonder if he'll be embarrassed. But then I think, maybe he'll stick up for me.

The issue of how children respond to a mother's disability came up in a number of interviews and focus groups. One woman related a conversation she overheard just the other day as she came to pick up her son from day care:

> He said something yesterday. I went to pick him up from day care. I was just watching him play with other kids in the sandbox and he was getting up to leave. One of the little girls whom I didn't recognize said, "Why is your mom in a wheelchair?"

And he just said, "Oh, she broke her back as a kid." That's all he said. It was sort of like matter of fact. I was so proud of him the way he said that, you know, I thought, you couldn't give a better answer to another kid than that. It was just so matter of fact.

This mother, and several others, emphasized the importance of mothers with disabilities being visible and involved in children's schools and activities. A few mothers came to their children's class to speak about disabilities. In one case this put an end to the teasing of an 11-year-old boy by some classmates. Of course, the inaccessibility of some venues restricts disabled parents from full participation in their children's lives: one mother attributed her husband's greater involvement in extracurricular activities to accessibility issues.

Contrary to the above indications of acceptance and comfort with mother's disability, another participant recounted a phase when her daughter refused to be out in public with her:

I had the scooter then. She'd sit on my lap but she'd never go for a walk. You know, my husband could take her to the park but I couldn't. I think she was embarrassed even when she was 4 years old.

This is the same little girl who had frequent and unexpected changes in caregivers for the first few years of her life, a factor to which the mother attributes various difficulties throughout the years. Being disagreeable and uncooperative as a young child she became somewhat distant as a teenager preferring to spend most of her time at friends' houses.

The participant whose now adult children spent time in foster care during her hospitalizations reflected on the impact of these separations on their emotional well-being. She noted with sadness the somewhat distant nature of her relationship with her adult children:

They will call and ask how I feel. But if I need help, I definitely won't pick up the phone and call my kids. This is where I phone my friends.

Her frequent hospitalizations as a young mother provided a formidable barrier to the formation of a close alliance with her children. Having spent a lot of time in hospital as a young child, she drew the following parallels between her relationship with her siblings and her children:

The bonding that I was talking about when I went away to the hospital and I didn't bond with my siblings, I think the same thing pretty much happened with my kids, depending on which kid and what operation.... And with them being pulled away all the time, I don't think they had a chance to bond with anybody either because they were going to different homes and everything. So we really both lost.

In the two cases noted above, the mother's impairment was a precursor to some degree of inconsistency in the children's care. Hence, it is not the impairment itself but the context in which it is embedded that can have a potentially adverse effect on the relationship between mothers with disabilities and their children. Where the contact with mother is stable and continuous, and the children receive consistent and nurturing care in her absence, the relationship has a greater chance of being a close and fulfilling one. Furthermore, it is important to emphasize the obviously complex and dynamic relationship between all parents and their children, regardless of disability status. By their very nature, relationships go through ebbs and flows, peaks and valleys. Even the closest of relationships experience periods of greater distance and lessened intimacy. Clearly, maternal disability is but one of many factors that could affect the relationship between mother and child.

DISCUSSION

Women who participated in this study provide us with a glimpse into the lived experience of parenting with a physical disability. As one would expect in any group of mothers, a range of parenting practices, experiences, and relationships were reported. This diversity cannot be attributed to any specific factor pertaining to the nature, severity, or age of onset of the mother's disability. The variability of experiences notwithstanding, participants' life stories demonstrate a strong commitment to children, actions to ensure their care and well-being in different circumstances, and attempts to shield them from any burden related to the maternal disability. While challenges and barriers were candidly reported, by and large, they do not overshadow the joy and fulfillment that these women derive from motherhood.

The issue of children caring for disabled parents was noted in the theoretical overview. The present study did not find any indication of this phenomenon among the children and families of participants. If anything, there were indications of participants' desire to shield their children from the burden of care. There is little doubt that being burdened with excessive, developmentally inappropriate responsibility and worry is not conducive to children's well-being. Nonetheless, there is a price to be paid for a hedonistic, self-indulgent upbringing where reciprocating and contributing to the well-being of others is not fostered.

Children whose lives are restricted by caring for a parent with a disability deserve our attention and concern. However, there is a big difference between a teenager who has little choice about providing intimate care to a parent and one who may be expected to assist more with household chores than some of his peers. Both the quality and quantity of tasks need to be considered, as well as the child's age and the overall dynamic of the parent-child relationship. Even when assistance in personal care is provided, this does not mean that a reversal of roles has occurred.

Research on young carers clearly indicates that this is rarely seen as an acceptable solution by parents themselves (Aldridge & Becker, 1996). Hence, the fact that this phenomenon exists at all is a reflection of the inadequacy and insufficiency of funded services to meet the personal-care needs of parents with disabilities. Of course, there may well be situations where children are expected to carry out tasks that are inappropriate, burdensome and restricting. Just as the presence of a disability does not impair the ability to function as a responsible parent, neither does it safeguard anyone from poor decision-making and possible deficits in parental competence. Without minimizing the plight of some children who may be overburdened with caring tasks, I am concerned about the possible equating in some people's minds of parental disability with overworked, emotionally burdened children.

Related to the topic of enhancing children's well-being is participants' accounts of the child-rearing practices they utilize and their overall relationship with their children. The emphasis on consistent parenting practices, and reliance on verbal explanations and instructions was noted by a number of mothers. This is consistent with narrative accounts found in the literature suggesting that such children tend to respond to verbal instructions from an early age. I began to take my (now 16-year-old) son out on my own as soon as he was able to climb into the car seat on his own. Although he was assertive and strong willed from a young age and would frequently negotiate parental limits, I knew I could count on his following my verbal instructions even as a young child.

In my work as a counselor and a psychologist I have often come across parents who struggle with how to enforce limits with teenagers. Clearly, physical strength is irrelevant in getting older children to respond to limit setting. Solid and consistent parenting practices from a young age go a long way toward preventing unmanageable situations and disregard for parental authority. Indeed, a number of participants showed a good deal of ingenuity in fostering an enjoyable yet manageable family atmosphere. These mothers can be a source of knowledge and inspirations to disabled and nondisabled parents alike.

An important consideration is the relationship between child-rearing practices, and level of formal and informal supports. One woman noted the difficulty with being consistent, and following through in the context of fatigue and limited supports. In other cases, insufficient, inadequate or nonexistent supports were implicated in adversely affecting the ability to handle behavioral issues. In extreme situations, this can have a lasting effect on the overall nature of the relationship between parents and children. Relationships are not formed and maintained in a vacuum, nor can they be nourished by good intentions alone. Although the people involved in the relationship enact the lived experience of being together, their behaviors are not just a reflection of personal intentions, but of extraneous forces as well. Negative distal and proximal factors like economic deprivation, crowded housing, and insufficient formal and informal supports penetrate the interactions between otherwise loving individuals. These powerful influences can slowly erode ties created by much individual effort on the part of parents and children. Indeed, one particular case exemplified the lasting impact that these factors can have on the relationship between a mother and her children

I believe that this study can advance our understanding of the relationship between parental disability and child well-being. The experience of study participants suggests that the welfare of children need not be compromised due to parental disability. Study participants gave numerous examples from their daily lives that describe their attempts to ensure their children's welfare. They also described loving relationships and positive communication with the children, as well as their pride in children who are well adjusted, caring, and appreciative of human diversity. Along side these accounts, and sometimes intertwined with them, are indications of how stressors such as poverty and lack of support can compound difficulties related to the disability. It is safe to say that in the presence of internal and external resources and supports, parental disability in and of itself need not present a significant risk factor. On the other hand, the high rate of poverty, single parenthood, and attitudinal barriers that characterize the lives of many women with disabilities may indeed, if unmitigated, present a risk to family well-being.

ACKNOWLEDGMENT

This research was supported by a scholarship from the Social Sciences and Humanities Research Council of Canada.

REFERENCES

Aldridge, J., & Becker, S. (1993). Punishing children for caring. *Children and Society, 7*(4), 277–278.
Aldridge, J., & Becker, S. (1996). Disability rights and the denial of young carers: The dangers of zero-sum arguments. *Critical Social Policy, 48*(16), 55–76.
Blackford, K. (1990). A different parent. *Healthsharing,* 20–25.
Blackford, K. (1999). A child's growing up with a parent who has multiple sclerosis: Theories and experiences. *Disability & Society, 14*(5), 673–685.
Booth, W., & Booth, T. (1994). Working with parents with mental retardation: Lessons from research. *Journal of Physical and Developmental Disabilities, 6*(1), 23–41.
Buck, F. M., & Hohmann, G. W. (1981). Personality, behavior, values, and family relations of children of fathers with spinal cord injury. *Archives of Physical Medical Rehabilitation, 62,* 432–438.
Buck, F. M., & Hohmann, G. W. (1982). Child adjustment as related to severity of paternal disability. *Archives of Physical Medical Rehabilitation, 63,* 249–253.
Campion, M. J. (1995). *Who's fit to be a parent?* London: Routledge.

Crist, P. (1993). Contingent interaction during work and play tasks for mothers with multiple sclerosis and their daughters. *American Journal of Occupational Therapy, 47*(2), 121–131.

Gill, C., Kewman, D., & Brannon, R. (2003). Transforming psychological practice and society: Policies that reflect the new paradigm. *American Psychologist, 58*(4), 305–312.

Glesne, C., & Peshkin, A. (1992). *Becoming qualitative researchers.* White Plains: Longman.

Greer, B. G. (1985). Children of physically disabled parents: Some thoughts, facts and hypotheses. In S. K. Thurman (Ed.), *Children of handicapped parents: Research and clinical perspectives.* Orlando: Academic Press.

Hough, E. E., Lewis, F. M., & Woods, N. F. (1991). Family response to mother's chronic illness: Case studies of well and poorly adjusted families. *Western Journal of Nursing Research, 13*(5), 568–596.

Keith, L. (1992). Who cares wins? Women, caring and disability. *Disability, Handicap & Society, 7*(2), 167–175.

Keith, L., & Morris, J. (1996) . Easy targets: A disability rights perspective on the 'children as carers' debate. In J. Morris (Ed.), *Encounters with strangers: Feminism and disability.* London: Women's Press.

Kelley, S., Sikka, A., & Venkatesan, S. (1997). A review of research on parental disability: Implications for research and counselling. *Rehabilitation Counseling Bulletin, 41*(2), 105–116.

Kennedy, K. M., & Bush, D. F. (1979). Counselling the children of handicapped parents. *Personnel and Guidance Journal, 58*(4), 267–270.

Kirshbaum, M. (1996). Mothers with physical disabilities. In D. M. Krotoski, M. A. Nosek, & M. A. Turk (Eds.), *Women with physical disabilities: Achieving and maintaining health and well-being.* Baltimore: Paul Brooks Publishing.

Kirshbaum, M., & Olkin, R. (2002). Parents with physical, systemic or visual disabilities. *Sexuality & Disability, 20*(1), 65–80.

Kocher, M. (1994). Mothers with disabilities. *Sexuality & Disability, 12*(2), 127–133.

LeClere, F. B., & Kowalewski, B. M. (1994). Disability in the family: The effects on children's well-being. *Journal of Marriage and the Family, 56*(May), 457–468.

Lewis, F. M., Woods, N. F., Hough, E. E., & Bensley, L. S. (1989). The family's functioning with chronic illness in the mother: The spouse's perspective. *Social Science Medicine, 29*(11), 1261–1269.

Lloyd, M. (2001). The politics of disability and feminism: Discord or synthesis? *Sociology, 35*(3), 715–723.

Meadow-Orlans, K. P. (2002). Parenting with a sensory or physical disability. In M. H. Bornstein (Ed.). *Handbook of parenting, volume IV. Social conditions and applied parenting.* Mahwah, NJ: Lawrence Erlbaum Associates.

Merriam, S. B. (1988). *Case study research in education.* San Francisco: Jossey-Bass.

Morris, J. (2001). Impairment and disability: Constructing an ethics of care that promotes human rights. *Hypatia, 16*(4), 1–16.

Olkin, R. (1999). *What therapists should know about disability.* New York: Guilford Press.

Olsen, R. (1996). Young carers: Challenging the facts and politics of research into children and caring. *Disability & Society, 11*(1), 41–54.

Olsen, R., & Parker, G. (1997). A response to Aldridge and Becker—'Disability rights and the denial of young carers: The dangers of zero-sum arguments'. *Critical Social Policy, 50*(17), 125–133.

Peters, L. C., & Esses, L. M. (1985). Family environment as perceived by children with a chronically ill parent. *Journal of Chronic Diseases, 38*(4), 301–308.

Power, P. W. (1985). Family coping behaviours in chronic illness: A rehabilitation perspective. *Rehabilitation Literature, 46*(3–4), 78–82.

Prilleltensky, O. (2003). A ramp to motherhood: The experiences of mothers with physical disabilities. *Sexuality & Disability, 21*(1), 21–47.

Prilleltensky, O. (2004). *Motherhood and disability: Children and choices.* New York: Palgrave Macmillan.

Seidman, I. E. (1991). *Interviewing as qualitative research.* New York: Teachers College Press.

Sidall, R. (1994). Lost childhood. *Community Care,* 9–15 June, 14–15.

Thomas, C. (1997). The baby and the bath water: Disabled women and mother-hood in social context. *Sociology of Health & Illness, 19*(5), 622–643.

Thorne, S. E. (1991). Mothers with chronic illness: A predicament of social construction. *Health Care for Women International, 11,* 209–221.

Wates, M. (1997). *Disabled parents: Dispelling the myths.* Cambridge: National Childbirth Trust Publishing.

Wates, M., & Jade, R. (1999). *Bigger than the sky: Disabled women on parenting.* London: Women's Press.

ADDITONAL READING

Young Carers Research Project. (2002). *Final report: A carers Australia Project.* Available online at www.carers.asn.au

15

Parenting a Child With a Chronic Medical Condition

JANE CASE-SMITH

*T*he demands and responsibilities of caring for children who have disabilities appear to be different from those of parents with typical children (Burke, Harrison, Kauffmann, & Wong, 2001; Gallimore, Coots, Weisner, Gamier, & Guthrie, 1996; Innocenti & Huh, 1992; King, King, & Rosenbaum, 1996). Although most researchers agree that caregiving for children with disabilities can be stressful (Dyson, 1996; Smith, Oliver, & Innocenti, 2001), the overall effect on families' well-being seems to vary across time and across individual families (Knafl, Breitmayer, Gallo, & Zoeller, 1996; Scorgie, Wilgosh, & McDonald, 1998; Tak & McCubbin, 2002). Early research (e.g., Tizard & Grad, 1961) focused on the psychological effects and the social isolation and adversity associated with raising a child with a disability (Barnett & Boyce, 1995). More recent studies have demonstrated that families with children with disabilities face complex issues; however, the overall impact on the family is not necessarily negative (Harris & McHale, 1989; Patterson & Blum, 1996; VanLeit & Crowe, 2002). For some families, the impact is positive, strengthening the family as a unit. To implement a model of family-centered care in pediatric practice, professionals need to acknowledge and understand how a child's disability affects the entire family.

Turnbull and Turnbull (1997) use a family systems model to examine how a child's disability affects family functions. The economic function of the family is affected because parents generally work fewer hours outside the home in order to care for their child and costs for treatment and medication are high. Therefore, parents' earning ability decreases at the same time that their costs for treatment and medication increase. Additionally, the child care demands on parents' time increases as daily care of the child rises above that required for typical children (Dunlap & Hollingsworth, 1977; Harris & McHale, 1989; Helitzer, Cunningham-Sabo, VanLeit, & Crowe, 2002). For example, parents may regularly implement numerous therapeutic procedures, engage in feeding for long periods of time or frequently throughout the day, administer medications or medical procedures (e.g., suctioning, gastrostomy, and feedings), and attend therapy and clinic appointments. Because more time is spent in daily care activities, less time is available for other activities, such as recreation and socialization (Helitzer et al., 2002; Turnbull & Turnbull, 1997). Barnett and Boyce (1995) found that mothers with children with Down syndrome were unable to maintain employment and spent less time in social

From "Parenting a child with a chronic medical condition," by J. Case-Smith. *The American Journal of Occupational Therapy, 58*(5), 551–560. Reprinted with permission of *The American Journal of Occupational Therapy.*

activities. Their survey results demonstrated that socialization and work activities were replaced with child care activities. Fathers also reported more child-care time and less time in social activities.

Turnbull and Turnbull (1997) explain that when parents' socialization is limited, the entire family is affected. Families are the bases from which children learn to interact with others; therefore, children's first experiences with friends and family are vital to their social skill development. Loss of social activity opportunities early in life can have long-term implications for building friendships and social supports.

Other researchers have investigated the types of accommodation that the family system must make when it includes children with developmental disabilities (Gallimore et al., 1996). These authors define accommodation as the family's functional responses or adjustments to the demands of daily life with a child with special needs (Gallimore et al., 1996; Gallimore, Weisner, Kaufman, & Bernheimer, 1989). Every accommodation is presumed to have costs as well as benefits to the individuals of the family and to the family as a whole. The types of accommodations that families make change throughout the life cycle. Some investigators report that adjustments are greatest when first learning about the disability (Weisner, 1993); other authors propose that coping becomes more difficult and greater adaptations are needed as children get older and performance discrepancies increase (Bristol & Schopler, 1983; Suelzle & Keenan, 1981). Examples of accommodations made by families are that the mother arranges for flexibility in work or works at home, the family's home is altered to improve safety or accessibility, and the caregiving responsibilities of both parents increase (Gallimore et al., 1996; Helitzer et al., 2002).

A few studies have examined the impact of children with medical diagnoses who require ongoing intervention and medical technology on parents (see Patterson & Blum, 1996 for a review). Caring for a child who requires routine use of medical technology, such as respirators, gastrostomy pumps, suctioning equipment, can be socially isolating for parents. Some parents report that they are virtually housebound (Andrews & Nielson, 1988). For example, parents may not be able to find babysitters, the child's behaviors may create uncomfortable social situations, the logistics of leaving the house for nonessential events may be overwhelming, as when equipment, medical supplies, and medical technology needs to be packed and unpacked. Kirk (1998) and Murphy (1997) reported that most families with children with chronic medical problems must rely on nurses and other health care professionals for respite care. In addition, the home environment is not as conducive to social activities when it is filled with medical technology and supplies, taking on the appearance of an intensive care unit (ICU). Although parents seem to accommodate to the presence of medical technology, friends and extended family may feel less comfortable. Concerns about the child's exposure to viruses and bacteria may also limit social opportunities.

Parents have reported that their experiences with a child who requires continual medical care is exhausting and at times overwhelming (Jennings, 1990; Kirk, 1998). The uncertainty of chronic illness and the child's prognosis can produce ongoing anxiety for parents (Andrews & Nielson, 1988; Murphy, 1997). The stress associated with a child's chronic illness can create problems in the mother's relationships with her other children and in the marriage (Kirk, 1998; Murphy, 1997).

Other areas of family function that are often affected when a child has chronic medical problems are parents' self-identity and social-emotional well-being (Turnbull & Turnbull, 1997). When all or most family activities revolve around the exceptionality (e.g., therapies, meetings with professionals, caregiving, hospitalizations), the exceptionality may become the major identifying characteristic to the parents (Patterson & Blum,

1996). For example, the parents may introduce themselves as the parents of a child with a congenital heart condition or a neurological syndrome.

The degree of family stress appears to partially relate to the amount of support available. Families without access to respite and services are more likely to feel over-burdened, emotionally exhausted, and socially isolated (Kirk, 1998; Murphy, 1997; Tak & McCubbin, 2002). Support in the form of friends, extended family, financial security, professional services, and community resources can help families maintain healthy, balanced lives (Gallimore, Weisner, Bernheimer, Guthrie, & Nihira, 1993; Humphry & Case-Smith, 2001; Turnbull & Turnbull, 1997; VanLeit & Crowe, 2002).

Understanding how parents' occupations and experiences differ when they include a child with chronic medical problems can help occupational therapy practitioners focus on the issues that matter most to families. Professionals need a deep understanding of the experiences of these families in order to fit their interventions into the family's daily life and to help them make accommodations that are of low cost and high benefit. The purpose of this study was to examine in depth the caregiving, social occupations, and self-identities of parents with children with significant disabilities and chronic medical conditions. We examined these occupational areas because the literature suggests that these family functions are substantially affected by young children with serious medical issues and intense caregiving needs (Barnett & Boyce, 1995; Crowe, 1993; Kirk, 1998; Patterson, Jernell, Leonard, & Titus, 1994).

METHOD

Design

We implemented an ethnographic approach to examine the caregiving, social occupations, and self-identities of families with preschool-age children with chronic medical conditions and disabilities. The design used multiple sources for data about the families, including in depth interviews with the parents and extended observations of the families. The informants were mothers and fathers, and almost all observations included the entire nuclear family. As part of an interdisciplinary early intervention training project in a Midwest university, the parents consented to allow graduate students to participate with them in 60 hours of family activities and outings. I selected data from 8 of the 22 participating families for analysis because their children had ongoing and complex medical concerns, were dependent on technology, or had significant disabilities that affected all areas of development, or all. Each graduate student conducted an in-depth interview with one set of parents, transcribed the interview, and subsequently participated in 60 hours of activities with the family over a 6-month period. The students described the family outings and activities in depth and detail, generating between 12 and 15 field notes. Following description of the activity and the interactions, each student wrote journal entries that interpreted their experiences based on coursework readings on family occupations and interactions.

Participants

The training project coordinator, who is the mother of a child with cerebral palsy, recruited the families (*n* = 22) with children with disabilities from her school and hospital contacts. Each signed informed consent to participate in the study. The eight families in this study had children with combinations of complex medical issues and significant developmental delays. The children were 4 to 6 years of age. All of the families were married couples and six of the eight had other children. Two of the children with disabilities

TABLE 15.1 Medical Diagnoses of Children With Chronic Medical Conditions

Name	Participants' Medical Diagnoses and Risk Factors
Annie	Twin, anoxia at birth, cerebral palsy, seizures, cortical blindness
Sean	Congenital heart defect, digestive problems, on transcutaneous peritoneal nutrition (TPN), genetic syndrome
Katie	Premature birth, gastrostomy tube, blind, seizures
Michael	TPN, jejunostomy tube, gastrostomy tube, genetic syndrome: velocardiofacial disorder, heart defects
Carlie	Premature, gastrostomy tube, hypersensitive to sounds and oral stimulation
Jeremy	Near strangling, severe brain injury, cortically blind, seizures, severe cerebral palsy
David	Hypoplastic left heart, cerebral vascular accident following heart surgery
Kevin	Severe spastic quadriparesis cerebral palsy, seizures, mental retardation

Note: All names are pseudonyms.

were adopted at birth. All of the families were Caucasian and middle class. Five of the eight children received 40 or more hours per week of nursing services. The graduate students who interviewed and observed the families were four occupational therapists, one nurse, one special educator, and two speech pathologists. Table 15.1 lists the diagnoses of the children whose families participated in the study.

Instrumentation/Procedures

The faculty and staff of the training project designed the interview guide based on family systems concepts defined in Turnbull and Turnbull (1997). Parents were asked to describe a typical day, their family routines, social supports, interventions and their satisfaction with those interventions, and their hopes and dreams for the future. The interviews were transcribed verbatim. Field notes regarding nonverbal responses and the environment during the interviews were recorded. During the 60 hours that the students spent with the families, they accompanied the family to therapy, clinic, and physician visits, individualized educational program meetings, family outings, respite, and typical activities as defined by the family. Examples of family outings and activities were touring the science museum, eating at restaurants, swimming, and bowling. The students attended baseball games, picnics, birthday parties, and church events with their families. Each student described his or her experiences, focusing on the family's occupations and their interactions with medical and educational professionals.

Data Analysis

Following several readings of the interviews, field notes, and journals, I coded each statement or group of statements with a label that defined its theme. These labeled sections were combined and organized into common and related themes. Data within the thematic categories were analyzed to identify concepts. An iterative process was implemented to reorganize the themes and concepts to obtain the best fit using all of the data. The concepts were interpreted using related literature and reflection based on my experiences with families over 25 years in early intervention programs. Two mothers from the study reviewed the themes and concepts to provide member checks and validate the findings. Two graduate students and three project faculty served as peer reviewers by examining the data and the interpretation. The peer reviewers and member checks resulted in slight modification of the themes and reorganization of the data; this process also served to confirm the truth-value of the themes.

RESULTS

Three themes emerged related to caregiving. "The challenge of always being there" describes mothers' constant efforts to provide for their children's medical, educational, and recreational needs given their total dependency on their parents. "Change in career plans" describes how in each family, one parent gave up his or her career plans to stay home and care for the child with special needs. "Making decisions and tolerating compromises" describes compromises that the parents made in caring for their children. The themes that emerged related to the families' social lives were "Where do we find a sitter?" which describes the lack of resources for respite care and the difficulties the parents experienced when leaving the house, and "anticipating the unanticipated," which describes the elaborate planning required when families did venture from their homes. A third set of themes described issues in the families' self-identify and illustrated how each family's identity was defined by the child with special needs. The parents explained how their experiences with their children helped them to appreciate life and demonstrate more sensitivity to and tolerance of individual differences. They had become strong advocates for their children and other children with similar needs.

Managing Caregiving Responsibilities

Each parent described a typical day, revealing the level of caregiving required of the child with a medical condition. In most of the families, the parents maintained a rigorous, highly scheduled day of medical procedures and caregiving responsibilities. Sean's father describes their typical routine:

> We get up at 6:15. We get ready for work. Sean gets up by 7:00 and gets unhooked from his TPN [transcutaneous peritoneal nutrition]. He gets a bottle and his diaper changed. When the nurse is not there, we drawup his meds. ... It takes about an hour to get all the medications together for the day and then we lay them out. All of the meds are given over the course of the day. ... He probably gets some meds every half hour or so. Then he gets a break [at 3:30]. We start the evening meds around 7:00 He gets insulin at 9 a.m., 3 p.m., and again at 9:00 p.m. We put him down to bed between 9:00 and 9:30.

Michael is the youngest of five children. He has "a G-tube [gastrostomy], a J button [jejunostomy], and a broviak [for the TPN], and a trach." His mother describes her day of caregiving:

> During the week, Michael gets up between 7:00 and 7:30. I have already taken my shower, two of the kids are already gone, two of the kids are getting ready. We kind of sponge him down because he wakes up soaking wet from his diaper. We disconnect his TPN, give him his breathing treatments, his meds, change dressings. ... After the first wet diaper, we put his pants and shoes on him and hook up his pump, and then we get ready for school.

> He gets tube fed for 4 hours a day. ... Then he comes home, and he gets more medicine, more breathing treatments, another diaper change, goes to bed for a nap. Then we have to wake him up for therapy ... so we get him up, change him again, and it's either speech, OT or PT, depending on which day of the week it is. Some days it's doctor's appointments. ... We do that and then usually between 4:00 and 7:00 we're driving everyone else to their stuff, taking them to piano lessons or choir or scouts or whatever it is, ice skating lessons. ... A couple times a week we give him a bath in the evening, and when we do that, we have to go through changing all of the dressings, which takes about an hour. About 8:30 he goes to bed. I'm usually up two or

three times in the night suctioning him or something like that … so that is a typical Michael day.

These descriptions reveal highly structured days, filled with many caregiving tasks. Although most families with young children lead busy, highly scheduled days; these families' activities revolved around caregiving tasks and medical procedures, not recreational and social activities. The five families who received nursing care expressed how grateful they were to have professional assistance in caregiving, yet numerous medical and therapeutic procedures remained to be administered by the parents. The families seemed to have incorporated these intensive caregiving responsibilities into their daily lives.

The Challenge of Always Being There

The children's medical issues seemed to require the constant attention and energy of the families. Five of the children cycled through infections brought on by their immobility, shallow breathing, and suppressed immune systems. The parents expected periods of illness and relied heavily on their nurses for care during these periods. When the children were ill, therapies and routine appointments had to be put on hold. The parents' activities were also cancelled, so that they could be home with their children. These times were discouraging because often the children would lose skills, and the progress in learning new skills was put on hold.

Beyond the medical procedures and caregiving routines, the parents were concerned about their children's developmental growth and their abilities to engage in interaction with others. This concern about the child's involvement in play seemed to present the greater challenge to the parents. The parents recognized that time spent with the child in caregiving and medical procedures did not fulfill the child's need to play and socially interact.

Because these children had limited ways of expressing their feelings, interaction and communication required constant effort by the parents. Jeremy's mother said, "Our biggest challenge with him right now is trying to find a way for him to interact more independently and to communicate with us." The student with this family observed that when the mother played physical games with Jeremy, it was important, "to look for subtle signs, like a slight furrow of his brow or the pursing of his lips" to know when he was tired and ready to stop.

One student explained with empathy how Annie's mother worried about how she felt when she showed signs of illness:

> I was struck by the stress of wondering what was wrong with Annie. It is so hard to know since her communication is so impaired. She can't answer questions, speak, or communicate her thoughts using a device. She can activate switches with voice output … but her understanding of language seems to be limited to a small set of familiar words and phrases. I wonder if it would be beneficial to some how to teach her words related to pain and discomfort … I would find this [lack of communication] upsetting and terribly frustrating, knowing that a seizure was likely on the way and being unable to do anything to stop it.

Perhaps because Jeremy, Annie, and Katie could not play independently, their parents expressed that they felt guilty when their children were left alone. They tried many methods to engage them in independent play given their severely limited movement and vision. For example, several families had borrowed or owned switch-activated toys and easy-to-activate toys. Despite these efforts, the families had yet to discover methods for their children to play independently.

Katie's mother explained, "[the challenge is] keeping her entertained because she can not do anything for herself … she likes to be entertained. … We're trying to find something that she can do independently. …" The student noted that Jeremy's "participation in the world is through his family members." At age 6, "he is completely dependent on them for his every need."

The literature has identified the importance of a balance between meeting the child's developmental needs and managing the illness (Patterson & Blum, 1996; Tak & McCubbin, 2002; Turnbull & Turnbull, 1997). The parents seemed to make great efforts to maintain this balance, keeping the child's developmental skills a priority.

Change in Career Plans

Primarily due to their children's frequent medical appointments, illness, and hospitalizations, the parents changed their career goals. In six of the eight families, the mother left paid employment to become a full-time mother. In the family with five children—one of which had a rare genetic disorder—the father held three jobs to help pay for the medical expenses and allow his wife to stay home. In another family, the mother left her job to be home full time, and the father changed jobs to be home more of the time. One mother explained that she did not work outside the home because, "When [my daughter] is sick … everything stops because we don't know how sick she's going to get … she has seizures and sometimes she ends up in the hospital for a couple days, and if the respite worker calls off, I don't have anyone to watch her." These unpredictable events were not compatible with maintaining a job.

In one exception, a mother held a part-time position that allowed her and her husband to alternate days at home so that one or the other was at home with their child everyday. In a second exception, the father left his work to become a stay-at-home dad while his physician wife continued her practice. This father stated, "There were three people trying to deal with Carlie's feeding issues. So we made a decision that one of us had to stay home so that she would have a little more consistency." Both parents were pleased with the progress she had made since her father has been at home full time.

As in previous research (Barnett & Boyce, 1995; Crowe, VanLeit, Berghmans, & Mann, 1997; Dunlap & Hollingsworth, 1977; Helitzer et al., 2002), these eight families had shifted their family occupations, devoting more time and energy to caregiving and less to socialization and work. When caregiving for children with specific needs requires that one parent stay home, the family's financial well-being, and the parents' social network and self-identity can be negatively affected (Barnett & Boyce, 1995; Turnbull & Turnbull, 1997).

Making Decisions and Tolerating Compromises

Parents in this study were asked to make difficult decisions for their children on a regular basis—decisions about services, medications, and treatments that had important effects on their children. The parents were also frequently given advice and offered alternative treatments. Sometimes when asked to make decisions about treatments, they did not always feel that they were knowledgeable about the potential effects, risks, and benefits. Generally these decisions involved compromise that weighed the costs and benefits of several options.

For example, Jeremy had intractable seizures that needed to be controlled by medication. However, the medication made him drowsy, lethargic, and nonresponsive; therefore, his parents asked for less potent medication. As a result Jeremy was more alert, responsive, and communicative; however, he also had 30 to 40 seizures a day. His parents valued the ability to have daily positive interaction with their son at the risk of possible long-term consequence of the seizure activity.

Kevin's parents and physician agreed to the insertion of a baclofen pump to decrease his spasticity. By decreasing his muscle tone, his parents could easily position him with good alignment in his wheelchair. Unfortunately, the muscle tone inhibitor also affected his arm movement, such that he could no longer use his arms to reach and hold objects. Despite his loss of strength, his mother decided to continue the baclofen and hoped that he would regain some of his arm strength.

Another context for family decision making was the Individualized Education Program (IEP) meeting. In Kevin's IEP meeting, his mother decided that due to his seizure meds, sleep needs, and endurance, she would bring him to school late, that is, between 9:30 or 10:00. Although this later arrival time meant that Kevin would miss 2 hours of instruction, his mother negotiated this arrangement because she knew that if he became overly tired, his seizures would increase, and he would not benefit from the instruction he did receive.

In family-centered intervention, professionals recognize that parents are the primary decision makers when planning services for their child (Dunst, Trivette, & Deal, 1994; Humphry & Case-Smith, 2001). The Individuals with Disabilities Education Act Amendments (1997) reinforce this concept by specifically including the parents in every educational decision that is made for the child. Although professionals recognize that parents have these rights, they also acknowledge that good decision making requires deep understanding of the issues. At times, the parents felt that they were being asked to weigh options without adequate information and without knowledge of the costs associated with each option. The parents in our study discussed the compromises that they had needed to make when planning medical and educational interventions. These decisions seemed to weigh on the parents and they expressed anxiety regarding whether or not they had made the best choice.

Maintaining a Social Life

As discussed in the previous section, socialization was affected by the parents' inability to find a sitter and the lack of respite care. When families, including the child with a medical condition, attended recreational or social events outside their home, extraordinary planning and creative adaptability were required.

Where Do We Find a Sitter?

Most of the families did not use child-care providers given the extensive caregiving demands of their children; therefore, the parents had limited options for leaving home. Five of the children had poorly controlled seizures, four had compromised immune systems, two vomited frequently, and two had very low endurance for activity. In several of the families, one extended family member took care of the child for short periods if the parents needed some respite. For Annie's parents, "Basically the only people that help are Dan's parents … no one else has taken the time to learn how to do the medicines."

Although several of Jeremy's extended–family members had indicated an interest in learning his medical treatment to help care of him, these arrangements had not been made. Sean's family also did not have any help with respite other than nurses; "I would say the only extended family that really helps is [my husband's] mother, and mostly when we are not home and people need to drop off supplies. When we are in the hospital [with Sean], she will watch our daughter … so the only respite that we have had is the nurse." In general, the families only attended community activities in which the entire family could participate.

These parents, like those described by Kirk (1998) and Murphy (1997), rarely accessed respite. The parents did not complain about lack of respite and seemed to accept their situations. In some cases, the child's care could be taught to others, but the parents seemed reluctant to take the chance that problems may occur.

Anticipating the Unanticipated

Because the children in this study had multiple and often unpredictable needs, parents felt that they had to carefully and extensively plan each activity outside the home. Unanticipated events and preparing for them was a dominant theme in each family's social life.

When Jeremy's family went swimming or bowling, the parents had to check the facilities' accessibility before the visit. His father prepared for a bowling outing by researching the facility's accessibility and its least busy times. This family organized the equipment and supplies needed before every event. They developed plans "A" and "B"—"A" hoping that Jeremy would tolerate the activity or "B" fearing that he would not and they would need to return home. Carlie's reflux required that her parents take two to three changes in clothes with them on outings. They always had an "escape plan" in case she began to vomit. Carlie had a very low tolerance to noise so her parents used headphones at birthdays and in restaurants. The headphones allowed Carlie to enjoy the activity without being overwhelmed.

David's parents often had to curtail social events and outings because his endurance was poor. "We mainly have problems because David gets tired faster, he gets colds easier, and if he gets any type of cold we pretty much have to stay in the house. We have to do what he can do. So if he gets worn out we just have to go home ... he has asthma and when you can't breathe and you have a weak heart, it is double trouble." David's mother further explained:

> You make plans with friends, but you really don't know if you're going to be there until you're there ... because he can get sick, he can have a seizure, his respite provider may not show up ....

In general the families made careful decisions about their outings and the social events they attended. They weighed the costs and benefits, they decided whether or not they had the energy, then they planned carefully what supplies and equipment would be needed. Each had mastered packing all of the equipment and supplies that may be needed, including headphones, medications, extra clothing, and medical supplies. As well supplied as they were, they also prepared to return home quickly, curtailing their attendance when problems arose. Several parents voiced that they hoped that relatives and friends understood their frequent early departures.

Perhaps these parents persevered in making efforts to participate in social events in order to maintain a balance and a semblance of typical family functioning. Gallimore et al. (1996) discussed the ongoing importance of family flexibility and adaptability to balance family functions when children have developmental disabilities or medical chronic conditions.

Maintaining a Self-Identity

With the level of care required by these children, it is not surprising that the disability became a prominent aspect of the family's identity and social–emotional selves. Through many of the conversations with the parents, it became apparent that the families viewed their self-identity in a positive way, to the extent that they made opportunities to support others in similar situations.

Celebrating Life

An important element of the parents' attachment to and feelings about their child was that each had faced the very real possibility that the child would die. Each child, at some point, and usually not at the time of birth, had reached a state of critical medical condition. These times, when their children were critically ill and in ICUs, left the parents with indelible memories. Although the students did not specifically ask about these traumatic times, the parents provided detailed accounts of medical crises when they thought they would "lose" their child.

David's parents described his heart surgeries during his first 2 years. During the last heart surgery, he had a stroke and was in a coma for several days. Michael's genetic disorder is known to result in early death, and he has been critically ill a number of times. Carlie spent the first 2 months in the neonatal ICU "barely holding on to life." Jeremy had been a typically developing infant until an accident in which he was almost strangled by slipping through his highchair. He was very close to death in the 24 hours following the accident.

Parents seemed to respond to these experiences of critical illness or severe injury by vowing to be continually grateful for their child's survival and life. Several of the parents referred to their child as a gift who allowed them to appreciate life. About half of the parents continued to live with the knowledge that they may yet lose their child. However, rather than grieving, this knowledge seemed to make them to appreciate the time that they had with their child and the joys that he or she brought to the family. Michael's mother explained; "Michael has given us so much. His brothers and sisters love him. They've learned about what it's like to be different. … They've changed. My husband and I have changed … because Michael has these issues, we enjoy every little thing he does."

The parents described ways that they had become more sensitive to and tolerant of individual differences. They seemed to appreciate life more, having almost lost a child and knowing how tenuous life is.

Becoming an Advocate

The families actively participated in advocacy for children with disabilities and had joined advocacy organizations or support groups. For example, Sean's mother belonged to two support groups, a transcutaneous peritoneal nutrition support group and a support group for children with genetic disorders.

Two other mothers worked part-time for advocacy groups. Mary, Jeremy's mother, worked part-time for a state family advocacy agency. Her role was to maintain a Web site for families with children with disabilities. She also belonged to a parent organization that matched parents throughout the United States who had similar children and established long-distance communication. Michael's mother also worked a few hours a week for an advocacy group. "You know, I finally feel like I have a purpose. I'm on the family advisory council at the hospital."

Helitzer et al. (2002) suggested that mothers of children with disabilities assume roles that bridge the world of medical and educational professional with everyday home life. These support groups may replace some of the social activities that the parents have lost or cannot sustain. The personal satisfaction that they achieve through their advocacy occupations may fulfill their interests in leadership and professional interaction that they may have otherwise experienced in a career.

The findings of this study suggest that the identities of these parents revolved around their preschool children with chronic medical conditions. The parents felt competent in caring for their children, who had survived life-threatening trauma or illness. They had accessed a full range of services and had joined advocacy and support groups. Each family felt that sharing their stories and their experiences was important as they told their stories in detail to the students and opened their homes to the students for 6 months. Parents communicated that the child had a positive effect on family members who had become more sensitive to and accepting of disabilities. They also seemed to feel more appreciative of each other and of life itself.

Occupational Therapy Practice Implications

Practitioners can help families maintain a balance of family functions by problem solving to find ways to enable children with severe disabilities to play and interact and suggesting efficient ways for parents to manage their daily caregiving routines. For example, recommending use of assistive technology, such as adapted switches or augmentative communication devices, can allow children with limited motor function to access toys that provide auditory and visual stimulation. Assistive technology is most helpful when it fits well into the families' values and style of communication and provides meaningful play to the child (Deitz & Swinth, 1997).

The medical and educational decisions these parents faced were difficult to make, and often the parents felt that they were without one clearly best choice. Sometimes these parents had to choose the least detrimental option among several potentially negative scenarios. Professionals can support parents in their decision making by providing them accurate, relevant information (King et al., 1996; Patterson et al., 1994) and supporting their decision once it has been made. Parents should be prepared and informed as much as possible when asked to prioritize intervention and treatment options. Once parents have made a decision, professionals should not only honor it, but embrace and implement the decision so that it can serve the best interests of the child and family. Parents in early intervention have expressed that they wished professionals were nonjudgmental and would think the best of the choices they made as parents (McWilliam, Tocci, & Harbin, 1998).

To help parents balance their caregiving responsibilities with social and recreational activities, practitioners can identify sources of respite that parents can use, acknowledging that competence in nursing and medical procedures would be necessary. Professionals can encourage parents to teach the child's care to extended family members. Extended family often want to help but do not know how. When they participate in the child's care, they gain a better understanding of the parents' experiences and can offer more emotional support.

Practitioners should encourage families to participate in recreational and social activities (Dunst et al., 1994). Practitioners can help by identifying community recreational facilities that are accessible and suggest methods to make outings successful. An occupational therapist's role is to listen and provide parents with information on support and advocacy groups, including those on the Internet. They can also encourage families to establish identities in organizations and with social groups beyond those focused on disability (Dunst et al., 1994; Turnbull & Turnbull, 1997).

Limitations

This sample of families was homogeneous across a number of dimensions, including race, socioeconomic status, and composition. The homogeneity allowed for in-depth exploration of their similar experiences and functions. The strong cohesion among family members may be unique to the participants who were studied and who volunteered to participate in a graduate student training project. All of the families had financial resources and medical insurance; the study's findings can not be generalized to families without these resources.

Recommendation for Future Research

Inclusion of a larger and more heterogeneous group of participants would increase the generalizability of the study's findings. Future qualitative research should explore family occupations when children have other types of disabilities, such as behavioral problems. The siblings' experiences should also be explored because the research literature investigating sibling experiences is minimal. The shifts in parents' roles and their methods of adapting to their children's caregiving needs should be further analyzed using quantitative research methods. Analysis of measures of coping strategies, social supports, perception of stress, and adaptability in parents with children with chronic conditions can produce predictive models of family adaptation and resiliency to further extend and validate the findings of this study.

CONCLUSIONS

These families had round-the-clock demands and responsibilities to care for children with significant chronic medical conditions and developmental disabilities. The parents had shifted their occupations from work outside the home and social activities to caregiving activities and frequent interaction with health care professionals. When children have chronic medical conditions, practitioners can help families balance the child's medical needs and developmental needs. They can also support families in balancing caregiving responsibilities with social and recreational activities. Resilient families, such as those who participated in this study, give us lessons to pass onto other families in similar circumstances.

ACKNOWLEDGMENTS

I appreciate the families' willingness to share their lives with The Ohio State University IMPACTS graduate students and faculty. I thank the IMPACTS students and families who allowed me to use the data from their experiences together. I also acknowledge the IMPACTS faculty for their assistance in collecting and interpreting the data. This study and the IMPACTS project were funded by a U.S. Office of Special Education and Rehabilitative Services personnel preparation grant, H325A010114.

REFERENCES

Andrews, M. M., & Nielson, D. W. (1988). Technology dependent children in the home. *Pediatric Nursing, 14,* 111–114.

Barnett, W. S., & Boyce, G. C. (1995). Effects of children with Down syndrome on parent's activities. *American Journal on Mental Retardation, 100,* 115–127.

Bristol, M. M., & Schopler, E. (1983). Stress and coping in families with autistic adolescents. In E. Schopler & G. B. Mesibov (Eds.), *Autism in adolescent and adults* (pp. 251–278). New York: Plenum.

Burke, S. O., Harrison, M. B., Kauffmann, & Wong, C. (2001). Effects of stress point intervention with families of repeatedly hospitalized children. *Journal of Family Nursing, 7*(2), 128–158.

Crowe, T. K. (1993). Time use of mothers with young children: The impact of a child's disability. *Developmental Medicine and Child Neurology, 35,* 621–630.

Crowe, T. K., Van Leit, B., Berghmans, K. K., & Mann, P. (1997). Role perceptions of mothers with young children: The impact of a child's disability. *American Journal of Occupational Therapy, 51,* 651–661.

Deitz, J. C., & Swinth, Y. (1997). Accessing play through assistive technology. In L. D. Parham & L. S. Fazio (Eds.), *Play in occupational therapy with children.* St. Louis, MO: Mosby.

Dunlap, W. R., & Hollingsworth, J. S. (1977). How does a handicapped child affect the family? Implications for practitioners. *The Family Coordinator, 26,* 286–293.

Dunst, C. J., Trivette, C. M., & Deal, A. G. (Eds.). (1994). *Supporting and strengthening families: Methods, strategies, and practices.* Cambridge, MA: Brookline.

Dyson, L. L. (1996). The experiences of families of children with learning disabilities: Parental stress, family functioning, and sibling self-concept. *Journal of Learning Disabilities, 29,* 280–286.

Gallimore, R., Coots, J., Weisner, T, Gamier, H., & Guthrie, D. (1996). Family responses to children with early developmental delays II: Accommodation intensity and activity in early and middle childhood. *American Journal on Mental Retardation, 101,* 215–232.

Gallimore, R., Weisner, T., Bernheimer, L., Guthrie, D., & Nihira, K. (1993). Family responses to young children with developmental delays. Accommodation activity in ecological and cultural context. *American Journal of Mental Retardation, 98,* 185–206.

Gallimore, R., Weisner, T., Kaufman, S., & Bernheimer, L. (1989). The social construction of ecological niches. Family accommodation of developmentally delayed children. *American Journal of Mental Retardation, 94,* 216–230.

Harris, V. S., & McHale, S. M. (1989). Family life problems, daily caretaking activities, and the psychological well-being of mothers and mentally retarded children. *American Journal on Mental Retardation, 94,* 231–239.

Helitzer, D. L., Cunningham-Sabo, L. D., VanLeit, B., & Crowe, T K. (2002). Perceived changes in self-image and coping strategies of mothers of children with disabilities. *Occupational Therapy Journal of Research, 22,* 25–33.

Humphry, R., & Case-Smith, J. (2001). Working with families. In J. Case-Smith (Ed), *Occupational therapy for children* (4th ed.). St. Louis, MO: Mosby.

Individuals With Disabilities Education Act Amendments (1997). Pub. L. 105–117, 34 C.ER.

Innocenti, M. S., & Huh, K. (1992). Families of children with disabilities: Normative data and other considerations on parenting stress. *Topics in Early Childhood Special Education, 12,* 403–427.

Jennings, P. (1990). Caring for a child with a tracheostomy. *Nursing Standard, 4*(32), 38–40.

King, G. A., King, S. M., & Rosenbaum, P. L. (1996). How mothers and fathers view professional caregiving for children with disabilities. *Developmental Medicine and Child Neurology, 38,* 397–407.

Kirk, A. (1998). Families' experiences of caring at home for a technology-dependent child: A review of the literature. *Child Care, Health, and Development, 24,* 101–114.

Knafl, K., Breitmayer, B., Gallo, A., & Zoeller, L. (1996). Family response to childhood chronic illness: Description of management styles. *Journal of Pediatric Nursing: Nursing Care of Children and Families, 11,* 315–326.

McWilliam, R. A., Tocci, L., & Harbin, G. L. (1998). Family centered services: Service providers' discourse and behavior. *Topics in Early Childhood and Special Education, 18,* 206–221.

Murphy, K. E. (1997). Parenting a technology assisted infant: Coping with occupational stress. *Social Work in Health Care, 24,* 113–126.

Patterson, J., & Blum, R. W. (1996). Risk and resilience among children and youth with disabilities. *Archives of Pediatric and Adolescent Medicine, 150,* 692–698.

Patterson, J., Jernell, J., Leonard, B., & Titus, J. C. (1994). Caring for medically fragile children at home: The parent-professional relationship. *Journal of Pediatric Nursing, 9,* 98–106.

Scorgie, K., Wilgosh, L., & McDonald, L. (1998). Stress and coping in families of children with disabilities: An examination of recent literature. *Developmental Disabilities Bulletin, 26,* 22–42.

Smith, T. B., Oliver, M. N., & Innocenti, M. S. (2001). Parenting stress in families of children with disabilities. *American Journal of Orthopsychiatry, 71,* 257–261.

Suelzle, M., & Keenan, V. (1981). Changes in family support networks over the life cycle of mentally retarded persons. *American Journal of Mental Deficiency, 86,* 267–274.

Tak, Y. R., & McCubbin, M. (2002). Family stress, perceived social support and coping following the diagnosis of a child's congenital heart disease. *Journal of Advanced Nursing, 39,* 190–198.

Tizard, J., & Grad, J. C. (1961). *The mentally handicapped and their families.* New York: Oxford University Press.

Turnbull, A. P., & Turnbull, H. R. (1997). *Families, professionals, and exceptionality: A special partnership* (2nd ed.). Columbus, OH: Merrill.

VanLeit, B., & Crowe, T. K. (2002). Outcomes of an occupational therapy program for mothers of children with disabilities: Impact on satisfaction with time use and occupational performance. *American Journal of Occupational Therapy, 56,* 402–410.

Weisner, T. S. (1993). Siblings in cultural place. Ethnographic and ecocultural perspectives. In Z. Stoneman, & P. Berman (Eds.), *Siblings of individuals with mental retardation, physical disabilities, and chronic illness* (pp.51–83). Baltimore, MD: Brookes.

16

In the Midst of a Hurricane: A Case Study
of a Couple Living With AIDS

LYDIA P. BUKI, PATTI UMAN, LORI KOGAN, AND BETHANNE KEEN

That is the big thing I have learned from this illness. The time is now, *if you have*
people that you love and care about, you take that time. You have to live each
day like you have a lifetime, and each day like you have just a short period of
time. It's now, *it's* today.

—Rosalie

*A*t least 1 million people in the United States are living with human immunodeficiency
virus (HIV) infection (Centers for Disease Control and Prevention [CDC], 2010b). Of
these, approximately half a million live with AIDS (CDC, 2010a). As a result of highly active
antiretroviral drug therapies (HAART), the life expectancy of these individuals has increased
steadily from years to decades (Mitchell & Linsk, 2004; Palmer & Bor, 2001). In comparison
to previous treatments, these new drug therapies often have fewer side effects and require
both a lower number of pills and smaller dosages (Wagner, Remien, Carballo-Dieguez, &
Dolezal, 2002). However, the transition from living with the HIV virus to dealing with
AIDS, and the resultant physical and mental deterioration, brings numerous changes in the
patient's lifestyle (Palmer & Bor, 2001). It also places extra burdens on intimate partners,
such as safety, disclosure, and anticipation of disability and death, as well as caregiving concerns (Derlega, Winstead, Oldfield, & Barbee, 2003). Partners, friends, spouses, and other
family members often become the primary caregivers to the person with AIDS; informal
family caregivers are now considered the frontline of home care (McNamera & Rosenwaxa,
2010). It is not uncommon for partners to provide in-home care for 10 years or more, and
for caregivers to feel that they have little choice about fulfilling that role (Kalichman, 2000;
Stajduhar & Davies, 2005).

Although the data still confirm that gay and bisexual men, as well as men who have
sex with men (MSM), bear the brunt of the condition, those who become infected through
high-risk heterosexual contact account for 31% of all new infections (CDC, 2008). In fact,
the number of heterosexual AIDS cases has nearly doubled since the mid-1990s and continues to rise (CDC, 2008). However, there is much less information and research on the
impact of HIV/AIDS on heterosexuals than on gays, bisexuals, or MSM. Heterosexual couples are too often overlooked, despite the fact that they represent a group with distinctive
needs. Thus, their needs are not always addressed, and they are often unprepared to cope
with the realities of the illness (Pomeroy, Green, & VanLaningham, 2002).

From "In the midst of a hurricane: A case study of a couple living with AIDS," by L. Buki, L. Kogan,
B. Keen, and P. Uman, 2005, *Journal of Counseling & Development*, 83, 470–479. Reprinted with
permission from the American Counceling Association (ACA).

Research shows that heterosexual persons with AIDS (PWAs) and their partners are at great risk of detrimental mental health outcomes. Heterosexual PWAs report higher levels of depression and less available social support than their homosexual counterparts (Mosack et al., 2009). Other concerns faced by heterosexual couples include uncertainty, worry about confidentiality issues, changes in personal relationships, and feelings of loneliness, isolation, and discrimination (Bogart et al., 2008; Pomeroy et al., 2002). In the ever-expanding HIV literature, only a handful of research studies explore how heterosexual serodiscordant couples experience and manage HIV in their relationships (Persson, 2008), a limitation we sought to overcome in this study by interviewing not only a man with AIDS but also his wife (who was his full-time caregiver).

One of the most prevalent stressors serodiscordant couples face is coping with changes in their social support system (Mosack et al., 2009; Somlai & Heckman, 2000). Studies show that many patients, as well as their immediate families, are rejected or abandoned by other family members, friends, and partners when they disclose their illness (Bogart et al., 2008). Thus, families living with HIV/AIDS often experience limited social support, isolation, and prejudice due to the stigma and fear associated with the disease (Bogart et al., 2008; Jarman, Walsh, & DeLacey, 2005; Vanable, Carey, Blair, & Littlewood, 2006). For example, Brashers et al. (2003) found that people avoid contact with PWAs because they associate the disease with homosexuality, IV drug use, and promiscuity. In fact, gay patients in gay communities are usually more informed, experience less stigma, and have greater social support than heterosexual individuals living in communities in which AIDS is not as prevalent (Brashers et al., 2003; Mosack et al., 2009; Wagner et al., 2002).

An additional source of stress for PWAs is uncertainty in their medical, personal, and social lives, as well as the cycle of sickness and health experienced with this illness (Brashers et al., 2003; Kalichman, 2000). This cycle is often marked by periods of uncertainty, renewed hope, and readjustments (Brashers et al, 2003; Trainor & Ezer, 2000). Thus, uncertainty is a constant stressor that often impairs quality of life (Brashers et al., 2003). In addition, despite medical advances that have improved management of the illness (Mitchell & Linsk, 2004; Wagner et al., 2002), the HIV replication process and adaptive qualities of the virus may require concurrent use of numerous medications and frequent changes in the medical regimen to manage symptoms. This forces PWAs to make changes in their daily routine to accommodate medication schedules and the side effects their medications cause (Trainor & Ezer, 2000). In this effort, their partner's involvement in treatment can positively influence medication adherence (Palmer & Bor, 2001; Remien et al., 2005; Wagner et al., 2002).

Despite these stressors, PWAs may experience positive changes as a result of their illness. Many infected persons develop new coping skills, find positive personal growth, and develop a renewed outlook on life (Baumgartner, 2007; Brashers et al., 2003). Their relationships have the potential to deepen as they feel an urgency to make the most of their time together with loved ones and improve the quality of their relationships (Palmer & Bor, 2001). Although some relationships become strained, others may bring couples together in a mutually supportive and emotionally engaged partnership in which HIV is a jointly shared and managed experience (Persson, 2008). In fact, in one study, 72% of couples felt that their commitment to each other was stronger after the diagnosis (Beckerman, 2002). However, Palmer and Bor (2001) noted a definite difference between patient and caregiver in their understanding of time and construct of the future.

As the illness advances, caregiving needs of PWAs increase and become more taxing (McNamera & Rosenwaxa, 2010; Stetz & Brown, 2004). Thus, caregivers have to drastically shift their lives to fulfill their obligation to care for the PWA (Stajduhar & Davies, 2005). Higher levels of external support can help caregivers deal with daily stressors. However, when caregivers feel that they do not receive enough help or support, they experience pain, depression, and anger, as well as feel diminished coping after their partner's death (McNamera & Rosenwaxa, 2010; Palmer & Bor, 2001). In contrast to friends and other family members, partners and spouses appear to be least likely of all caregivers to receive informal assistance with daily activities (McNamera & Rosenwaxa, 2010; Meeker, 2004; Stajduhar & Davies, 2005). Perhaps visitors and friends offer less help to partners and spouses, feeling that it is that person's unique role to care for the patient. The burden on caregivers is further enhanced when the PWAs, knowing that their requests for assistance will not be avoided, seek more support from the partner and friends than from others (Derlega et al., 2003). Likewise, caregivers who live with the PWA may perceive their activities as a duty or assumed because they live with the patient, and may find less gratification and meaning in those daily activities than caregivers who experience their work as nurturing and reciprocal (Ayres, 2000; Stajduhar & Davies, 2005).

Further stress ensues when caregivers experience conflict with the PWA. Conflict often arises when the PWA and caregiver disagree about the handling of side effects from medication, the medication regimen to follow, or how much autonomy to allow the PWA in certain situations. Caregivers often struggle between honoring a patient's self-determination and acting beneficially, trying to provide both care and respect (Meeker, 2004). This conflict can be particularly distressing to a caregiver for whom the patient was an important source of support prior to the onset of the illness (Turner, Pearlin, & Mullan, 1998). The combination of minimal external support, reduced gratification, and conflict can put tremendous strain on the caregiving relationship (Kalichman, 2000; Turner et al., 1998).

To reduce stress, PWAs and their caregivers must develop coping strategies. One such strategy is the solace offered by spiritual practices (Cotton et al., 2006; Ironson et al., 2002; Trevino et al., 2010). The majority of PWAs engage in some sort of daily spiritual activity, usually in the form of prayer, meditation, or breathing exercises (Somlai & Heckman, 2000). Both PWAs and caregivers rely on their spirituality (organized and nonorganized spiritual or religious beliefs and behaviors) to provide emotional and cognitive resources during stressful times and to bring a sense of meaning to their lives (Ayres, 2000; Ironson et al., 2002). Enhanced meaning can often bring a sense of hope, equilibrium, and resolution to daily challenges (Trainor & Ezer, 2000). In addition, spiritual beliefs and behaviors have been associated with a longer survival rate and better health outcomes, less depression, higher quality of life, and greater self-esteem in PWAs (Cotton et al., 2006; Ironson et al., 2002; Trevino et al., 2010). Caregivers also find comfort in their spiritual beliefs during and after the death of their loved one insofar as spirituality provides solace during the grieving process (Richards, Acree, & Folkman, 1999).

Given the prevalence of HIV in heterosexual individuals, the many stressors experienced by the population, the limited supports available to them to buffer the stress, and the limited data about their experiences, in this article we present a case study of a couple living with AIDS. We discuss the daily activities, challenges, coping strategies, and relationship dynamics of a heterosexual, HIV-serodiscordant (mixed HIV status) couple in which the male partner has AIDS and the female partner is his primary caregiver. Rather than looking for specific determinants of behavior, our goal was to gain a holistic understanding of what it meant to this couple to live with AIDS. Lastly, we sought to identify specific counseling recommendations for individuals who work with HIV-serodiscordant couples.

METHOD

Participants

At the time of the interviews, John was 42 years old and in the advanced stages of AIDS. Rosalie, who was not infected with HIV, was John's primary caregiver. He and Rosalie had been married for 22 years and had two children, a 19-year-old son and a 17-year-old daughter. John had begun to show physical signs of his illness approximately 4 years after his diagnosis, and when his physical condition deteriorated, Rosalie left her job to care for him. Subsequent to this life change, Rosalie received some training and financial compensation for working as John's hospice caregiver. The couple was referred to us by a local psychotherapist who worked with AIDS patients and their families. We had no preexisting relationship with John and Rosalie prior to our assessment of their interest in this study.

Design and Analysis

Using predetermined variables to test established hypotheses can sometimes influence the outcome of the research and fail to uncover meaningful events (Coyle, 1998; Glachan, 1998; Polkinghorne, 1991). Although counseling psychology has tended to underutilize qualitative research, increasingly researchers are recognizing it as the preferable way of obtaining in-depth knowledge and insights regarding the human experience (e.g., Morrow, 2007; Ponterotto, 2005). It may be said that we developed the study methodology in collaboration with John and Rosalie, insofar as the couple not only requested that their real names be used in the study, but also agreed to be interviewed only under the condition that their stories be published to help others in similar circumstances. As described by many PWAs (e.g., Funk & Stajduhar, 2009; Trainor & Ezer, 2000) and clearly stated by John and Rosalie, people have a need to tell their stories. We felt that the best way to communicate their stories was through a case study.

Case studies are used in the social sciences because of their power to convey vividly the "dimensions of a social phenomenon or individual life" (Reinharz, 1992, p. 174). Typically, a case study is conducted to present uniqueness; our choice to conduct a case study was based on the relatively little attention focused on the experiences of HIV-serodiscordant, heterosexual couples. Three semi-structured interviews were conducted with each participant over a period of one week, each interview taking place on a different day of the week. We (i.e., the first and fourth authors) developed a tandem interview session in which John and Rosalie were interviewed at the same time in their home, in different rooms. This procedure was preferred for a variety of reasons: (a) it allowed each of the participants freedom to express his or her own story; (b) it reduced the possibility of Rosalie answering questions for John, given that he had physical difficulty talking; (c) both respondents could feel that their stories were equally valued; and (d) perceptions of events could be presented from both the husband's and wife's points of view. Also, having two researchers interview both members of the couple, as opposed to John or Rosalie only, allowed for investigator triangulation of the data (Huberman & Miles, 1998). In other words, it allowed for verification of the data collected from both informants (i.e., by obtaining two perspectives on the phenomenon), as well as for convergence between the two researchers regarding interpretation of the data.

Independently, we prepared an interview guide with questions to ask our assigned informant (i.e., John or Rosalie). We adopted a nondirective, nonevaluative Rogerian (Rogers, 1951) stance, as recommended by Flick (1998), "to prevent the interviewer's frame of reference being imposed on the interviewee's viewpoints" (p. 77). We introduced structured questions as required to attain conversational depth and understanding of the impact or meaning of living with AIDS for the interviewees (see Flick, 1998). Because of our experience as crisis counselors, we felt comfortable eliciting sensitive material. This allowed the informants' accounts to go beyond general statements and delve into multiple levels of experience. Toward the end of each interview, we verbally summarized key themes that emerged during that meeting and invited feedback from our informant that would ensure an accurate understanding of his or her experience. Therefore, patterns began taking shape during the data collection process, and, in turn, informed the questions we developed for our next interview (see Patton, 2002).

We developed both sets of interview questions based on the literature on living with AIDS and caregiving and from a professional consultation with a nurse who had extensive experience with caregiving and end-of-life issues. The questions John's interviewer prepared for him inquired about his daily activities, such as: "What do you do each day?" and "How do you organize your life?" We discovered early on, however, that following an interview guide was generally ineffective with John, because the prepared questions seemed to miss the point of the story he wished to tell. For example, he was perplexed by the question "What is a typical day like for you?" He responded: "Do you mean what do I *do*? Well, the first thing is try to get in touch with my Higher Power." John's interviewer began to see that his life was not about *doing* anymore; rather, it was about *being*—living with pain, meditating and praying, and feeling the loving presence of Rosalie. Consequently, John's interviewer adjusted the questions, with the goal of learning what was important to John in his life. Although the prepared questions did not address John's experience, the flexibility of the qualitative process allowed us to adjust the questions and thereby open the way for him to present a more relevant story.

Rosalie's interviewer also prepared questions to guide her interviews with Rosalie. The theme of inquiry centered on learning about a partner's diagnosis with HIV and caregiving. For example, questions included: "How did you find out about the diagnosis, and how did you feel then?," "What keeps you going?," and "Has your ability to cope changed as the disease progressed?"

All interviews were audiotaped taking about 1.5 hours each. Themes were extracted by listening to the audiotapes and asking questions about the data, such as "What aspects of the experience of AIDS are salient to the informant?," "How has the informant reacted to these experiences?," "What challenges were identified by the informant?," and "What is the meaning of the experiences to the informant?" These questions follow the structure proposed by Denzin (1989) to understand the "existentially problematic moments in the lives of individuals" (p. 129).

Initially, we each analyzed the series of interviews we had conducted with our informant (i.e., either John or Rosalie), and subsequently weaved together the two analyses for the writing of this chapter.

RESULTS

Four common themes emerged from John and Rosalie's narratives: the emotional impact of learning about the diagnosis, new roles and experiences in daily life, the need for social support, and the spiritual journey.

Emotional Impact of the Diagnosis

Six years before the interviews, and after 16 years of marriage, John and Rosalie initiated a marital separation. They were separated for approximately nine months. During this time, John contracted the HIV virus where he learned of his diagnosis eight months after he and Rosalie reunited to rebuild their marriage. Rosalie was tested for the virus shortly after learning of John's diagnosis. At the culmination of the most terrifying two weeks of her life she found out with great relief that she was not infected.

John told Rosalie about the diagnosis the same day he found out. Rosalie received a phone call at work and John asked her to come home. He said he had something to tell her. Although Rosalie had no reason to suspect that he could be HIV positive she explained that when she saw his face, she intuitively knew what he was going to tell her. John said, "I told my wife the very first day that I found out. She said she knew already for some reason. She accepted me right off the bat....She let me know that there's no difference, nothing's changed." Rosalie remembered how she felt when she heard about the diagnosis: "How I see it is like a big puzzle that was kind of tossed in the air and all these puzzle pieces are now falling into place. The closer those pieces get down to the bottom, the more there is an understanding of what is happening."

Soon after receiving the diagnosis, John was forced to resign from his job, resulting in the loss of his health insurance coverage. For the first time in her life, Rosalie, who worked as a staff member in a home for developmentally disabled children, became the primary breadwinner in the household. She recalls this period as a very difficult time in which the family was "scattered." Just beginning to learn how to deal with the intensity of her feelings, Rosalie often cried in the shower or on her way to work. In contrast, John experienced feelings so overwhelming that they led to several suicide attempts. Convinced that his illness would rob Rosalie of the best years of her life, John recalled:

> I wanted her to divorce me because she could never have a full life as long as I was alive. But she wouldn't see it, which caused a lot of grief in my heart. Just knowing that she could not live out her most fruitful years with her husband, or a husband, or—another way of looking at it—a dysfunctional husband, which I am. So, I guess she must have evaluated...what she thought was [highest] on her list, and keeping me on was the better decision. And it was, for me [also]. But it took me a long time, of hurt and guilt on my part, to overcome...I know if you do something wrong, you feel guilty. But this was years before, and I can't even single out what event occurred, you know. So I bear the brutality of it..., but not the guilt any longer.

The most significant change in the marriage was the shifting roles Rosalie and John experienced because of the illness. Prior to the illness, John had played the traditional role of head of the household. As John's illness progressed and Rosalie was forced to take on more responsibility in supporting the family, it was difficult for her to accept that John could not work anymore. She wondered, "Why couldn't he? He looked fine, didn't he?" In time, she developed a greater understanding of the fatigue that accompanies the experience of AIDS:

> You couldn't visually see how physically sick he was, so a lot of times our nature says, "Well, you are okay, you are all right. Why don't you get a little job?," or "Why don't you try to do things around the house? Why don't you do something? Don't just lay there." That was how my intellect was until I could really get an understanding of this disease. This is just a real physical sickness, that even if you didn't look sick, you really have this horrible, horrible tiredness in your body that just zonks you out and just doing small things take a lot of energy out of you.

Learning how to care for John was not easy. According to Rosalie, John was stubborn and when he had trouble doing simple physical tasks such as lifting a glass, he refused help. Although she understood that he was still capable of making his own decisions, she often had to remember to respect her husband's right to think and act for himself:

> He won't want any help, unless he asks for it. And that is something I've become sensitive to. And I think that's really been the whole thing. Just really respecting John...respecting his wants and his needs....And also I find myself not only being his wife, but this person that helps him, his caregiver. [When it comes to his health,] it's not my decision. It's John's decision. And that's something that has really come to me in the last couple of months. It's not what I want. It's what John wants. Because

I kind of think, what would I do for myself if I try to put myself in that position? But I'm not in that position, *John* is in that position and I have to go by what he thinks.

Intimacy between John and Rosalie changed during the course of his illness. Although the relationship deepened and the bond between them strengthened, they floundered for a period of time not knowing how to replace the sexual intimacy that had necessarily been stripped from their marriage. They learned together how to increase the intensity of the other kinds of love they had for each other. John explained:

> It's unfortunate that we have just one word for so many [kinds of love] because we get things twisted. The Greeks had four or five words for love. . . . The loves that [I'm referring to] are fulfilling in a very miraculous way. They seem to kick into gear in a greater way, to compensate, you know. But you have to cultivate them, too.

One of their favorite things to do together was to play a tape of meditative music and quietly hold each other.

John could not remember a time when Rosalie wasn't taking care of him in his illness. Even before she was being paid as a hospice nurse, she was always there for him. At the time of the interview when she wasn't administering to his physical needs she was often tending to his emotional and spiritual needs. Rosalie noted that "in a situation like this you can really lose yourself in the other person and their needs, but I am going to be here and I am going to stay here."

John expressed that what he wanted most for Rosalie's future was happiness, and he did not want her to grieve for him. "Maybe she'll be lucky enough to find the man of her dreams," he said, "and get remarried." When the interviewer asked if it was hard for him to imagine her being with another man, John responded, "No, it is been hard with me sick, and her being alone."

Rosalie and John's experience with his illness did not occur in isolation. Their two teenage children, a daughter and a son, were also deeply affected by the news of John's diagnosis. When Rosalie tested negative for the HIV virus she was relieved, but her first thought was for her children. She said,

> There was also the problem of, okay, was *I* HIV positive? And we had to go through that turmoil for a while. But I'm not HIV positive, you know. So that was the hardest thing for me. Because I knew the kids were eventually going to lose their father, and I didn't want to do it to them too. I didn't want to be HIV positive and have the children lose me too.

Rosalie soon realized she would be the surviving parent of their two children. She noted that it was a rough transition for the family. At first the kids believed John would die right away. After several years passed and they saw him recover from a number of crises, they started to take his illness more in stride. Life became a little more normal for them, and their friends often came by to visit. As John became more ill, however, the children began to realize that he would not be with them much longer. One night their son broke down. Rosalie and John helped him begin the grieving process, offering him comfort as he realized the painful reality that his father would soon die. As a family, they confronted these challenging times successfully, and Rosalie felt that the family was finally able to come together because there was no more denying that the illness was taking John's life. "We've kind of come to this place, John and I, of being in harmony with each other and in harmony with our family and with our children. Just real bonding between us."

Daily Life: New Roles, New Experiences

Upon entering John and Rosalie's home, one would not have guessed all of the challenges they had experienced in the past five years. Their home was in a modest neighborhood and was warm and cozy. Furnished in soft colors, it seemed very lovingly cared for. In the living room, the sofa was covered with a lovely spread made up of fabrics with various designs and pictures were displayed in frames of various types and sizes. Often some of the children's friends were visiting when the interviewers arrived and the home was filled with a sense of life and anticipation. Few would have realized that this home was officially John's hospice during his illness.

At the time of the interviews, John was a small man who was emaciated and fragile. He walked in a slow teetering manner as if in pain from slow starvation. Although his hair was thinning it was long and woven into a pencil-thin braid at the back of his neck. He and his interviewer spoke in a small room that appeared to have been furnished for his comfort during the illness. It included a hospital bed, a leather recliner, a small television, and a set of bookshelves. The shelves held books on a wide variety of topics including psychological, literary, scientific, inspirational, and medical titles. This room also housed a multitude of reminders that John's life was medically bound by numerous prescription bottles occupying various places in the room. There were many pills in different shapes and sizes with menacing-looking machines near the bed which had lights, knobs, and hoses. A volume of the *Physician's Desk Reference* was also noted.

Although Rosalie was his primary caretaker a nurse visited John in their home twice a week to take vital signs and check on his general health. John explained, "I have flare-ups about twice a year. Each time I have a flare-up it takes three or four months to recover. So you might say that I'm always recovering and on the brink of [being] sick." Together, John and his doctor had endlessly adjusted, and gradually whittled down, his assortment of prescription drugs. John could not remember exactly all of the pills he was taking. He admitted that, over time, he had come to devalue knowledge of what drugs his doctor had prescribed to him because the list was so long and had changed so frequently.

As his pain increased John began taking morphine. Initially he had not wanted to use morphine because he considered it to be a dangerous drug and was concerned that it would affect the functioning of his mind. By the fifth year of his illness the pain in his bones and joints had become so intense, especially upon awakening in the morning, that he needed the morphine "just to take the edge off." Other daily challenges included the ability to balance when standing or walking, as the bottoms of his feet were often numb, and watching his gums shrink and his teeth deteriorate.

John's wife Rosalie presented as a very gentle and kind woman with beautiful sparkling eyes. Pleasant and smiling, she had a lively enthusiasm in her voice. Although to the casual observer everything might have seemed fairly normal, Rosalie shared with the interviewer her feeling that much of her life was "up in the air":

> When everything is over, I think I will be able to really sum up a lot of the feelings that I have inside that I find hard to express or I don't have the words for. When everything is over, I think I'll probably have a lot of things inside of me. Isn't that what happens? Like when you are in the midst of a hurricane it's real hard to kind of...figure out everything. But once you are out of it, you can kind of go, "hey, yeah, I was in the middle of that hurricane, and this is what happened." So it's just real hard for me to kind of sum up...or really express a lot of the things I have inside of me. And...and I keep saying that will happen once everything is over.

Knowing that even small tasks exhausted John, Rosalie spent a great part of her day administering to his physical needs. She helped him eat, take his medicine, and communicate (often by telephone) with doctors, friends, and family.

John explained that he mostly read, slept, watched television, and spent time with Rosalie. He hadn't felt hungry lately, but tried to heed the doctor's advice about drinking lots of fluids. He also tended to family matters around the home. However, when speaking to John, it was clear that his life wasn't about *doing* anymore; it was about *being*. On difficult days, John felt drained and was in severe pain. He had trouble staying awake due to the amount of morphine he was taking, thus, he would search for the Higher Power within himself. He would meditate and recall the many good things that had happened in his life and he would pray for help in weathering the storm.

The Need for Social Support

Like many PWAs, John experienced a decline in social relationships as his illness progressed. He explained that maintaining contact with people was important to him, but even though a number of good friends stayed in touch, others had stopped visiting or making contact. He wondered if it had something to do with his physical appearance. John recognized that he had "that look" which publicly identified him as an AIDS patient: sunken eyes, an emaciated frame, an unbalanced walk. At the time of the interviews he weighed 94 pounds. When he had first seen that number on his scale a few months earlier he could not believe it. Five years prior to when John received what he stated was "the news" about his illness, he weighed about 145 pounds. Having lost in excess of 50 pounds from his 5' 7" frame, more than one-third of his total body weight; it was not surprising that he said he felt astonished when he saw himself in the mirror. He commented that he did not see a reflection of himself, but rather the face and body of a concentration camp victim.

Rosalie also experienced social support difficulties often feeling judged by others. In particular, she did not like being questioned about how John contracted HIV. When people asked "How did he get it?" she would reply, "Who cares how he got it?! He is HIV positive and that is all that matters." There was friction also with visitors who did not know John very well. For example, John often struggled with simple tasks like walking or lifting a glass. Others would look at Rosalie as if to say, "Do something!," when in fact Rosalie was caring for John by allowing him the independence he desired. She respected his need for autonomy and his ability to make decisions about what he could or could not do.

Despite these difficulties John and Rosalie strove to remain as socially active as possible. John and his pastor worked together to create a coffee house which was a place where AIDS patients could gather one day a week, enjoy free coffee and food, and socialize with one another. Close to the time of the interviews John and Rosalie went to the coffee house speculating that it might be his last visit. The reality of his illness and of his anticipated death were emphasized by the absence of those who had once been companions in weathering the storm, but now had made peace with the hurricane.

> We did drop in last Thursday, just at the right time. We stayed for a half hour and saw that, of everybody that was there when we started the program, we had three still alive. Almost everybody I knew was dead. It kind of makes you feel like a survivor. However, you are bonding with people who die, and it happens over and over again. Pretty soon, you'd just like to side-step the AIDS people. But I can't do that, because by facing them now, I'm facing my own situation.

John admitted his desire to "side-step the AIDS people" in an effort to flee from the face of death, yet he knew that confronting such fear was necessary for him to reach acceptance and inner peace.

The Spiritual Journey

John's spiritual journey consisted of coming to terms with his own mortality and coping with his illness. When asked how he got through the difficult days, John said he was always searching for the Higher Power within himself by practicing meditation and prayer.

He explained, "I have to look at this as a spiritual adventure, for my own sanity; because if I didn't, it would be morbid." During meditation he tried to recall the many good things that had happened in his life. Meditating brought him to a place where he could "place a face" on his spirituality and his Higher Power. He explained that he no longer prayed for a healing or cure as he first did. Instead, he prayed for help in "weathering the storm." Comparing himself to Paul the Apostle, John attained some peace of mind "in God's words to Paul, 'My grace is sufficient unto you'." As Paul prayed three times that the thorn be removed from his flesh, John felt as well, "I've been told [for] the third time these last few years [that healing would not come]. Now I am set, accepted and relaxed." Actually, John considered himself lucky, in a way. "You don't know when you are going to die," he said to the interviewer, "but I have a far clearer idea."

Rosalie also drew strength from spirituality as she cared for John and prepared herself for life after John's death. Rosalie explained that God helped her survive all the changes she had endured. She took comfort "in the scripture that assures 'all works out for those who love God and act according to His purpose'." She felt she had been called on by God to care for John, and therefore she knew everything would work out for good. Several times each day Rosalie set aside a few minutes for her to read, meditate, or listen to inspirational music. Her goal was to quiet herself, listen to what was inside, and to get in touch with her present experience. Rosalie explained,

> That is the big thing I have learned from this illness. The time is *now*, if you have people that you love and care about, you take that time. You have to live each day like you have a lifetime, and each day like you have just a short period of time. It's *now*, it's *today*.

In her own words, Rosalie experienced "a profound realization" when she understood that her relationship with John was not really ending with his death. She felt that the illness was taking John's life, "but [it isn't] taking John, just his body. This is a short time in a real existence."

DISCUSSION

The relationship between John and Rosalie was a dominant theme in both of their interviews. The couple was just in the midst of reestablishing their relationship after a short time apart, and had to bear the weight of John's diagnosis. Decisions about caregiving are strongly dependent on the relationship status prior to an AIDS diagnosis, as often the seronegative partner assumes the role of primary caregiver (Palmer & Bor, 2001). Caregivers can feel left out by health service providers who often fail to recognize a family caregiver when making decisions for the PWA (Meeker, 2004; Stetz & Brown, 2004). Stetz and Brown (2004) found that because health care providers are more focused on the patient's health, family members who may be equally stressed can be overlooked. These preexisting difficulties are then compounded by the role changes that often mark PWAs' relationships, as the caregiver struggles between honoring the PWA's self-determination and acting beneficially (Meeker, 2004). Rosalie alluded to some of the challenges they encountered when she discussed John's stubbornness and her initial resistance to letting him struggle, for example, as he picked up and drank from a glass. Yet her strong commitment to John and to their relationship eventually led her to understand John's need to do what he could for himself. Subsequently, she remained respectful of his choice despite the effort it took for her to adopt this observer role.

In addition to role changes, couples often struggle with alternative ways to demonstrate intimacy and affection when sexual contact is no longer possible (Beckerman, 2002;

Bradley, Remien, & Dolezal, 2008; Palmer & Bor, 2001; Pomeroy et al., 2002). For many couples, physical intimacy, rather than sexual activity, is a great comfort to both partners (Palmer & Bor, 2001). As the couple dealt with the dilemma of wanting to be sexual but not being able to do so (except at great risk of infecting Rosalie with HIV, a chance they were not willing to take), they turned to alternatives and reframed the meaning of love, broadening its definition to fit their new reality.

As partners struggle to adapt to their new roles when a partner is diagnosed with AIDS, children of parents with AIDS likewise experience turmoil. Schuster and colleagues (2000) found that most children generally stay with their parents even through the most severe symptoms and therefore experience circumstances that may be especially challenging. In addition, children often assumed more adult roles and even caretaking of their parent. Despite these challenges, researchers have found that as long as parents model a positive parental attitude during the illness, most children of parents with AIDS do well later in life (Stein, Rotheram-Borus, & Lester, 2007). Therefore, it is important for parents to remain committed to their parenting roles, help their children understand the illness, and support the children as they initiate the grieving process This will help them develop coping strategies and skills in emotional regulation (Stein et al., 2007). John and Rosalie, despite their own difficulties adjusting to AIDS, remained committed to meeting their children's needs and continued to be a source of strength and learning for them. The parenting role appeared to remain stable in the midst of many other role changes.

John, like many PWAs, struggled to redefine himself after learning about his illness. No longer able to contribute to society and his family in traditionally accepted ways (e.g., through work and by providing financial support), he fought strong feelings of inadequacy. Compounded by the necessary changes in the couple's sexual expression, John reported feeling like a "dysfunctional" husband. He did make several suicide attempts. This is consistent with previous research which has suggested that PWAs have elevated rates of depressive disorders and are especially vulnerable to feelings of despair and guilt (Brashers et al., 2003; Eller et al., 2005; Perez, et al., 2009). In time, John was able to focus his cognitions on positive aspects of his life, not dwell on the negative, and take control whenever possible (e.g., making decisions about medication in conjunction with his doctor). Consistent with previous research indicating that PWAs' cognitive appraisal of their situation is an important predictor of coping success (Pakenham & Rinaldis, 2001). Overall, John experienced an improvement in his quality of life and relationships after he changed the negative way in which he was appraising his situation. In redefining himself and reprioritizing what was important, day-to-day living became John's focus and educating himself about pills or other such tasks became unimportant. Although this could be interpreted as learned helplessness, we believe that John would have seen it as reflective of a shift in priorities.

Similarly, a host of overwhelming feelings (e.g., anger, guilt, depression, grief) often accompanies the initial news of a partner's diagnosis (Stetz & Brown, 2004). Caregivers often repress these feelings and outwardly remain optimistic in order to protect the PWA from stress or because these feelings are seen as "inappropriate" (Meeker, 2004; Stajduhar & Davies, 2005). This was true of Rosalie, who cried in the shower as a way to grieve privately, even secretly, particularly upon finding out that John was infected with HIV and she was not. The presence of children added complexity to Rosalie's emotional reaction, given her initial fear that she might also die, leaving the children alone.

Rosalie also contended with the reality of becoming the sole family provider for the first time in 22 years of marriage. Many caregivers report developing new confidence, gaining additional competencies, taking better care of themselves, and becoming advocates for others in similar situations as they assume new responsibilities (Brown & Stetz, 1999; Viney, Allwood, Stillson, & Walmsley, 1992). The role changes that Rosalie was forced to make illustrate both positive and negative aspects of this type of challenge. Within a short period of time she was forced to perform new roles for which she was ill prepared (i.e., primary breadwinner, full-time hospice caregiver), requiring her to gain many new skills and make radical changes in her daily life. However, this shift in responsibilities helped her gain the confidence that she would be able to take care of her family after John's death, allowed her to strengthen her spiritual beliefs, and prompted her to learn to take better care of herself. Perhaps most importantly, Rosalie felt that she had learned what was important to her in life, suggesting that she underwent a kind of value-clarification process that would have a positive impact on her psychological well-being for the foreseeable future.

Facing the reality of an AIDS diagnosis demands significant adjustment to extra burdens associated with having the disease (Brashers et al., 2003; Derlega et al., 2003). Initial changes often occur unnoticed by people outside the home. Even though a lack of outwardly apparent illness can help couples maintain a sense of normalcy, it also creates difficulties (Trainor & Ezer, 2000). Like Rosalie, some people may struggle to understand why an outwardly healthy PWA cannot work or assume other responsibilities. Through educational experiences, she came to understand that although many physical symptoms (e.g., tiredness) were not apparent, they impaired John's ability to perform mundane tasks. During the developmental adaptation process, PWAs and their caregivers also come to understand that AIDS does not progress as a gradual decline of physical health, but is an illness marked by a succession of ups and downs. Until fairly recently, people diagnosed with AIDS prepared to die within a relatively short period of time. With the advances in medical care such as HAART, PWAs are living longer thereby dealing with an unavoidable cycle of opportunistic infections (Mitchell & Linsk, 2004; Trainor & Ezer, 2000). This forces PWAs and their partners to face death several times throughout the course of the disease. John's physical "flare-ups" illustrate this phenomenon. The downward cycle with small plateaus of stability presents unique challenges, yet it can also help people develop new adaptive habits and coping skills. During these times, John and Rosalie learned how to talk about John's illness and at the same time, how to talk about the future. The couple's house, a combination of life and death artifacts, was symbolic of these two diametrically opposed realities taking place under one roof.

A caregiver's contact with family and friends usually decreases as the illness progresses, even as the need for support increases (Bogart et al., 2008; Vanable et al., 2006). John and Rosalie both reported that contact with people outside the family had slowly decreased over the course of his illness. Despite these changes in the support system John and Rosalie employed some common coping strategies to reduce their social isolation. For example, they discussed the importance of talking and sharing their perspectives with other people who were also struggling to live with AIDS. The coffee house that the couple frequented (created by John and his pastor) was a place where PWAs could gather and socialize. This type of gathering may also have been a vehicle for other therapeutic elements more traditionally associated with support groups or group therapy (e.g., Brashers et al., 2003; Burgoyne & Renwick, 2004; Mosack et al., 2009). For instance, John's discussion about feeling like a "survivor" when most of the initial members of the coffeehouse group had died was possibly a reflection of downward comparison, in which people compare themselves to others who are in a worse state. This cognitive strategy has been put forth as one way in which people can feel more positive about their own standing (Trainor & Ezer, 2000). Moreover, being with others who struggle with parallel issues can help reduce feelings of isolation and improve overall health (Burgoyne, 2005; Burgoyne & Renwick, 2004). As John explained, there are both positive and negative aspects to connecting with other PWAs. Although it is important for PWAs to feel understood and connected to others undergoing similar experiences, it is painful to experience losses when these companions die. Facing these losses, as well as many other concurrent losses experienced by the couple (e.g., changing roles, physical deterioration, erosion of social support system), added complexity to their grieving process.

Many PWAs and their caregivers draw peace and strength from their spiritual beliefs (Cotton et al., 2006; Ironson et al., 2002; Trevino et al., 2010). Both organized and nonorganized religion and spirituality can help people derive meaning from their experiences as they attempt to come to terms with their own mortality (Ironson et al., 2002). This coping strategy is clearly depicted in John's discussion of the relationship with his Higher Power, and in Rosalie's meaningful and comforting "breakthrough" that her relationship with John will continue after his death. Their shift in priorities, by which the depth of their feelings toward each other assumed the greatest position and other more mundane issues (i.e., material possessions) shifted to the background, was viewed as a positive spiritual change by both.

Contributions and Limitations of the Study

As traditional avenues of contributing to society are curtailed, PWAs and their caregivers often feel the desire to comfort and counsel others who are experiencing similar situations as one way to find meaning in their own pain (Funk & Stajduhar, 2009; Mitchell & Linsk, 2004). The couple felt these sentiments strongly as expressed by John who stated: "I would very much like to make a contribution to the world's knowledge about what it is like to live with AIDS, and see publication of this report as an opportunity to do this."

Every person's experience of living with AIDS is unique. All of us handle challenging situations differently, drawing from our past experiences, our personality characteristics, our current relationships, and the various environmental contexts in which our lives are embedded. Moreover, we may heed social desirability to different degrees. Therefore, John's and Rosalie's subjective experiences will not be representative of the subjective experiences of all other HIV-serodiscordant, heterosexual couples. In particular, our findings may not reflect the experiences of couples who are willing to discuss the mode of HIV transmission. John alluded to having only a very vague sense of how he became infected, and Rosalie felt strongly that this information was irrelevant. Therefore, we cannot ascertain the impact of the mode of transmission on their adaptation to living with AIDS. Their stories, however, have given us a glimpse into distinct themes as perceived by a couple going through a unique life-changing experience. There is much we can learn from what they have told us, as was suggested by their intention to share their story so that others may profit from it.

Working With PWAs and Their Caregivers: Our Personal Reflections

Witnessing our informants' experiences and documenting their journeys had a profound effect on us, the interviewers, as well. Our assumptions about the grieving process and about living with a chronic and often fatal disease were challenged. We marveled at the strength of the human spirit, particularly the affirming way in which Rosalie and John learned to live within the context of the disease. To observe their zest for life in the middle of death was very moving.

As investigators and observers we helped create their reality, and we were changed by it in the process. Although this type of empathy is a common element of the counseling process, it was compounded in this situation because of the particularly intimate views and complete honesty offered by both Rosalie and John. We were honored to be a part of the process by which they would leave a legacy. Unavoidably, we examined our own spiritual beliefs, our comfort levels in dealing with life and death, and our own life priorities during various stages of this project. By acknowledging and honoring our emotional reactions we gained better insight into the issues that arise for counselors working with PWAs and their caregivers.

Recommendations for Counselors Working With PWAs and Their Caregivers

As counselors, we help PWAs and their caregivers weather the winds of the hurricane. We help PWAs reconstruct the self and reprioritize their lives to improve their quality of life. We aid caregivers during both the caregiving and grieving processes. We provide communities of PWAs with the education and support needed to embrace families living with AIDS, thus helping communities to enhance the quality of life of PWAs and their families. Several recommendations for counselors working with PWAs and their caregivers emerged from our interactions with John and Rosalie and our experience with the research process. These recommendations address the needs of PWAs, their caregivers, families, and communities.

1. Consider the benefit of including the entire family in the therapy process. Members of a PWA's family have specific needs due to their own personality traits, ways of coping and grieving, and the intensity of their relationship with the PWA.

2. Due to the uncertainty brought about by the nature of the disease, be cautious when setting therapeutic goals with PWAs and their caregivers. Goals should be crafted as a cooperative effort with the couple, carefully choosing time frames with which the couple is comfortable.

3. Assist couples in renegotiating roles within the marriage, especially if new roles challenge that couple's gender and/or cultural norms. For couples with children, it is important to retain the parenting role as a critical collaborative task.

4. Remain aware of where people are in the stages of the disease and help them explore how much information and responsibility they can handle (or desire) in terms of making decisions about their medical status and other personal issues.

5. Bear in mind the inherent risk involved when couples living with AIDS tell others about their disease. Discuss with clients their expectations of disclosure as well as ways to address possible negative reactions from others.

6. Recognize that partners of PWAs may need some period of time to adjust to the diagnosis. They may benefit from normalizing the amount of time they need to accept news of this nature, and should not be forced to make any immediate decisions that would affect either themselves or others.

7. Support caregivers' efforts to care for themselves. Although caregivers for people with short-term illnesses can sometimes delay taking time for themselves until after a patient's death, this is not practical for caregivers of PWAs. Due to the cyclic and prolonged nature of the illness, caregivers should be encouraged to discover and maintain self-care habits early in the adaptation process.

8. Provide additional guidance and support as caregivers' responsibilities shift from caring for a chronically ill partner to supporting a partner as he or she dies.

9. Recognize that most PWAs and their caregivers desire the opportunity to talk about their feelings, either one-on-one or in a group setting. Assist them in finding avenues for expression, such as creating a "coffeehouse" setting or through writing, painting, or other creative outlets.

10. Help couples learn how to express intimacy in new ways, when sexual intimacy is no longer possible.

Living with AIDS is an unremitting challenge for PWAs and their caretakers. As John and Rosalie so eloquently demonstrated, it does not have to be a dark and lonely journey. It can in fact be a transcendental one, allowing for a tremendously enriching spiritual experience. John and Rosalie exemplify the unlimited potential of the human spirit in the face of adversity. As counselors, it is our responsibility to help PWAs, their caregivers, and families tap into their inner resources and gain strength from their unique histories and interpersonal relationships. Let us utilize the growing knowledge and research in this area to help PWAs and their caretakers realize this potential.

REFERENCES

Ayres, L. (2000). Narratives of family caregiving: The process of making meaning. *Research in Nursing & Health, 23*(6), 424–434.

Baumgartner, L. M. (2007). The incorporation of the HIV/AIDS identity into the self over time. *Qualitative Health Research, 17*(7), 919–931.

Beckerman, N. L. (2002). Couples coping with discordant HIV status. *AIDS Patient Care & STDs, 16*(2), 55–59.

Bogart, L. M., Cowgill, B. O., Kennedy, D., Ryan, G., Murphy, D. A., Elijah, J., et al. (2008). HIV-related stigma among people with HIV and their families: A qualitative analysis. *AIDS & Behavior, 12*(2), 244–254.

Bradley, M. V., Remien, R. H., & Dolezal, C. (2008). Depression symptoms and sexual HIV risk behavior among serodiscordant couples. *Psychosomatic Medicine, 70,* 189–191.

Brashers, D. E., Neidig, J. L., Russell, J. A., Cardillo, L. W., Haas, S. M., Nemeth, S., et al. (2003). The medical, personal, and social causes of uncertainty in HIV illness. *Issues in Mental Health Nursing, 24,* 497–522.

Brown, M., & Stetz, K. (1999). The labor of caregiving: A theoretical model of caregiving during potentially fatal illness. *Qualitative Health Research, 9*(2), 182–197.

Burgoyne, R. (2005). Exploring direction of causation between social support and clinical outcome for HIV-positive adults in the context of highly active antiretroviral therapy. *AIDS Care, 17,* 111–124.

Burgoyne, R., & Renwick, R. (2004). Social support and quality of life over time among adults living with HIV in the HAART era. *Social Science & Medicine, 58*(7), 1353–1366.

Centers for Disease Control and Prevention. (2008). *Estimates of New HIV Infections in the United States.* Retrieved from http://www.cdc.gov/hiv/topics/surveillance/resources/factsheets/pdf/incidence.pdf

Centers for Disease Control and Prevention. (2010a). *Basic Statistics.* Retrieved from http://www.cdc.gov/hiv/topics/surveillance/basic.htm#lwa

Centers for Disease Control and Prevention. (2010b). *HIV in the United States.* Retrieved September 28, 2010, from http://www.cdc.gov/hiv/resources/factsheets/us.htm

Cotton, S., Puchalski, C. M., Sherman, S. N., Mrus, J. M., Peterman, A. H., Feinberg, et al. (2006). Spirituality and religion in patients with HIV/AIDS. *Journal of General Internal Medicine, 21,* S5–S13.

Coyle, A. (1998). Qualitative research in counseling psychology: Using the counseling interview as a research instrument. In P. Clarkson (Ed.), *Counseling psychology: Integrating theory, research and supervised practice* (pp. 57–73). London: Routledge.

Denzin, N. K. (1989). *Interpretive interactionism.* Newbury Park, CA: Sage.

Derlega, V. J., Winstead, B. A., Oldfield, E. C., & Barbee, A. P. (2003). Close relationships and social support in coping with HIV: A test of sensitive interaction systems theory. *AIDS * Behavior, 7*(2), 119–129.

Eller, L. S., Bunch, E. H., Kemppainen, J., Holzemer, W., Nokes, K., Portillo, C., et al. (2005). Self-care strategies for depressive symptoms in people with HIV disease. *Journal of Advanced Nursing, 51*(2), 119–130.

Flick, U. (1998). *An introduction to qualitative research.* London: Sage.

Funk, L. M., & Stajduhar, K. I. (2009). Interviewing family caregivers: Implications of the caregiving context for the research interview. *Qualitative Health Research, 19*(6), 859–867.

Glachan, M. (1998). Balancing the qualitative and the quantitative in counseling psychology research. In P. Clarkson (Ed.), *Counseling psychology: Integrating theory, research and supervised practice* (pp. 182–188). London: Routledge.

Huberman, A. M., & Miles, M. B. (1998). Data management and analysis methods. In N. K. Denzin & Y. S. Lincoln (Eds.), *Collecting and interpreting qualitative materials* (pp. 179–210). Thousand Oaks, CA: Sage.

Ironson, G., Solomon, G. F., Balbin, E. G., O'Cleirigh, C., George, A., Kumar, M., et al. (2002). The Ironson-Woods spirituality/religiousness index is associated with long survival, health behaviors, less distress, and low cortisol in people with HIV/AIDS. *Annals of Behavioral Medicine, 24*(1), 34–48.

Jarman, M., Walsh, S., & DeLacey, G. (2005). Keeping safe, keeping connected: A qualitative study of HIV-positive women's experiences of partner relationships. *Psychology & Health, 20*(4), 533–551.

Kalichman, S. C. (2000). Couples with HIV/AIDS. In K. B. Schmaling & T. G. Sher (Eds.), *The psychology of couples and illness: Theory, research, and practice* (pp. 171–189). Washington, DC: American Psychological Association.

McNamera, B., & Rosenwaxa, L. (2010). Which carers of family members at the end of life need more support from health services and why? *Social Science & Medicine, 70*(7), 1035–1041.

Meeker, M. A. (2004). Family surrogate decision making at the end of life: Seeing them through with care and respect. *Qualitative Health Research, 14*(2), 204–225.

Mitchell, C., & Linsk, N. (2004). A multidimensional conceptual framework for understanding HIV/AIDS as a chronic long-term illness. *Social Work, 49*(3), 469–477.

Morrow, S. L. (2007). Qualitative research in counseling psychology: Conceptual foundations. *The Counseling Psychologist, 35*(2), 209–235.

Mosack, K. E., Weinhardt, L. S., Kelly, J. A., Gore-Felton, C., McAuliffe, T. L., Johnson, M. O., et al. (2009). Influence of coping, social support, and depression on subjective health status among HIV-positive adults with different sexual identities. *Behavioral Medicine, 34*(4), 133–144.

Pakenham, K. I., & Rinaldis, M. (2001). The role of illness, resources, appraisal, and coping strategies in adjustment to HIV/AIDS: The direct and buffering effects. *Journal of Behavioral Medicine, 24*(3), 259–279.

Palmer, R., & Bor, R. (2001). The challenges to intimacy and sexual relationships for gay men in HIV sero-discordant relationships: A pilot study. *Journal of Marital & Family Therapy, 7,* 419–431.

Patton, M. Q. (2002). *Qualitative research and evaluation methods* (3rd ed.). Thousand Oaks, CA: Sage.

Perez, J. E., Chartier, M., Koopman, C., Vosvick, M., Gor-Felton, C., & Spiegel, D. (2009). Spiritual striving, acceptance coping, and depressive symptoms among adults living with HIV/AIDS. *Journal of Health Psychology, 14,* 88–97.

Persson, A. (2008). Sero-silence and sero-sharing: Managing HIV in serodiscordant heterosexual relationships. *AIDS Care, 20*(4), 503–506.

Polkinghorne, D. E. (1991). Qualitative procedures for counseling research. In C. E. Watkins, Jr. & L. J. Schneider (Eds.), *Research in counseling* (pp. 163–204). Hillsdale, NJ: Erlbaum.

Pomeroy, E. C., Green, D. L., & VanLaningham, L. (2002). Couples who care: The effectiveness of psychoeducational group intervention for HIV serodiscordant couples. *Social Work Practice, 12*(2), 238–252.

Ponterotto, J. G. (2005). Qualitative research in counseling psychology: A primer on research paradigms and philosophy of science. *Journal of Counseling Psychology, 52*(2), 126–136.

Reinharz, S. (1992). *Feminist methods in social research*. New York: Oxford University Press.

Remien, R. H., Stirratt, M. J., Dolezal, C., Dognin, J. S., Wagner, G. J., Carballo-Dieguez, A., et al. (2005). Couple-focused support to improve HIV medication adherence: A randomized controlled trial. *AIDS, 19*(8), 807–814.

Richards, T., Acree, M., & Folkman, S. (1999). Spiritual aspects of loss among partners of men with AIDS: Post-bereavement follow-up. *Death Studies, 23*(2), 105–127.

Rogers, C. R. (1951). *Client-centered therapy*. Boston: Houghton Mifflin.

Schuster, M. A., Kanouse, D. E., Morton, S. E., Bozzette, S. A., Miu, A., Scott, G. B., et al. (2000). HIV-infected parents and their children in the United States. *American Journal of Public Health, 90*(7), 1074–1081.

Somlai, A. M., & Heckman, T. G. (2000). Correlates of spirituality and well-being in a community sample of people living with HIV disease. *Mental Health, Religion, & Culture, 3*(1), 57–70.

Stajduhar, K. I., & Davies, B. (2005). Variations in and factors influencing family members' decisions for palliative home care. *Palliative Medicine, 19*(1), 21–32.

Stein, J. A., Rotheram-Borus, M. J., & Lester, P. (2007). Impact of parentification on long-term outcomes among children of parents with HIV/AIDS. *Family Process, 46*(3), 317–333.

Stetz, K. M., & Brown, M. A. (2004). Physical and psychosocial health in family caregiving: A comparison of AIDS and cancer caregivers. *Public Health Nursing, 21,* 533–540.

Trainor, A., & Ezer, H. (2000). Rebuilding life: The experience of living with AIDS after facing imminent death. *Qualitative Health Research, 10*(5), 646–660.

Trevino, K. M., Pargament, K. I., Cotton, S., Leonard, A. C., Hahn, J., Caprini-Faigin, C. A., et al. (2010). Religious coping and physiological, psychological, social, and spiritual outcomes in patients with HIV/AIDS: Cross-sectional and longitudinal findings. *AIDS & Behavior, 14*(2), 379–389.

Turner, H. A., Pearlin, L. I., & Mullan, J. T. (1998). Sources and determinants of social support for caregivers of persons with AIDS. *Journal of Health & Social Behavior, 39*(6), 137–151.

Vanable, P. A., Carey, M. P., Blair, D. C., & Littlewood, R. A. (2006). Impact of HIV-related stigma on health behaviors and psychological adjustment among HIV-positive men and women. *AIDS & Behavior, 10*(5), 473–482.

Viney, L. L., Allwood, K., Stillson, L., & Walmsley, R. (1992). Caring for the carers: A note on counseling for the wider impact of AIDS. *Journal of Counseling & Development, 70*(3), 442–444.

Wagner, G. J., Remien, R. H., Carballo-Dieguez, A., & Dolezal, C. (2002). Correlates of adherence to combination antiretroviral therapy among members of HIV-positive mixed status couples. *AIDS Care, 14,* 105–109.

17

Parental Illness, Family Functioning, and Adolescent Well-Being: A Family Ecology Framework to Guide Research

SARA PEDERSEN AND TRACEY A. REVENSON

*P*arental illness is a stressful experience for young people, constituting a potential threat to physical and mental health and normative development. Although it is difficult to obtain statistics, available data suggest that a substantial number of young people, approximately 13 to 14% of adolescents, experience serious parental illness (Centers for Disease Control and Prevention, 2001; Masten, Neeman, & Andenas, 1994). Still, research literature examining the effects of parental illness on the child's development and well-being remains underdeveloped in contrast to the substantial literatures on families adjusting to a child's illness (see, Barakat & Kazak, 1999) and on the relation of stressful life events to child and adolescent pathology (see review by Grant et al., 2003).

Living with a physically ill parent may be especially challenging for adolescents. An adolescent's greater cognitive development enables an understanding of the implications of the illness for oneself and one's family, which may result in greater psychological distress than would be experienced by a younger child. Further, an adolescent's ability to take on additional family responsibilities or roles during parental illness may compromise the normative development of social ties and competencies outside the home. Despite this heightened risk, there are few studies of adolescents' adaptation to serious parental illness.

One explanation for this gap may be the absence of a comprehensive theoretical framework to guide research. This chapter proposes such a framework, as well as a research agenda based on that framework.

We offer a *family ecology framework* that illustrates the interrelationships among parental illness characteristics, family functioning, and adolescent well-being. To provide a foundation for this frame work, the existing research literature in developmental, clinical, and community psychology, and in family medicine were viewed. Because of the dearth of studies on families coping with parental illness, we also turned to theoretical, clinical, and empirical work on families with ill children, particularly research that is grounded in family systems and developmental perspectives. In particular, Kazak's (1989) family systems model of family adaptation in the context of childhood illness guided our thinking (see also Kazak, Simms, & Rourke, 2002). Using the family ecology framework, we describe a set of mediating and moderating pathways through which serious parental illness affects adolescent well-being and family functioning, reviewing the available evidence for each pathway. In the final section, we present guidelines to direct future research on parental illness in adolescence that is consistent with the family ecology framework.

The experiences of childhood and parental illness have many similarities but are not identical. There are critical differences in the coping tasks, role redistribution, and long-term sequelae for families coping with parental versus childhood illness. Thus, we do not review the literature on families coping with a child's illness although we acknowledge the conceptual contribution that research on families who are coping with a child's illness has made to researchers' thinking about the effects of parental illness on adolescent well-being and family functioning.

FAMILY ECOLOGY FRAMEWORK

The proposed family ecology framework finds its underpinnings in general systems theory (e.g.,von Bertalanffy, 1968) and human ecology (e.g., Bronfenbrenner, 1977). Four basic principles underlie the framework: (a) individual behavior can only be understood within its social context; (b) individuals exist within a number of interdependent systems or contexts; (c) the *reciprocal* relationships between individuals and the social systems with which they interact are essential for understanding development and adaptation; and (d) variables beyond the level of individual attributes (i.e., social and cultural variables), particularly those that specify the relations between individuals and systems, must be included in order to understand adaptational processes (Revenson, 1990). The framework is loosely based on stress and coping theories (e.g., Lazarus, 1999; Scheier & Carver, 2003) but does not adhere to them strictly. That is, the concepts of stress, cognitive appraisal, and coping are invoked, but because the framework involves the interplay of the adolescents' and other family members' appraisals and reactions to the illness, it goes beyond the traditional individual-level stress and coping approach (see also Degotardi, Revenson, & Ilowite, 1999; Revenson, 1994, 2003).

The specific pathways by which parental illness is expected to affect adolescent well-being and family functioning are depicted in Figure 17.1. In general, characteristics of the parent's illness, such as type and severity of illness, are hypothesized to affect family functioning and adolescent well-being (distal effects) indirectly through a number of individual- and family-level mediators (proximal effects). More specifically, illness severity is expected to impact appraisals of stigma and threat, physiological stress responses, the distribution of roles and responsibilities within the family, and daily hassles. These processes, in turn, will shape family functioning and adolescent well-being. The individual- and family-level mediators also interact with each other; for example, the nature of the parent's illness may create particular perceptions of stigma, which may affect the adolescent's and the family's life in the form of increased physiological stress responses, which ultimately affect health and well-being. It is also important to note that within this framework, the adolescent's illness appraisals or coping strategies may not be congruent with those of other family members', creating additional stress and family dysfunction.

The mediational, or indirect, pathways in the framework may be affected by a number of contextual or moderator variables that will alter the direction or magnitude of illness effects on the mediating variables. Contextual moderator variables include whether the parent and adolescent are the same gender, the family's attachment style, and cultural norms concerning emotional responses to stress. Table 17.1 presents a more complete list of potential moderator variables. Although we have chosen not to include moderational processes in Figure 17.1, the proposed moderators affect specific and multiple pathways in the Figure 17.1 and are more interlinked than we have depicted graphically. For example, the youth's developmental stage and gender may moderate the path between parental illness severity and family role redistribution (Path c), which is itself a mediator of the relationship

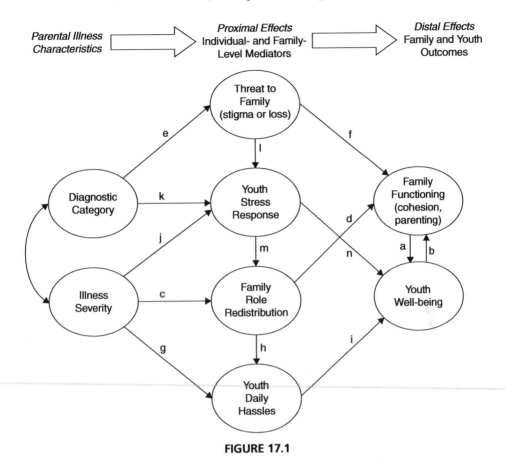

FIGURE 17.1

Mediating pathways within a family ecology
framework for research on parental illness.

between parental illness severity and family functioning (Paths c–d). The mediating and moderated pathways proposed in the framework are not exhaustive but reflect a wide range of intra- and extra familial factors that may elucidate the underlying processes. In the next section we will review studies that have tested the major pathways in the family ecology framework, noting the strength of the evidence, the types of illnesses that have been studied, and whether the evidence is based on child, adolescent, or mixed-aged samples.

**TABLE 17.1 Proposed Moderators of Parental Illness
Effects on Families and Adolescents**

Level of Analysis	Moderator
Individual	Youth developmental stage Parent's age at onset of illness Ill parent's gender Ill parent's family role Individual (youth and parent) coping style Other youth and parent psychological resources
Dyadic and family	Parent-youth gender congruence Marital relationship quality Family coping style Family attachment style
Extrafamilial/societal	Social support Cultural norms Access to care

Note. Not all of the potential moderators listed in Table 17.1 are discussed in detail in the text. We chose to highlight those that have received the least attention in the literature to date.

SUPPORTING EVIDENCE FOR THE FAMILY ECOLOGY FRAMEWORK: STUDIES OF THE EFFECT OF PARENT ILLNESS ON YOUTH DEVELOPMENT AND FAMILY FUNCTIONING

Scope and Organization of the Evidence

In this section, we review those studies that provide support for the major pathways in the family ecology framework. We started with four existing literature reviews of how parental illness impacts family functioning and adolescent well-being (Armistead, Klein, & Forehand, 1995; Finney & Miller, 1999; Korneluk & Lee, 1998; Worsham, Compas, & Ey, 1997) and the studies that composed those reviews. We then turned to *PsycINFO*, the psychology database, to search for published, peer-reviewed literature using the following terms and combinations of these terms: *parental illness, maternal illness, paternal illness, chronic, physical, disease, family functioning, adolescent functioning*, and *adolescent well-being*. We also searched using the specific illness terms *cancer, HIV, AIDS, diabetes, heart disease*, and *spinal cord injury*.[1] We then checked the references of the sources identified using this search procedure for any relevant keywords. Publications containing the keywords in their titles were also retrieved.

Although we drew on the literature examining family and parental reactions to a child's illness in building the theoretical framework, we excluded these studies from the current literature review. We also excluded studies that sampled only parents with a mental illness or an acute illness with no long-term health implications. Although we targeted empirical articles for review, we also retrieved theoretical articles, literature reviews, and clinical reports. In addition, because research that specifically addresses the effects of parental illness effects on families with adolescents was limited, we included studies of parental illness in families with young children when they addressed an underresearched area.

In the following section, we describe the ways in which the central construct of interest—parental illness—has been conceptualized. We then review the literature that examines direct effects of parental illness on two outcomes: family functioning and adolescent well-being. Although the family ecology framework is explicitly transactional (i.e., it assumes that family functioning and youth development are mutually influential), the effects of parental illness on family functioning and on adolescent well-being are considered separately in an effort to highlight the state of the research on each pathway within the proposed model. The final part of the section reviews evidence for the mediating and moderated pathways in the family ecology framework.

Defining and Measuring Parental Illness

For the most part, researchers have relied on two dimensions to characterize parental illness: type of illness (diagnosis) and severity (Patterson & Garwick, 1994; Rolland, 1999).[2]

---

[1] These illnesses and conditions were chosen because the Centers for Disease Control (Kochanek & Smith, 2004) has identified them as 5 of the 10 most common causes of death for adults in the age ranges during which they are most likely to raise children (25–44 years and 45–65 years). Unlike other common causes of death, such as accidents, homicide, and suicide, the illnesses that we selected are associated with chronic disability and may impair one's ability to maintain daily routines. Spinal cord injury was added to the list in an effort to adjust for any gender bias in the targeted illnesses, which mostly affect women. This bias remains in the literature and the current review, however, as very few articles have addressed familial adjustment to parental heart disease or spinal cord injury—conditions that are more likely to affect men.

[2] On the basis of earlier work by Rolland (1984), Kazak (1989) proposed that an analogous set of illness characteristics—onset, course, and outcome—affect family adaptation in the context of childhood illness.

Contrasting the experiences of families in which the ill parents have different diagnoses suggests that one illness impacts family life more negatively or in a different way than another, regardless of cross-cutting dimensions such as prognosis or level of disability. The dimensions of diagnosis and severity are not orthogonal, however; some diagnoses may be less stigmatizing or threatening in part because these illnesses are associated with less disability than other illnesses, for example, diabetes compared with AIDS.

Studies that operationalize parental illness as diagnosis and those that operationalize illness as severity require different sets of assumptions about the causal mechanisms linking parental illness to adjustment. For example, a cancer diagnosis generally carries more life threat than diabetes, although many forms of cancer are less life threatening because of advances in treatment and detection. Thus, most youth coping with a parent's cancer are coping with the issue of parental loss to some degree and in a qualitatively different fashion than youth coping with a parent's diabetes or arthritis. Moreover, no diagnosis is monolithic; for example, different types or stages of cancer pose different degrees of life threat, so even the label "cancer" tells little about potential parental loss. Unless the adaptive tasks of particular diagnoses are spelled out (Moos & Schaefer, 1984), using diagnosis as a marker of stress is limited.

Conceptualizing parental illness by its severity, rather than diagnostic type, implies a different mediating mechanism, one that involves familial role redistribution (Reiss, Steinglass, & Howe, 1993). Irrespective of diagnosis, more severe illnesses have a greater impact on the parent's ability to fulfill familial roles and responsibilities, placing greater demands on family members. For example, a mother diagnosed with breast cancer at an advanced stage may not only experience more debilitating symptoms of illness but also undergo more frequent treatments over a longer period of time—interfering to a greater degree with parenting tasks and thus affecting the child's well-being—than a mother diagnosed with early-stage breast cancer.

One particularly important aspect of severity is onset, or the rapidity with which the illness symptoms develop. The adaptive tasks demanded of a family facing a parental illness with a sudden and traumatic onset, such as spinal cord injury resulting from an accident, may be different from those faced by a family in which a parent is diagnosed with an illness that also results in physical debilitation but develops gradually over a long period of time, such as Parkinson's disease. To complicate matters, many of the chronic illnesses addressed in the literature that we used to build our framework, such as breast cancer and HIV/AIDS, have both gradual and rapid aspects to their onset. For example, a mother may experience symptoms such as exhaustion and frequent infections that lead her to request an HIV test. A positive result on the test may result in a rapid change in the life of the mother and her family as they cope with the diagnosis and a complex regimen of medications and doctor visits. The progression of the illness symptoms in this case is gradual, but the diagnosis and the treatment-related life changes that ensue are rapid and traumatic.

Empirical work rarely contrasts these different illness dimensions. Perhaps because of convenience, most study a single parental illness in an effort to establish the association between illness severity and adjustment (e.g., Armistead, Tannenbaum, Forehand, Morse, & Morse, 2001; Compas et al., 1994; Compas, Worsham, Ey, & Howell, 1996; Dutra et al., 2000; Ell, Nishimoto, Mantell, & Hamovitch, 1988; Grant & Compas, 1995; Lewis, Hammond, & Woods, 1993; Murphy, Steers, & Dello Stritto, 2001; Rotheram-Borus & Stein, 1999; Steele, Forehand, & Armistead, 1997). Only a few studies have compared family functioning across different illnesses (e.g., Dura & Beck, 1988; Lewis, Woods, Hough, & Bensley, 1989; Stetz, Lewis, & Primomo, 1986; Yates, Bensley, Lalonde, Lewis, & Woods, 1995), compared physical versus mental illnesses (e.g., Anderson & Hammen, 1993; Hirsch, Moos, & Reischl, 1985;

Johnson & Lobo, 2001; Mikail & von Baeyer, 1990; Pelton, Steele, Chance, Forehand, & the Family Health Project Research Group, 2001; Peters & Esses, 1985), or compared families with illness to families without known illness (e.g., Harris & Zakowski, 2003; Kotchick et al., 1997).

Association Between Parental Illness and Family Functioning

In the family systems literature, families characterized as well-functioning are described as cohesive, flexible, and self-reflective (Walsh, 2003). Markers of positive family functioning during parental illness include high levels of communication, a family identity that is not defined by the illness, and the ability to redistribute family roles in ways that do not compromise the development of individual members (Patterson & Garwick, 1994; Reiss et al., 1993; Rolland, 1999). In contrast, poorly adapting families have been characterized as those that use extensive family reorganization as a coping response. Reorganization is defined as the extent to which the intrafamilial transactions are altered to meet the needs of the sick individual. Although short-term reorganization during acute illness or a crisis phase of a chronic illness is adaptive, maintaining a family structure, organization, and identity that revolve around the ill parent for an extended length of time compromises the family's ability to meet the developmental needs of other members, especially children (Reiss et al., 1993). Reiss et al. (1993) provided support for this in a case study of one family's response to the father's end-stage renal disease, where reorganization contributed to increased psychological distress in each family member.

Few empirical studies of parental illness, however, have assessed reorganization directly. One cross-sectional study that compared family organization among impoverished families in which the mother was HIV− to impoverished families in which the mother was HIV+ revealed no association between maternal HIV serostatus and the extent to which family routines were consistent and organized (Kotchick et al., 1997).

A greater number of studies have assessed aspects of family functioning, such as cohesion and conflict. In a series of interrelated studies of the families of women with either breast cancer, fibrocystic breast disease, or diabetes, family functioning was measured using self-report scales assessing family adaptability, cohesion, and/or the family's satisfaction with the quality of the family's interactions (Lewis et al., 1989, 1993; Yates et al., 1995). These measures of family functioning were modestly related to illness severity, with some families at risk for low cohesion and increased conflict when the illness was more severe. In a study that used only the subsample of families with maternal breast cancer, Lewis et al. (1989) found a negative correlation between illness severity (operationalized as frequency of illness demands on the family) and spousal reports of family functioning. However, this significant finding was not replicated when the women's reports of functioning were substituted for their husbands' reports (Lewis et al., 1993). In addition, women's reports of family functioning did not differ among the three diagnoses (breast cancer, fibrocystic breast disease, and diabetes; Yates et al., 1995).

Two additional studies suggest that more severe illnesses are associated with poorer family functioning. In a study of parents with chronic headaches, parental perceptions of the extent to which the illness interfered with daily life were inversely associated with perceptions of family cohesiveness, and perceptions of pain severity were inversely associated with family organization (Mikail & von Baeyer, 1990). Dura and Beck (1988) found that families with maternal diabetes or chronic pain reported lower cohesiveness than families with no illness although only families in which the mothers had chronic pain reported greater conflict than the families without illness. The authors suggest that these findings are best explained not by diagnosis, however, but by levels of disability. Mothers with chronic pain reported the most disability—particularly in the area of family and home responsibilities—followed by mothers with diabetes, and mothers with no illness reported the least disability.

Not all studies, however, have identified a negative relation between illness severity and family functioning. Kotchick et al.'s (1997) study of HIV+ mothers and their children found that disease severity was unrelated to either parent-child relationship quality or parental monitoring, although mothers who were HIV+ tended to score lower than mothers who were HIV– on these measures of parenting. It should be noted, however, that the socioeconomic conditions under which the impoverished, inner-city participants in this study lived are substantially different from samples in many of the other studies were viewed, which may have limited the variance in the variable tapping the organization of family routines. In sum, although how parental illness is conceptualized (diagnosis vs. severity), who is reporting on the quality of family functioning, and other unstudied dimensions (e.g., level of disability) are critical constructs in understanding the effects of parental illness on family well-being, the nature and extent of the impact of parental illness on family functioning remains undetermined.

Association Between Parental Illness and Adolescent Well-Being

Some scholars have suggested that parental illness exerts devastating effects on the behavioral and psychosocial well-being of adolescents (Hollingsworth, 1982; Patenaude, 2000). Yet only a relatively small number of empirical studies have considered the unique challenges posed by parental illness to families with adolescents. We examine three domains of youth well-being that have been addressed in the empirical literature: psychological distress, problem behaviors, and positive well-being.[3]

Psychological Distress

Contrary to Hollingsworth's (1982) expectations that adolescents' advanced cognitive development would protect them from psychological distress during parental illness, the empirical evidence suggests that adolescents are at *greater* risk than young children (Armistead et al., 1995; Worsham et al., 1997). A substantial proportion of adolescents with HIV+ mothers have been observed to exhibit high levels of depression (Gardner & Preator, 1996). In several studies, illness severity has been associated with internalizing symptoms among youth whose fathers had hemophilia or both hemophilia and HIV/AIDS (Steele et al., 1997), urban adolescents whose parent (usually the mother) was diagnosed with AIDS (Rotheram-Borus & Stein, 1999), and middle childhood youth whose mothers were HIV+ (Hough, Brumitt, Templin, Saltz, & Mood, 2003). Illness severity also was related to externalizing symptoms of psychological distress in the Hough et al. (2003) study. Another study of parent-adolescent pairs in which the parent was HIV+ found that parental distress associated with illness-related pain positively predicted adolescent reports of somatic symptoms (Lester, Stein, & Bursch, 2003). Finally, one study of the children (ages 9–17) of chronic headache sufferers found that these young people experienced more symptoms of anxiety and depression than a comparison sample of adolescents with no parental illness (Mikail & von Baeyer, 1990).

Adolescent children of parents with cancer—particularly girls whose mothers are ill—may also be at greater risk for anxiety and depression than younger children (Compas et al., 1994, 1996; Grant & Compas, 1995). In the series of studies by Compas and colleagues, the

---

[3]This chapter provides evidence for unidirectional effects of parental illness on adolescent and family functioning. It is equally important, however, to test the competing hypothesis that families with members susceptible to physical illness are also families with members susceptible to psychological dysfunction over the course of that illness.

severity of the parent's illness was associated with a heightened stress response (character-ized by intrusive thoughts, anxiety, and depression) among adolescents. Another group of researchers examining the psychological symptoms (including anxiety and depression) of adult daughters of women with breast cancer failed to find a significant difference between these daughters and a matched sample with no maternal history of breast cancer. However, daughters of women with breast cancer were more likely to feel uncomfortable about their involvement with the mother's illness *if* the illness had occurred during childhood or ado-lescence (Wellisch, Gritz, Schain, Wang, & Siau, 1991, 1992). Harris and Zakowski (2003), however, found no evidence of risk among adolescents experiencing parental cancer. In this study of 50 youth, adolescents experiencing parental cancer reported lower anxiety and fewer PTSD symptoms than a comparison group of adolescents with no history of parental cancer.

Problem Behavior

The effect of parental illness on conduct problems, drug use, and other risk-taking behaviors has rarely been addressed, and the existing literature is equivocal. Patenaude (2000) sug-gested that children of parents with cancer would react by acting out. In contrast, Christ, Siegel, and Sperber (1994) argued that acting out occurs only if the adolescent exhibited problem behaviors prior to the illness. Gardner and Preator (1996) similarly concluded that increased conduct problems among children of parents with HIV/AIDS stems from the accumulation of risk factors associated with the illness rather than the illness per se. For example, young people experiencing maternal HIV/AIDS may be at risk for dysfunction because of the cumulative impact of other stressors, such as poverty. Women diagnosed as HIV+ and their families tend to live in economically disadvantaged circumstances, exacer-bating illness-related stress on the family and, potentially, the economic ramifications of parental loss (Gardner & Preator, 1996).

In the empirical literature, one study of mothers with HIV found that HIV-related stres-sors on the mother (e.g., HIV-related physical symptoms, opportunistic infections, and CD4 counts) were directly related to child behavior problems among youth aged 7 to 14 (Hough et al., 2003). In contrast, in another study of maternal HIV/AIDS, Rotheram-Borus and Stein (1999) did not find an association between maternal health status and adolescent problem behaviors, such as drug use, sexual risk, and conduct problems. Maternal risk behaviors and substance use were associated with youth problem behaviors, suggesting that adolescents with ill parents may exhibit greater risk behaviors than youth whose parents are not ill only to the extent that parental illness co-occurs with parental risk behaviors. Thus, youth risk behaviors are not a direct outcome of parental illness, but they result from the modeling of parental risk behaviors. In contrast, studies on younger children find that parental illness is associated with problem behaviors. Armistead et al. (2001) observed a significant cor-relation between illness severity and aggressive behavior in children aged 6 to 11 whose mothers were HIV+. A more in-depth analysis of 15 mothers in this sample found that mothers perceived increased behavior problems following disclosure of their HIV status to their children (Shaffer, Jones, Kotchick, Forehand, & the Family Health Research Project Research Group, 2001).

Positive Well-Being

Four studies identified differences in self-esteem (one aspect of positive well-being) between children and adolescents facing parental illness and children and adolescents who were not experiencing parental illness. Hirsch et al. (1985) conducted a study of ado-lescents whose parents were diagnosed with either physical illness (arthritis) or mental illness (depression) and compared them with adolescents of parents with no known health disorder. Adolescents with an arthritic or depressed parent reported lower self-esteem than comparison youth. Armsden and Lewis (1994) similarly found that, among youth in middle childhood, those experiencing maternal breast cancer and diabetes reported lower self-esteem than a comparison sample with no known parental illness. One study on children of parents with coronary heart disease found that boys, but not girls, of parents with coronary heart disease reported lower self-esteem than a matched comparison sample (Räikkönen, Keltikangas-Järvinen, & Pietikäinen, 1991). Finally, Siegel, Raveis, and Karus (2000) found that the self-esteem of young people experiencing parental cancer (40% of whom were adolescents) tended to be lower than that which is found in surveys with normative samples of youth.

Other aspects of positive well-being are rarely addressed in the parental illness literature. In particular, personal growth associated with the parental illness experience has not been studied, despite empirical support for the hypothesis that many young people report psychosocial benefits following a traumatic experience (e.g., Milam, Ritt-Olson, & Unger, 2004). Milam et al. (2004) also identified individual differences in the extent to which the adolescents in their cross-sectional study reported that they had experienced growth following a negative life event. For example, older adolescents endorsed the growth measure more highly than younger adolescents. In contrast, substance use was negatively associated with scores on the post-traumatic growth scale. These findings suggest that not only young people can use a negative event to enhance their skills or psychological resources but also individual and contextual characteristics may influence the degree to which adolescents capitalize on the opportunity for growth through the challenge of parental illness.

It should be noted that we had hoped to find evidence to support the hypothesis that some young people would find the parental illness experience to be a challenge that leads to personal growth. The small empirical literature in this area, however, focuses almost exclusively on negative outcomes associated with parental illness. Thus, we were unable to include studies that examined competence development or positive growth in our review. We hope that such outcomes will be addressed in future empirical research with families living with parental illness.

Summary

The literature provides support for the hypothesis that parental illness negatively impacts some aspects of adolescent well-being. Adolescent children of ill parents are at greater risk for anxiety, depression, and low self-esteem (Compas et al., 1994; Hirsch et al., 1985; Siegel et al., 2000). Parental illness may also lead to increased problem behaviors among youth evidencing such behaviors before diagnosis (Christ et al., 1994). Empirical research in this area, however, is limited and often does not address conflicting hypotheses reported in theoretical and clinical research. For example, Christ et al. (1994), Gardner and Preator (1996), and Patenaude (2000) disagree regarding the extent to which adolescents are at risk for problem behaviors during parental illness. Only one empirical study, however, examined problem behaviors among adolescents with ill mothers (e.g., Rotheram-Borus & Stein, 1999), and although the findings support Gardner and Preator's (1996) observations, the extent to which these results generalize to other populations of youth experiencing parental illness is unknown. The literature also rarely examines how adolescents may view parental illness as a challenge from which they may learn more about themselves and their skills and abilities. Finally, few studies take into account moderating variables—such as cognitive development, gender, and age of onset of parental illness—that may buffer or exacerbate illness effects on adolescent outcomes.

MEDIATING MECHANISMS

In the following section, we propose a series of mediating mechanisms to account for the observed associations among parental illness, family functioning, and adolescent well-being. In particular, we focus on mediating pathways that can be incorporated into interventions. These mediators are the alphabetically labeled paths in Figure 17.1. Mediators of illness effects on family functioning include familial role redistribution and threat to the family's identity through stigma and potential loss. Mediators of illness effects on youth well-being include daily hassles and the stress response. Family functioning and adolescent well-being are also assumed to be mutually influential, although these pathways are not described explicitly below (see Paths a and b in Figure 17.1).

Mediators of Illness Effects on Family Functioning
Role Redistribution

Stetz et al. (1986) observed that role redistribution was the most common coping mechanism used by families experiencing parental illness. If an ill parent is incapable of fulfilling the roles that he or she previously filled, other family members may be required to adopt those roles (see Path c). Whether or not roles are reassigned fairly (with clear communication and with concern for well family members' developmental needs) may affect family functioning (see Path d; Patterson & Garwick, 1994; Rolland, 1999).

For example, one parent in a family may be responsible for picking the children up from after-school activities. If that parent develops a movement disorder or if medications and other treatments affect the parent's cognitive and perceptual functioning, that parent may no longer be able to operate a car safely, interfering with this role. The family may utilize a number of behavioral strategies to cope with this role limitation. In the case of a two-parent family, the well parent may adjust his or her schedule to accommodate the children's transportation needs. Arrangements may be made for another adult to bring the children home, an older sibling may become responsible for bringing the children home, or the children may stop engaging in after-school activities in order to take the school bus home. None of these solutions automatically results in family dysfunction. Some teens may be happy to assist, gaining new responsibilities and respect. Familial relationships may be adversely affected, however, when one or more family members feel overly or unfairly burdened by the family's response to the illness.

The role redistribution mediational hypothesis is supported by a few empirical studies. In one study of HIV+ mothers, maintaining stable family routines was associated with better parent-child relationship quality (Dutra et al., 2000). Lewis et al. (1989), in one study of maternal breast cancer, also implicitly assessed a role redistribution hypothesis. The family's use of introspective coping mediated the association between illness demands and family functioning although the statistical significance of the indirect effect was not reported. This finding could imply that families that use more introspective coping techniques are more successful in readjusting to the demands of the parent's illness without compromising the development of well family members; however, our ability to interpret this finding is limited because the relations among illness demands, introspective coping, and family reorganization have not been tested in other studies.

Threat to the Family's Identity

Weihs and Reiss (2000) suggested that illness in a family member threatens the "life course of the family" (p. 19). The family's relational processes are shaped by the extent to which that system is threatened by the potential loss of the ill family member. If the family views the illness as a serious threat to the ill member's life (see Path e), family functioning may be affected such that the patterns of transactions among family members will become reorganized around the illness (see Path f). In this way, illness may compromise the normative identity development and transactional processes of the family system (Reiss et al., 1993). Illnesses that are stigmatized may also threaten the family's belief systems—the shared conceptions of the qualities that define the family's identity (see Path e; Reiss et al., 1993)—and, in turn, family functioning.

No empirical studies have examined changes in family identity brought about by parental illness, nor have investigators elucidated how such changes relate to family functioning. More specifically, no empirical studies have examined the stigma or level of life threat associated with an illness as a mediator of the association between illness and family functioning.

Mediators of Illness Effects on Youth Well-Being
Daily Hassles

Parental illness may impact youth well-being by creating a surplus of daily hassles experienced by the adolescent. Daily hassles are "stresses and strains of daily life" (Rowlison & Felner, 1988, p. 433; DeLongis, Folkman, & Lazarus, 1988) and have been associated with depression, anxiety, antisocial behavior, and academic achievement (DuBois, Felner, Meares, & Krier, 1994; Masten et al., 1994; Rowlison & Felner, 1988). To the extent that parental illness increases the difficulties associated with daily life (e.g., increased chores, nagging from parents), greater dysfunction among youth with ill parents should be observed.

We hypothesize that daily hassles mediate the effects of parental illness on youth well-being and that this individual-level pathway is related to the family-level process of role redistribution in the context of parental illness (Patterson & Garwick, 1994; Rolland, 1999). Illness demands may lead directly to increased hassles when youth are asked to adopt new roles associated with the illness, such as accompanying the ill parent to medical appointments (see Path g). Alternately, the redistribution of existing family roles, such as household responsibilities, may lead to greater daily hassles for adolescents (see Path h). These new or increased familial responsibilities may then affect adolescent well-being by interfering with the development of peer relationships and attachment to important others outside the family system (see Path i; Compas et al., 1994; Feeney & Ryan, 1994; Rolland, 1999; Weihs & Reiss, 2000). Indeed, Lewis et al. (1989) observed that husbands' perceptions of maternal illness demands on the family were inversely associated with the quality of the child's peer relationships.

Grant and Compas (1995) most explicitly addressed the issue of perceived hassles by asking adolescents with ill parents to report the stressors associated with their family responsibilities. An earlier publication with the same sample found that girls with ill mothers reported greater anxiety and depression than girls with ill fathers and boys with ill mothers or fathers (Compas et al., 1994). Later analyses indicated that greater family responsibilities fully accounted for this interaction (Grant & Compas, 1995), suggesting that adolescent girls bear the burden of role restructuring in families experiencing illness.

Stress Response

The stress response pathway suggests that parental illness contributes to youth maladjustment to the degree that parental illness represents, and is appraised as, a discrete, negative, and uncontrollable life event (Compas, 1987; Masten et al., 1994). Appraisals of the event's stressfulness create feelings of threat and helplessness and even decreased immune function (McEwen, 1998). In other words, the mediating process driving the association between parental illness and youth well-being is cognitive–emotional. Perceived stress among the adolescent children of ill parents may arise because of worry about parental death associated with a very severe illness (see Path j), worry about the child's own risk of illness, and death if the parent's illness is associated with genetic susceptibility (see Path k), or the family-level perceived stigma associated with particular diagnoses (see Path l). Finally, perceived stress may result from illness demands associated with familial role redistribution that the adolescent perceives as adversely affecting his or her peer, school, and family relationships (see Path m; Compas et al., 1994). The extent to which the adolescent appraises the parent's illness as stressful determines his or her response to the illness (see Path n; Contrada & Guyll, 2000), including emotions, coping behaviors, or both.

Few studies have tested the perceived stress hypothesis in the context of parental illness. In a study on children of cancer patients, Compas et al. (1994) found that perceived stress attributed to the parent's illness predicted adolescents' anxiety, depression, and stress-response symptoms. In contrast, studies examining disclosure effects on children's well-being in families with maternal HIV/AIDS—which could constitute an approximate measure of perceived threat or stigma associated with diagnosis—have not found differences between children who know about their mothers' health status and those who do not (e.g., Armistead et al., 2001; Murphy et al., 2001) although one study found that mothers perceived increased child behavior problems and decreased parent-child relationship quality following disclosure (Shaffer et al., 2001). Similarly, in a study of families in which the father had hemophilia and was HIV+, although bivariate analyses revealed that disclosure of the father's HIV+ status was related to lower grades and greater depression among the children in the sample, no association between disclosure and child well-being was observed after adjusting for parent-child relationship quality (Armistead, Klein, Forehand, & Wierson, 1997).

The children in these studies of adjustment to parental HIV, however, tended to be in middle childhood, rather than adolescence, raising the possibility that cognitive development may moderate the association between parental illness and perceived stress. Alternately, the children in the disclosure and nondisclosure samples may have appeared similar on the outcomes studied because the youth nondisclosure samples were aware of the parent's diagnosis—or, at least, that the parent was seriously ill—without having been told and subsequently experienced levels of threat and stress similar to that of youth in the disclosure samples.

Parenting

Parental illness may also affect youth well-being through its impact on family functioning. One aspect of family functioning that has received attention in the empirical literature is parenting. Illness may affect parenting in two ways. First, as a chronic illness becomes more serious, the illness may impact the parent's ability to fulfill his or her usual role responsibilities (see Path c). The subsequent redistribution of family roles may affect the family's functioning as a whole and, specifically, the parent's relationship with the child (see Path d). Second, a particular diagnosis may lead the parent to experience perceived stigma and threat (see Path e). The distress associated with this experience may also interfere with parenting.

Kotchick et al. (1997) suggested that illness may affect aspects of the parent–child relationship, such as the quality of that relationship, and the extent to which the parent monitors the child's behaviors. Indeed, in their study, poor, urban HIV+ mothers rated themselves lower on indices of positive parenting, including mother–child relationship quality and monitoring, than a comparison sample of poor, urban mothers who had not been diagnosed as HIV+. Reyland, McMahon, Higgins-Delessandro, and Luthar (2002) similarly found that inner-city adolescents (ages 11–16) living with an HIV+ mother experienced less positive mother–child relationships (e.g., more hostility and indifference from the mother) than a comparison sample from the same community. Although mediation analyses assessing the significance of the indirect effect of HIV serostatus on youth outcomes were not conducted in these studies, other analyses using the same sample of children and mothers, as in the Kotchik et al. (1997) study, found that the children of HIV+ mothers had more externalizing and internalizing symptoms and lower social and cognitive competence than children from the comparison sample (Forehand et al., 1998).

Summary

The theoretical literature suggests that daily hassles and perceived stress mediate the effects of parental illness effects on adolescent well-being, but very few empirical studies have tested mediators of parental illness effects on family functioning. Studies that examine perceived stress as a mediator yield mixed results, suggesting that this pathway is conditional on other variables, such as cognitive development. Finally, there is some evidence to suggest that parental illness impacts youth adjustment through aspects of family functioning, such as parenting.

Contextual Moderating Factors

Are the associations among parental illness characteristics, family functioning, and youth well-being the same or different across populations and contexts? Developmental theorists have emphasized the importance of developing models that incorporate factors that could alter the nature of the associations among the variables studied (Rutter, 1990). Identifying intra- and extrafamilial factors that color the family's experience of a parent's illness is a crucial step in the development of a framework to guide research. In this section, a number of potential family- and individual-level moderators of the relations among parental illness, family functioning, and youth well-being are proposed, and empirical evidence for these moderators is presented.

Developmental Stage

The developmental stage at which a young person experiences parental illness represents a critical yet understudied moderator of the association between illness and youth well-being. Older children may experience greater threat of loss because they are more knowledgeable about the potential consequences of disease and more capable of conceptualizing death. Further, older children are more capable of adopting additional household responsibilities. Such responsibilities may prohibit involvement in extrafamilial contexts that promote positive development and in which youth become more interested as they age, such as their peer group (Berndt, 1996).

Alternately, older children may adapt to the illness experience more easily because of greater cognitive resources and prior exposure to stressors. They may also accomplish tasks that require a high level of responsibility with more ease and less stress than younger children would experience when confronted with the same task. Thus, older children may find additional familial responsibilities associated with parental illness to be a challenge that promotes positive growth, rather than an impediment to the development of peer ties. Indeed, Milam et al. (2004) found that age was associated with positive growth following a negative life event in a large sample of Latino adolescents. Older adolescents were more likely than younger adolescents to identify benefits associated with their traumatic experience. One potential explanation for this finding is that older youth are more equipped by their maturity, social development, and cognitive development to view negative experiences as opportunities for personal growth.

Only the studies on children of cancer patients by Compas and his associates (e.g., Compas et al., 1994, 1996; Grant & Compas, 1995) bring developmental stage into the equation. Their findings suggest that adolescent and young adult children of people with cancer exhibit greater anxiety and depression than preadolescent children. These associations are further moderated by other variables, such as gender.

Ill Parent's Gender or Family Role

The ill parent's gender has seldom been studied as a moderator. Most studies sample ill parents of only one gender—usually mothers (e.g., Dura & Beck, 1988; Lewis et al., 1989, 1993; Yates et al., 1995). One study of cancer patients and their spouses (Compas et al., 1994) revealed that the perceived seriousness of the illness varied by the adult's gender and status as patient versus (healthy) spouse. Women perceived the cancer as more stressful than men, as did spouses (vs. patients). A study of coronary heart disease patients and their spouses also found that women were more distressed than men and that this gender difference was more pronounced among spouses than patients (Rohrbaugh et al., 2002). In other studies, wives of rheumatic disease patients were more likely to bear the burden of familial role redistribution than ill women, ill men, or husbands of patients (Revenson, 1994, 2003).

Of course, family role rather than—or in addition to—gender per se is likely a strong contributing factor to any differences in family or youth adjustment to parental illness. In a more traditional two-parent family in which the mother has assumed most of the caretaking responsibilities and the father is primarily responsible for the family's income, maternal illness may necessitate the father and children assuming more childcare and housekeeping roles. Paternal illness may result in other family members seeking out new employment situations to maintain the family's economic solvency. For families in which both parents are of the same gender, the effect of the illness on the family and child would likely depend more on the family roles adopted by the ill parent than on the parents' gender. In a single-parent family, parental illness could require reassignment of both caretaking and breadwinner roles within the family.

Parent and Youth Gender Congruence

The congruence between the gender of the ill parent and that of the child may moderate the association between parental illness and youth well-being. When the ill parent is the same gender as the child, the child would be more likely to assume some of the parent's roles; for example, daughters of ill mothers might be more likely than sons to take on housekeeping chores (Compas et al., 1994). Only studies by Compas and his colleagues address this explicitly. Compas et al. (1994) found support for the hypothesis that the gender of the sick parent and his or her child interacts to predict child well-being: Adolescent girls reported greater anxiety and depression than adolescent boys, and this finding was most robust among girls with sick mothers. This finding was accounted for by the increased household responsibilities adopted by girls experiencing maternal illness (Grant & Compas, 1995).

It is also possible that poorer adjustment by same-sex dyads is colored by perceived risk. Some illnesses—for example, certain types of breast cancer—may be partially determined by genetic factors such that same-sex children are more likely to develop the illness themselves. Research on healthy adult women's breast-cancer-related distress indicates that a maternal history of breast cancer puts a woman at risk for heightened breast-cancer-related distress, particularly, if she cared for her mother during the illness and if her mother died of the illness (Erblich, Bovbjerg, & Valdimarsdottir, 2000).

Family Coping Style

Coping has rarely been conceptualized at a family level. Instead, this construct has most often been viewed as reflective of an internal cognitive–emotional process of decision-making that culminates in behavior designed to ameliorate the perceived stress associated with a particular situation or experience (Lazarus, 1999). Only recently has coping been conceptualized and studied as an interpersonal or dyadic process (e.g., Bodenmann, 1997; Lyons, Mickelson, Sullivan, & Coyne, 1998; Revenson, 1994, 2003; Revenson, Kayser, & Bodenmann, 2005; Schmaling & Sher, 2000). When family-level coping is examined in the context of illness, researchers most often study families with an ill child rather than an ill parent (e.g., Degotardi, 2000; Hauser, DiPlacido, Jacobson, Willett, & Cole, 1993).

No studies could be found that explicitly examined individual- or family-level coping as a moderator of the association between parental illness and family functioning. The results of one study on families with adolescents experiencing juvenile rheumatoid arthritis, however, support the hypothesis that family coping moderates illness effects on family functioning and youth well-being (Degotardi, 2000). Still, if parental illness leads to a redistribution of roles in the family (affecting the balance of relationships established among family members), family coping style may determine the extent to which adolescents are the recipients of "unfair" redistributions that leave them feeling overburdened or resentful. Open dialogue about the illness also may make families less likely to view the illness as a threat to the family's development.

Intervention research suggests that coping plays an important role in determining youth adjustment during parental illness. An evaluation of a 24-session cognitive–behavioral intervention targeting the coping skills of parents living with HIV/AIDS and their adolescent children found both short-term and long-term benefits associated with participation in the intervention. The intervention was successful at reducing youth rates of childbearing over 4 years and resulted in short-term reductions in youth problem behaviors and emotional distress, relative to a randomized control group (Rotheram-Borus, Lee, Gwadz, & Draimin, 2001; Rotheram-Borus et al., 2003).

Family Attachment Styles

Weihs and Reiss (2000) suggested that fear of separation from the ill parent depends on the quality of the attachment relationships in the family. Families may exhibit secure or insecure styles of attachment in their relationships (Ainsworth, 1979) just as individuals. Attachment at the family level is defined as the holistic pattern of attachment exhibited within the intrafamilial relationships over time (Weihs & Reiss, 2000). Families may be securely attached or may exhibit ambivalent, avoidant, or disorganized patterns of attachment among members. To date, the empirical literature has not examined family-level attachment styles in studies of parental illness experiences.

Social Support

Support from both within and outside of the family system may moderate the mediational processes described in Figure 17.1. A wealth of research over the past 2 decades has demonstrated that the quality of interpersonal relationships is a strong predictor of adjustment to illness among adult populations (Sarason, Sarason, & Gurung, 2001; Schmaling & Sher, 2000; Stanton & Revenson, in press; Wills & Fegan, 2001). Most of the coping tasks of illness require help from others. Thus, people faced with a serious illness need an available network of interpersonal relations on which they can count for both emotional sustenance and practical help during periods of pain, disability, and uncertainty. Children of ill parents serve on this frontline. In essence, then, they occupy a dual role in the adjustment process: as a primary provider of emotional and instrumental support to the ill parent and as a family member who needs additional support in the face of a major and often long-lasting life stressor.

Support received by the adolescent may come from many sources, including the ill parent, other family members, peers, teachers, religious mentors, and other adolescents in a similar situation. Such support may involve demonstrations that the adolescent is loved, valued, and cared for, as well as the provision of helpful information or tangible assistance. Receiving support should enable adolescents to use effective coping strategies by helping them come to a better understanding of the problem faced, increasing motivation to take instrumental action, and reducing emotional stress, which may impede coping.

As described earlier, many adolescents take over parental responsibilities, particularly during acute or early phases of illness, reducing the amount of time adolescents spend socializing with their own peer networks, one potential source of support. Further, even long-standing peers may not understand the challenges the adolescent faces. Support groups or Internet chat groups can be helpful at these times. Discussing stressful events in a supportive, uncritical social environment allows people to process emotions, maintain or reestablish a positive self-concept, and find meaning (Lepore, 2001). Disclosure of stressful experiences may regulate emotion by changing the focus of attention, increasing habituation to negative emotions, or facilitating positive cognitive reappraisals of threats (for adolescents facing parental illness with a genetic component, the threat associated with the fear of developing the same illness as the parent). Recent research, however, suggests that support groups are not uniformly effective (e.g., Helgeson, Cohen, Schulz, & Yasko, 2000).

Within a family ecology framework, it is important to remember that adolescents living with parental illness occupy many social roles in addition to family member and parent caregiver—they are friends, students, athletes, and community members. Especially, when there is a great amount of role restructuring in the family, role conflict is likely to occur, and the amount of support the child is able to provide to either the ill parent or to the healthy spouse, who may be falling apart, may be limited by the need to perform well or derive satisfaction from other social roles. Thus, role conflict and role overload, a result of familial role restructuring, may not only interrupt ongoing social relationships but also increase daily hassles and the physiological stress response. Clearly, social support may operate to bisect many of the arrows in Figure 17.1.

Cultural Norms

Most studies have been conducted on samples of White, middle-class, two-parent families. The "universal" models of family-level effects of parental illness that support this research ignore the influence of cultural background on the way in which individuals and families perceive illness and disabilities (Landrine & Klonoff, 1992). Family and youth expectations of the youth's emotional and instrumental contributions to family life are also related to cultural norms (Fuligni & Pedersen, 2002). Cultural norms may influence the extent to which the adolescent's family responsibilities increase during parental illness and the extent to which the responsibilities contribute to youth maladjustment or distress. Cultural norms may also shape coping, emotional expression, and other aspects of the response to illness.

Access to Care

Much of the health psychology and prevention literatures have identified striking racial and socioeconomic disparities in morbidity, mortality, and the use of health-related services. Research has documented that access to care is one of the major contributors to these differences in health care use and health-related outcomes (Smedley, Stith, & Nelson, 2003). Such discrepancies are apparent across a variety of forms of health care, including both treatment and prevention. In particular, racial or ethnic background, education, income, and health insurance are related to the receipt of services that may prevent the onset of chronic health conditions or allow for early intervention that minimizes the effect of the health condition on the individual and his or her family (Sambamoorthi & McAlpine, 2003). Although we were unable to identify any examples of research that specifically addressed issues related to access to care and family or adolescent adjustment to parental illness, we suggest that this is one potentially important moderator of illness effects on the family. We expect that greater access to care and access to the highest quality of care would both minimize the inconvenience of treatment (reducing the extent to which families must adjust their daily routines to accommodate the illness) and minimize the functional disability associated with the illness (reducing the extent to which the illness impedes the parent's ability to fulfill his or her role in the family).

Summary

Research on parental illness conducted within a family ecology framework requires a greater understanding of how aspects of the family's experience may alter the effects of the illness on family and youth well-being. However, moderator or contextual variables have seldom been studied. Gender—of the ill parent and of the adolescent—seems to play a crucial role in determining the effects of the illness. Other factors at the family and extra-familial levels, including coping style, culture, social support, and access to care, may also affect the direction and magnitude of the association between parental illness and family/youth well-being.

BLUEPRINT FOR FUTURE RESEARCH ON ADAPTATION TO PARENTAL ILLNESS

Reviewing the literature on parental illness does not simply suggest that the field needs more research in this area—which it does—and that prospective, longitudinal studies are needed to disentangle the directionality of effects—which they are—but that future studies should move from asking *whether* there is an effect toward uncovering variables that mediate or moderate the association between parental illness and adjustment. We offer some more specific guidelines for researchers who are interested in designing studies of youth and family adaptation to parental illness. These guidelines stem from limitations in the existing literature, as well as the multiple, interconnected mediational and moderational pathways suggested by the family ecology framework.

1. *Measures must capture the quality of family-level processes.* Few studies assessed family-level constructs, such as reorganization, that may elucidate the nature of the illness effects or integrate data from multiple family members. Most studies used single- or dual-informant reports of illness effects, which may not be sufficient to capture family-level processes and may present different perceptions of "reality." Differences between mothers', fathers', and children's reports of family functioning suggest that individuals view the family environment differently depending on age, gender, or role in the family. For example, men and women perceive illness severity differently (Revenson, 1994, 2003). Research that uses multiple informants—mothers, fathers, and children—may begin to capture processes occurring at the family level (Compas et al., 1994; Degotardi, 2000; Dura & Beck, 1988; Hauser et al., 1993). An important first step toward this goal is the design and validation of reliable, multiple-informant measures of family-level processes critical to the illness response, such as cohesion, adjustment, and role redistribution. The work by Hauser and his colleagues (Hauser et al., 1993) is a first step.

2. *Comparisons within and across illnesses should be more nuanced, focusing on the adaptive tasks and cascading set of changes in the family's transactions necessitated by the illness.* Comparisons across illnesses may yield more fruitful information than single illness studies for several reasons. First, they allow researchers to disentangle the confounded effects of illness severity and diagnosis. Second, multiple-illness studies may illustrate both common coping tasks of chronic illness and those that

are specific to particular diagnoses. Both general and illness-specific coping tasks are important to understanding how an illness leads to particular outcomes (Moos & Schaefer, 1984). Third, multiple-illness studies provide an indication of the generalizability and specificity of research findings across diagnoses.

Other aspects of any particular diagnosis, such as rapidity of onset and disease progress, degree of illness intrusion (Devins, Edworthy, Guthrie, & Martin, 1992), and life threat also may affect the family's adaptational process and warrant greater attention in future research. Family and adolescent adjustment may be shaped by the length of time that a parent experiences physical symptoms of an illness without a diagnosis, the prognosis of the illness at the point of diagnosis, how fast or slow the disease worsens, and whether there are symptomatic and asymptomatic periods and how long they last. Family adaptation to an illness may be smoother in cases in which the disease progresses steadily and slowly, as each family member has time to adjust to his or her new roles and tasks and anticipate mechanisms for coping with future problems. Families may find the rapid readjustment required by an illness with cyclical symptomatic and asymptomatic stages more challenging. Alternately, cycles of relative health may make the cycles marked by greater disability easier for some families to bear. These are all hypotheses that could be—but have not yet been—tested empirically.

3. *Studies of ethnically, racially, and economically heterogeneous samples of families are needed to disentangle the confounded effects of socioeconomic status, ethnic group membership, and illness.* Most studies of cancer patients are conducted with White, middle-class samples, and most studies of HIV/AIDS patients are conducted with economically disadvantaged African American samples. Therefore, it is impossible to determine whether differences in study findings are observed because the types of illnesses studied affect families and youth differently, because members of different racial/ethnic categories view illness differently, or because the samples experience differing levels of social and economic disadvantage independent of the illness. The far-reaching changes in population demographics that are expected to occur over the next decade have important implications for psychological research (Yali & Revenson, 2004). Ignoring the historic, economic, and sociocultural contexts in which individuals are situated limits our knowledge and our ability to create effective, culturally anchored research, interventions, and policy for families with parental illness.

4. *Studies should include more positive or growth-related outcomes in addition to traditional indices of psychopathology.* Parental illness and other forms of adversity may offer families and young people the opportunity to develop strengths and competencies (Walsh, 2003). No studies to date have examined positive outcomes among adolescents experiencing parental illness although many studies show that adults facing severe life stressors, such as illness, find benefits or growth in their experience (e.g., Tennen & Affleck, 2002). Some adolescents may find that parental illness allows them to acquire skills, such as self-reliance, that promote positive development. It is important not only to document these positive outcomes but also to identify factors that may enhance such outcomes (Seligman & Csikszentmihalyi, 2000). One of the major limitations of the existing literature is that studies of youth outcomes associated with parental illness tend to focus on indicators of negative development or maladjustment. The literature in this area would benefit from a refocusing of efforts toward understanding the situations under which adolescents are able to use the challenge of parental illness as a springboard to positive growth and development. Conducting qualitative studies of adolescents' parental illness experiences and using the results to develop and pilot measures of positive growth through parental illness are necessary first steps toward

incorporating valid and reliable measures of positive adaptation into large-scale, longitudinal empirical studies.

5. *Research efforts should have a distal goal of prevention and intervention.* Given the strong public health implications of research in the area of parental illness and family and youth adjustment, it is important for researchers to design studies with their "eyes on the prize." It is given that the literature on parental illness would benefit from more well-designed, prospective, and longitudinal studies. Such studies would help identify the most effective targets for intervention by action-researchers seeking to enhance posttraumatic growth and ameliorate any negative effects of parental illness on youth and families. We do not suggest, however, that action-researchers should wait for those studies to be published before developing and evaluating interventions in this area of research. Rather, preventive interventions and other forms of action-research are essential complements to basic and developmental research in areas with strong clinical and public health implications, such as parental illness. Rigorously evaluated interventions, developed on the basis of well-constructed theory and existing research, not only have the potential to help young people challenged by parental illness but, if the interventions incorporate a random-assignment strategy, could also elucidate the hypothesized causal mechanisms underlying our proposed frame-work. For example, an evaluation of an intervention designed to reduce stigma and threat may reveal fewer negative youth outcomes among a randomly assigned intervention group, relative to a treatment-as-usual control group. Such a finding would not only help the youth who received the intervention but also provide supporting evidence for one major pathway in our proposed framework. Alternately, the intervention could reveal null findings or no convincing evidence that the intervention was effective in enhancing youth outcomes by reducing stigma or threat. In this situation, researchers could begin to test alternate pathways in the proposed framework that may yield more fruitful results.

CONCLUSION

Theories in health psychology, child development, and family medicine, as well as a small body of empirical and clinical research, indicate that adolescents appear to be at heightened risk for maladjustment as a result of parental illness. These findings have both conceptual and methodological limitations that impede the translation of research findings into practice. We advocate that research is needed to identify the mediating mechanisms by which parental illness affects families and youth, as well as moderating contextual factors that may shape those mediating processes. The family ecology framework presented here has the potential to serve as a blueprint for research in this area, elucidating the causal pathways linking illness to family and youth well-being while remaining sensitive to variation in individual families' needs and experiences. As empirical support is found for some of the framework's pathways and disconfirming evidence is found for others, a more comprehensive understanding of the parental illness experience will emerge. Such knowledge will aid researchers and clinicians in the design and implementation of effective interventions that can achieve the ultimate goal of assisting atrisk youth and families cope with and learn from the experience of parental illness.

ACKNOWLEDGMENT

We thank Diane L. Hughes, Anne E. Kazak, and Edward Seidman for their helpful feedback on previous versions of this chapter.

REFERENCES

Ainsworth, M. S. (1979). Infant-mother attachment. *American Psychologist, 34,* 932–937.

Anderson, C. A., & Hammen, C. L. (1993). Psychosocial outcomes of children of unipolar depressed, bipolar, medically ill, and normal women: A longitudinal study. *Journal of Consulting and Clinical Psychology, 61,* 448–454.

Armistead, L., Klein, K., & Forehand, R. (1995). Parental physical illness and child functioning. *Clinical Psychology Review, 15,* 409–422.

Armistead, L., Klein, K., Forehand, R., & Wierson, M. (1997). Disclosure of parental HIV infection to children in the families of men with hemophilia: Description, outcomes, and the role of family processes. *Journal of Family Psychology, 11,* 49–61.

Armistead, L., Tannenbaum, L., Forehand, R., Morse, E., & Morse, P. (2001). Disclosing HIV status: Are mothers telling their children? *Journal of Pediatric Psychology, 26,* 11–20.

Armsden, G. C., & Lewis, F. M. (1994). Behavioral adjustment and self-esteem of school aged children of women with breast cancer. *Oncology Nursing Forum, 21,* 39–45.

Barakat, L. P., & Kazak, A. E. (1999). Family issues. In R. T. Brown (Ed.), *Cognitive aspects of chronic illness in children* (pp. 333–354). New York: Guilford Press.

Berndt, T. J. (1996). Transitions in friendships and friends' influence. In J. A. Graber, J. Brooks-Gunn, & A. C. Petersen (Eds.), *Transitions through adolescence: Interpersonal domains and context* (pp. 57–84). Hillsdale, NJ: Erlbaum.

Bodenmann, G. (1997). Dyadic coping: A systemic-transactional view of stress and coping among couples: Theory and empirical findings. *European Review of Applied Psychology, 47,* 137–141.

Bronfenbrenner, U. (1977). Toward an experimental ecology of human development. *American Psychologist, 32,* 513–531.

Centers for Disease Control and Prevention. (2001). *Morbidity and Mortality Weekly Report, 50,* 120–125.

Christ, G. H., Siegel, K., & Sperber, D. (1994). Impact of parental terminal cancer on adolescents. *American Journal of Orthopsychiatry, 64,* 604–613.

Compas, B. E. (1987). Stress and life events in childhood and adolescence. *Clinical Psychology Review, 7,* 275–302.

Compas, B. E., Worsham, N. L., Epping-Jordan, J. E., Grant, K. E., Mireault, G., Howell, D. C., et al., (1994). When mom or dad has cancer: Markers of psychological distress in cancer patients, spouses, and children. *Health Psychology, 13,* 507–515.

Compas, B. E., Worsham, N. L., Ey, S., & Howell, D. C. (1996). When mom or dad has cancer: II. Coping, cognitive appraisals, and psychological distress in children of cancer patients. *Health Psychology, 15,* 167–175.

Contrada, R. J., & Guyll, M. (2000). On who gets sick and why: The role of personality and stress. In A. Baum, T. A. Revenson, & J. E. Singer (Eds.), *Handbook of health psychology* (pp. 59–84). Mahwah, NJ: Erlbaum.

Degotardi, P. B. (2000). Stress, family coping and adjustment in adolescents with juvenile rheumatoid arthritis (Doctoral dissertation, City University of New York, 2000). *Dissertation Abstracts International, 61,* 22–40B.

Degotardi, P. J., Revenson, T. A., & Ilowite, N. (1999). Family-level coping in juvenile rheumatoid arthritis: Assessing the utility of a quantitative family interview. *Arthritis Care and Research, 12,* 314–324.

DeLongis, A., Folkman, S., & Lazarus, R. S. (1988). The impact of daily stress on health and mood: Psychological and social resources as mediators. *Journal of Personality and Social Psychology, 54,* 486–495.

Devins, G. M., Edworthy, S. M., Guthrie, N. G., & Martin, L. (1992). Illness intrusiveness in rheumatoid arthritis: Differential impact on depressive symptoms over the adult lifespan. *The Journal of Rheumatology, 19,* 709–715.

DuBois, D. L., Felner, R. D., Meares, H., & Krier, M. (1994). Prospective investigation of the effects of socioeconomic disadvantage, life stress, and social support in early adolescent adjustment. *Journal of Abnormal Psychology, 103,* 511–522.

Dura, J. R., & Beck, S. J. (1988). A comparison of family functioning when mothers have chronic pain. *Pain, 35,* 79–89.

Dutra, R., Forehand, R., Armistead, L., Brody, G., Morse, E., Morse, P. S., et al., (2000). Child resiliency in inner-city families affected by HIV: The role of family variables. *Behaviour Research and Therapy, 38,* 471–486.

Ell, K., Nishimoto, R., Mantell, J., & Hamovitch, M. (1988). Longitudinal analysis of psychological adaptation among family members of patients with cancer. *Journal of Psychosomatic Research, 32,* 429–438.

Erblich, J., Bovbjerg, D. H., & Valdimarsdottir, H. B. (2000). Looking forward and back: Distress among women at familial risk for breast cancer. *Annals of Behavioral Medicine, 22,* 53–59.

Feeney, J. A., & Ryan, S. M. (1994). Attachment style and affect regulation: Relationships with health behavior and family experiences of illness in a student sample. *Health Psychology, 13,* 334–345.

Finney, J. W., & Miller, K. M. (1999). Children of parents with medical illness. In W. K. Silverman & T. H. Ollendick (Eds.), *Developmental issues in the treatment of children* (pp.433–442). Needham Heights, MA: Allyn & Bacon.

Forehand, R., Steele, R., Armistead, L., Morse, E., Simon, P., & Clark, L. (1998). The Family Health Project: Psychosocial adjustment of children whose mothers are HIV infected. *Journal of Consulting and Clinical Psychology, 66,* 513–520.

Fuligni, A. J., & Pedersen, S. (2002). Family obligations and the transition to adulthood among youths from Asian, Latin American, and European back-grounds. *Developmental Psychology, 38,* 856–868.

Gardner, W., & Preator, K. (1996). Children of seropositive mothers in the U.S. AIDS epidemic. *Journal of Social Issues, 52,* 177–195.

Grant, K. E., & Compas, B. E. (1995). Stress and anxious-depressed symptoms among adolescents: Searching for mechanisms of risk. *Journal of Consulting and Clinical Psychology, 63,* 1015–1021.

Grant, K. E., Compas, B. E., Stuhlmacher, A. F., Thurm, A., McMahon, S. D., & Halpert, J. A. (2003). Stressors and child and adolescent psychopathology: Moving from markers to mechanisms of risk. *Psychological Bulletin, 129,* 447–466.

Harris, C. A., & Zakowski, S. G. (2003). Comparisons of distress in adolescents of cancer patients and controls. *Psycho-Oncology, 12,* 173–182.

Hauser, S. T., DiPlacido, J., Jacobson, A. M., Willett, J., & Cole, C. (1993). Family coping with an adolescent's chronic illness: An approach and three studies. *Journal of Adolescence, 16,* 305–329.

Helgeson, V. S., Cohen, S., Schulz, R., & Yasko, J. (2000). Group support interventions for women with breast cancer: Who benefits from what? *Health Psychology, 19,* 107–114.

Hirsch, B. J., Moos, R. H., & Reischl, T. M. (1985). Psychosocial adjustment of adolescent children of a depressed, arthritic, or normal parent. *Journal of Abnormal Psychology, 94,* 154–164.

Hollingsworth, C. (1982). Adolescents' reactions to parental illness or death. In R. O. Pasnau (Ed.), *Psychosocial aspects of medical practice: Children and adolescents* (pp. 201–209). Menlo Park, CA: Addison Wesley.

Hough, E. S., Brumitt, G., Templin, T., Saltz, E., & Mood, D. (2003). A model of mother-child coping and adjustment to HIV. *Social Science & Medicine, 56,* 643–655.

Johnson, M. O., & Lobo, M. L. (2001). Mother-child interaction in the presence of maternal HIV infection. *Journal of the Association of Nurses in AIDS Care, 12*(1), 40–51.

Kazak, A. E. (1989). Families of chronically ill children: A systems and social-ecological model of adaptation and challenge. *Journal of Consulting and Clinical Psychology, 57,* 25–30.

Kazak, A. E., Simms, S., & Rourke, M. T. (2002). Family systems practice in pediatric psychology. *Journal of Pediatric Psychology, 27,* 133–143.

Kochanek, K. D., & Smith, B. L. (2004). Deaths: Preliminary data for 2002. *National Vital Statistics Reports, 52*(13), 28.

Korneluk, Y. G., & Lee, C. M. (1998). Children's adjustment to parental physical illness. *Clinical Child and Family Psychology Review, 1,* 179–193.

Kotchick, B. A., Forehand, R., Brody, G., Armistead, L., Morse, E., Simon, P., et al., (1997). The impact of maternal HIV infection on parenting in inner-city African American families. *Journal of Family Psychology, 11,* 447–461.

Landrine, H., & Klonoff, E. A. (1992). Culture and health-related schemas: A review and proposal for interdisciplinary integration. *Health Psychology, 11,* 267–276.

Lazarus, R. S. (1999). *Stress and emotion: A new synthesis.* New York: Springer Publishing.

Lepore, S. J. (2001). A social-cognitive processing model of emotional adjustment to cancer. In A. Baum & B. L. Andersen (Eds.), *Psychosocial interventions for cancer* (pp. 99–116). Washington, DC: American Psychological Association.

Lester, P., Stein, J. A., & Bursch, B. (2003). Developmental predictors of somatic symptoms in adolescents of parents with HIV: A 12-month follow-up. *Journal of Developmental and Behavioral Pediatrics, 24,* 242–250.

Lewis, F. M., Hammond, M. A., & Woods, N. F. (1993). The family's functioning with newly diagnosed breast cancer in the mother: The development of an explanatory model. *Journal of Behavioral Medicine, 16,* 351–370.

Lewis, F. M., Woods, N. F., Hough, E. E., & Bensley, L. S. (1989). The family's functioning with chronic illness in the mother: The spouse's perspective. *Social Science & Medicine, 29,* 1261–1269.

Lyons, R. F., Mickelson, K. D., Sullivan, M. J., & Coyne, J. C. (1998). Coping as a communal process. *Journal of Personal and Social Relationships, 15,* 579–605.

Masten, A. S., Neeman, J., & Andenas, S. (1994). Life events and adjustment in adolescents: The significance of event dependence, desirability, and chronicity. *Journal of Research on Adolescence, 4,* 71–97.

McEwen, B. S. (1998). Protective and damaging effects of stress mediators. *New England Journal of Medicine, 338,* 171–179.

Mikail, S. F., & von Baeyer, C. L. (1990). Pain, somatic focus, and emotional adjustment of children of chronic headache sufferers and controls. *Social Science & Medicine, 31,* 51–59.

Milam, J. E., Ritt-Olson, A., & Unger, J. B. (2004). Posttraumatic growth among adolescents. *Journal of Adolescent Research, 19,* 192–204.

Moos, R. H., & Schaefer, J. A. (1984). The crisis of physical illness. In R. H. Moos (Ed.), *Coping with physical illness: Vol.2. New perspectives* (pp.3–25). New York: Plenum Press.

Murphy, D. A., Steers, W. N., & Dello Stritto, M. E. (2001). Maternal disclosure of mothers' HIV serostatus to their young children. *Journal of Family Psychology, 15,* 441–450.

Patenaude, A. F. (2000). A different normal: Reactions of children and adolescents to the diagnosis of cancer in a parent. In L. Baider, C. L. Cooper, & A. K. De-Nour (Eds.), *Cancer and the family* (pp. 239–254). Chichester, England: Wiley.

Patterson, J. M., & Garwick, A. W. (1994). The impact of chronic illness on families: A systems perspective. *Annals of Behavioral Medicine, 16,* 131–142.

Pelton, J., Steele, R. G., Chance, M. W., Forehand, R., & the Family Health Project Research Group. (2001). Discrepancy between mother and child perceptions of their relationship: II. Consequences for children considered within the context of maternal physical illness. *Journal of Family Violence, 16*(1), 17–35.

Peters, L., & Esses, L. (1985). Family environment as perceived by children with a chronically ill parent. *Journal of Chronic Diseases, 38,* 301–308.

Räikkönen, K., Keltikangas-Järvinen, L., & Pietikäinen, M.http://www.sciencedirect.com/science/article/pii/002239999190081X—COR1#COR1http://www.sciencedirect.com/science/article/pii/002239999190081X—AFF2#AFF2 (1991). Type A behavior and its determinants in children, adolescents and young adults with and without parental coronary heart disease: A case-control study. *Journal of Psychosomatic Research, 35,* 273–280.

Reiss, D., Steinglass, P., & Howe, G. (1993). The family's organization around the illness. In R. E. Cole & D. Reiss (Eds.), *How do families cope with chronic illness?* (pp. 173–213). Hillsdale, NJ: Erlbaum.

Revenson, T. A. (1990). All other things are *not* equal: An ecological perspective on the relation between personality and disease. In H. S. Friedman (Ed.), *Personality and disease* (pp. 65–94). New York: Wiley.

Revenson, T. A. (1994). Social support and marital coping with chronic illness. *Annals of Behavioral Medicine, 16,* 122–130.

Revenson, T. A. (2003). Scenes from a marriage: Examining support, coping, and gender within the context of chronic illness. In J. Suls & K. A. Wallston (Eds.), *Social psychological foundations of health and illness* (pp. 530–559). Malden, MA: Blackwell.

Revenson, T. A., Kayser, K., & Bodenmann, G. (Eds.). (2005). *Emerging perspectives on couples coping with stress.* Washington, DC: American Psychological Association.

Reyland, S. A., McMahon, T. J., Higgins-Delessandro, A., & Luthar, S. S. (2002). Inner-city children living with an HIV+ mother: Parent-child relationships, perceptions of social support, and psychological disturbance. *Journal of Child and Family Studies, 11,* 313–329.

Rohrbaugh, M. J., Cranford, J. A., Shoham, V., Nicklas, J. M., Sonnega, J. S., & Coyne, J. C. (2002). Couples coping with congestive heart failure: Role and gender differences in psychological distress. *Journal of Family Psychology, 16,* 3–13.

Rolland, J. S. (1984). Toward a psychosocial topology of chronic and life threatening illnesses. *Family Systems Medicine, 2,* 245–262.

Rolland, J. S. (1999). Parental illness and disability: A family systems framework. *Journal of Family Therapy, 21,* 242–266.

Rotheram-Borus, M. J., Lee, M. B., Gwadz, M., & Draimin, B. (2001). An intervention for parents with AIDS and their adolescent children. *American Journal of Public Health, 91,* 1294–1302.

Rotheram-Borus, M. J., Lee, M., Leonard, N., Lin, Y., Franzke, L., Turner, E., et al. (2003). Four-year behavioral outcomes of an intervention for parents living with HIV and their adolescent children. *AIDS, 17,* 1217–1225.

Rotheram-Borus, M. J., & Stein, J. A. (1999). Problem behavior of adolescents whose parents are living with AIDS. *American Journal of Orthopsychiatry, 69,* 228–239.

Rowlison, R. T., & Felner, R. D. (1988). Major life events, hassles, and adaptation in adolescence: Confounding in conceptualization and measurement of life stress and adjustment revisited. *Journal of Personality and Social Psychology, 55,* 432–444.

Rutter, M. (1990). Psychosocial resilience and protective mechanisms. In J. Rolf, A. S. Masten, D. Cicchetti, K. H. Nuechterlein, & S. Weintraub (Eds.), *Risk and protective factors in the development of psychopathology* (pp. 181–214). New York: Cambridge.

Sambamoorthi, U., & McAlpine, D. D. (2003). Racial, ethnic, socioeconomic, and access disparities in the use of preventive services among women. *Preventive Medicine, 37,* 475–484.

Sarason, B. R., Sarason, I. G., & Gurung, R. A. R. (2001). Close personal relationships and health outcomes: A key to the role of social support. In B. R. Sarason & S. Duck (Eds.), *Personal relationships: Implications for clinical and community psychology* (pp. 15–41). Chichester, England: Wiley.

Scheier, M. F., & Carver, C. S. (2003). Self-regulatory processes and responses to health threats: Effects of optimism on well-being. In J. Suls & K. A. Wallston (Eds.), *Social psychological foundations of health and illness* (pp. 395–428). Malden, MA: Blackwell.

Schmaling, K. B., & Sher, T. G. (2000). *The psychology of couples and illness.* Washington, DC: American Psychological Association.

Seligman, M. E. P., & Csikszentmihalyi, M. (2000). Positive psychology: An introduction. *American Psychologist, 55,* 5–14.

Shaffer, A., Jones, D. J., Kotchick, B. A., Forehand, R., & the Family Health Project Research Group. (2001). Telling the children: Disclosure of maternal HIV infection and its effects on child psychosocial adjustment. *Journal of Child and Family Studies, 10,* 301–313.

Siegel, K., Raveis, V. H., & Karus, D. (2000). Correlates of self-esteem among children facing the loss of a parent to cancer. In L. Baider, C. L. Cooper, & A. K. De-Nour (Eds.), *Cancer and the family* (pp. 223–238). Chichester, England: Wiley.

Smedley, B. D., Stith, A. Y., & Nelson, A. R. (Eds.). (2003). *Unequal treatment: Confronting racial and ethnic disparities in health care.* Washington, DC: National Academies Press.

Stanton, A., & Revenson, T. A. (2010). Progress and promise in research on adaptation to chronic illness. In H. S. Friedman & R. C. Silver (Eds.), *The Oxford handbook of health psychology.* New York: Oxford University Press.

Steele, R., Forehand, R., & Armistead, L. (1997). The role of family processes and coping strategies in the relationship between parental chronic illness and childhood internalizing problems. *Journal of Abnormal Child Psychology, 25,* 83–94.

Stetz, K. M., Lewis, F. M., & Primomo, J. (1986). Family coping strategies and chronic illness in the mother. *Family Relations, 35,* 515–522.

Tennen, H., & Affleck. G. (2002). Benefit-finding and benefit-reminding. In C. R. Snyder & S. Lopez (Eds.), *Handbook of positive psychology* (pp. 584–597). New York: Oxford University Press.

von Bertalanffy, L. (1968). *General systems theory: Foundations, developments, applications.* New York: Braziller.

Walsh, F. (2003). Family resilience: A framework for clinical practice. *Family Process, 42,* 1–18.

Weihs, K., & Reiss, D. (2000). Family reorganization in response to cancer: A developmental perspective. In L. Baider, C. L. Cooper, & A. K. De-Nour (Eds.), *Cancer and the family* (pp. 17–40). Chichester, England: Wiley.

Wellisch, D. K., Gritz, E. R., Schain, W., Wang, H., & Siau, J. (1991). Psychological functioning of daughters of breast cancer patients. Part I: Daughters and comparison subjects. *Psychosomatics, 32,* 324–336.

Wellisch, D. K., Gritz, E. R., Schain, W., Wang, H., & Siau, J. (1992). Psychological functioning of daughters of breast cancer patients. Part II: Characterizing the distressed daughter of the breast cancer patient. *Psychosomatics, 33,* 171–179.

Wills, T. A., & Fegan, M. F. (2001). Social networks and social support. In A. Baum, T. A. Revenson, & J. E. Singer (Eds.), *Handbook of health psychology* (pp. 139–173). Mahwah, NJ: Erlbaum.

Worsham, N. L., Compas, B. E., & Ey, S. (1997). Children's coping with parental illness. In S. A. Wolchik & I. N. Sandler (Eds.), *Handbook of children's coping: Linking theory and intervention* (pp. 195–213). New York: Plenum Press.

Yali, A. M., & Revenson, T. A. (2004). How changes in population demographics will impact health psychology: Incorporating a broader notion of cultural competence into the field. *Health Psychology, 23,* 147–155.

Yates, B. C., Bensley, L. S., Lalonde, B., Lewis, F. M., & Woods, N. F. (1995). The impact of marital status and quality on family functioning in maternal chronic illness. *Health Care for Women International, 16,* 437–449.

18

My Life With Muscular Dystrophy: Lessons and Opportunities

ROBERT P. WINSKE

I am 41 and the middle son of three boys born with a rare form of muscular dystrophy known as nemaline rod myopathy. To date there is still little information known about the disease, as was the case at the time when we were born in the early to mid-1960s, though it is clear that it is a progressive condition and is passed from mother to son. At the time of each of our births, what made the case more baffling to the doctors was how this occurred. As I stated, muscular dystrophy is a congenital impairment that is passed through the X-chromosomes of the mother. To my mother's knowledge, however, she herself didn't have the disability.

When my older brother was born, the doctors requested that my parents check the family tree and see if there was anyone on either side of the family who may have had muscular dystrophy. However, as requested, my parents with the assistance of their parents did check each side and their efforts proved unsuccessful. To their knowledge, no one on either side of the family had ever been diagnosed and treated for any form of the impairment. Though my mother did have a physical disability, to her knowledge it was polio not muscular dystrophy. She became sick as a young child in the late 1940s, which was at the height of the polio epidemic that extended into the early fifties. Growing up, my mother always talked about being a young girl getting sick in which her muscles got weak, especially in her lower extremities and was told by her parents that it was polio. She had no reason to doubt this information because her mother was a registered nurse. She was also treated in hospital wards where several children her age were being treated for the same condition and some were worse than she was. My mother was still able to walk, which was not so for most of the children.

As there were no signs of the disease found on either side of the family, the doctors believed the occurrence of muscular dystrophy was a fluke. There was no reason why it occurred, and they informed my parents that to their understanding, the odds to their having another child with the birth defect were unlikely. This led them to decide to have another child. Like my brother, I also was born with the same form of muscular dystrophy. This really perplexed the doctors not only because my parents had another baby with the disease but also because I wasn't as severely impacted by its limitations.

However, following the birth of a second child with the neuromuscular condition, the doctors again insisted that someone on one side of the family had to have had the condition. They even wondered if a family member had a baby with the same or similar condition, but

Reprinted from *Families Living With Chronic Illness and Disability,* by P.W. Power and A.E. Dell Orto, 2004. New York: Springer Publishing.

never took the baby home. This was common at that time as children with birth defects were generally institutionalized because it was an embarrassment to families to have children with impairments. It was also believed that parents couldn't provide the needed, specialized care. If this were the case, the doctors believed that whoever in the family may have had a child with muscular dystrophy wouldn't want to admit to it, being ashamed or embarrassed, along with the belief that everyone wants the perfect baby.

Following the doctor's recommendation, my parents again went back to their parents to examine both sides of the family. It was emphasized that it was important to know if there was any family history of muscular dystrophy so the doctors could more efficiently treat me and my brother. Again, as with the previous search the second attempt to identify anyone in the family who may have had the same or similar condition also proved unsuccessful. No one in the family reported having any family members with any physical disabilities. Because of the absence of any disclosure, it was suggested that my parents not have any more children because it couldn't be guaranteed that they wouldn't have another child with the physical impairments. With each of our births, it was also recommended that they not bring us home, as the doctors attempted to tell my parents that we would never grow up to be anything, to have independent lives, and would demand a lot of care. Such communication was especially true after I was born. The doctors tried to explain that my parents already had their hands full with taking care of a child with a severe physical impairment. Trying to take care of two would be too much and too overwhelming. In both cases, my parents opted not to listen to the doctors, so they took me home with them; about two years later, they had their third child. Again, a boy was born with the same physical impairments, but with less impairment than I had.

Following the birth of my parents' third child, the physicians were perplexed as to how parents who had no history of muscular dystrophy on either side of the family could have three children with the condition. The only thing they were left to believe was that my mother as a child had been misdiagnosed as having polio. They believed that it could have been an easy mistake because at the time many children were getting sick with polio, and the symptoms my mother recalled experiencing as a child were similar to the impairments experienced with polio. This perception existed for several years until my younger brother was 15 years old. Around that time, my mother and he had, concurrently, a muscle biopsy, a process in which they had a small piece of muscle removed from their thigh to be analyzed. This analysis revealed that each had the same condition, and then these results were compared to biopsy results my older brother and I had as young children. Thus, as had long been expected, my mother did in fact have muscular dystrophy.

But our lives continued, and my parents successfully raised three children with muscular dystrophy. Each of us completed high school and went on to college. My older brother obtained a job as an advocate of individuals with various impairments after leaving Boston University, I was a senior at Northeastern University, and my younger brother entered the first year at University of Massachusetts at Amherst after earning an AA degree from Newbury Junior College. However, after my brothers and I had begun to move forward with our lives, my mom found that her mother started to have slight problems with memory, which in the early days was minimal but then slowly progressed. This would eventually lead her to bring her mother to be seen by a doctor because she was concerned that there may be something more serious than that of aging. She was told that her mother did in fact have major health problems and that she was in the early stages of Alzheimer's.

As the disease would progress, my mom would be faced with one of the most difficult decisions that no child ever looks forward to making regarding one's parent. She would realize that despite existing support systems, her mother was no longer safe living on her own, and my mom would have to make the decision that she was unable to care for her mother's needs and would have to put her in a nursing home. She knew her mother wouldn't want that as she'd always made it clear that she wanted to remain and die in her own home with her dignity. However, my mom knew a nursing home was the only real option available, fearing that not acting so would result in her mother doing something that would result in serious injury or worse yet, put a neighbor at risk in the elderly housing complex where she was living.

During this process of placing her mother in a nursing home, my mother needed to obtain a variety of information about her mother for the nursing home, which included a determination of eligibility for Medicaid, which is the insurance company that covers the nursing home expenses. One item needed was my grandmother's birth certificate, leading my mother to call the city hall in the town of Kennebunkport, Maine. That is the town where my grandmother had always reported as being born and raised. However, this was unsuccessful because when speaking with the town's city hall administrator, my mother was told that there was no record of anyone with the name my mother had provided. A bit confused, my mother followed the recommendation of the city hall employee, which was to check neighboring towns in the event my grandmother had been mistaken. Though my mother found it difficult to believe her mother wouldn't know the town where she'd been born, she wondered whether she had been born in a different city and just raised in Kennebunkport. My mother spent days calling numerous city halls in those cities and towns surrounding Kennebunk port. All of these calls were unsuccessful, as none of the cities or towns had any record of anyone being born there with her mother's name.

After days of numerous phone calls, feeling frustrated, my mother contacted her mother's sister to ask for assistance inquiring where her mother was born. To my mother's shock, she found out that her mother was adopted as a child. This frustrated my mother. She could only think of why her mother never mentioned this, especially, during the early years in which she and my father were checking both of their family's background to see if there was any history of muscular dystrophy on either side of the family. In further conversation with her aunt, my mother indeed discovered that her mother was aware that she did in fact have muscular dystrophy. But for reasons my own mother will never understand, her mother was apparently embarrassed by this diagnosis, and her mother told the doctors treating my mother as child to tell her it was polio, not muscular dystrophy.

After this revelation, my mother was extremely confused, understandably frustrated, and angry that her mother kept this information from her. Her mother was a registered nurse and should have known that muscular dystrophy is a genetic disorder and not the result of something she or my mother had done wrong that resulted in this impairment. Even more aggravating for my mother was how her mother could remain silent about this information when she, my father, and the doctors were working with both sides of the family to explore if there was any history of the impairment. My mother found herself not knowing how she should feel or how to approach this topic with her mother. Her mother probably wouldn't have a clear understanding of her reasoning behind the decision or understand the frustration my mother was dealing with. Alzheimer's had robbed her mother of an ability to comprehend anything beyond simple child-like questions and reasoning. She had to figure out herself how to deal with the anger and frustration she had toward her mother, which she knew would be difficult. My mom was unable to resolve questions regarding her mother's decision making, as well as how to set aside these feelings. She knew she had to do this, because she could see her mother quickly withering away day by day as the Alzheimer's progressed, and knew that things were only going to get worse. Therefore, for her mother to be properly cared for at that time and in the later years of her life, and knowing the effects Alzheimer's would continue to have, she had to put these feelings aside if she were to make sure that her mother's needs were met.

Though my mother didn't—and probably never would—totally understand or forgive her mother for what she did at that time, my mother was able to put these feelings aside and put her mother into a nursing home where she was properly cared for during the final few years of her life. I don't know how my mother was able to do this as I knew how she felt, though I do know it took a great deal of strength. She would have drawn on the same strength and courage it took to raise three children with physical impairments during a time when most parents would have had their children placed in an institution, which was recommended when my brother and I were born.

During my lifetime, I've gone through numerous changes due to the progression of my impairment. I started as an individual who was able to walk, then to one who walked and used a manual wheelchair when having to go for any distances or when my legs were sore and weak due to fatigue, then to one who used a manual chair at all times because I was no longer able to walk, though I was able to perform all activities of daily living. Currently, I require the use of an electric wheelchair for mobility and rely on a personal care attendant to assist me with all activities of daily living.

Though I have dealt with and will continue to deal with rough times that are associated with a progressive form of a physical impairment, I truly can't complain about my life. I have completed both bachelor's and master's degrees from two major universities in Boston and have always had a great job. In most instances, such accomplishments are not true for individuals with major impairments. When people first meet me, whether they are personal care attendants, colleagues, students, or clients, they tend to be surprised at my positive outlook on life. I think they believe they probably would be angry if they were in my situation. But, perhaps, they would not be angry, since I believe that most people with various limitations learn to make the most out of life. Of course, there will always be some people who will never be able to accept their life, choosing instead to be bitter and angry about their situation and wishing they were dead. Some of these people will indeed die, whether through willing themselves to die or from self-induced or assisted suicide.

Concerning my positive outlook on life, I attribute most of this attitude to my parents. They wouldn't allow me or my two brothers to sit back and feel sorry for ourselves, or use our disability as an excuse for not doing something. My mother particularly served as a personal inspiration for us. Though she also has muscular dystrophy, she taught us through example how to live and make the most out of life. She believes that having a disability doesn't entitle one to look for pity from others, or to feel sorry for oneself.

My mother even advocated early in my life, fighting with the local school board, that my brothers and I be integrated and mainstreamed into regular classes with our nondisabled peers, years before the Massachusetts public law, Chapter 766, was enacted guaranteeing equal public education for children with disabilities.

Feeling sorry for ourselves was not an option. While in high school, it was instilled in us that we were expected to go to college, and to get ahead in life and to get a good job. Continued education was a necessity. Though I received social security benefits as an individual with a disability, my parents made it clear it was only while in school that I would collect benefits and would not do so for life. Having a job was an important value for my parents, and they insisted that my brothers and I were to have jobs every summer, with a majority of the money to be set aside to pay for college. This value is one that stuck with me. Since earning a bachelor's degree, I've always had a job, even when, because of a dramatic change in my impairment, I had to take time off from work. Each time I knew I would return to work. Not working was never an option in my mind though the doctors would have preferred that I only collect disability benefits. I believe that having a job is important because it allows people to understand that individuals with disabilities are capable of working and can be productive members of society who shouldn't feel sorry for themselves because of their limitations.

Another belief I value that allows me to have a positive outlook on life is that there is always someone worse off than myself. When I was 11 years old and had recently undergone surgery for scoliosis, I was sent to a residential school for children with disabilities for 4 years. This school was wired via television cameras to the classrooms, which allowed me to participate in the school curriculum while recuperating from the surgery. Because the local junior high school where I was born and raised was inaccessible to individuals with physical impairments, I attended this "hospital school." While attending the school, I went home on weekends and holidays. I realized that half of the students lived there like myself because their family wanted nothing to do with them, choosing to make them wards of the state and to be forgotten about. But as a young boy I hated to be away from my family, and during this time I gained an appreciation of how fortunate I was. I realized that my parents cared for and loved me and only sent me to this "hospital school" because it was the only viable option for my junior high education.

Many at this school had no one and would be there until they were 21. Then they would leave the school and at that time not know what would happen to them. I also feel fortunate because I was born with my disability and it's the only life I've known. Compared to those who acquire an impairment due to a traumatic event or an illness, I've always said that if I had to have a disability, I'm glad I was born with it. Yes, there have been changes in my condition resulting in a loss of independence. But I grew up knowing that I was going to experience exacerbations with this neuromuscular impairment. The only thing I had to live with was not knowing when the condition would get worse, and to what extent the change would be. If an individual acquires his or her impairment later in life, with one's life turned upside down with no warning that the life they were used to is suddenly taken away, for that person the adjustment is extremely difficult if they do make any adjustment at all.

In addition, I've always been thankful that my impairment affects my body and not my mind. I do not consider myself better than someone else with a different condition. But I'd rather have it the way that I am even though I depend a great deal on assistance from others. Importantly, despite my physical limitations, I'm able to understand my needs and direct others on how to assist me with my needs, and with my intact cognitive functions I have earned two college degrees and maintain a great job. These are just my personal beliefs, and I do not ever intend to insult those who have severe, cognitive impairments, such as traumatic brain injuries or Alzheimer's disease.

My final belief that has allowed me to maintain a positive attitude is the conviction that God doesn't put more on one's plate than one is able to manage. Though I am not a very religious individual, I do not want to convey the impression that I've never been angry about my situation or bitter, and depressed wishing that I was dead. There have been numerous times when I wonder why I don't understand what it's all about, and why it happened to me; I can't wait to ask God what it was all about. However, in time I always come around to the beliefs that have allowed me to adjust and make the most out of my life and realize how lucky I am.

I have always been asked, "If there was a cure for muscular dystrophy would I take it?" People are usually amazed when I state that I would decline. Why I decline a hypothetical cure is because this is the only life I know and I feel, because of the reasons discussed, that I am truly blessed for my life. I believe that having this impairment allows me, despite my limitations, to serve as an example that one is still able to have a happy and productive life.

III

Family Issues in Illness and Disability: Conclusion

DISCUSSION QUESTIONS

1. The chapter by Prilleltensky on "My Child is Not My Carer" discusses the author's personal experience as being a mother with a physical neuromuscular disability (muscular dystrophy) and the well-being of her children. Discuss the following: (a) How would raising hildren be both the same and different for mothers with and *without* disabilities during parenting responsibilities? (b) Would there be any differences if the father (instead of the mother) had a disability?
2. The chapter by Case-Smith on parenting a child with a chronic medical illness suggests that the demands and responsibilities on families are much different than parenting children without disabilities. Discuss some unique cultural differences in parenting children with chronic medical conditions. What would be the overall psychosocial impact on the well-being of the family that was raising children with disabilities?
3. As rehabilitation professionals, what would be some of the essential and necessary services and resources to utilize in working with families that have children with disabilities? Considering the developmental stage of adolescents, what would be some essential and necessary services and resources for this age group?
4. Some scholars suggest that in parental illness, family systems theory many times does not generalize to the unique cultural differences that challenge families with disabilities, whether it be the parent or a child with the disability. Accordingly, how are family systems theories both the same and different when dealing with disability within the family? Are there particular theories or approaches that may work better than others?
5. In Buki et al.'s chapter relating to one heterosexual HIV-serodiscordant (i.e., one HIV-positive and one HIV-negative partner) couple's experience with AIDS, what are some of the unique caregiver stressors associated this specific disability?
6. In this same chapter by Buki et al., discuss the emotional, social, interpersonal, and spiritual effects on an individual living with HIV or AIDS.
7. Discuss issues related to the philosophy that "families are better able to cope with a seriously ill child during the early years of a marriage."
8. Regardless of the disability, pick one or more of the disabilities found in Part III and discuss the impact that the disability would have early on in the individual's career decision making and how it would affect their future occupation.
9. Given the unique characteristics associated with children who have chronic illnesses and disabilities, provide an argument for *and against* home-schooling such children.
10. How much responsibility, if any, do parents and families have to develop and cultivate their children's spiritual and/or religious beliefs and practices in dealing with illness or disability?

PERSONAL PERSPECTIVE

Adding another perspective on the family is the personal perspective by Janet Lingerman. Janet carefully describes what happens to a married couple when the sudden event of a medical crisis with a newborn occurs. Her story identifies the many coping methods utilized when unexpected traumas associated with illness and disability emerge. Sibling dynamics are also discussed. Importantly, Janet Lingerman's family journey shows that despite the many serious disruptions and crises a family can survive and even grow in spiritual health and maturity.

Maintaining a balanced attitude as a family member while experiencing the continued impact of a chronic illness or severe disability is crucial to effective coping. Achieving this balanced outlook while confronting the many realities associated with a serious medical condition is an endless struggle. In this chapter, these realities have been conceptualized as perspectives, such as vulnerability, family challenges, stress, family change, and relationships with health care professionals. In turn, these realities also become a foundation for family understanding, resilience, and affirmation. The mother's story in the following account identifies the many perspectives highlighted in the chapter and illustrates how the awareness of changes, stressors, and one's vulnerability can stimulate understanding and resilience.

DEALING WITH SPINA BIFIDA: A MOTHER'S PERSPECTIVE

Janet Lingerman

Maintaining a Balanced Attitude

Both my husband and I have come from upper-middle-class families of four children; he is the youngest of four boys, and I am the oldest child in my family. Each of us has also compensated for a mild form of disability. Although I remember almost no direct conversations regarding my congenital hearing loss, I was taken regularly to Boston for tests and treatments. Probably before my school years, I had taught myself to read lips and to stay close to people whose words I wanted to hear. Reading difficulties plagued my husband during his school years, and he received tutoring and summer help. He, too, was able to succeed in school, intellectually able to fine-tune his auditory learning abilities. Both of us made a practice of "passing" as normal, choosing instead to work around the difficulties.

At the time of our marriage I was 21½ years old and my fiancé was 29. Our courtship had been a relatively short, 10 months. Although we attempted to expand our family shortly after marriage, there were problems. Pregnancy difficulties over 6 years were the first problems that either of us had really come across that could not be resolved by working harder. Action oriented, we tried all medical possibilities from tests to surgeries, capitalizing on the hope of each other. We became closer than most couples, I think, but the closeness was largely nonverbal as we rarely discussed our disappointments but could see it in each others' faces, especially, during the many times in the hospital, sitting quietly, sometimes holding hands. We considered it a sign of strength that we could maintain our optimistic facade, especially with others, even members of our families of origin who visited but were not overly attentive.

The most difficult trial during our early marriage occurred when I had to have emergency surgery for a ruptured ectopic pregnancy that could have ended my life. I was more

From *The Psychological and Social Impact of Disability*, 2007, 5th edition, pp. 408–417. Springer Publishing.

concerned that the surgery ended not only the pregnancy but also our chances for having children at all. Aware only of a sense of defeat and questions about what to do with my life, I sought no further than my husband and the doctor for support for my bruised self-esteem. Initiating adoption procedures and keeping busy did help to fend off some of the discouragement.

The following fall another pregnancy began against all medical odds. This pregnancy, like the others, got off to a troublesome start, and we didn't dare hope it would continue. It did continue, however, even without any medical intervention, for which we would later be glad. As each month passed, and we could feel the baby moving, we became more and more sure that our troubles were over. By 7 months we felt as if we were home free, because even babies born that early often survived unscathed. We went through Lamaze classes together. Those months in the last half of the pregnancy will probably always be remembered as our happiest, closest, and most deliciously carefree with both of us wrapped up in the event to come. Beth's delivery was "medically unremarkable." For us, it was a most remarkable achievement, all the more worthy because we had warded off all anesthesia and even the threatened forceps. Yet, even as we congratulated each other and snapped a photo or two in the delivery room, we registered the silence of the staff that came only moments before the doctor told us what he had just discovered: Beth had been born with a meningomyelocele (open spine).

The obstetrician was kind and gentle, putting his hand on my arm as he told us of the meningomyelocele. He told us nothing more, and my strong biology background registered a thud in the back of my mind, but did not connect. All I could ask was whether Beth would be all right, and whether she would live, to which I received affirmative answers. On a maternal high, I found the nurses to be annoyingly business like and was glad to finally return to my room to make phone calls. My husband was back with me when we were told the baby would be sent by ambulance to Boston, and even then we assumed that Beth would be hospitalized for whatever was necessary and would come home later fine. The pediatrician arrived and began the jumble of what was to be our introduction to spina bifida. Although I recall that he gave a long description of the many organs and functions affected by the condition, I remember little else except his kindness and brutal honesty. A voice in my head kept repeating, "My baby won't be like that," and I was worrying about my husband, who had also been up all night and was expected to accompany the baby to Boston.

My husband will never forget that trip to Boston, being asked whether to treat the baby, a decision, really, whether to let her live. He was told that she was paralyzed from the waist down, would never walk, and would be retarded if she lived at all and then he had to return to me to go through it all again. With essentially no guidance from anyone, we were asked to make a decision regarding a child for whom we had waited for 6 years and about a condition we had never heard of until just hours earlier. Coming to an agreement was only the first of many extreme difficulties, as we juggled our high value on this child against a future we could not begin to imagine. Beth's back was closed at the age of 24 hours. With this commitment, I resolved that if she were to be disabled, at least I would see to it that she maximized every potential.

In those early days we did not cope; we existed. Minute followed minute, and crisis followed crisis. We tried to keep up with our social life in an effort to maintain some semblance of an old reality, but I found those times dreamlike and irrelevant, because I was unable to think of anything but Beth and us. My husband appeared to me to be intensely emotional, but he kept it in tight control; it was too big for us to discuss in anything but small snatches.

Our families were in their own shock and did not know how to help. Nor did we know how to ask for help. Our mothers visited Beth and me in the hospital, and I was grateful, especially, sensing that they were ill equipped to deal with the horror stories of others packed in around us at the nursery. I at least had had a medical background and could better understand both the hope and the limits of care given in answer to the insistent beeping of monitors. Meanwhile, our siblings received contradictory misinformation and tended either to minimize or exaggerate the facts of Beth's condition. Many people, family included, came to us with success stories about other children with spina bifida. Although I acknowledged their intent to help with hope, I also made a very conscious effort to put out of my mind these other stories, knowing that Beth was an individual and would be in her own way different from the others.

Within days of Beth's birth, our entire value system changed abruptly. All issues, problems, and questions were related to matters of life and death. Nothing seemed more important than survival. Concurrently, the value we placed on friendship skyrocketed, as there seemed so few people who could even begin to understand what we were going through. I seemed to live at a layer many levels deeper and more vulnerable than ever before and became acutely sensitive, while at the same time attempting an incongruous facade of strength. We learned quickly that others needed to be put at ease with us, because they felt inadequate to help. Most did not know whether to send us a baby gift or flowers for condolence, whereas what was really important was that they cared enough to send anything. As time went on, I found, and still find, more and more people with problems of many kinds turning to me for solace, because they know somehow that I have grown sensitive ears.

In her first 18 months, Beth had nine operations, including brain surgery for a shunt and two revisions for the hydrocephalus that developed at 3 weeks. She seemed to spend more time in the hospital than out of it. Two or three times when she had severe urinary tract infections, I opted to keep her at home and give her injections around the clock to avoid another hospitalization. Carrying out a relentless litany of medical procedures, equipment applications, exercises, treatments, and medication administrations, I have never ceased to be amazed at what one can learn to consider an ordinary part of life. Part of what was most difficult was keeping track of the constant changes. When she first came home at the age of six weeks, I initially had little confidence in caring for this small girl. It felt as if she belonged more to the hospital than to us. The staff had been very supportive in teaching me, though, and by the end of the first year I had gained some considerable expertise. My life was lived more moment to moment than day to day, with a motto of, "Tomorrow may not be any better, but at least it'll be different," or, "At least I'll never be bored." Planning even a day in advance was difficult because there were so many appointments and changes. But by the end of the first year, I had developed a technique called "putting my worries on hold." I was able to make an observation of impending crisis, set a reasonable time for a new evaluation of the problem, and mentally put aside anxiety on the issue until the appointed time and the new information. I would then (1) act, (2) decide it was a false alarm, or (3) go back on hold until the next assessment. I was determined to "accept" her condition and to avoid foisting my hang-ups on her, and to the extent that even at my worst I have managed to keep her independence in sight as my first priority for her, I have been fairly successful in maintaining an attitude of optimism and open honesty. Emotionally speaking, however, the first year was relatively easy, with numbness and denial carrying me along.

My husband, meanwhile, pulled together after the initial weeks into a stable strength. His attitude is generally more pessimistic and fatalistic than my complementary optimist activism. To this day, he starts with the worst possibilities and works toward reality, whereas I look to the most hopeful, backtracking toward reality where we meet minds. Although I do not entirely understand his ability to mentally analyze a problem and work toward a solution alone, I do see that this method works for him. He says about problems: "I think about them alone, in the car, uninterrupted, and I break the cycle" of going round and round on the same issue. On the other hand, he does not entirely understand my need to, as he puts it, "Sit around and talk about the same things."

When Beth was 18 months old, she had to have double hip surgery, necessitating use of a spica cast and a Bradford frame for 2 months. Concurrently, my husband was laid up with what was later diagnosed as a broken back, which could have left him a paraplegic as well. Both were in body casts at the same time. It was then that I began to seriously doubt my ability to continue. We had also just begun Beth's program of intermittent catheterization primarily to avoid what we considered to be destructive surgery on her bladder. Although I became tied to the schedule and even the urologist was skeptical, Beth had far fewer infections. More tired than I ever knew was possible, I also felt especially lonely with my husband seeming to be someone else when he was on high doses of painkillers. My life seemed to consist of nothing besides constant nursing duties, and I knew that I was not functioning well at all.

Until this time I had had very little in the way of external support besides medical expertise and a few select baby-sitters on whom I depended heavily for some time out. My husband and I have insisted on maintaining some semblance of a social life, with some time set aside for just the two of us. We have both found it essential to our sanity and to our marriage in spite of financial pressures and hassles in getting sitters. We have had extraordinarily good luck with training students in high school or college. I hide nothing from them and describe what is involved to check their reactions before actually teaching them and putting them to work. For privacy's sake, we have insisted on having only girls involved with the catheterization and found that once they have matured a bit beyond their own self-consciousness over puberty, they accept our medical regime as a matter-of-fact.

Through our Lamaze teacher, I became involved with an organization of parents of special-needs children. I had, of course, met many other parents of disabled children and had had meaningful conversations at clinics, in hospital corridors, and occasionally on the phone, but there was no sense of continuity with these people who were not otherwise parts of our lives. After a lecture sponsored by Parent to Parent on the subject of birth defects, I discovered a sense of warm, interested, understanding community spirit among the local parents in over an hour of conversation. The parents were as varied as the special needs their children represented. It was exhilarating to be face-to-face with a group of sane people who could cope (something I very much needed to know how to do), people who were just as much in awe of my situation as I was of theirs. Parent to Parent also helped open many doors to worlds of assorted resources. Even though I had, since the beginning, specialized in becoming an expert on the subjects of spina bifida and hydrocephalus from a medical standpoint, through the parent group, I began to learn of consumer services, sources of adaptive equipment and clothing, and helpful hints to facilitate the translation of medical treatment into individual family living.

By the time Beth was 2½, our lives had stabilized—with my husband back on his feet and Beth home for a whole year without hospitalization. I went to an exercise class and became satisfyingly involved with Parent to Parent, matching families for phone support. With assistance through an early intervention program, Beth had begun to walk with a walker and braces to the waist, and her developmental age was gaining on her chronological age. During this time, we got a call from the adoption agency telling us that they had a 3-week-old baby girl for us to pick up in just 4 days. She was adorable and very much wanted, even so suddenly, but those first months were awfully hectic for me, because Lindsey had her own set of problems; colic from the start, pneumonia requiring hospitalization at the age of 10 weeks, 4 months of incessant crying, and finally the discovery of her allergy to milk that lasted until she was over 2 years old. Actually, now I am glad for these problems because they established immediately a place for Lindsey in our family, which might otherwise have tended to put aside her needs for Beth's, which still seemed so urgent. Always, even during the hardest times, I knew that Lindsey's assertive presence was beneficial to all of us although I worried about whether she got enough attention. I felt somewhat saddened and slightly cheated that Lindsey and I would never be as intimately involved as Beth and I had been. It was my husband who helped me see that I was overinvolved with Beth, not that Lindsey was lacking my attention. Both girls were thriving, Beth as the oldest and Lindsey with the attentions of a big sister.

Once I gained some time and the distance that Beth's schooling provided at age 3½, I was able to see our enmeshment more clearly. I had not been prepared for the sense of responsibility I would feel toward a child, perhaps even an able-bodied one. The enmeshment had been understandably born out of our desires for a child and the related needs of this particular one. Enmeshment was also fostered by the system that taught me all the care and treatments. I once realized that I was expected to carry out 9 hours of assorted treatments per day, while meals, baths, groceries, a social life, laundry, errands, and recreation were to come out of the little remaining time. The diluting effect of Lindsey's arrival had been very healthy. My husband's role and mine did not change a great deal, but they expanded instead to include more tasks, some of which were traded or shared. He spent many hours on the paper work and financial mix-ups of insurance, handicapped license plates, taxes, and the like.

By the time Beth was 5 and Lindsey 2½, I was mired in depression. My previously optimistic ability to make the most of a hard situation had burned out in negative musings on how badly we would lose this game of life with a disabled child in spite of all the hard work. To my credit, I knew even then that Beth's disability was far from the whole problem (scapegoating), but I also knew that I needed professional help. I had read many times about the grief surrounding the birth of a child with defects, but the literature did not ring true for me. My life certainly included denial, anger, bargaining, depression, and acceptance. But for me, these were not milestones on a timeline but were aspects of every day, sometimes every hour. Furthermore, there was little grief attached to the "expected baby." The grief was tied up in the whole mental picture I had had for my family, our future, and myself. Feeling I had failed myself, my husband, Beth, the family, and even society itself, what I really had lost was my whole sense of self-worth, which I defined in terms of what I could do.

The most significant help came to me through a fine clinical psychologist who worked individually with me, primarily on the issue of self-esteem, helping me to better integrate my thinking with my feelings. From the start he offered me respect, as if I had as much to teach him as he had to teach me, and he responded with compassion and human reactions, from time to time with tears in his eyes. His positive regard for me supported his assumption that I could grow through this, and that, indeed, I already had. I was certain that I had crossed the line into insanity, wishing I could quietly evaporate. He got me an antidepressant, which helped me to go on and see that all of the overwhelming things I was feeling were, even in all their intensity, normal reactions to abnormal circumstances. The counselor taught me a whole new perspective on worth and value, one that rested on who I am, not on what I do. From this viewpoint then, failures or disapproval could not change my value as a person.

Crucial to the counseling was my somewhat private but strong faith in God, a faith shared by the counselor but not by my husband. Rigidly clinging to various misconceptions, I was less able to utilize effectively the resources of my faith. For instance, guilt was not an issue for me intellectually or even spiritually, because I believe in forgiveness. But emotionally, I felt I deserved this disaster, not realizing I also had to forgive myself. I learned about peace and pacing, as well as about my own human limitations, and I relearned a sense I had had long ago that there is something to be learned in every situation. Knowing I was doing the best I could under the circumstances, I could let God take over the responsibility for the end results and put aside long-term worries. The counselor helped me gain a perspective, a broader sense of time and meaning for my life. Contemplating the biblical concept of unconditional love also helped bolster my sense of self-esteem. By the time we terminated, I was able to see myself as a special and unique individual, equipped with my own set of strengths and weaknesses, grown and growing. These gifts could actually be used for the benefit of others, and a future began to form for the first time in 5 years. I had never before seen myself in this light, and it was a monumental turning point for me. Also, a growing involvement with our local church provided not just spiritual sustenance but practical assistance and a warm, new support network as well.

The interaction between the girls has been decidedly normal although frequently they seem closer than do many sisters, sharing well and at times showing surprising consideration for each other. Beth's time in school has given me a chance to be with just Lindsey and to delight in her development, which, although less studied than Beth's, has been remarkable in its own right. The two of them fight and squabble like any other siblings and also gang up against us. It is a loud, irritating nuisance, but I realize a sense of gratefulness that they can be so normal, that each has an effect on the other is clear. In a burst of independence and, perhaps, competition with her sister, Beth learned to catheterize herself last fall, but tries on occasion to go "like Lindsey" without a catheter. Lindsey in the meantime was very slow in toilet training, and I wondered if she craved the attention Beth got at the toilet. Although I have made a concerted effort to help each view herself as an individual, I am seldom sure of how life looks from their angle.

I have also tried to direct disability-related anger at the equipment or the spina bifida itself, as opposed to Beth herself. I don't know yet whether she can herself make the distinction. She said several months ago, "I hate meatballs, applesauce, and myself," then paused while my ears pricked up and added, "I don't know why I said that, Mummy." As casually as I could, I asked her what she didn't like about herself. "Oh," she thought, "casts and braces and catheters and stuff." We talked it out, cried it out, as I tried to help her separate these things from whom she is. A few weeks later she asked, "Mummy, how come you always like to talk to me about braces and crutches and spina bifida?" Perception is perhaps Beth's greatest strength, and I knew as I chuckled that I'd been had. Yet it wasn't much later that she said, "You know, Mum, there are some good things about spina bifida. I get lots and lots of extra attention."

In the meantime, Lindsey is becoming quite the athlete, and I have wondered how Beth would take to her sister's prowess on bikes, skis, and roller skates. Beth has opted to try each to the best of her ability with our help, and since Lindsey's first steps "without anything," Beth has so far been quite proud of her sister. In a thousand little ways, such as grocery shopping (Who rides in the cart? Who walks?), my husband and I have also had to face Lindsey's passing Beth in abilities, and we are reminded that it is personhood that is important, not abilities. With this in mind, I can freely encourage Lindsey's weekly swimming with more enthusiasm that I might otherwise have.

My husband and I, like Beth and Lindsey, lead parts of our lives together and other parts more separately. We have mustered a fairly united front in house rules and discipline. Now that I am out of the house more, having returned to school with the goal of eventually rejoining the workforce, my husband has to pick up more of the childcare and household chores. Conversely, I hope, in time, to provide some income to offset the pressures on him. Although it is still difficult to predict the future for either of our children, we have a hopeful coinciding picture of independence for each. We may be wrong, but we have probably considered a full spectrum of possible outcomes although we don't look too far ahead. The more I study, the more I come to the comforting conviction that, despite some asynchrony, our family is indeed generally functional. It is far from perfect, and nothing is ever that simple. However, a strong alliance in our marriage, our flexibility, and the healthy dyads in each direction can all help build our coping strengths. These years, although frequently overwhelming, have been a challenge to growth for each of us. Frankly, I am proud of the maturity we have both gained. I become more and more convinced that the lessons most worth learning are also the most painful ones. The pain will undoubtedly continue, but so, too, I think, will the growth.

IV

Interventions and Resources: Introduction

Since the first edition of this book was published in 1977, there has been a significant growth in the literature on topics related to the issues presented in this section, Part IV. Topics chosen for this section reflect the growing need in counseling, psychology, rehabilitation, and other social sciences to prepare professionals for the diagnosis, treatment, prevention, and the coordination of important resources to help persons with chronic illnesses and disabilities achieve optimal levels of independent functioning.

The first chapter in this section relates to the all-important topic of substance abuse disorders where the need for treating this mental health condition has involved partnering with programs and services that reach beyond the traditional rehabilitation, mental health, or the criminal justice systems. For instance, state, regional, and locally operated mental health programs, health care prevention and wellness programs, community support, disability benefits, and the state-federal system of vocational rehabilitation all must work in concert. Reid and Barrera report the incidence and prevalence of substance abuse disorders through the large data collection from the National Survey on Drug Use and Health (Lowinson, Ruiz, Millman, & Langrod, 2005). The reader will be informed of issues related to key terms and definitions; prevalence data; patterns of use; socioeconomic, ethnic, and gender differences; and the dual diagnosis of coexisting mental and physical disabilities. There is a brief description of drug categories and their effects on the body including stimulants, hallucinogens, marijuana, depressants, opioids, psychotherapeutics, psychotropics, prescription medications, and nicotine. Indeed, this chapter accentuates the fact that substance abuse disorders affect the mind, body, and spirit of individuals, families, and other groups.

The chapter by Jackson, Thoman, Alina, Surís, and North on working with active duty military and their trauma-related mental health needs is a particularly timely topic. The conflicts in Iraq and Afghanistan have become the longest sustained U.S. military operation since the Vietnam War and the first extended conflict to rely on an all-volunteer military, at a time when there are fewer available active duty military personnel than in previous conflicts. This situation has created a different military climate compared with previous sustained military operations, with greater dependence on National Guard and reservists, longer deployment durations, multiple deployments, and shorter intervals between deployments. As a consequence, there are a significant number of combat veterans who have unique social, cultural, medical, physical, and psychological issues.

More than one million service members have been deployed to Iraq or Afghanistan with nearly half of all soldiers having been deployed more than once. As a consequence of multiple deployments, this exposes service members in this high-risk occupation to more psychological and physical injury. In fact, more than 43,000 service members have been wounded since this conflict began. The most common injuries reported are blast wounds and soft tissue and orthopedic injuries including amputations, burns, hearing loss, and traumatic brain injury (TBI). With regard to fatalities, the Department of Defense reports that more than 6,000 soldiers have been killed in action as a result of mortar, rocket, and artillery fire; small-arms fire; multiple high-intensity blasts; roadside bombs; improvised explosive devices; and surprise sniper attacks.

Indeed, the military and their family members are a cultural unto themselves, which require specific knowledge and skills to work within this culture, as well as an understanding of the within-group differences. Military personnel are fundamentally different from the personnel of previous military operations such as the Gulf War and the Vietnam War in a number of ways. For example, women make up a larger percentage of deployed forces than ever before, comprising 14% of deployed military personnel. Compared to their civilian counterparts, military mothers are three times more likely to be single parents and five times more likely to be married to a military and deployable spouse. Many deployed female soldiers are also mothers of young children and suffer long periods of separation from their children and spouses. For deployed women, especially those who are mothers, family disruptions and family-related concerns are superimposed on the other stresses of deployment.

One of the primary issues dealt with in this particular chapter is the transition back to civilian life for active duty personnel. Overall for our service members, there are significant challenges medically, physically, socially, emotionally, psychologically, vocationally, and in many other ways. Working with individuals and family members of active duty military, as well as veterans, requires a special set of knowledge, awareness, and skills to work within this cultural group. The chapter by Jackson and colleagues focuses on the mental health problems among active duty military, as well as veterans. Special attention has been given to post-traumatic stress disorder, other psychiatric disorders, and TBI.

The next chapter by Brodwin, Sui, and Cardoso discusses the all-important topic of assistive technology (AT). The use of AT is a growing area that has made a profound impact on the quality of the lives and employment opportunities for individuals with disabilities. Brodwin et al. discuss how AT has provided greater independence in all life areas for persons with disabilities, which has enabled them to perform activities not possible in the past. For example, AT enhances social functioning, recreational activities, and work opportunities, thus decreasing client/consumer functional limitations. Overall, AT helps by "leveling the playing field" between people with disabilities and those without disabilities.

When utilizing AT, a consumer's self-worth, sense of belonging, and the attitudes of others play a dynamic role. Therefore, consumer involvement is imperative to the process. Initially, in the assessment/evaluation phase of rehabilitation, the rehabilitation counselor should help the consumer identify the priorities and motivation for requesting AT. These should be in the forefront throughout the entire process as they are key to successful implementation and use of AT. By carefully defining achievement goals with the consumer, the counselor will be able to clearly identify what he or she wants to accomplish by using technology. This involves the activities that motivate a consumer to use AT and is crucial to successful adaptation and use.

Brodwin, Sui, and Cardoso suggest that AT can also improve self-esteem, self-efficacy, and motivation, which are central elements in increasing client/consumer confidence and belief in self. These authors present the case that the use of AT leads to good person-centered outcomes, efficacy of the individual, and a strong motivation for engaging in other life areas not believed possible before. Additionally, this chapter does an excellent job presenting the human side to the use of technology and the relationship between client/consumers and these technological devices and equipment. Overall, recommendations are offered by the authors to assist rehabilitation professionals in helping consumers with accepting, utilizing, and benefiting from technology.

The chapter "Dance of Disability and Spirituality" by Boswell, Hamer, Glacoff, Knight, and McChesney employs Knight and a qualitative methodology where face-to-face interviews assess emerging themes that characterize the role of spirituality in the lives of men and women with severe disabilities. Issues of spirituality are commonly discussed in the alcohol and substance abuse literature and in materials relating to support systems such as alcoholics and narcotics anonymous. However, within the last decade, the literature concerning spirituality has expanded into a wide range of health care contexts. For example, the role of spirituality has been a mainstay research topic in the fields of oncology, traditional and mind-body medicine, energy psychology, cardiac care, and psychosocial issues related to death, dying, loss, and grief.

What makes this particular study unique is that the authors utilized an interdisciplinary team of five researchers representing different areas of expertise that included exercise and sport science, health education and promotion, recreation and leisure, and English. Also unique in the present study are the expanded findings of earlier work done by these authors that specifically focused on the spiritual experiences of women with disabilities. For instance, this study has included the perspectives of male participants with disabilities for the purpose of exploring spiritual issues. These authors accentuate the fact that spirituality plays a major role for people with disabilities in healing severe, chronic suffering and losses.

The authors further suggest there continues to be inadequate information on the perspectives of spirituality and the person's spiritual belief system. Spiritual beliefs enable people with disabilities and family members to establish meaning for the disability, which many times requires extraordinary psychosocial support. Accordingly, the authors of Chapter 22 encourage professionals to pay attention to the benefits of listening to the individual's spiritual beliefs that extend beyond one's religious beliefs. Ultimately, rehabilitation and other counseling professionals who truly want to work within a cultural context of their clients must then attend to issues of spirituality.

Rehabilitation and other counseling professionals will find Brodwin and Sui's chapter very beneficial in helping them work with women with disabilities who have been victims of abuse. This conceptual chapter is directed at informing and sensitizing counseling professionals to the critical issues of abuse, pointing to the fact that the most common type of violence against women is between intimate partners. Females constitute the vast majority of victims, while males comprise the majority of perpetrators. This crime, commonly referred to as domestic violence, intimate partner violence, spousal abuse, or wife abuse, occurs at much higher rates for women with disabilities than for women without disabilities.

Additionally, this chapter synthesizes relevant literature by presenting issues that are unique and challenging to women with disabilities. The authors provide an overview of the phenomenon of abuse, a description of specific types of abuse issues that challenge women as clients/consumers of rehabilitation counseling services, sociopathic characteristics of batterers and perpetrators, the long-term psychosocial effects of being abused, and recommendations for counselors who seek to improve the quality of life for abused women who have disabilities.

Lastly, James Herbert provides his personal perspective on the recovery and rehabilitation of his quintuple by-pass, open-heart surgery that was done in November 2002. Dr. Herbert illustrates how tapping into one's spiritual beliefs at a critical time in life can build coping and resiliency for handling the day-to-day stressors of postsurgery life. Through this experience, he shares with the reader his renewed appreciation of the ordinary, extraordinary, and unexpected outcome originating from his recovery experience.

19

Substance Use and Substance Use Disorders

CHUCK REID AND MARIA BARRERA

*T*his chapter is a basic primer on substance use disorders (SUD). SUD typically include a wide range of information; however, the material presented will focus primarily on key terms and definitions; prevalence data; patterns of use; socioeconomic, ethnic, and gender differences; and the dual diagnosis of SUD with coexisting mental and physical disabilities. There will be a brief description of drug categories and their effects on the body including stimulants, hallucinogens, marijuana, depressants, opioids, psychotherapeutics, psychotropics, prescription medications, and nicotine. Other major areas presented will be state-of-the-art treatment modalities and future directions for SUD treatment.

PREVALENCE

Today, when trying to get an overall picture of the prevalence of drug use in American society, we find that accurate information is often difficult to obtain. One issue involves the number of different data collection techniques and different reporting methods. Survey methodology is one of the most widely used techniques to report drug use. However, it is difficult to compare data and get accurate rates in terms of prevalence, when statistical techniques vary so much. Sources for prevalence data on drug use include the National Survey on Drug Use and Health (NSDUH), Monitoring for the Future, the National Alcohol Survey, the Behavioral Risk Factor Surveillance System, the Youth Risk Behavior Survey, the Drug Abuse Warning Network, and Arrestee Drug Abuse Monitoring. Prevalence data for this chapter is taken mainly from the NSDUH (Lowinson, Ruiz, Millman, & Langrod, 2005).

Illicit Drug Use

According to the NSDUH, in 2010 approximately 21.8 million Americans, age 12 and older, were users of illicit drugs. The most commonly used illicit drug was marijuana with approximately 17 million current users in the month prior to survey administration. Another 5.1 million used marijuana and another drug including psychotherapeutic drugs, pain relievers, tranquilizers, stimulants, and sedatives. Besides marijuana, there were another 9.2 million Americans who used the above-listed drugs illegally.

Age

The NSDUH developed a number of categories to indicate different rates of illicit drug use. Table 19.1 represents the basic age categories as documented in the report.

TABLE 19.1 Different Rates of Illicit Drug Use by Age

Ages	Classification of Drug (Illicit) (%)	Psychotherapeutics (%)
12–17	10.0	3.1
18–25	21.2	6.3
26 and older	6.3	2.1
50–59	6.2	None reported

Source: National Survey on Drug Use and Health (NSDUH, 2010).

Gender

Over the years, the rate of illicit drug use among males has been higher than that among females. The NSDUH (2010) stated that 10.8% of males and 6.6% of females reported using illicit drugs in the month prior to taking this survey. With regard to psychotherapeutics, 3.1% of males and 2.4% of females engaged in the nonmedical use of psychotherapeutics the month prior to responding to their survey. The difference in illicit substance use for men increases with age. Overall for females, high school seniors, college students, and young adults use illicit substances less frequently and less heavily than men.

Race/Ethnicity

The reported rate of illicit drug use among persons ages 12 years and older varied by race and ethnicity in 2009. The data report that the highest group of illicit drug users include Native American or Alaska Indians (18.3%). The following racial and ethnic groups who were illicit drug users and who considered themselves biracial include Blacks (9.6%); Whites (8.8%); Hispanics (7.9%); and Asians (3.7%). Two races, age 12 years and older, that had an increase in the rate of illicit drug use from 2008 to 2009 were American Indians or Alaska Natives (from 9.5% to 18.3%) and Hispanics (from 6.2% to 7.9%). According to Lowinson et al. (2005), these rates are inconsistent with the rates at which these racial/ethnic groups appear in treatment or prison.

Disability/Comorbidity

Approximately 54 million Americans live with a disability. People with disabilities are unemployed or underemployed at higher rates compared to the general population. This problem persists for people who have graduate and professional degrees and is compounded for persons with mental and physical disabilities and SUD. Studies indicate that people with disabilities and SUD experience greater social, employment, and educational barriers (Hollar, 2008).

Dual diagnosis (comorbidity) has been an issue for people who use substances; one aspect of comorbidity or dual diagnosis is a person who has a mental illness and SUD. It is estimated that 8% of patients with psychiatric disabilities have chemical dependency issues. In the past, there has been conflict in the treatment community concerning what treatment modality would best serve this population. More recently, the concept of dual diagnosis has been more refined, and the two disorders are being addressed simultaneously (Lowinson et al., 2005). Dual diagnosis also represents persons who have physical disabilities and SUDS. Research indicates that people with disabilities and SUD incur at a much higher rate than the general population. Prevalence data vary. Some studies report the prevalence with SUD as low as 12% and others a high of 60% depending on the type of disability (West, Graham, & Cifu, 2009).

A myriad of issues exist for people with SUD within the state/federal system of vocational rehabilitation. These issues include, but are not limited to, lower success with case closure, a lack of staff knowledge of problems relating to this population, negative staff perceptions of this population, specialized transportation needs, and social and interpersonal relationship issues (Hollar, 2008). More detailed information regarding prevalence data, group information, demographic information, and geographic data can be found in the NSDUH (2010).

SUD: TERMS AND DEFINITIONS

Before addressing drugs used and treatment issues that are important for individuals with SUD, it is necessary to provide some definitions that will assist in understanding the concepts that will be addressed in the treatment section of this chapter. Hart and Ksir (2011) provide an excellent appendix of drug (product and generic) names, as well as a glossary of terms and definitions commonly used in SUD. The information provided is in a clear, concise manner and covers terms used in the prevention and treatment of SUD. The terms and definitions provided in this chapter were taken from this work.

- **Abstinence.** Refraining completely from the use of alcohol or another drug. Complete abstinence from alcohol means no drinking at all. Abstinence syndrome.
- **Additive effects.** When the effects of two different drugs add up to produce a greater effect than either alone. As contrasted with antagonistic effects, in which one drug reduces the effect of the other, or synergetic effects, in which one drug greatly amplifies the effect of the other.
- **Affective education.** In general, education that focuses on emotional content or emotional reactions in contrast to cognitive content. In drug education, one example is learning how to achieve "feelings" (of excitement or belonging to a group) without using drugs.
- **Alcohol.** Generally refers to grain alcohol, or ethanol, as opposed to other types of alcohol (for example, wood or isopropyl alcohol), which are too toxic to be drinkable.
- **Alcohol abuse.** In the *Diagnostic and Statistical Manual of Mental Disorders, 4th ed., Text Revision (DSM-IV-TR)*, alcohol abuse is defined as a pattern of pathological alcohol use that causes impairment of social or occupational functioning. Compare with alcohol dependence.
- **Alcohol dependence.** In the *DSM-IV-TR*, alcohol dependence is considered a more serious disorder than alcohol abuse in that dependence includes either tolerance or withdrawal symptoms.
- **Alcoholics Anonymous (AA).** A worldwide organization of self-help groups based on alcoholics helping each other to achieve and maintain sobriety.
- **Alcoholism.** The word has many definitions and therefore is not a precise term. Definitions might refer to pathological drinking behavior (e.g., remaining drunk for two days), to impaired functioning (e.g., frequently missing work), or to physical dependence.
- **Blood alcohol concentration (BAC).** Also called blood alcohol level. The proportion of blood that consists of alcohol. For example, a person with a BAC of 0.10% has alcohol constituting one tenth of 1% of the blood and is legally intoxicated in all states.
- **Behavioral tolerance.** Repeated use of a drug can lead to a diminished effect of the drug (tolerance). When the diminished effect occurs because the individual has learned to compensate for the effect of the drug, it is called "behavioral tolerance." For example, a novice drinker might be unable to walk with a BAC of 0.20%, whereas someone who has practiced while intoxicated would be able to walk fairly well at the same BAC.

- **Biopsychosocial**. A theory or perspective that relies on the interaction of biological, individual psychological, and social variables.
- **Brand name**. The name given to a drug by a particular manufacturer and licensed only to that manufacturer. For example, Valium is a brand name for diazepam. Other companies may sell diazepam, but Hoffman-LaRoche, Inc. owns the name Valium.
- **Chemical name**. The name that is descriptive of a drug's chemical structure. For example, the chemical name sodium chloride is associated with the generic name table salt, of which there may be several brand names, such as Morton's.
- **Controlled drinking**. The concept that individuals who have been drinking pathologically can be taught to drink in a controlled, nonpathological manner.
- **Delirium tremens**. Alcohol withdrawal symptoms, including tremors and hallucinations.
- **Drug**. Any substance, natural or artificial, other than food that by its chemical nature alters structure or function in the living organism.
- **Drug abuse**. The use of a drug in such a manner or in such amounts or in situations such that the drug use causes problems or greatly increases the chance of problems occurring.
- **Drug dependence**. A state in which a person uses a drug so frequently and consistently that the individual appears to need the drug to function. This may take the form of physical dependence, or behavioral signs may predominate (e.g., unsuccessful attempts to stop or reduce drug use).
- **Drug misuse**. The use of prescribed drugs in greater amounts than, or for purposes other than, those prescribed by a physician or dentist.
- **Generic name**. For drugs, a name that specifies a particular chemical without being chemically descriptive or referring to a brand name. As an example, the chemical name sodium chloride is associated with the generic name table salt, of which there may be several brand names, such as Morton's.
- **Medical model**. With reference to mental disorders, a model that assumes that abnormal behaviors are symptoms resulting from a disease.
- **Narcotic**. Opioids (in pharmacology terms), or a drug that is produced or sold illegally (in legal terms); in the United States, a "controlled substance."
- **Side effects**. Unintended drug effects that accompany the desired therapeutic effect.
- **Withdrawal syndrome**. The set of symptoms that occur reliably when someone stops taking a drug; also called "abstinence syndrome."

SUBSTANCES: CATEGORIES AND EFFECTS

The court system, physicians, chemists, psychologists, addictionologists, psychopharmacologists, and criminologists all have different ways of categorizing substances and their effects. For the purpose of this chapter, we will use the basic categories presented in Hart and Ksir (2011). According to Hart and Ksir, the seven main categories of psychoactive drugs are stimulants, hallucinogens, marijuana, depressants (including alcohol), opioids, psychotherapeutics, and nicotine. Nicotine and psychotherapeutics will not be discussed in this chapter.

Stimulants

The major stimulant drugs of abuse are amphetamines, cocaine, and methamphetamines. These drugs have similar effects on the brain, central nervous system, and physiology.

Stimulant drugs produce wakefulness and a sense of energy and well-being at moderate doses. Acute effects at low and moderate doses have certain physiological and behavioral effects on human beings. Except for duration, the effects of the amphetamines and cocaine are similar. The physiological effects of these substances include increased blood pressure and heart rate, sweating, and respiration. Other physiological effects are an increase of blood flow to the large muscle groups and the brain and a decrease in flow to the internal organs and extremities. Also noted was the dilation of pupils and elevated body temperature. Amphetamines and cocaine also suppress appetite (anorectic effects). Because of the side effects of amphetamines in particular, some individuals may take this class of drug as diet pills. Those who lose weight typically must take larger doses to maintain the weight loss. After the person terminates its use, then they typically gain weight again. However, the negative side effect of amphetamines is drug dependency. Thus, the medical community rarely uses this drug for the treatment of obesity (Maisto, Galizio, & Connors, 2008).

According to Newton, De la Garza, Kalechstein, and Nestor (2005), the behavioral effects of stimulants are a major draw for those who use these drugs. Some behavioral effects of low and moderate doses of amphetamines and cocaine produce mood elevation and a sense of elation. Individuals showed increased sociability, talkativeness, arousal, and alertness. Insomnia also often develops in the individual. It has also been noted that these stimulants enhance performance on a number of physical and mental tasks. Stimulants decrease boredom and increase resistance to fatigue and are oftentimes used as a study aid (amphetamine-induced all-nighters). One issue with this type of stimulant use is that information learned under the influence of a drug is best remembered when an individual attempts to recall it in the same drug-induced state. This is called "state-dependent learning." This phenomenon suggests that people will have problems learning information when under the influence of a drug because the ability to retrieve the information will not be as good as when the person is sober (Poling & Cross, 1993).

Another popular myth about cocaine and methamphetamines deals with their ability to increase sexual prowess. While some users have reported strong sexual feelings and performance with stimulants, most people do not. For men, cocaine and methamphetamine use may increase sexual desire, but the drugs often cause impotence by causing erectile dysfunction (Maisto et al., 2008). Recently, a new trend in the gay community is to combine stimulant drugs with drugs designed to treat erectile dysfunction (e.g., Viagra, Levitra). This combination seems to allow the user to maintain an erection while under the influence of methamphetamines. The combination, however, has been associated with risky sexual behavior and increased probability of HIV with men and women who have unprotected sex (Halkitis, Shrem, & Martin, 2005).

Maisto et al. (2008) reported that there are a number of acute and chronic effects related to frequent and high doses of stimulants such as amphetamines, cocaine, and methamphetamines. High doses of stimulant drugs are known to produce a psychotic state and are often more serious than use of methamphetamines or crack cocaine itself. The most common symptom of stimulant psychosis is paranoid delusions. Another common symptom is compulsive stereotyped behavior such as hair pulling, chain smoking, or body rocking, as well as hallucinations. Additionally, there is a high risk of overdose with cocaine or amphetamine use.

Regular and long-term use of stimulants over time creates multiple problems. One problem is that users may develop a tolerance for the drug where higher doses are required to achieve the same effects. Many other users show physical signs of withdrawal, dependency, depression, changes in appetite, sleep disturbances, anxiety, and cravings for the drug (Doweiko, 2009).

Hallucinogens

Another class of drugs is the hallucinogens where over a hundred different hallucinogenic plants and mushrooms have been identified. This chapter will cover some of the more well-known hallucinogens. As many of these drugs have similar effects, the most widely used hallucinogens such as mescaline/peyote, LSD, and psilocybin (mushrooms), and effects of amphetamine-like drugs will also be covered.

According to the NSDUH (2010), 1.3 million persons aged 12 or older reported using hallucinogens for the first time within the past 12 months. Compared to the number of people who use alcohol and marijuana, the users of hallucinogens are not as prevalent. Hallucinogens that are most commonly abused can be divided into four main groups: phenylalkylamines such as mescaline and MDMA; ergot alkaloid derivatives such as LSD; indolealkylamines such as psilocybin and DMT; and atypical hallucinogenic compounds such as ibogaine (Glennon, 2004).

According to Fields (2010), major hallucinogenic effects are influenced by the personality of the user, the expectations of the drug, the user's overall general experience with taking illicit drugs, the state of mind of the individual and, most important, the setting in which the individual uses. The adverse effects of hallucinogens can sometimes add to existing neuroses and personality disorders, and can produce transient waves of mild anxiety, paranoia, or severe panic. Users of hallucinogens often report a wide range of reactions. Low to moderate doses of hallucinogens produce alterations in mood and perception. They distort space and time perception and induce hallucinations. Some users report a sense of insight and expanded awareness, while others report discomfort or a fear of loss of control.

Hallucinogens that act on serotonin receptors have comparable effects although they differ in potency, duration of action, and other pharmacological variables. The most potent of this class is LSD. Doses as low as 25 µg can produce effects. Doses range from about 12 µg to as much as 350 µg as found on the street. Street preparations include windowpane, tablets, and blotter (Dal Cason & Franzosa, 2003). Hawks and Chiang (1986) noted that LSD is absorbed rapidly and effects are felt within 20 to 60 minutes after administration. These effects last for 8 to 12 hours, and the drug is quickly metabolized and eliminated from the body. Seventy-two hours after use, neither LSD nor its metabolites can be detected by urine tests.

According to Grinspoon and Baker (1979), psilocybin and mescaline are less potent than LSD. Psilocybin is about 1% as potent as LSD. Tolerance builds with most serotonergic drugs, and there is also cross-tolerance among them. Mescaline is consumed by eating peyote buttons. Five to 20 buttons provide the user with about 200 to 800 mg of mescaline, with effects lasting about 12 to 14 hours. The lowest effective dose is about 200 mg. Overall, it is reported that mescaline is about 1/3000 as potent as LSD (Strassman, 2005).

There have been a number of adverse effects attributed to serotonergic hallucinogens. It was once claimed that these substances caused damage to chromosomes resulting in birth defects in the children of users. Research in this area showed no credible evidence of increased childhood disabilities when the drug was taken in normal doses. In higher doses, there may be a possible risk of fetal damage if taken by pregnant women (Grinspoon & Baker, 1979). Grinspoon and Baker identified panic reactions and acute panic reactions to serotonergic hallucinogens as another issue of concern. These issues could lead to a psychotic state where the person may cause harm to self or others. In order to avoid "bad trips," users should stay in a comfortable place, be reminded that they are on a drug, and use lower doses of the drug. However, even with these precautions, problems could occur.

Abraham, Aldridge, and Gogia (1996) addressed the issue of flashbacks with the use of serotonergic hallucinogens. Flashbacks may be brought on by marijuana use, fatigue, stress, or when the person is in a dark environment. Re-experiencing flashbacks can occur months or years after use and can manifest as visual trails, visual perceptions, intensified colors, halos around objects, or color flashes. Halpern and Pope (2003) stated that in most instances, the flashbacks caused little or no problem, but in a small number of users they may be life disrupting. In extreme cases, individuals may be given the *DSM-IV-TR* diagnoses of hallucinogen persisting perception disorder. The accepted treatment for this disorder is with the use of benzodiazepines (BZ) or with antipsychotics.

Serotonergic hallucinogens have been associated with long-term psychiatric disorders. It is often difficult to decide whether the drug caused the psychosis or if the person was predisposed to psychosis before taking the drug. Another issue is that users of serotonergic hallucinogens often have histories with using other drugs as well. A consensus of the research seems to indicate that when psychiatric problems arise following the use of serotonergic hallucinogens, it usually involves people who have already been diagnosed with psychotic symptoms or manifested prepsychotic symptoms before using the drugs (Halpern & Pope, 1999; Meyer & Quenzer, 2005).

Marijuana

Marijuana, also known as cannabis sativa, is a hemp plant that grows freely throughout the world. According to the NSDUH (2010), marijuana is the most commonly used illicit drug. Data gathered as part of the 2009 NSDUH revealed 16.7 million reported that they used marijuana within the past month of being surveyed. A breakdown by age of current marijuana users reports that among those aged 12 to 17, 7.3% are users; among those aged 18 to 25, 18.1% are users; and among those aged 26 and older, 4.6% are users.

Marijuana is a relatively popular drug, yet the mechanism by which it affects normal brain functioning is not fully known (Sussman & Westreich, 2003). According to Hart and Ksir (2011), there are at least 400 different compounds in the cannabis plant of which 70 are unique to cannabis, while 61 of these have psychoactive effects.

The single compound in marijuana, Δ9-tetrahydrocannabinol (THC), is the most active ingredient, which was first identified in 1964 (Nicoll & Alger, 2004). Once THC is in the body, it is transformed into a metabolite that seems to cause its effects on the central nervous system. THC mimics the effects of at least one naturally occurring neurotransmitter, anandamide, but is 4 to 20 times as more potent (Martin, 2004). According to Maisto et al. (2008), THC is highly lipid soluble and is almost entirely insoluble in water. THC is deposited in various organs after being carried through the bloodstream. Metabolization occurs mainly in the liver, but the substance can be metabolized in other organs as well. The THC metabolites are execrated through the urine and feces. THC can be detected in the urine for more than 30 days, depending on the level of use.

According to Maisto et al. (2008), the evidence as to the development of tolerance in humans with the use of cannabis is unclear. Studies have been conflicting. What researchers do know is that if tolerance does exist it occurs with higher doses over longer periods of use. To date, the mechanisms by which tolerance occurs are still unknown. Another issue involving cannabis is the concept of physical dependence. Smith (2002) indicated that there is no identifiable withdrawal syndrome. Jones (1980) describes several aspects associated with dependence. These aspects included sleep disturbance, nausea, irritability, and anxiety. At the current time, it seems that aspects of physical dependence most likely are associated with sustained heavy use of cannabis.

Over the past few decades, there have been efforts to legalize cannabis. This effort has been promoted by an increased use of cannabis by HIV/AIDS patients. Medical researchers claim that cannabis decreases the vomiting and nausea associated with their disease. They also note that cannabis stimulates the appetite and assists them in regaining weight. A number of states have passed laws allowing the use of cannabis for medical purposes. There have also been successful efforts to create cannabis clubs in a number of cities. Cannabis has also been used to treat cachexia, a disorder associated with HIV infection or cancer where an individual physiologically wastes away (Maisto et al., 2008). Cannabis has also been used successfully in the treatment of glaucoma (Joy, Watson, & Benson, 1999).

Acute and long-term effects of cannabis include the effects on cardiovascular, immune, respiratory, and reproductive systems. The short-term physiological effects on people who are in good health are not remarkable. These short-term effects include, but are not limited to, bloodshot eyes, slow reaction to light, increased heart rate and pulse, increased hunger, and decreased motor activity. There is no evidence to date suggesting long-term use of cannabis produces any significant threat to the cardiovascular or immune systems in healthy adults. There is the possibility that heavy and prolonged use of cannabis may result in irreversible damage to the respiratory system. Another area of potential concern with long-term heavy use of cannabis is the effects on the reproductive system. Some male users show decreases in the mobility of sperm and the number of sperm, and heavy use by women can affect the menstrual cycle. Pregnant women should avoid the use of cannabis. More research is needed to obtain more accurate information on the short- and long-term effects of cannabis use (Lowinson et al., 2005; Maisto et al., 2008).

Psychological effects of cannabis include cognitive, behavioral, emotional, social, and environmental effects. The major cognitive effects of cannabis are short-term memory impairment, the perception of time moving slowly, and the inability to attend and focus on ideas. Cannabis has behavioral effects on a person's psychomotor activity and impairs motor coordination when driving a motor vehicle. Individuals who use cannabis often times have certain emotional effects that can be positive or negative depending on the users past experiences and expectancies. For example, positive emotional effects consist of the user feeling a carefree or relaxed experience depending on the cannabis dose. The negative emotional effects of cannabis use are associated with anxiety or dysphoria and can occur more frequently than anticipated. The social and environmental effects generally associated with cannabis use are known as the "amotivational syndrome." Amotivational syndrome has been described by McGlothin and West (1968) as the decrease of ambition, loss of goals, and apathy of the user. The occurrence of amotivational syndrome is more prevalent among the younger population of cannabis users.

Depressants

The depressant category of psychoactive drugs as classified by Hart and Ksir (2011) includes alcohol, barbiturates, sleeping pills and other sedatives, and inhalants. These substances for the most part are central nervous system depressants, with alcohol being the most predominate and widely used in our society.

Although there has been a great deal of research addressing the neurobiology of alcohol, those findings are beyond the scope of this chapter. The focus here will be on the clinical aspects of alcohol. For a comprehensive overview of the research, see Lowinson et al. (2005). Alcohol dependence is classified as a disease and is caused by a combination of social, cultural, genetic, and environmental factors. Alcohol dependence is not a single disorder; it consists of subtypes with varying degrees of psychosocial and biological origins (*DSM-IV-TR,* 2000). There is no set pattern identified for the progression of this disease ranging from moderate, heavy, alcohol dependence. Yet, there seems to be some well-defined characteristics of the progression to alcohol dependence.

Lowinson et al. (2005) postulates that binge drinking to the point of intoxication may be an early sign of alcohol dependence, as well as some emotional factors indicating a craving for this substance. The peer culture of drinking seems to play a part in the progression of this disorder as does the concept of tolerance, which suggests that the person who craves the need for more alcohol must drink larger quantities to achieve the same effect. When drinking to intoxication becomes a behavior pattern, alcohol-related problems tend to increase. These problems include, but are not limited to, losing days at work, driving while intoxicated, interpersonal relationship issues, blackouts, hangovers, impaired performance in a number of life areas, feelings of remorse or guilt, and alcohol-dependence syndrome. Medical problems such as alcohol-induced psychotic disorder, Wernicke's encephalopathy, liver disease (liver cirrhosis and fatty liver), peripheral neuropathy, and Korsakoff's syndrome are also prevalent. Finally, for long-term heavy drinkers, alcohol withdrawal can be a serious problem. Symptoms of withdrawal vary in intensity from signs of over activity, sweating and heart palpitations, to the syndrome of delirium tremens. Delirium tremens can manifest as visual, auditory, and tactile hallucinations. Anywhere from 5% to 15% of people with delirium tremens die from the syndrome.

Another class of depressants is the barbiturates. All the substances in this class share the compound barbituric acid. The chemical differences in the compounds effect the time of absorption, biotransformation, distribution, and excretion from moderate to heavy. The lipid solubility manifests in their potency and onset of action. More lipid-soluble compounds have a faster onset and greater potency (Ropper & Brown, 2005). According to Doweiko (2009), duration of action is one way to classify barbiturates. The first group is the ultrashort barbiturates. Their effects start in seconds and last for less than 30 minutes. This class includes drugs such as Brevital and Pentothal. The short-acting compounds, of which Nembutal is an example, act rapidly with effects lasting from 3 to 4 hours. Amytal and butisol are examples of the most common intermediate-duration barbiturates. These compounds take effect in about an hour and last from 6 to 8 hours. The most common long-acting barbiturate is phenobarbital. This class is absorbed slowly and lasts from 6 to 12 hours. Ciraulo, Ciraulo, Sands, Knapp, and Sarid-Segal (2005) stated that low-dose users of barbiturates reported feeling a sensation of euphoria, reduced anxiety, sedation, decreased motor activity, difficulties coordinating movement, disinhibition, excitement, and rage. Users also reported side effects such as mental slowness, dizziness, and nausea. Barbiturates are often used to induce sleep, but research by Drummer and Odell (2001) pointed out that these substances are not effective for sleep after a few days of continued use and tolerance develops quickly.

Charney, Mihic, and Harris (2006) identified the rapid eye movement (REM) rebound effect where loss of REM sleep causes the person to have vivid and at times nightmarish dreams. These dreams can lead the person to resume the drug use to avoid the dreams. Because barbiturates often have a long half-life, users often experience a drug-induced hangover the day after use as noted by Wilson, Shannon, and Shields (2007). Finger, Lund and Slagel (1997) showed that the use of barbiturates could cause sexual problems such as decreased sexual desire, delayed ejaculation, and erectile problems in men. Other issues with barbiturates are tolerance and dependence and unintentional overdose as noted by Charney et al. (2006). Barbiturate-like drugs such as Miltown, Quaalude, Soper, Doriden, Placidyl, and Noludar were thought to be safe and effective replacements for barbiturates. However, researchers have shown that they are similar to barbiturates in their potential for abuse (Doweiko, 2009).

Opiates

The frequency of opiate abuse has had a major impact on the production and consumption of this substance. The availability of pure and very potent heroin has increased the number of individuals dependent upon the substance to 900,000 in the United States (Inciardi, 2002). Some of the major opiate compounds include morphine, heroin, hydrocodone, hydromorphone, codeine, and oxycodone. The illicit use of opiate prescription such as Oxycontin has become very prevalent among young people. Oxycontin pills can be taken at 20-, 40-, and 80-mg tablets and are administered by crushing the pill to produce a powder that can be injected or snorted. There are opiate drugs that are also known as "designer" drugs. Designer heroin also known as "China White" is more likely to increase the chances of death or overdose because it is often made by compounds that are untested (Maisto et al., 2008).

Opiate drugs can be administered nasally, intravenously, or subcutaneously, or can be smoked. When the opiate reaches the bloodstream, it passes into the body and accumulates in the kidneys, lungs, liver, spleen, digestive tract, muscles, and brain. The strength of heroin and its lipid solubility allow for saturation in the blood–brain barrier. The emission of opiates is a fast process that happens in the liver through the kidneys into the urine within 2 to 4 days after use. Opiate use produces acute psychological and physiological effects. Some psychological effects opiate users experience include vivid dreams otherwise known as pipe dreams and the feeling of heavy limbs. Unlike depressants, opiates have acute physiological effects that cause respiratory depression and low body temperature. Most opiate users also experience nausea, vomiting, and constriction of the pupils (Maisto et al., 2008).

Inhalants

Inhalants are another group of abused substances. It is difficult to ascertain the prevalence of inhalant abuse and that is particularly true in the adult population. It has been estimated that approximately one in ten people from eighth graders to adults have used solvents/gases to alter their consciousness (Lowinson et al., 2005). The vast majority of these people are adolescents. Most of them will use inhalants a few times, stop, and do not develop other problems (Crowley & Sakai, 2005). Spray paint and gasoline are the most widely used compounds; they account for approximately 61% of inhalants that are abused (Spiller & Krenzelok, 1997). Patterns of inhalant abuse were identified by Hernandez-Avila and Pierucci-Lagha (2005). The four patterns are transient social use, chronic social use, transient isolated use, and chronic isolated use. Transient social use involves users of 10 to 16 years of age and only occurs for a brief period of time. The chronic social users are 20 to 30 years of age and have daily use that can result in brain damage. A transient isolated user is 10 to 16 years of age and has a brief history of secluded inhalant use. An individual considered to have chronic isolated use typically is aged 20 to 29, abuses this drug alone, and has a pattern of continuous abuse for more than 5 years.

The methods of administration for inhalants predominantly consist of sniffing or snorting the chemical from the container. Other users have a process called "bagging" where they will place the bag of glue over his or her mouth and inhale. Another practice for users of inhalants is described as "huffing." The individual will place a rag that has been wet with inhalant chemicals over his or her mouth and nose for absorption. Finally, a recent method of administration has been found by Nelson (2000), where the individual boils the inhalant and attempts to inhale the fumes. According to Doweiko (2009), there are certain complications from inhalant abuse that may result in the user experiencing toxicity or death. Worcester (2006) reported that some of the consequences include liver and kidney damage, respiratory conditions, depression, reduction in blood cell production possibly from aplastic anemia, and permanent muscle damage. Because the use of inhalants is so prevalent among young adults, the profound effects usually occur on the central nervous system. There is a continuum of inhalant abuse that can lead to death because this can happen on the first-time use or the 200th time. Depression and suicidal ideation have been associated with the abuse of inhalants among adolescents (Espeland, 1997).

The abuse of varied forms of nitrates includes amyl nitrate, butyl nitrite, and isobutyl nitrite. Both butyl nitrite and isobutyl nitrite are sold legally at mail-order houses or in specialty stores, depending on the state laws. Amyl nitrite, obtained through prescription, may cause dizziness, giddiness, or rapid dilation of blood vessels in the head (Schwartz, 1989).

Benzodiazepines and Similar Sedative Hypnotics

BZ and similar sedative hypnotics have largely replaced barbiturates in medical therapeutics and in incidences of abuse (Lowinson et al., 2005). Gitlow (2007) reported that BZs are safer than barbiturates and have been found to be effective in the treatment of a number of disorders such as the control of seizures, symptoms of anxiety, insomnia, and muscle strains. They are the most widely prescribed psychotropic medications in the world. Yearly in the United States, BZ use and abuse result in hundreds of millions of dollars in unnecessary medical costs (Doweiko, 2009).

As stated above, BZs have a number of medical uses and this often leads to overprescribing by doctors. In particular, psychotherapists are often opposed to treating anxiety with tranquilizers because they are concerned that treatment with these drugs will undermine patients' motivation to do therapeutic work (Lowinson et al., 2005). Lowinson et al. also state that drug abuse counselors oppose medication of any kind and particularly the sedative hypnotics. They view all mind-altering drugs as a risk factor for addicts because these drugs may trigger a return to drug-seeking behavior.

All BZs have similar effects with the difference in their duration of action. BZs are classified using pharmacological characteristics, which are often based on their therapeutic half-lives (Charney et al., 2006):

1. Ultra-short acting (<4 hours or less)
2. Short acting (<6 hours)
3. Intermediate acting (6 to 24 hours)
4. Long acting (24+ hours)

BZs are compared with barbiturates, but they have a larger safety margin than barbiturates and are more selective in their action. BZ molecules bind to gated chloride channels in the neuron wall that is normally activated by gamma aminobutyric acid. Although these medications have been used for over 50 years, there is disagreement about their effectiveness long term. Some researchers believe that the antianxiety effects are not useful in treating continuous anxiety over a long period of time, while others view the BZs as being effective in the long-term control of anxiety. Most evidence suggests that patients become tolerant to the antianxiety effects of the BZs, although they may reach therapeutic limits in which the drug seems to be less effective. Caution should be exercised when increasing dose levels to avoid patients seeking relaxation rather than just the relief of anxiety (Doweiko, 2009). Lowinson et al. (2005) found some adverse effects with the use of BZs. There is also the issue of addiction, dependence, and tolerance. Additionally, some behaviors reported with higher doses used for extended periods of time includes hostility, rebound insomnia, major depression, amnesia, and aggressive or violent behavior. BZs can produce toxic psychosis, a type of organic brain syndrome and changes in cognition. BZs may present some reinforcing or desirable effects in people who have abused other drugs. Most nondrug abusers or nonanxious people do not report these desirable effects. In case drug dependence does develop, the classic treatment is a gradual withdrawal from the drug (BZ).

There is another set of compounds that are unrelated to BZs or barbiturates. These include buspirone, Rohypnol, zolpidem, zaleplon, and Rozerem. Currently, there is active and ongoing research to ascertain the benefits and liabilities of these medications (Doweiko, 2009).

TREATMENT

The purpose of this section is to briefly describe the major components treatment for people with substance abuse issues. A brief description of assessment, diagnosis, prevention, and treatment modalities will be discussed. The number of theoretical models and treatment modalities is vast. A thorough presentation is beyond the confines of this chapter. Thus, some of the major theoretical concepts in substance abuse treatment are presented.

Substance abuse issues are complex and multidimensional. When counselors equate abstinence with being healthy and nonabstinence with being unhealthy, treatment becomes simplistic. This view, however, does not take into consideration that abstinence is not the only goal of treatment and does not allow for individualized treatment approaches. Further, it ignores ongoing research that indicates that chemical dependency can have many patterns of use, misuse, and abuse. There can be many causes for chemical dependency, so treatment should be multimodal to address the individualized needs of each client in order to address the person's unique pattern of use or abuse. With this broader view of substance abuse, it is possible to better understand, assess, diagnose, and treat the person with a more individualized approach (Lewis, Dana, & Blevins, 2002).

Lewis et al. (2002) noted that assessment is a way of finding the causes and nature of the client's issues. It is a way to collect information, allow the clients the opportunity to ask questions, clarify client's and counselor's roles, and increase the counselor's understanding of the client's needs. Hansen and Emrick (1985) pointed out the importance of avoiding predetermined ideas about the client and determine treatment decisions based on data collected from the assessment and other available information. These decisions should take into account the client's background and culture. Lack of sensitivity to these issues and a simplistic view of treatment can seriously limit the counselor's effectiveness. Lewis et al. (2002) listed a number of assessment instruments that can be used in clinical settings. These instruments include the Comprehensive Drinking Profile, the Michigan Alcoholism Screening Test, the Substances Abuse Problem Checklist, the Questionnaire on Drinking and Drug Abuse, the Alcohol Dependence Scale, the Addiction Severity Index, and the Time-line Follow-Back Assessment Method. They also described instruments to assess cognitive-behavioral factors. These included the Inventory of Drinking Situations, the Cognitive Appraisal Questionnaire, and the Situational Confidence Questionnaire.

The *DSM-IV-TR* (2000) is the main diagnostic tool in the United States for the diagnosis of psychiatric disorders attributable to usable substances. It is comparable to the ICD-10, which is used in Europe. The disorders in the *DSM-IV-TR* (2000) are separated into two types. The first type identifies disorders that relate to the pattern of use and/or consequences of substance use itself, such as abuse or dependence. The second type includes disorders caused by the pharmacologic effects of the substances, such as intoxication, withdrawal, and substance-induced mental disorders (Lowinson et al., 2005). For a more complete description, see the *DSM-IV-TR* (2000).

Prevention relates to actions that decrease the incidences of substance abuse or at least stabilizes the number of cases of substance abuse. The goal of prevention programs is a point of disagreement for many counselors. An older view sees the purpose of prevention as a means to maintain or achieve abstinence, while a newer view focuses on harm reduction and responsible use. Specific abstinence goals such as minors not using substances have been shown to be more successful than total prohibition. The success of specific abstinence models and the failure of total abstinence approaches have led to the increased support for the harm reduction model. Proponents of harm reduction emphasize the reduction of the harm caused to society and the individual by drug or alcohol use rather than blanket abstinence. A number of prevention programs have been shown to be effective. These programs include mass media programs, educational programs, economic control, legal restrictions, parenting programs, drug-free workplaces, drug abuse resistance education, community peer-based programs, community-based programs facilitated by licensed professionals, and combined psychoeducational and treatment programs. These community-based education and treatment programs may be the state-of-the-art in prevention and treatment for people with substance use or abuse issues. In a personal communication with Reynaldo Vela (director) (personal communication, June 10, 2011) of A Helping Hand (AHEAD), he stated that "the provision of services must be client centered and administered in a holistic manner. The Helping Hand (AHEAD) agency assists clients by providing multiple services in one location and helping the clients conserve resources."

Research has shown that the majority of people with substance abuse issues resolve them without treatment. Sobell and Sobell (1993) reported that 57% of participants in their studies weighed the costs and benefits of their substance use and as the disadvantages of their abuse grew, therapeutic change took place. Change was immediate for 29% of the participants in their studies. Kessler et al. (2001) noted that remission without treatment happens often but that many individuals with substance abuse disorders do seek the help of treatment resources.

One treatment resource is self-help groups. These groups are usually run by peers although practitioners often include the use of these groups in their treatment. Established in 1935, AA is the oldest self-help group as noted by Emrick, Lassen, and Edwards (1977). The basis of AA is alcohol and drug recovery through group participation following the twelve-step program, which guides people on the road to recovery. Group meetings facilitate recovery with the use of peer association, learning through the experiences of others, and building social relationships with others that do not use substances.

According to Miller and Hester (1980), there are numerous models and theories to explain substance abuse behaviors. Miller and Hester use five basic categories. These categories are the moral model, the American disease model, the biological model, the social learning model, and the sociocultural model. The American disease model postulates that substance dependence is a progressive, irreversible disease with psychological, physical, and spiritual causes. People with the disease need to be identified, confronted, and helped so they may accept that they have the disease. Once this is done, they are persuaded to abstain from substances. The hallmark of the biological model is that substance dependence is seen as a result of physiological or genetic processes. The pharmacology of drug actions falls under this category. The treatment in this model warns those who may be at risk and counsels them to avoid substances. The concept that SUDs are caused by complex learning from the interaction of a person with the environment identifies the social learning theory model. This type of treatment is straightforward, rewards nondrug–using behaviors, and punishes drug–using behavior. The sociocultural model states that culture and societies influence substance-use patterns. Treatment interventions here are societal in nature. The concept of a combination of these models, the biopsychosocial model, has been proposed and has been widely researched with much support in recent years.

Maisto et al. (2008) identified a number of treatment settings. The main categories here were hospital settings, intermediate settings, and outpatient settings. Thombs (2006) discussed the application of different psychotherapies to the treatment of people with chemical dependency issues. Thombs addressed ways that psychoanalytic models, conditioning models, and cognitive models could be modified to address the specific needs of substance-abusing clients. He also addressed ways of modifying the family system model for use with chemical dependency issues, as well as the inclusion of social and cultural factors in the treatment of chemical dependency.

Perhaps the goal of all treatment for people with chemical dependency issues is the same. That goal may be to assist people in functioning well in society. The purpose of treatment should be to assist people in increasing their level of functioning and reducing their use of substances and preventing harm to themselves and to society.

Motivational interviewing can be defined as any clinical strategy designed to enhance client motivation for change. There are a number of effective motivational interventions. These interventions include FRAMES (feedback, responsibility, advice, menu, empathy, self-efficacy) approach, personal contact with clients not in treatment, flexible pacing, decisional balance exercises, and discrepancies between personal goals and current behavior. The FRAMES approach consists of six elements: responsibility for change, feedback regarding personal or risk impairment, advice about changing, empathetic counseling, menus of self-directed change option, and self-efficacy or empowering the client to believe that change is possible (Miller & Sanchez, 1994).

According to Miller and Rollnick (1991), motivational interviewing is a process where the counselor becomes a helper and expresses acceptance of the client. Motivational interviewing is a journey in which even clients with low readiness to try can benefit from the process. The following assumptions are based on motivational interviewing as a counseling style. These assumptions are ambivalence about change; ambivalence is solved by working on client values, collaborative partnership between counselor and client, showing empathy, support, and a directive counseling style that points out cognitive dissonance or contradictory client statements with being argumentative.

Noonan and Moyers (1997) concluded that motivational interviewing is a useful clinical intervention and is an effective, efficient, and adaptive therapeutic style worthy of further development, application, and research. Motivational interviewing can be used effectively in managed care because it is cost-effective, time efficient, effective, mobilizes client resources, and emphasizes client motivation to enhance adherence. Table 19.2 shows the template for change using motivational interviewing, according to Miller and Rollnick (1991).

TABLE 19.2 Stage-Specific Motivational Conflicts

Stage of Change	Client Conflict
Precontemplation	I don't see how my cocaine use warrants concern, but I hope that by agreeing to talk about it, my wife will feel reassured.
Contemplation	I can picture how quitting heroin would improve my self-esteem, but I can't imagine never shooting up gain.
Preparation	I'm feeling good about setting a quit date, but I'm wondering if I have the courage to follow through.
Action	Staying clean for the past 3 weeks really makes me feel good, but part of me wants to celebrate by getting loaded.
Maintenance	These recent months of abstinence have made me feel that I'm progressing toward recovery, but I'm still wondering whether abstinence is really necessary.

Source: Adapted from Miller & Rollnick, 1991.

CONCLUSION

Although the recidivism rates for SUD depend on a number of factors, knowing whether clients are mentally prepared versus precontemplating the need for a change becomes important. As the United States begins for the first time in its history to consider legislation to legalize marijuana, it does not appear that a substantial decrease in SUD itself is on the horizon anytime soon. Illegal substances' availability, cost, and altering state of euphoria often achieved will remain important for individuals who desire an escape from the stresses and strains of daily life.

REFERENCES

Abraham, H. D., Aldridge, A. M., & Gogia, P. (1996). The psychopharmacology of hallucinogens. *Neuropsychopharmacology, 14,* 285–298.

Charney, D. S., Mihic, S. J., & Harris, R. A. (2006). Hypnotics and sedatives. In J. G. Hardman, L. E. Limbird, & A. G. Gilman (Eds.), *The pharmacological basis of therapeutics* (pp. 401–427). New York: McGraw-Hill.

Ciraulo, D. A., Ciraulo, J. A., Sands, B. F., Knapp, C. M., & Sarid-Segal, O. (2005). Sedative hypnotics. In H. R. Kranzler & D. A. Ciraulo (Eds.), *Clinical manual of addiction psychopharmacology.* Washington, DC: American Psychiatric Publishing.

Crowley, T. J., & Sakai, J. (2005). Inhalant-related disorders. In B. J. Sadock & V. A. Sadock (Eds.), *Kaplan & Sadock's comprehensive textbook of psychiatry* (pp.12–47). New York: Lippincott, Williams & Wilkins.

Dal Cason, T. A., & Franzosa, E. S. (2003). Occurrences and forms of the hallucinogens. In R. Lang (Ed.), *Hallucinogens: A forensic drug handbook* (pp. 37–66). London: Academic Press.

Doweiko, H. E. (2009). *Concepts of chemical dependency.* Belmont, CA: Brooks/Cole Cengage Learning.

Drummer, O. H., & Odell, M. (2001). *The forensic pharmacology of drugs of abuse.* New York: Oxford University Press.

Emrick, C. D., Lassen, C. L., & Edwards, M. T. (1977). Nonprofessional peers as therapeutic agents. In A. S. Gurman & A. M. Razin (Eds.), *Effective psychotherapy: A handbook of research* (pp. 120–161). New York: Pergamon Press.

Espeland, K. E. (1997). Inhalants: The instant, but deadly high. *Pediatric Nursing, 23*(1), 82–86.

Gitlow, S. (2007). *Substance use disorders* (2nd ed.). New York: Lippincott, Williams & Wilkins.

Glennon, R. A. (2004). Neurobiology of hallucinogens. In M. Galanter & H. D. Kleber (Eds.), *Textbook of substance abuse treatment* (pp.181–190). Washington, DC: American Psychiatric Press.

Fields, R. (2010). *Drugs in perspective.* New York: McGraw-Hill.

Finger, W. W., Lund, M., & Slagel, M. A. (1997). Medications that may contribute to sexual disorders: A guide to assessment and treatment in family practice. *Journal of Family Practice, 44,* 33–44.

Halkitis, P. N., Shrem, M. T., & Martin, F. W. (2005). Sexual behavior patterns of methamphetamine—using gay and bisexual men. *Substance Use and Misuse, 40,* 703–719.

Halpern, J. H., & Pope, H. G. (1999). Do hallucinogens cause residual neuropsychological toxicity? *Drug and Alcohol Dependence, 53,* 247–256.

Halpern, J. H., & Pope, H. G. (2003). Hallucinogen persisting perception disorder: What do we know after 50 years? *Drug and Alcohol Dependence, 69,* 109–119.

Hansen, J., & Emrick, C. D. (1985). Whom are we calling alcoholic? In W. R. Miller (Ed.), *Alcoholism: Theory, research and treatment* (pp.164–178). Lexington, MA: Gin Press.

Hart, C. L., & Ksir, C. (2011). *Drugs, society & human behavior.* New York: McGraw-Hill.

Hawks, R. L., & Chiang, C. N. (1986). *Urine testing for drugs of abuse.* Research Monograph 73. Washington, DC: National Institute on Drug Abuse.

Hernandez-Avila, C., & Pierucci-Lagha, A. (2005). Inhalants. In H. R. Kranzler & D. A. Ciraulo (Eds.), *Clinical manual of addiction psychopharmacology* (pp. 269–303). Washington, DC: American Psychiatric Publishing.

Hollar, D. (2008). The relationship between substance use disorders and unsuccessful case closures in vocational rehabilitation agencies. *Journal of Applied Rehabilitation Counseling, 39*(2), 25–27.

Inciardi, J. A. (2002). *The war on drugs III: The continuing saga of the mysteries and miseries of intoxication, addiction, crime, and public policy.* Boston: Allyn & Bacon.

Jones, R. T., (1980). Human effects: An overview. In R. C. Peterson (Ed.), *Marijuana research findings* (pp. 54–80). Rockville, MD: National Institute on Drug Abuse.

Joy, J. E., Watson, S. J., & Benson, J. A. (1999). *Marijuana and medicine: Assessing the science base.* Washington, DC: National Academy Press.

Kessler, R. C., Aguilar-Gaxiola, S., Bergland, P., Caraveo-Anduago, J. J., Dewit, D. J., Greenfield, S. F., et al. (2001). Patterns and predictors of treatment seeking after the onset of a substance use disorder. *Archives of General Psychiatry, 58,* 1065–1071.

Lewis, J. A., Dana, R. Q., & Blevins, G. A. (2002). *Substance abuse counseling* (3rd ed.). Pacific Grove, CA: Brooks/Cole.

Lowinson, J. H., Ruiz, P., Millman, Robert B., & Langrod, J. G. (2005). *Substance abuse: A comprehensive textbook.* Philadelphia: Lippincott Williams & Williams.

Maisto, S. A., Galizio, M. & Connors, G. J. (2008). *Drug use and abuse.* Belmont, CA: Thomson Corporation.

Martin, B. R. (2004). Neurobiology of marijuana. In M. Galanter, & H. D. Kleber, (Eds.) *Textbook of substance abuse treatment* (pp.201–206). Washington, DC: American Psychiatric Press.

McGlothin, W. H., & West, L. J. (1968). The marihuana problem: An overview. *American Journal of Psychiatry, 125,* 370–378.

Meyer, J. S., & Quenzer, L. F. (2005). *Psychopharmacology: Drugs, the brain, and the behavior.* Sunderland, MA: Sinauer Associates Inc.

Miller, W. R., & Hester, R. K. (1980). Treating the problem drinker: Modern approaches. In W. R. Miller & R. K. Hester (Eds.), *The addictive behaviors: Treatment of alcoholism, drug abuse, smoking, and obesity* (pp. 11–141). New York: Plenum Press.

Miller, W. R., & Rollnick, S. (1991). *Motivational interviewing: Preparing people to change addictive behavior.* New York: Guilford Press.

Miller, W. R., & Sanchez, V. C. (1994). Motivating young adults for treatment and lifestyle change. *Alcohol use and misuse by young adults.* Notre Dame, IN: University of Notre Dame Press.

Nelson, T. (2000). *Pharmacology of drugs of abuse.* Seminar presented by the Division of Continuing Studies, University of Wisconsin-Madison, Madison, WI.

Newton, T. F., De La Garza, R., Kalechstein, A. D., & Nestor, L. (2005). Cocaine and methamphetamine produce different patterns of subjective and cardiovascular effects. *Pharmacology, Biochemistry and Behavior, 82,* 90–97.

Nicoll, R. A., & Alger, B. E. (2004). The brain's own marijuana. *Scientific American, 291*(6), 68–75.

Noonan, W. C., & Moyers, T. B. (1997). Motivational interviewing. *Journal of Substance Misuse 2,* 8–16.

Poling, A., & Cross, J. (1993). State-dependent learning. In F. van Haaren (Ed.), *Methods in behavioral pharmacology* (pp. 245–256). Amsterdam: Elsevier.

Ropper, A. H., & Brown, R. H. (2005). *Adams and Victor's principles of neurology* (8th ed.). New York: McGraw-Hill.

Schwartz, R. H. (1989). When to suspect inhalant abuse. *Patient Care, 23*(10), 39–50.

Smith, N. T. (2002). A review of the published literature into cannabis withdrawal symptoms in human users. *Addiction, 97,* 621–632.

Sobell, M. B., & Sobell, L. C. (1993). *Problem drinkers: Guided self-change treatment.* New York: Guilford Press.

Spiller, H. A., & Krenzelok, E. P. (1997). Epidemiology of inhalant abuse reported to two regional poison centers. *Journal of Toxicology: Clinical Toxicology, 35,* 167–174.

Strassman, R. (2005). Hallucinogens. In M. Earlywine (Ed.), *Mind-altering drugs: The science of subjective experience* (pp. 49–85). Oxford, UK: Oxford University Press.

Sussman, N., & Westreich, L. (2003). Chronic marijuana use and the treatment of mentally ill patients. *Primary Psychiatry, 19*(9), 73–76.

Thombs, D. L. (2006). *Introduction to addictive behaviors* (3rd ed.). New York: The Guilford Press.

West, S. L., Graham, C. W., & Cifu, D. X. (2009). Rates of persons with disabilities in alcohol/other drug treatment in Canada. *Alcoholism Treatment Quarterly, 27,* 253–264.

Worcester, S. (2006). Survey: Teens use inhalants more, worry about risks less. *Clinical Psychiatry News, 34*(6), 28.

Wilson, B. A., Shannon, M. T., Shields, K. M., & Stang, C. L. (2007). *Prentice-Hall nurse's drug guide, 2007.* Upper Saddle River, NJ: Prentice Hall.

20

Working With Trauma-Related Mental Health Problems Among Combat Veterans of the Afghanistan and Iraq Conflicts

JAMYLAH JACKSON, LISA THOMAN, ALINA M. SURÍS,
AND CAROL S. NORTH

The ongoing conflicts in Iraq and Afghanistan are bringing large numbers of returning combat veterans home with social, cultural, and psychological issues unique to this cohort. Operation Enduring Freedom (OEF) began in Afghanistan in 2001, Operation Iraqi Freedom (OIF) began in Iraq in 2003, and Operation New Dawn (OND) began in Iraq (a new phase following the end of OIF) in 2010. OEF/OIF/OND veterans are military personnel enlisted or activated after 2001. Of the more than one million service members deployed to Iraq or Afghanistan, nearly half have been deployed more than once. More than 43,000 service members have been wounded, with the fatality count approaching 6,000 (U.S. Department of Defense [U.S. DoD], 2011). Traumatic combat exposures in Iraq and Afghanistan include mortar, rocket, and artillery fire; small arms fire; multiple high-intensity blasts; roadside bombs; improvised explosive devices (IEDs); and surprise sniper attacks (Mental Health Advisory Team 5 [MHAT-V], 2008; Seal, Bertenthal, Miner, Sen, & Marmar, 2007). Commonly sustained injuries are blast wounds and soft tissue and orthopedic injuries including amputations, burns, hearing loss, and traumatic brain injury (TBI) (Grieger et al., 2006).

The OEF/OIF/OND conflicts are the longest sustained U.S. military operations since the Vietnam War and the first extended conflicts to rely on an all-volunteer military (Institute of Medicine [IOM], 2010) at a time when there are fewer active-duty military personnel available than in the previous conflicts. This situation has created a different military climate compared with previous sustained military operations, with greater dependence on National Guard and reservists, longer deployment durations, multiple deployments, and shorter intervals between deployments. These more numerous deployments coupled with the shorter intervals between them are destined to increase the need for transition and readjustment time for returning soldiers and their families.

Medical advances have increased the survival rates of soldiers with significant injuries. Improvements in body armor and emergency medical care have reduced combat fatality-to-injury ratios to their lowest level in history (1:7.2 for OIF, 1:5.0 for OEF, 1:2.6 in Vietnam, and 1:1.7 in World War II) (Leland & Oboroceanu, 2010; U.S. DoD, 2011). Therefore, more veterans from the OEF/OIF conflicts than ever before are returning home with severe combat-related injuries requiring specialized care. Accompanying these physical wounds are the mental wounds of war. Hoge, Auchterlonie, and Milliken (2006) found that 19% of troops returning from Iraq and 11% of Afghanistan veterans come home to face mental health problems; rates are higher among those with repeated deployments.

OEF/OIF military personnel are fundamentally different from those of previous military operations such as the Gulf War and Vietnam War in a number of ways. There has been much discussion regarding the uniqueness of the OEF/OIF conflicts in their heavy use of National Guard and reservist personnel. Deployed soldiers within today's reservist units are older and more likely to have families than in the Vietnam War era. Reservists and National Guard units also differ in many ways from active-duty military. Reservists are less likely to be part of a cohesive unit with the high levels of camaraderie and trust that active component service members who live and train together experience. Reservists generally function as civilians except during monthly weekend trainings and actual deployment. The transition back to civilian life for reservists occurs more abruptly than for active-duty personnel and may thus be more difficult. Family members of reservists are less connected to the military community and do not receive the support of interactions with other families of deployed soldiers in the way that regular military families do.

Women make up a larger percentage of deployed forces than ever before comprising 14% of deployed military personnel (Women in Military Service for America Memorial Foundation, 2010). Between 2002 and 2006, 50% of deployed women using veteran health care had been activated from Reserve or Guard units. Compared with their civilian counterparts, military mothers are three times more likely to be single parents and five times more likely to be married to a military and deployable spouse (Joint Economic Committee U.S. Congress, 2007). National Guard and reservist mothers who are primary caregivers may find it more difficult to arrange for alternative child care than do mothers who are active-duty personnel. Many deployed female soldiers are also mothers of young children and suffer long periods of separation from their children and spouses. For deployed women, especially those who are mothers, family disruptions and family-related concerns are superimposed on the other stresses of deployment.

Although women have typically been excluded from direct combat operations, expansion of support functions (e.g., mechanic, military police, transportation) performed by female military personnel coupled with the nature of the OEF/OIF conflicts (insurgency warfare) has increased traumatic exposures among female troops in the war zone (Street, Vogt, & Dutra, 2009). In Iraq, like their male counterparts, female soldiers are frequently exposed to surprise ambushes of their convoys, mortar and grenade attacks, gunfire exchange, IEDs, witnessing serious injury or death, and personal threat of serious injury or death (Street et al., 2009). Female soldiers are also more likely than male soldiers to experience discrimination and harassment, with half or more acknowledging some form of sexual harassment each year in the military (Lipari, Cook, Rock, & Matos, 2008).

To inform the provision of mental health interventions for OEF/OIF veterans, a thorough understanding of the mental health problems in this population is a necessary first step. This chapter will thus first review research on the prevalence and types of mental health problems among OEF/OIF veterans, associated risk factors, and other psychosocial issues. Following this, empirical evidence for treatment in this population will be provided. This material will provide guidance to clinicians working with mental health and psychosocial problems of veterans of the OEF/OIF conflicts.

PSYCHIATRIC AND READJUSTMENT PROBLEMS OF RETURNING OEF/OIF VETERANS

Mental health problems among OEF/OIF veterans may be divided into post-traumatic stress disorder (PTSD), other psychiatric disorders, and TBI. In addition to all the problems that are known to affect returning military personnel from previous wars, they may also experience a variety of psychosocial issues, many of which may be unique to this special population.

Exposure to Military Trauma

PTSD may develop in relation to a number of different types of trauma such as physical and sexual assault, combat exposure, natural disasters, motor vehicle collisions, and other kinds of accidents. The types of traumatic events most likely to be associated with PTSD represent human acts of intentional physical harm such as combat, assault, and sexual assault (Breslau et al., 1998). Exposure to trauma is difficult to define for military combat. The combat theater differs from many other kinds of trauma situations in which the danger is ongoing and recurrent. Some types of threats also vary from one war to another. The types of combat-related traumatic incidents experienced by OEF/OIF veterans have been enumerated based on previous research, including a RAND study by Tanelian et al. (2008) building on previous work by Hoge et al. (2004) in OEF/OIF veterans and earlier work of Castro, Bienvenu, Hufmann, and Adler (2000) with soldiers deployed to Kosovo. The list of traumatic combat incidents can be found in Table 20.1.

Missing from this list of combat experiences, however, is the possibility of prolonged exposure (PE) to potential threats that are outside of any of the 11 types of trauma identified. The type of warfare in the Iraq and Afghanistan conflicts differs from that of prior conflicts and wars in several ways that pertain to the types of trauma faced by today's soldiers. There are no front lines because it is uncertain when and from where the next attack may come. Thus, the threat is constant and ongoing. Especially in Iraq, many of the operations occur in largely urban areas where large crowds make identification of the enemy difficult. Any travel presents ongoing threats of encountering IEDs. Suicide bombers may infiltrate purportedly "safe" zones, creating a sense of prolonged potential for risk even on post in primarily non-combat-related positions. While this ongoing potential threat is part of the stressful environment of today's combat theater, it does not clearly fulfill the requirement of experiencing an immediate threat described in criterion A for PTSD (*DSM-IV-TR*, 2000). Regardless, this type of stressor was found to be associated with post-traumatic symptoms (Kolkow, Spira, Morse, & Grieger, 2007).

TABLE 20.1 Traumatic Combat Incidents

Serious injury or death of a friend

Viewing dead or seriously injured noncombatants

Witnessing an accident resulting in serious injury or death

Smelling decomposing bodies

Being physically moved or knocked over by an explosion

Sustaining an injury not requiring hospitalization

Sustaining a blow to the head from any accident or injury

Sustaining an injury requiring hospitalization

Engaging in hand-to-hand combat

Witnessing brutality toward detainees/prisoners

Being responsible for the death of a civilian

Killing enemy combatants

Handling or uncovering human remains

Being attacked or ambushed

Receiving incoming artillery, rocket, or mortar fire

Experiencing a close call

Another established list of traumatic combat incidents (MHAT-IV, 2006) includes 30 different types of OEF/OIF combat experiences. The lack of standardization in the literature regarding what does and does not qualify as combat trauma and the lack of a consistent system of evaluating the severity of combat experiences leaves much to be resolved by clinical judgment. Although psychiatric syndromes associated with combat-related stressors that do not meet criterion A cannot, by definition, be determined to represent PTSD, the possibility that the symptoms may represent another psychiatric disorder should not be overlooked.

While combat trauma is the type of trauma traditionally identified in association with military experience, OEF/OIF veterans are also at risk of exposure to military sexual trauma (MST), both while deployed and stateside. MST as defined by the Department of Veterans Affairs (VA) includes both sexual harassment and sexual assault during a military service (Surís & Lind, 2008). National VA statistics from 2002 to fiscal year 2009 indicate that 21.9% of female and 1.1% of male veterans seeking VA health care acknowledged a history of MST (Surís & Smith, in press). The larger proportion of male service members, however, yields nearly equal numbers of men and women in this population who have a history of MST (Surís & Lind, 2008). The number of women with MST is expected to grow substantially as the number of women serving in the military increases.

Post-Traumatic Stress Disorder

PTSD is the psychiatric disorder most likely to arise after OEF/OIF deployments (Seal et al., 2007). According to the *Diagnostic and Statistical Manual of Mental Disorders*, fourth edition (*DSM-IV-TR*; American Psychiatric Association, 2000), the diagnosis of PTSD requires exposure to a traumatic stressor representing a threat to life or limb. The diagnostic criteria allow for three types of qualifying exposures to the traumatic event: direct experience of the event, directly witnessing the event, or learning of the experience of a traumatic event by a loved one or a close associate. Additionally, trauma-related symptoms that impair functioning or cause clinically significant distress must be present for more than 1 month. These symptoms must include at least one re-experiencing symptom (Group B: e.g., intrusive recollections, nightmares, flashbacks, emotional, or physiological distress in response to reminders of trauma), at least three avoidance/numbing symptoms (Group C: e.g., avoidance of reminders of the trauma, restricted range of affect, feeling isolated from others, psychogenic amnesia for parts of the trauma, loss of interest or participation in usual activities, and/or sense of a foreshortened future), and at least two hyperarousal symptoms (Group D: e.g., sleep disturbance, concentration problems, hypervigilance, exaggerated startle response, jitteriness, irritability).

A recently published literature review noted that studies vary widely in their estimates of the prevalence of PTSD among OEF/OIF veterans (Ramchand et al., 2010), with most studies reporting rates between 5% and 20%. For example, in a review of psychiatric diagnoses in VA medical records of OEF/OIF veteran patients, Sayer et al. (2010) found that PTSD was diagnosed in 26%, and 39% had a positive PTSD screen. Erbes, Westermeyer, Engdahl, and Johnsen (2007) reported that 12% of OEF/OIF veterans enrolled in treatment were diagnosed with PTSD. This variability in reported prevalence may relate in part to substantial methodological variability and limitations in the design of many of these studies. Major methodological limitations in this research include the use of screening instruments rather than diagnostic assessment, inconsistent time frame of assessment (e.g., current diagnosis in the last month, versus cumulative prevalence across the entire period since return from war, versus lifetime prevalence), cross-sectional and retrospective design, and selection bias with underrepresentation of those most severely wounded or removed from duty. The above prevalence estimates of psychiatric illness in OEF/OIF veterans can be compared with estimates among military veterans of other eras, 2% to 10% for Persian Gulf

War veterans (Kang & Bullman, 1996) and 15% for Vietnam-era veterans (Schlenger et al., 1992). The lifetime prevalence of PTSD in the general population is 7.5% (Kessler, Sonnega, Bromet, Hughes, & Nelson, 1995). PTSD would be expected to be substantially more prevalent in treatment populations than in more general populations (Ramchand et al., 2010).

Other Psychiatric Disorders

PTSD is not the only clinically important outcome of combat trauma. It is typically accompanied by at least one other disorder and often several disorders, especially major depressive disorder, substance-use disorders, and other anxiety disorders (Seal et al., 2007).

A large study of OEF/OIF veterans receiving VA health care identified psychiatric disorders in 25% of the veterans, with more than half (56%) of these cases having at least two disorders (Seal et al., 2007). Of those with more than one disorder, 29% had two disorders and 27% had three or more disorders. The most common disorders identified were PTSD (13%), other anxiety disorders (6%), adjustment disorder (6%), depressive disorders (5%), and substance-use disorders (5%). In a survey of previously deployed military OEF/OIF service members, Tanelian et al. (2008) identified "probable" major depression in 14% overall and in about two-thirds of those with probable PTSD. Reviewing VA records of OEF/OIF veterans presenting for treatment, Sayer et al. (2010) found higher rates of diagnosed psychiatric disorders: depressive disorders in 28%, other anxiety disorders in 10%, and substance-use disorders in 5% (with an additional 35% screening positive for potential drug or alcohol disorders). Studies using screening instruments have reported even higher rates of psychiatric disorders. In a study of Iraq war soldiers, Maguen et al. (2010) found positive screens for depression in 32% and alcohol abuse in 25%.

Several studies have focused on alcohol problems. Erbes et al. (2007) reported that 33% of OEF/OIF veterans enrolled in the treatment screened positive for hazardous levels of alcohol use, including one-half of the veterans with a positive PTSD screen. A study of OEF/OIF veterans seeking treatment through a VA primary care clinic found that more than one-fourth acknowledged hazardous drinking behavior (McDevitt-Murphy et al., 2010). A study of OEF/OIF veterans seeking health care through a VA postdeployment health clinic found that nearly one in four indicated at least one problematic drinking behavior (Jakupcak, Luterek, Hunt, Conybeare, & McFall, 2008).

Statistics on suicide show an alarming increase in completed suicides in recent years among OEF/OIF-era active-duty service members and veterans. Research has identified several risk factors for suicide among OEF/OIF military personnel and veterans. Indicators of elevated suicide risk include exposure to military combat, significant stressors such as prolonged deployment-related separation from loved ones, relationship problems, PTSD, alcohol and other substance-use disorders, TBI, and impulsivity (Kang & Bullman, 2008; Martin, Ghahramanlou-Holloway, Lou, & Tucciarone, 2009; MHAT-V, 2008). A recent survey of OEF/OIF veterans found that 12.5% had experienced thoughts of suicide during the 2 weeks prior to the interview (Pietrzak et al., 2010). The veterans who reported suicidal ideation also had higher rates of positive PTSD and depression screens and reported more psychosocial problems. The avoidance symptom cluster was specifically associated with suicidal ideation. Postdeployment social support and a sense of purpose and control were protective. In a larger study of OEF/OIF veterans registered with the VA, Lemaire and Graham (2010) found that depressive disorders, PTSD, and psychotic disorders were all significantly associated with suicidal ideation. Suicidal ideation was most prevalent among those with depression and second in prevalence among those with PTSD, but the risk was highest among veterans with both these disorders. These findings underscore the importance of conducting a thorough assessment for mental disorders in addition to PTSD for veterans exposed to trauma.

Traumatic Brain Injury

TBI is considered a "signature injury" of the Iraq and Afghanistan wars. TBI is defined as a traumatically induced structural injury and/or physiological disruption of brain function resulting from an external force, immediately followed by new onset or worsening of at least one of the following clinical signs: any period of loss or a decreased level of consciousness; loss of memory for events immediately before or after the injury (post-traumatic amnesia); alteration in mental state at the time of the injury (e.g., confusion, disorientation, slowed thinking); and neurological deficits (e.g., weakness, loss of balance, change in vision, praxis, paresis/plegia, sensory loss, aphasia) that may or may not be transient (VA/DoD, 2009, p. 16).

Mild TBI is also referred to as "a concussion." Mild TBI symptoms range from minor transient symptoms to enduring, severe problems (VA/DoD Practice Guidelines, 2009). TBI commonly involves cognitive difficulties such as problems with attention and concentration, memory, and executive function. Physical symptoms may include headaches, fatigue, sleep problems, and sensitivity to light and noise. Behavioral and emotional symptoms may include depressed or anxious mood, irritability, impaired impulse control, and aggressive behavior. Most symptoms typically resolve within a month (McCrea, 2007), and full recovery from mild TBI typically occurs (McCrea, 2007) within 3 to 12 months (Carroll, Cassidy, Holm, Kraus, & Coronado, 2004).

Postconcussional disorder is defined by *DSM-IV-TR* (in Appendix B: Criteria Sets and Axes Provided for Further Study) as a syndrome occurring after a head trauma causing significant cerebral concussion. To meet diagnostic criteria, neuropsychological testing or quantified cognitive assessment must document evidence of problems of attention or memory. Additionally, there must be at least 3 months' duration of at least three of eight possible symptoms (fatigue, disordered sleep, headache, vertigo or dizziness, unprovoked irritability or aggression, anxious/depressed/labile mood, personality change, and apathy/lack of spontaneity) beginning after the injury and causing significant impairment in social or occupational functioning.

TBI has been found to be quite prevalent among OEF/OIF veterans. A survey of postdeployment service members found that 19% screened positive for "probable TBI" (Tanelian et al., 2008). In a recent review of VA administrative data (Carlson et al., 2010), 22% of OEF/OIF veterans had a positive TBI screen and 37% of them had confirmed TBI. Mild TBI is often comorbid with PTSD and other psychiatric disorders, which may in part reflect difficulties in differentiating it from other disorders or problems. In the study by Carlson et al. (2010), 85% of veterans with confirmed TBI also met criteria for at least one psychiatric diagnosis and 64% met criteria for at least two: 64% had PTSD, 46% had major depression, 35% had another anxiety disorder, 34% had adjustment disorder, and 26% had substance-related disorders. A study of OIF soldiers assessed at 3 months postdeployment for mild TBI found that loss of consciousness in the incident was associated with screening positive for PTSD (44%) and major depression (23%) (Hoge et al., 2008). In a review of VA records of OEF/OIF veterans presenting for treatment, TBI was diagnosed in 4% overall but 19% of patients with positive screens for probable PTSD or comorbid drug or alcohol disorder (Sayer et al., 2010).

Risk Factors for Mental Health Problems in OEF/OIF Veterans

There is considerable evidence that the degree and type of trauma exposure experienced by a service member during deployment increase the likelihood of developing deployment-related mental health problems. The degree of exposure to combat, as represented by the number of firefights, for example, is associated with subsequent development of PTSD (Hoge et al., 2004). Severity of both combat exposure and combat injuries has been found to be associated with psychiatric disorders among OEF/OIF veterans (Tanelian et al., 2008). In a study of wounded army soldiers recovering at Walter Reed Army Medical Center, 4% had PTSD in the first month after arrival, with the rate increasing to 12% at 4 and 7 months (Grieger et al., 2006). The severity of the soldiers' physical problems was associated with greater likelihood of both PTSD and depression, although the degree of combat exposure they had experienced was not associated with psychiatric illness in this study.

A postdeployment study of OIF soldiers found that 40% had to kill during combat. Even after controlling for other types of combat exposure, the experience of having to kill in combat was associated with the likelihood of screening positive for PTSD, alcohol abuse, problems with anger and relationships, and impaired psychosocial functioning (Maguen et al., 2010). Multiple deployments also increase the risk for PTSD, presumably due to cumulative effects of exposure to trauma and other deployment stress experienced over a period of time. One study found that 27% of veterans deployed three or four times had problems with depression, anxiety, or acute stress, compared with 12% of those deployed only once (MHAT-V, 2008).

Exposure to MST is especially likely to be associated with postdeployment psychiatric problems, and the mental health consequences of MST may combine additively as well as interactively with mental health effects of other traumas experienced during deployment. Kimerling et al. (2010) found that female veterans exposed to MST while deployed were 3.5 times more likely to have a psychiatric disorder than other female veterans. MST is found to be associated specifically with PTSD, depression, and substance-use disorders as well as with various psychological symptoms (Surís & Lind, 2008) and impaired functioning (Street et al., 2009). Women assaulted during military service may feel trapped in their environment, as they may be reluctant to report the incident for fear of negative career consequences—especially if the perpetrator is a senior officer. The victim of MST has been betrayed by a person she was supposed to be able to trust, and she may have no choice but to continue to work alongside this person (because military personnel cannot readily transfer their duty station; Street et al., 2009; Surís & Smith, in press). The victim is thus placed in a position of having to depend on people whom she cannot trust, while at the same time she may also feel distanced from the camaraderie of her fellow soldiers. Military environments create intense camaraderie (e.g., willingness to sacrifice one's life for one's comrades) and trust that are vital for mutual protection and safety of the unit and its members. The sense of betrayal of trust and the alienation from colleagues that accompany MST are thus likely to be even more pronounced than with sexual trauma experienced in civilian environments.

Age, ethnic group membership, military rank, and branch of military have also been found to be associated with risk of PTSD and other psychiatric disorders among OEF/OIF veterans (Kang & Hyams, 2005). Veteran subgroups with increased risk of psychiatric illness are women, teenagers, ethnic minorities, divorced/separated veterans (Tanelian et al., 2008), enlisted personnel compared with officers, and members of the Army and Marines who are three times more likely than Navy and Air Force personnel to have PTSD (Kang & Hyams, 2005). PTSD has also been found to be more prevalent among reservist personnel than among active-duty soldiers (25% vs. 17%; Milliken, Auchterlonie, & Hoge, 2007).

Fontana and Rosenheck (2010) recently found that newly returning veterans appear to have a greater burden of PTSD, although less-comorbid substance abuse, than veterans whose deployment ended years ago. Substance abuse among today's returning soldiers is associated with impaired social functioning and is further associated with greater substance abuse, suggesting the potential for a spiraling downward trajectory among veterans with dual diagnoses.

Veterans entering treatment shortly after service in the war zone have been found to have less psychopathology than veterans entering treatment many years postdeployment

(Fontana & Rosenheck, 2008, 2010). They have also been found to have better social functioning in terms of greater education, more employment, intact rather than broken marriages, and fewer legal problems. Based on this research, treatment providers can expect that veterans who seek treatment a long time after return from war may present with more severe psychopathology than those who enter treatment right after homecoming.

Psychosocial Problems and Emotional Distress

Although the majority of returning troops will not experience psychiatric illness after homecoming, many more will experience adjustment problems. The first adjustment for veterans returning home is the loss they may feel upon separation from the tight camaraderie of the military unit that some veterans describe as more like family than even their own families. Once home, veterans may experience difficulties reacclimatizing to the rapid transition from a combat zone to civilian life. They may face adjustment issues in relationships disrupted by deployment, problems redefining roles in the home, and other readjustment problems such as negotiating difficult vocational and occupational choices. Couples must navigate fluctuations from interdependence to independence and back again, which can create conflicts and role confusion. Marital relationships may become strained as veterans and their partners seek to renegotiate roles and re-establish intimacy.

In surveys of returning personnel conducted 1 month postdeployment, approximately 4% of both active duty and reserve service members reported problems with interpersonal conflict; by 6 months, however, 14% of active duty and 21% of reserve service members reported interpersonal conflict (Milliken et al., 2007). These increases in reported problems with more time elapsed suggest a process of deterioration in interpersonal relationships during the first several months back home. Immediately upon return home, many veterans enter a "honeymoon" period, experiencing relief and joy at being rejoined with their families as their predominant feelings, but these positive feelings apparently fade as readjustment to civilian life proceeds.

Veterans who are parents may face special challenges. For example, because the veteran's partner has had to assume all parenting functions, the returning veteran may feel left out of parent–child interactions. Until returning, veterans adjust to the developmental changes and the new level of maturity their children have achieved during their absence, they may continue to treat their children as if they were younger. Some returning veterans tend to interact with their children as if they were soldiers, creating distance in the parent–child relationship. Therefore, children may also be affected by deployment and readjustment of their parents or other close family members. Children with a parent returning from deployment may experience problems with regression and acting-out behaviors (Litz & Orsillo, 2011). The amount of family disruption following a combat-related injury to a family member during an OEF/OIF deployment has been found to be associated with higher levels of distress in children (Cozza et al., 2010).

One clinically important area that research appears to address only indirectly is how deployment and readjustment affect the developmental stages of life that returning veterans must negotiate. Veterans returning from deployment in their mid to late twenties may find themselves having to choose a new career, as military skills learned and achievements such as rank and leadership may not translate well into civilian jobs. Older veterans leaving military service after many years face a dilemma of whether to retire from work altogether or embark on a new career. Many veterans will therefore face stressful mid-life career changes that may necessitate returning to school after a long time away or having to start "at the bottom" in their careers. Injuries or health problems that develop during deployment may force some returning veterans to reconsider their previously chosen career paths. Veterans who opted to join the military and not attend college may be disadvantaged in competing for jobs with civilians who attained educational degrees and direct experience in their chosen line of work while the veteran was deployed. Repeated deployments are expected to be associated with greater financial and employment stress, especially with the greater composition of older, married soldiers in today's military reserve units.

Developmental issues of military deployments may also disrupt social relationships. Returning veterans may find that they are "out of sync" with same-aged peers and friends. Their friends may be at different life stages having moved on with their own careers, family involvements, friendships, and social activities. The veteran may feel disconnected from former friends in the civilian world who may not feel that they can understand the veteran. Older veterans who are medically retired from their military careers, or who have enough years of service to retire, return home to find that they do not have much in common with their civilian peers who will continue working for a number of years until they are of retirement age.

Given the many issues surrounding readjustment to civilian life, it is understandable that a substantial proportion of returning veterans may encounter difficulties with social and interpersonal functioning, decreased productivity, marital and family problems, occupational and school problems, lack of engagement in community and leisure activities, problems managing anger, and alcohol misuse (Sayer et al., 2010). In a review of VA records of OEF/OIF veterans, an average of 42 months postdeployment found that 40% of the veterans acknowledged problems readjusting to civilian life and 25% had difficulties in *all* areas of functioning (Sayer et al., 2010). The most frequently endorsed problem areas were those related to interpersonal functioning, such as confiding personal thoughts and feelings to others and getting along with spouses, children, and friends. The single most frequently reported problem was difficulty controlling anger. Occupational functioning problems, such as finding or keeping a job and doing what is needed for work or school were often endorsed. Problems were also reported in functioning at home, such as completing chores; in leisure functioning, such as enjoyment or making good use of free time; and in finding meaning and purpose in life. Increasing use of alcohol and other substances was another problem area identified among veterans after they had returned from deployment.

Several studies have found functioning problems to be associated with PTSD. Problems readjusting to civilian life-endorsed OEF/OIF veterans were found to be associated with screening positive for "probable PTSD" in a VA medical record study by Sayer et al. (2010), although many veterans without probable PTSD also reported having such problems. Impairment in psychosocial and occupational functioning and adjustment were found to be associated with PTSD in a study of National Guard and Reserve veterans (Shea, Vujanovic, Mansfield, Sevin, & Liu, 2010). Interpersonal and social problems were specifically associated with avoidance and numbing symptoms, but overall functional impairment and global distress was specifically associated with hyperarousal symptoms. Problems in physical functioning, role functioning, physical pain, and general health were found to be associated with PTSD in a study that reviewed intake data from OEF/OIF veterans seeking health care through a VA postdeployment health clinic (Jakupcak et al., 2008). Disruptions to relationships, especially family relationships, have been found to be more strongly associated with mental health functioning in female than in male veterans (Vogt, Pless, King, & King, 2005). It has been noted that interpersonal and other problems associated with PTSD may unfortunately further isolate veterans from the social support systems designed to help them (Erbes et al., 2007).

MENTAL HEALTH TREATMENT FOR TRAUMATIZED OEF/OIF VETERANS

Any major review of treatment for mental health problems of traumatized OEF/OIF veterans must be preceded by an understanding of the substantial barriers to engagement and retention in treatment faced by today's veteran population. Younger cohorts of veterans differ from Vietnam-and Persian Gulf–era veterans in important ways that may affect their ability to engage and remain in treatment, including gender composition, marital status, legal history, age, and deployment experiences (Fontana & Rosenheck, 2008). For example, many OEF/OIF veterans have young families and are employed. These two factors alone can create scheduling challenges that make it difficult for veterans to remain in treatment for long periods of time that requires them to take time off work or arrange for child care. In contrast, older veterans may have more seniority in their jobs or may be retired, and their children may be adults, thus allowing the veterans more flexibility with scheduling. It stands to reason that the recent OEF/OIF veteran cohorts may differ from previous cohorts in their treatment needs and responses to approaches geared toward meeting their current issues. A 2008 IOM report on PTSD treatment identified the need for research to determine which kinds of treatment and strategies for delivery will be most effective for this particular cohort.

An organizational barrier to mental health treatment might be its lack of capacity to accommodate veterans' limitations. For example, many veterans may be unable to leave work during hours that treatment is available; obtaining transportation to the service provider facility that may be inconveniently located for many veterans may be a hardship. VA PTSD Clinical Teams have historically accommodated Vietnam-era veterans who have more chronic and persistent symptoms than those of recently returning veterans (Erbes, Curry, & Leskela, 2009), whose treatment needs may be different and whose growing numbers may overwhelm existing service capacities. VA personnel have been added nationally to address the mental health treatment needs of the current OEF/OIF cohorts, but not all facilities received these additional resources.

Stigma has been a longstanding barrier to mental health care for those in the military. Soldiers with mental health problems have been found to be twice as likely as their peers to acknowledge concerns related to the stigma surrounding mental illness. In particular, they voice worries about embarrassment, damage to their careers, loss of confidence in them by members of the unit, and being perceived by their peers as weak if their mental illness is discovered (MHAT-V, 2008; Milliken et al., 2007). Many of these concerns may be well founded, as the military has historically maintained a policy of reporting substance abuse and other mental health problems to the soldier's superiors (IOM, 2010). These mandatory reporting rules may deflect many personnel who need treatment from accepting mental health and substance-abuse treatment referrals. Although a desired function of the mandatory reporting requirement is to identify impaired soldiers who could potentially endanger themselves and others, this practice unfortunately acts to reduce the likelihood that those needing treatment will receive it. Addressing this issue, the IOM encouraged the DoD to "actively promote an environment to reduce stigma and encourage treatment for mental health and substance use disorders in an effort to improve military readiness and ability to serve" (IOM, 2010, p. 6).

Recently, strategies have been employed to normalize the use of mental health services after combat exposure including postdeployment evaluations within the military and also at VA facilities upon discharge from the military. Despite these efforts, some veterans deliberately downplay symptoms in efforts to avoid detection of their mental health problems, either as an attempt to achieve faster discharge from military service or in hopes that their symptoms will abate without professional attention.

Engagement and retention in mental health treatment appear to be especially difficult for current cohorts of returning military veterans. A comparison of treatment adherence of OEF/OIF veterans and Vietnam-era veterans found OEF/OIF treatment dropout rates to be more than twice those of Vietnam veterans, and treatment attrition was independent of pretreatment distress level (Erbes et al., 2009). Evidence regarding the association of treatment adherence with occupational status has been mixed (Erbes et al., 2009; Fontana & Rosenheck, 2008). Possible explanations for higher treatment attrition rates within this cohort might be greater sensitivity of OEF/OIF veterans to stigma surrounding mental health problems or that treatment approaches designed for prior-era veterans may not adequately meet the needs of veterans of the current wars. Chard, Shumm, Owens, and Cottingham (2010) observed that the chronic PTSD does not generally respond as well to treatment as PTSD in newly returning veterans. Fontana and Rosenheck (2008) suggested that premature attrition from treatment may result in worsening symptoms over time, leading to decreased social functioning, particularly occupational functioning. Therefore, receiving effective treatment prior to the erosion of social support systems and before PTSD becomes persistent is likely to be a particularly important aspect of mental health care for returning veterans.

General Approach to Treatment of Trauma-Related Mental Health Problems

Mental health treatment of veterans begins with adequate psychiatric and psychosocial assessment. Accurate diagnosis of psychiatric disorders such as PTSD is needed to select the type of treatment most likely to be effective. Just as important, though, is the assessment of psychosocial problems that are likely to occur in association with psychiatric disorders such as PTSD but also commonly occur in the absence of psychiatric illness. Adjustment difficulties, distress, and isolated symptoms can create significant problems for veterans, and these issues should not be confused with psychiatric illness and clinicians should avoid pathologizing these kinds of difficulties. At the same time, clinicians should also take care to avoid minimizing the importance of psychosocial problems simply because these problems do not amount to a diagnosable disorder. Although reduction of symptoms is a worthy goal of treatment, restoring psychosocial functioning is also a vital consideration. Recognizing and providing assistance with these common problems can make an important difference in the lives of many veterans.

The mental health assessment of returning OEF/OIF veterans should provide a comprehensive evaluation of psychosocial functioning, including functioning prior to military service (Litz & Orsillo, 2011). Information should also be obtained regarding the veteran's coping behaviors, trauma history, and specific experiences of deployment that stand out for that veteran. Safety factors such as suicidality and homicidality should be carefully assessed as well as potential for domestic violence and child abuse. These safety factors and psychosocial functioning should continue to be evaluated along with symptom levels over the course of treatment, as all may change over time.

Treatment should not only be based on the psychiatric diagnosis but should also address specific symptoms. For example, veterans with PTSD who struggle with avoidance behaviors may benefit from therapy which specifically targets avoidance, such as PE therapy. Veterans with PTSD who express guilt and self-doubt about a decision they made in combat may benefit more from a therapy that focuses on negative thought patterns, such as cognitive processing therapy (CPT). Veterans with PTSD who are hyperaroused and cannot sleep may benefit from medication that has sedative side effects, and those with nightmares may benefit from administration of prazosin. The mental health treatment plan for returning veterans might include two or more therapeutic modalities.

Because mental health treatment approaches for OEF/OIF veterans have largely focused on PTSD, this review will begin with treatments for PTSD and then move to interventions for adjustment problems. Recently, the VA and DoD (2010) jointly published a set of Clinical Practice Guidelines outlining the most evidence-based treatment approaches for PTSD, recommended as "first-line" treatments. The IOM independently evaluated scientific evidence from 1980 to 2007 for pharmacologic and psychological treatment modalities for PTSD. These IOM and VA/DoD treatment reviews and recommendations played a significant role in determining the focus for the review of treatments provided later in this chapter. In general, time-limited therapy approaches may be most desirable for treating returning veterans, given the aforementioned barriers to treatment and relatively high therapy attrition rates in this veteran cohort. Randomized controlled trials (RCTs) are the current standard for determining the effectiveness of a treatment. Although RCTs specifically targeting OEF/OIF veterans' responses to traditional therapy approaches are increasingly populating the scientific literature, their numbers are still relatively sparse.

Established treatments for mild TBI are less well established. VA/DoD Clinical Practice Guidelines (2009) for mild TBI noted a lack of evidence establishing direct causality between the brain injury and postconcussive symptoms, and a lack of objective indicators of brain pathology. The recommendation set forth in those guidelines, therefore, was to treat these problems symptomatically.

Medication, Psychotherapy, or Both?

Research has provided substantial evidence of beneficial effects of both pharmacotherapy and psychotherapy in the treatment of PTSD. Controversy exists, however, on the comparative effectiveness of these two forms of treatment established by research. A 2007 IOM report concluded that existing evidence supporting psychopharmacologic approaches for the treatment of PTSD was not adequate. Other experts have interpreted the methods used in the IOM review as "overly conservative" (Stein et al., 2009, p. 30), concluding that the efficacy of medications in the treatment of PTSD is well established (Ravindran & Stein, 2010; Stein et al., 2009). Methodological differences in treatment studies are cited as likely explanations of differences in research findings on the relative effectiveness of psychological and pharmacological interventions for the treatment of PTSD (Stein et al., 2009).

Few studies have directly compared the efficacy of pharmacotherapy and psychotherapy for PTSD. A Cochrane review by Hetrick, Purcell, Garner, and Parslow (2010) found four studies comparing pharmacotherapy and psychotherapy, concluding from this review that there was not enough evidence to support or refute the effectiveness of combined medication and psychotherapy compared with medication or psychotherapy alone. Regardless, some experts (Friedman, 2008; Forbes et al, 2007; National Collaborating Centre for Mental Health, 2005) maintain that psychotherapy represents the best first-line treatment for PTSD and others maintain that pharmacotherapy represents the best first-line treatment for PTSD (Bandelow, Zohar, Hollander, Kasper, & Moller, 2002; Canadian Psychiatric Association, 2006; Stein, Ipser, & Seedat, 2006; Stein et al., 2009). Several experts recommend use of both medication and psychotherapy as likely to be most effective (Baldwin et al., 2005; Foa, Davidson, & Frances, 1999; Reeves, 2007; Ursano et al., 2004).

Pharmacotherapy

Antidepressant Agents

Selective serotonin reuptake inhibitors (SSRIs) such as paroxetine, sertraline, citalopram, and fluoxetine are considered a mainstay of treatment for PTSD as first-line pharmacotherapeutic agents (Ravindran & Stein, 2010; Stein et al., 2009). Although only paroxetine and sertraline are approved by the U.S. Food and Drug Administration for the treatment of PTSD, there is extensive evidence from numerous large RCTs of the efficacy of agents of this class (Ravindran & Stein, 2010; Stein et al., 2009). Long-term studies have further demonstrated evidence of benefit from SSRIs in maintaining acute-phase gains and preventing relapse (Ravindran & Stein, 2010; Roberts et al., 2010). Considerable evidence of efficacy has also accrued for other classes of antidepressants such as certain tricyclic antidepressants (e.g., amitriptyline, imipramine) and serotonin/norepinephrine-specific agents (SNRIs; especially venlafaxine), monoamine oxidase inhibitors (MAOIs, e.g., phenelzine), and alternate antidepressant agents (e.g., mirtazepine, nefazodone; Ravindran & Stein, 2010; Stein et al., 2009).

The strategies and procedures for treating PTSD with antidepressant medications are similar to treatment of major depression with these medications. The effectiveness of these medications is independent of their antidepressant properties. They ameliorate posttraumatic symptoms in all three PTSD symptom categories. They may also help with the management of common comorbid disorders (depressive disorders and other anxiety disorders such as panic disorder) and troublesome symptoms such as irritability, aggression, and suicidal ideation. The newer SSRIs and SNRIs have fewer adverse effects, favorable safety profiles, and simpler titration schedules compared with tricyclic antidepressants and other older psychotropic agents (Reeves, 2007). The advantages of these newer medications that nonpsychiatric physicians such as family practitioners and internists may be more ready to prescribe may improve patient access to psychotropic treatment of PTSD.

Several reviews of pharmacotherapy for PTSD (Cukor, Spitalnick, Difede, Rizzo, & Rothbaum, 2009; Davis et al., 2001; Ravindran & Stein, 2010; Stein et al., 2006 Cochrane review from Cukor, 2009) have noted that observed benefit from pharmacotherapy for PTSD in men and in combat veterans is not nearly as robust as that demonstrated in studies of civilian populations and women in particular. Stein et al. (2009), lamenting that many patients respond poorly to medication or show only partial reduction in symptoms, emphasized the need for development of better psychotropic agents for treatment of PTSD in the future. In response to incomplete or inadequate response of many patients to pharmacotherapy, augmentation strategies have been devised using agents from various psychoactive medication classes.

Anticonvulsants

Interest in the use of mood stabilizers to augment pharmacotherapy for PTSD arose in conjunction with theories that repeated traumatic experiences may lead to sensitization and kindling of limbic discharges (Reeves, 2007). Anticonvulsants, used in the treatment of seizure disorders in which kindling is implicated, have been demonstrated effective in the treatment of mood disorders as well. Despite a strong theoretical basis for the use of anticonvulsants in the treatment of PTSD and some suggestion of potential benefit from open-label studies, empirical evidence from RCTs is largely unavailable (Ravindran & Stein, 2010; Reeves, 2007).

Atypical Antipsychotics

Although psychotic symptoms are not part of the diagnostic criteria for PTSD, some patients with PSTD may experience brief episodes of psychotic-like symptoms and agitation that may be targeted by antipsychotic agents. The nonspecific sedating characteristics of this medication class may help reduce agitation and excessive arousal that may accompany PTSD, but even the newer, atypical antipsychotic agents (e.g., olanzepine, quetiapine, risperidone) that are free of many of the classical adverse effects of traditional antipsychotic agents (e.g., movement disorders and neuroleptic malignant syndrome) still pose significant long-term hazards in terms of adverse metabolic effects and unacceptable weight gain (Ravindran & Stein, 2010). Most support for the use of antipsychotic agents for the treatment of PTSD is derived from augmentation trials, and even in these studies, the evidence has been conflicting (Ravindran & Stein, 2010).

Antianxiety Agents

Although benzodiazepines are generally well tolerated, are relatively safe to use compared with other classes of sedatives, and have had extensive use in management of other anxiety disorders and for symptoms of anxiety, agitation, and sleep problems, their use in treatment of PTSD has been controversial. Evidence for efficacy of benzodiazepines in the treatment of PTSD is limited at best (Ravindran & Stein, 2010). Problems in the use of benzodiazepines may include oversedation, cognitive impairment, psychomotor incoordination, respiratory depression, and dangers of overdose. In particular, tolerance and dependence are well-established risks with prolonged use. In patients with substance abuse and certain personality problems that frequently accompany PTSD, benzodiazepines should be avoided. Dissociative and disinhibitory properties of benzodiazepines may cause problems in management of PTSD by further disinhibiting behaviors among patients with impulse control disorders and contributing to dissociative states that may accompany PTSD. In summary, there is little evidence for efficacy of benzodiazepines for treatment of PTSD, but there is considerable potential for problems emerging from the use of benzodiazepines in PTSD treatment and potential for worsening the PTSD (Ravindran & Stein, 2010; Reeves, 2007). Buspirone is a nonaddictive antianxiety medication that is widely used for treatment of anxiety, but there is no evidence for its efficacy in treating PTSD (Ravindran & Stein, 2010; Reeves, 2007).

"Emerging" Medications for PTSD

The pharmacologic agents of this category have some theoretical basis and some evidence of potential benefit, thus having garnered professional interest and popular support for their potential utility in the treatment of PTSD (Cukor et al., 2009). Agents in this category include prazosin, beta blockers, D-cycloserine, and ketamine.

Prazosin, an $\propto$-1-adrenergic blocker, which has been most frequently used as an antihypertensive agent, has seen increasing application to the treatment of PTSD in recent years, especially in the management of nightmares and related sleep disturbances in combat veterans. The role of central nervous system adrenergic activity involving norepinephrine metabolism implicated in PTSD provides a theoretical basis for the use of prazosin in the treatment of PTSD. Mounting evidence from case studies, retrospective chart reviews, and open-label trials suggest promise for prazosin as a promising adjunctive agent targeting specific sleep-related disturbances in PTSD, but more definitive evidence is needed from RCTs (Cukor et al., 2009).

Another antihypertensive agent, propranolol, which is a beta-blocker, has been studied for its potential to prevent the development of PTSD in traumatized individuals. The theoretical role of propranolol in prevention of PTSD is based on its known function on adrenergic activation that is involved in fear conditioning in the immediate aftermath of trauma (Cukor et al., 2009; Pittman et al., 2002 from Cukor, 2009). Reduction in reactivity to trauma reminders (although no differences in clinical outcomes) with administration of propranolol has been demonstrated in RCTs, and preliminary studies have suggested PTSD-preventive effects of propranolol. Further research is needed, however, to confirm efficacy of propranolol for treatment or prevention of PTSD (Cukor et al., 2009).

Ketamine is a nonbarbiturate anesthetic agent that acts as an antagonist at the *N*-methyl-D-aspartate (NMDA) receptor. Ketamine plays an essential role in learning and memory that is likely to be important to fear learning and extinction, processes implicated in the development of PTSD. Ketamine has been found to be associated with reduced rates of PTSD among burn patients and veterans who received the drug as part of medical care of their injuries (Cukor et al., 2009). Controlled trials are needed to determine whether ketamine is useful for PTSD treatment.

D-Cycloserine is a broad-spectrum antibiotic that is also functions as a partial NMDA receptor agonist. Research suggests the potential for D-clycloserine to facilitate generalized extinction of fear responses, but further study is needed in patients with PTSD (Cukor et al., 2009).

Psychotherapy

The VA's Office of Mental Health has initiated a national rollout of several evidence-based therapies targeting psychiatric and psychosocial problems, such as PTSD, depression, substance abuse, and family problems, commonly faced by returning veterans. The specific therapies being rolled out by the VA (described in the psychotherapies discussed below) are CPT, cognitive behavioral therapy (CBT), acceptance and commitment therapy, PE therapy, and integrative behavioral couple therapy (IBCT). Psychotherapies are deemed "evidence based" only after their efficacy has been supported by RCTs involving comparable groups with minimal attrition. These treatments require intensive therapist training and often include post-training consultation to assist with implementation. Many of these therapies have been studied in veteran populations, and more recent research has examined their utility with OEF/OIF veterans.

CPT for PTSD

CPT (Resick, Monson, & Chard, 2007) is a form of trauma-focused CBT employing both cognitive/behavioral and exposure techniques. Trauma-related beliefs regarding self, others, and the world are addressed with an emphasis on exploring issues of safety, trust, power/control, esteem, and intimacy.

As a manualized treatment, the CPT has 12 pre-set with sessions designed to build on one another although an additional session is provided when traumatic grief is prominent. CPT is offered in individual and group formats. It begins with psychoeducation focused on common psychological effects of trauma exposure. It frames PTSD as a disruption of the normal emotional recovery process following exposure to trauma. It then provides an explanation of the cognitive model and allows patients to practice identifying their own thoughts and resulting feelings related to specific traumatic and nontraumatic events. Throughout the therapy, maladaptive thoughts are gently challenged using Socratic questioning, and clients are taught cognitive/behavioral techniques to challenge their own negative thoughts. By considering alternate interpretations of events, clients can view their trauma(s) in a more realistic and balanced manner. Comparing treatment CPT outcomes between OEF/OIF and Vietnam veterans, Chard et al. (2010) found that both groups showed significant reductions in PTSD and depressive symptoms, but OEF/OIF veterans appeared to have less-severe PTSD at outcome when factors such as pretreatment symptom severity and number of sessions attended were taken into account.

PE Therapy for PTSD

There is far more evidence for the effectiveness of PE therapy than for any other therapy (Foa et al., 1999). PE targets the PTSD avoidance symptom cluster. PE therapy is thought to help decrease distress by allowing patients to approach the fearful memory in the presence of objectively safe reminders of the traumatic experience. Patients learn that the distress related to the memory will not last forever and they will eventually habituate to it. As anxiety surrounding the memory decreases, patients are able to gain fuller understanding and acceptance of their memory of the traumatic event. Likewise, patients practice "in vivo," such as, in real-life assignments to help them re-engage in activities they have been avoiding because they are reminders of the traumatic experience. Through these assignments, patients learn that feared situations such as a crowded shopping mall or watching a military documentary are objectively safe and can be tolerated. Repeated real-life practices in PE therapy result in habituation, with patients becoming less anxious and more actively engaged in their current lives.

PE therapy has four components. First, therapy begins with psychoeducation providing information about common trauma reactions and normalization of the patient's current avoidant coping strategies. The rationale of treatment and goals of treatment are explained. Second, patients learn breathing retraining to assist with relaxation. The third and fourth components are imaginal exposure (repeated retelling of the traumatic experience story) and *in vivo* exposure exercises. PE therapy is typically completed in 8 to 12 sessions.

Tuerk et al. (2011) conducted an RCT evaluating the effectiveness of PE with 65 OEF/OIF veterans. PE was demonstrated by this study to be as effective with OEF/OIF veterans as with other populations including civilians and veterans of other military eras.

Eye Movement Desensitization and Reprocessing for PTSD

Eye movement desensitization and reprocessing (EMDR) is another exposure-based therapy with considerable empirical support (Dodgson, 2009; Rothbaum, Astin, & Marsteller, 2005). This therapy involves identification of a troubling image of the most disturbing part of the trauma, a related bodily sensation, and a negative cognition connected to the most disturbing part of the trauma. Patients are instructed to hold an image and related sensations mentally for periods of 20 seconds while tracking movements of the therapist's finger in front of their eyes. It is believed that EMDR decreases distress by changing how the memory of the trauma is processed during the repeated eye-tracking episodes, but there is no empirical evidence to support this theory. Because EMDR is an exposure-based cognitive therapy, the exposure and cognitive aspects of the therapy likely provide the major operative components (Albright & Thyer, 2010).

Stress Inoculation Training for PTSD

Stress inoculation training (SIT) involves a combination of cognitive and behavioral approaches to anxiety and stress management. Skills learned in SIT include relaxation training (using breathing retraining, progressive muscle relaxation, and guided imagery), assertiveness training, role playing, cognitive restructuring, and thought-stopping techniques. The SIT approach is more present-centered than trauma-focused. In SIT, patients learn more adaptive strategies for managing and reducing their anxiety. Assertiveness and role-playing skills target difficult interpersonal interactions that can otherwise lead to avoidance and social isolation in veterans with PTSD. Through learning effective coping strategies, patients can engage in the situations they have tended to avoid, thereby improving relationships and their overall quality of life.

CBT for Depression

CBT is supported by substantial empirical evidence as a treatment of choice for PTSD (CPT, PE, EMDR, and SIT) and other mental health problems. Through cognitive restructuring techniques, CBT targets unrealistic cognitions that create or contribute to negative emotions. Patients learn to identify and change common patterns of negative thinking known as cognitive distortions. Relationships among thoughts, feelings, and behaviors are explored with an emphasis on using restructured cognitions and behavioral activation to improve mood states.

Acceptance and Commitment Therapy for Depression

Acceptance and commitment therapy (ACT) is a form of CBT that differs from traditional CBT in that its focus is not on examining or changing one's thoughts, feelings, or memories, but rather on simply recognizing and accepting them. This approach uses mindfulness and acceptance strategies along with commitment toward values-oriented behaviors to promote psychological flexibility and improvements in mood. ACT approaches have been used in the treatment of PTSD, although to date, RCTs evaluating its effectiveness for PTSD have not been conducted.

Seeking Safety

Seeking safety therapy was designed for simultaneous treatment of post-traumatic symptoms and comorbid substance misuse (Najavits, 2002). Seeking safety is recognized by the International Society for Traumatic Stress Studies as an effective treatment for coexisting PTSD and substance-use disorders, and it is widely used across a number of VA settings. This therapy is present-focused rather than trauma-focused. It is manualized with materials for both clinicians and patients. The primary theme throughout the treatment is *safety*: in interpersonal relationships and in management of emotions, thought processes, and behaviors. Seeking Safety incorporates a focus on ideals and values prior to the development of post-traumatic and substance use problems and their related behaviors. Seeking safety was designed to be adaptable to a number of formats, including group and individual therapy settings. This therapy provides content in case management, cognitive, behavioral, and interpersonal domains. The seeking safety materials provide 25 modules, such as safety, recovery cognitions, detaching from emotional pain, and community resources that can be presented in any order and as needed. Clinician self-care and therapeutic issues are also addressed. Modules have accompanying patient handouts with relevant psychoeducational materials and exercises for developing coping skills and practice assignments to be completed between sessions. The shorter time frame for seeking safety therapy may have practical implications for OEF/OIF veterans who have known problems with treatment retention.

Seeking safety has been applied in a variety of populations including male and female veterans, homeless individuals, and inmate populations. Outcome studies have demonstrated reduced post-traumatic stress symptoms, stronger problem-solving and coping skills, better social functioning, and an enhanced sense of meaning (see Najavits, 2009, for review). A small pilot study involving nine OEF/OIF veterans found improvements in PTSD symptoms and decreased frequency and amount of problematic alcohol consumption after a 10-session adaptation of the seeking safety protocol (Norman, Wilkins, Tapert, Lang, & Najavits, 2010).

Imagery Rehearsal Therapy for Nightmares

Imagery rehearsal therapy (IRT) for nightmares is a promising treatment that has been used in varying formats for many years and extensively implemented in VA settings. IRT research has demonstrated reduced trauma-related nightmares and other post-traumatic stress symptoms. A version of the therapy developed by Krakow and Zadra (2010) has been successfully implemented with veterans. This and similar protocols have been found to reduce nightmares and post-traumatic symptoms in mixed era veterans (including OEF/OIF veterans) as well as active duty soldiers (Forbes et al., 2001/2003; Lu, Wagner, Van Male, Whitehead, & Boehnlein, 2009; Moore & Krakow, 2007; Nappi, Drummond, Thorp, & McQuaid, 2010).

Family Therapies

Research clearly demonstrates that the stressors of deployment and the ensuing readjustment issues can negatively affect not only the veteran but also the veteran's family (Pietrzak, Goldstein, Malley, Johnson, & Southwick, 2009). The Veterans Health Administration (VHA) Uniform Mental Health Services Handbook (U.S. Department of Veterans Affairs, 2008) establishes guidelines for mental health care and integration of care across VA programs. The handbook recommends provisions for family involvement in treatment planning and care when requested by the veteran. Of particular relevance for returning veterans coping with post-traumatic or depressive symptoms or with adjustment concerns that also involve the family are two types of therapy: IBCT and a modified version of the Support and Family Education (S.A.F.E.) family group.

IBCT was developed by Jacobson and Christensen (1996) in response to research findings that traditional behavioral therapy for couples suffered from substantial relapse rates, and efficacy among various populations was variable (Jacobson & Margolin, 1979). IBCT retains the basic behavioral strategies of traditional behavioral couple therapy such as communication and problem-solving skills training and behavioral exchange interventions, but its primary and initial focus is on emotional acceptance. In this therapy, recurrent problematic interactions within couples are identified and couples are then encouraged to express underlying emotions of hurt and fear along with their anger during these interactions to promote empathy and intimacy. Christensen et al. (2004) and Jacobson, Christensen, Prince, Cordova, and Eldridge. (2000) demonstrated two distinct advantages of IBCT: (1) efficacy with a broader range of couples than served by traditional behavior therapy and (2) indications that the therapeutic benefits may be maintained.

Erbes, Polusny, MacDermid, and Compton (2008) developed an adaptation to IBCT that is especially tailored to the needs of returning OEF/OIF veterans and is briefer than standard IBCT, requiring 12 to 14 rather than 24 to 26 sessions. The adaptation of Erbes et al. provides an education component covering deployment-related concerns, PTSD, and various symptoms and incorporates motivational interviewing techniques such as identifying pros and cons of change as needed to enhance motivation to remain in treatment (Miller & Rollnick, 2002). Although this version of IBCT has not yet been empirically tested, Erbes et al. have suggested that reductions in relationship conflict and enhancement of partner empathy and intimacy, combined with education about effects of PTSD and use of skills training, may decrease the level of distress of both partners and improve relationship functioning after return from deployment.

S.A.F.E., developed at the Oklahoma City VA Medical Center (Sherman, 2003), is another form of family therapy designed to help family members cope with the psychological symptoms of the veteran in their family. The focus of the program is broad and deals with a number of mental illnesses including schizophrenia, depression, and bipolar disorder. The many topics covered require 18 sessions for completion of this program. In response to the recent influx of OEF/OIF veterans, Bowling, Doerman, and Sherman (2007) adapted and condensed the S.A.F.E. program to address issues specifically relevant to families of returning OEF/OIF veterans such as PTSD and general reintegration problems in a 12-session program with accompanying handouts of resource lists, psychoeducational materials, and exercises involving topics such as parenting, communicating with one's loved one, caring behaviors, and coping with PTSD. The developers of the program suggest two group meetings a month, one with veterans attending along with family members and the other for family members only, but facilitators are encouraged to adapt the program as appropriate. The response of families to this program has been overwhelmingly positive.

Virtual Reality Therapy

Virtual reality therapy (VRE) is a therapy that involves visualization, interaction, and/or manipulation of stimuli through use of computers. VRE utilizes technology to provide more consistent and controllable stimuli than what patients' imaginations can produce (Rizzo & Kim, 2005, Rizzo, Schulteis, & Kerns, 2004). VRE uses computer graphics in motion-tracked displays allowing vibrations, sounds, and scent deliveries to enhance the realism of the exposure. This approach has been used with some success to treat Vietnam veterans with PTSD (Rothbaum, Hodges, & Ready, 2001), World Trade Center survivors of the 9/11 attacks (Difede, Hoffman, & Jayasinghe, 2002), and Iraq veterans (Rothbaum, Rizzo, & Difede, 2010). Limitations of VRE involve associated costs, potential for malfunctioning equipment to disrupt the therapeutic process, and some clients being distracted by the realism. Research is needed to compare this type of exposure compares with more traditional therapies.

Treating General Postdeployment Adjustment Problems

Although psychosocial and adjustment difficulties on homecoming can be distressing (Shea et al., 2010), these difficulties by themselves do not constitute psychiatric illness and therefore warrant different kinds interventions. The first step in developing interventions for adjustment problems of returning veterans is a comprehensive assessment of psychosocial functioning that addresses areas identified above as well as safety issues, pending legal issues, and all other areas relevant for all service members (Litz & Orsillo, 2011). Because veterans recently returning from deployments are especially likely to have protective factors such as intact families, employment and educational aspirations, and fewer legal problems, clinical interventions for returning veterans should be designed to preserve the social assets already present.

An important area to assess is the level of functioning at work or in school. Occupational issues may vary from unemployment and difficulty finding a job to embarking on a new career after discharge or retirement from the military to problems of low productivity, anger, and interpersonal difficulties on the job. Veterans making a transition to a different career may benefit from vocational counseling that provides interest inventories and tests of skills and abilities, coaching for interviewing skills, assistance with resume writing, training in a new field, and emotional support and therapy to address potential impediments such as negative self-talk that can undermine confidence. Veterans who anticipate returning to school may need assistance at a case management level to help them identify and apply for educational benefits. These veterans may benefit from assistance in developing study skills and support as well as development of realistic expectations and management of stress associated with returning to school after a long period of time away and perhaps in a different context.

Assessment of family functioning may also identify problems in veterans after their return from deployment. Couples with relationship problems may benefit from marital therapy. Alternatively, special retreats designed for returning veterans and their spouses and offered by various organizations may allow the couple to bypass barriers to formal treatment such as stigma and inconvenience of multiple sessions. Family therapy and parenting classes may also be helpful. Specifically tailored programs have been developed to help children adjust to the deployment and return of a military parent. For example, Sesame Workshop (2010; the non-profit organization responsible for *Sesame Street*) has developed a collection of videos called the "Stop, Listen, and Connect" series to help children learn to cope with the topics of deployment and return of a parent, change in the family, and grief.

Relationships with friends and community involvement should also be assessed. Hypervigilance and anxiety around crowds is a common complaint of returning veterans, and these reactions may lead to withdrawal from activities in the community and isolation from the veteran's natural support systems. Participating in veterans' groups and community projects or volunteer activities of interest to the veteran may help decrease social isolation and provide meaning and a sense of purpose for the veteran. It may help the veteran to learn to make distinctions between "military self" and "home self."

Problems in the area of anger control may have repercussions across all domains of functioning. Assessment of anger-control problems should consider the potential for domestic violence and/or abuse toward children. An option for veterans with anger-control problems is referral to an anger-management group. Anger-management groups for returning veterans should address combat-specific issues, such as helping veterans understand that aggressive expression of anger that may have been adaptive in combat situations is not adaptive in civilian interactions.

Assessment of substance use is essential, given the very high rates of comorbid substance abuse problems in this population. Veterans who have difficulty controlling alcohol intake may feel that alcohol helps them cope with their symptoms and with distress. One focus of treatment for them will be the development of healthier alternative coping skills. Referral for formal alcohol treatment may be indicated.

Comprehensive resource and referral lists are essential for connecting this population with the myriad of interventions and resources to address the many psychosocial issues they face. Many veterans prefer to seek assistance with their reintegration difficulties through innovative sources such as the Internet (Sayer et al., 2010). Many organizations and agencies have developed websites that include links to resources for OEF/OIF veterans and their families and professionals who are treating this population. For example, the Defense Centers of Excellence for Psychological Health and Traumatic Brain Injury (2011) project supported by the National Center for Telehealth and Technology provides a website with information about relevant topics such as families and friendships, anger, stigma, and work adjustment. Self-assessments, informational podcasts and videos, and sections for family members and providers are also available on the website. A joint project of the Departments of Defense, Labor and Veterans Affairs created The National Resource Directory (2010), "a website for connecting wounded warriors, Service Members, Veterans, their families with those who support them." The site provides a number of resources at national and local levels that span a broad range of topics including information on education, training, and employment; housing and homelessness assistance; and support for caregivers. The National Center for PTSD (2011) offers a VA-sponsored website providing information for veterans and families with handouts on a number of subjects related to trauma and PTSD. It also disseminates tools, research data, and other information to support and educate providers who work with veterans.

CONCLUSIONS

This chapter has reviewed the mental health problems of returning veterans of the Iraq and Afghanistan conflicts and mental health treatments and other interventions for them. Returning combat veterans from the Iraq and Afghanistan wars represent a unique cohort of veterans. As their demographic characteristics and mental health issues may differ from previous veteran cohorts, their mental health treatment needs can also be expected to differ. Clinicians working with these veterans should be aware not only of the potential for psychiatric disorders such as PTSD, depressive and other comorbidities including TBI, but also the possibility of postdeployment readjustment problems. Many different modes of mental health treatment and other interventions are available for clinicians to use in efforts to help veterans with these problems. While research has provided considerable evidence of effectiveness for many of these treatments, further research into the comparative efficacy of various psychotherapies and psychopharmacologic agents is needed, as well as further development of even more effective and comprehensive treatments.

REFERENCES

Albright, D. L., & Thyer, B. (2010). Does EMDR reduce post-traumatic stress disorder? *Behavioral Interventions, 25*, 1–19.

American Psychiatric Association. (2000). *Diagnostic and statistical manual of mental disorders* (4th ed., text revision). Washington, DC: American Psychiatric Press.

Baldwin, D. S., Anderson, I. M., Nutt, D. J., Bandelow, B., Bond, A., Davidson, J. R. T., et al. (2005). Evidence-based guidelines for the pharmacological treatment of anxiety disorders: Recommendations from the British Association for Psychopharmacology. *Journal of Psychopharmacology, 19*, 567–596.

Bandelow, B., Zohar, J., Hollander, E., Kasper, S., & Moller, H. J. (2002). Task force on treatment guidelines for anxiety, obsessive-compulsive and posttraumatic stress disorders. World Federation of Societies of Biological Psychiatry (WFSBP) guidelines for the pharmacological treatment of anxiety, obsessive-compulsive and posttraumatic stress disorders. *World Journal of Biological Psychiatry, 3*, 171–199.

Bowling, U., Doerman, A., & Sherman, M. (2007). Operation enduring families: Information and support for Iraq and Afghanistan veterans and their families. Oklahoma City VA Medical Center Family Health Program. Retrieved February 1, 2011, from http://www.ouhsc.edu/oef

Breslau, N., Kessler, R. C., Chilcoat, H. D., Schultz, L. R., Davis, G. C., & Andreski, P. (1998). Trauma and posttraumatic stress disorder in the community. *Archives of General Psychiatry, 55*, 626–632.

Canadian Psychiatric Association. (2006). Clinical practice guidelines. Management of anxiety disorders. *Canadian Journal of Psychiatry, 51*(8 suppl 2), 9S–91S.

Carlson, K. F., Nelson, D., Orazem, R. J., Nugent, S., Cifu, D. X., & Sayer, N. A. (2010). Psychiatric diagnoses among Iraq and Afghanistan war veterans screened for deployment-related traumatic brain injury. *Journal of Traumatic Stress, 23*, 17–24.

Carroll, L. J., Cassidy, J. D., Holm, L., Kraus, J., & Coronado, V. G. (2004). Methodological issues and research recommendations for mild traumatic brain injury: The WHO Collaborating Centre Task Force on Mild Traumatic Brain Injury. *Journal of Rehabilitative Medicine, 43*, 113–125.

Castro, C. A., Bienvenu, R. V., Hufmann, A. H., & Adler, A. B. (2000). Soldier dimensions and operational readiness in U.S. Army forces deployed to Kosovo. *International Review of the Armed Forces Medical Service, 73*, 191–200.

Chard, K. M., Shumm, J. A., Owens, G. P., & Cottingham, S. M. (2010). A comparison of OEF and OIF veterans and Vietnam veterans receiving cognitive processing therapy. *Journal of Traumatic Stress, 23*, 25–32.

Christensen, .A, Atkins, D., Berns, S., Wheeler, J., Baucom, D. H., & Simpson, L. E. (2004). Traditional versus integrative behavioral couple therapy for significantly and chronically distressed married couples. *Journal of Consulting and Clinical Psychology, 72*, 176–191.

Cozza, S. J., Guimond, J. M., McKibben, J. B. A., Chun, R. O., Arata-Maiers, T. L., Schneider, B., et al. (2010). Combat-injured service members and their families: The relationship of child distress and spouse-perceived family distress and disruption. *Journal of Traumatic Stress, 23*, 112–115.

Cukor, J., Spitalnick, J., Difede, J., Rizzo, A., & Rothbaum, B. O. (2009). Emerging treatments for PTSD. *Clinical Psychology Review, 29*, 715–726.

Davis, L. L., English, B. A., Ambrose, S. M., & Petty, F. (2001). Pharmacotherapy for post traumatic stress disorder: A comprehensive review. *Expert Opinion on Pharmacotherapy, 2*(10), 1583–1595.

Defense Centers of Excellence for Psychological Health and Traumatic Brain Injury Project. (2011). Retrieved February 1, 2011, from http://www.afterdeployment.org/web/guest

Difede, J., Hoffman, H. G., & Jayasinghe, N. (2002). Innovative use of virtual reality technology in the treatment of PTSD in the aftermath of September 11. *Psychiatric Services, 53*, 1083–1085.

Dodgson, P. W. (2009). EMDR and PTSD. In A. Rubin & D. W. Springer (Eds.), *Treatment of traumatized adults and children: Clinician's guide to evidence-based practice* (pp. 257–348). Hoboken, NJ: Wiley.

Erbes, C. R., Curry, K. T., & Leskela, J. (2009). Treatment presentation and adherence of Iraq/Afghanistan era veterans in outpatient care for posttraumatic stress disorder. *Psychiatric Services, 6*, 175–183.

Erbes, C. R., Polusny, M. A., MacDermid, S., & Compton, J. S. (2008). Couple therapy with combat veterans and their partners. *Journal of Clinical Psychiatry, 64*, 972–983.

Erbes, C. R., Westermeyer, J., Engdahl, B., & Johnsen, E. (2007). Post-traumatic stress disorder and service utilization in a sample of service members from Iraq and Afghanistan. *Military Medicine, 172*, 359–363.

Foa, E. B., Davidson, J. R. T., & Frances, A. (1999). Treatment of posttraumatic stress disorder: The expert consensus guideline series. *Journal of Clinical Psychiatry, 60*, 1–76.

Fontana, A., & Rosenheck, R. (2008). Treatment-seeking veterans of Iraq and Afghanistan: Comparison with veterans of previous wars. *Journal of Nervous and Mental Disease, 196*, 513–521.

Fontana, A., & Rosenheck, R. (2010). War zone veterans returning to treatment: Effects of social functioning and psychopathology. *Journal of Nervous and Mental Disease, 198*, 699–707.

Forbes, D., Phelps, A. J., & McHugh, A. F. (2001). Imagery rehearsal in the treatment of posttraumatic nightmares in combat-related PTSD. *Journal of Traumatic Stress, 14*, 433–442.

Forbes, D., Phelps, A. J., McHugh, A. F., Debenham, P., Hopwood, M., & Creamer, M. (2003). Imagery rehearsal in the treatment of posttraumatic nightmares in Australian veterans with chronic combat-related PTSD: 12-month follow-up data. *Journal of Traumatic Stress, 16*, 509–513.

Friedman, M. J. (2008). Treatments for PTSD: Understanding the evidence. Pharmacotherapy. *PTSD Research Quarterly, 19*(1), 6–7.

Grieger, T. A., Cozza, S. J., Ursano, R. J., Hoge, C., Martinez, P. E., Engel, C. C., & Wain, H. J. (2006). Post-traumatic stress disorder and depression in battle-injured soldiers. *American Journal of Psychiatry, 163*, 1777–1783.

Hetrick, S. E. Purcell, R., Garner, B., & Parslow, R. (2010). Combined pharmacotherapy and psychological therapies for post traumatic stress disorder (PTSD). *Cochrane Database of Systematic Reviews, 7*, CD007316.

Hoge, C. W., Auchterlonie, J. L, & Milliken, C. S. (2006). Mental health problems, use of mental health services, and attrition from military service after returning from deployment to Iraq or Afghanistan. *Journal of the American Medical Association, 295*, 1023-1032.

Hoge, C. W., Castro, C. A., Messer, S. C., McGurk, D., Cotting, D. I., & Koffman, R. L. (2004). Combat duty in Iraq and Afghanistan, mental health problems, and barriers to care. *New England Journal of Medicine, 351*, 13-22.

Institute of Medicine. (2010). *Returning home from Iraq and Afghanistan: Preliminary assessment of readjustment needs of veterans, service members, and their families.* Washington, DC: The National Academies Press.

Jacobson, N. S., & Christensen ,A. (1996). *Integrative couple therapy: Promoting acceptance and change.* New York: Norton.

Jacobson, N. S, Christensen, A., Prince, S. E., Cordova, J., & Eldridge, K. (2000). Integrative behavioral couple therapy: An acceptance-based, promising new treatment for couple discord. *Journal of Consulting and Clinical Psychiatry, 68*, 351-355.

Jacobson, N. S., & Margolin, G. (1979). *Marital therapy: Strategies based on social learning and behavioral exchange principals.* New York: Bruner/Mazell.

Jakupcak, M., Luterek, J., Hunt, S., Conybeare, D., & McFall, M. (2008). Posttraumatic stress and its relationship to physical health functioning in a sample of Iraq and Afghanistan war veterans seeking postdeployment VA health care. *Journal of Nervous and Mental Disease, 196*, 425-428.

Joint Economic Committee U.S. Congress. (2007). *Happy Mother's Day? New JEC report reveals military moms face tough challenges to get mental health care, childcare, and family leave.* Washington, DC: Author. Retrieved February 1, 2011, from http://jec.senate.gov/public/index.cfm?p=PressReleases&ContentRecord_id=eb633779-7e9c-9af9-72ca-884578253e62&ContentType_id=66d767ed-750b-43e8-b8cf-89524ad8a29e

Kang, H. K., & Bullman, T. A. (1996). Mortality among US veterans of the Persian Gulf War. *New England Journal of Medicine*, 335, 1498-1504.

Kang, H. K., & Bullman, T. A. (2008). Risk of suicide among US veterans after returning from the Iraq and Afghanistan War Zones. *Journal of the American Medical Association, 300*, 652-653.

Kang, H. K., & Hyams, K. C. (2005). Mental health care needs among recent war veterans. *New England Journal of Medicine, 352*, 1289.

Kessler, R. C., Sonnega, A., Bromet, E., Hughes, M., & Nelson, C. (1995). Posttraumatic stress disorder in the National Comorbidity Survey. *Archives of General Psychiatry, 52*, 1048-1060.

Kimerling, R., Street, A. E., Pavao, J., Smith, M. W., Cronkite, R. C., Holmes, T. H., et al. (2010). Military-related sexual trauma among Veterans Health Administration patients returning from Afghanistan and Iraq. *American Journal of Public Health, 100,* 1409-1412.

Kolkow, T. T., Spira, J. L., Morse, J. S., & Grieger, T. A. (2007). Post-traumatic stress disorder and depression in health care providers returning from deployment to Iraq and Afghanistan. *Military Medicine, 172,* 451-455.

Krakow, B., & Zadra, A. (2010). Imagery rehearsal therapy: Principles and practice. *Sleep Medicine Clinics, 5,* 289-298.

Leland, A., & Oboroceanu, M. J. (2010). *American war and military operations casualties: Lists and statistics.* Washington, DC: Congressional Research Service. Retrieved February 1, 2011, from http://www.fas.org/sgp/crs/natsec/RL32492.pdf

Lemaire, C. M., & Graham, D. P. (2010). Factors associated with suicidal ideation in OEF/OIF veterans. *Journal of Affective Disorders, 130*, 231-238. doi:10.1016/j.jad.2010.10.021

Lipari, R. N., Cook, P. J., Rock, L. M., & Matos, K. (2008). 2006 Gender Relations Survey of Active Duty Members. DMDC Report No. 2007-002. Arlington, VA: Department of Defense Manpower Data Center.

Litz, B., & Orsillo, S. M. (2011). The returning veteran of the Iraq war: Background issues and assessment guidelines. In *The Iraq War Clinician Guide*, (2nd ed., pp. 21-32). White River Junction, VT: National Center for PTSD. Retrieved February 1, 2011, from http://www.ptsd.va.gov/professional/manuals/manual-pdf/iwcg/iraq_clinician_guide_ch_3.pdf

Lu, M., Wagner, A., Van Male, L., Whitehead, A., & Boehnlein, J. (2009). Imagery rehearsal therapy for posttraumatic nightmares in US veterans. *Journal of Traumatic Stress, 22*, 236-239.

Maguen, S., Lucenko, B. A., Reger, M. A., Gahm, G. A., Litz, B. T., Seal, K. H., Knight, S. J., & Marmar, C. R. (2010). The impact of reported direct and indirect killing on mental health symptoms in Iraq war veterans. *Journal of Traumatic Stress, 23*, 86-90.

Martin, J., Ghahramanlou-Holloway, M., Lou, K., & Tucciarone, P. (2009). A comparative review of US military and civilian suicide behavior: Implications for OEF/OIF suicide prevention efforts. *Journal of Mental Health Counseling, 31*, 101-118.

McCrea, M. (2007). *Mild traumatic brain injury and postconcussion syndrome: The new evidence base for diagnosis and treatment.* New York: Oxford University Press.

McDevitt-Murphy, M. E., Williams, J. L., Brackem, K. L., Fields, J. A., Monahan, C. J., & Murphy, J. G. (2010). PTSD symptoms, hazardous drinking, and health functioning among U.S. OEF and OIF veterans presenting to primary care. *Journal of Traumatic Stress, 23*, 108–111.

Mental Health Advisory Team 5 (MHAT-V). (2008). Office of the Surgeon Multi-National Force-Iraq and Office of the Command Surgeon and Office of the Surgeon General United States Army Medical Command. Retrieved from http://www.armymedicine.army.mil/reports/mhat/mhat_v/mhat-v.cfm

Miliken, C. S., Auchterlonie, J. L., & Hoge, C. W. (2007). Longitudinal assessment of mental health problems among active and reserve component soldiers returning from the Iraq war. *Journal of the American Medical Association, 298*, 2141–2148.

Miller, W. R., & Rollnick, S. (2002). *Motivational interviewing: Preparing people for change* (2nd ed.). New York: Guilford Press.

Moore, B. A., & Krakow, B. (2007). Imagery rehearsal therapy for acute posttraumatic nightmares among combat soldiers in Iraq. *American Journal of Psychiatry, 164*, 683–684.

Najavits, L. M. (2002). *Seeking safety: A treatment manual for PTSD and substance abuse.* New York: Guilford Press.

Najavits, L. M. (2009). Seeking safety: An implementation guide. In A. Rubin, & D. W. Springer (Eds.), *The clinician's guide to evidence-based practice.* Hoboken, NJ: Wiley.

Nappi, C. M., Drummond, S. P., Thorp, S. R., & McQuaid, J. R. (2010). Effectiveness of imagery rehearsal therapy or the treatment of combat-related nightmares in veterans. *Behavior Therapy, 41*, 237–244.

National Center for PTSD. (2011). Washington, DC: United States Department of Veterans Affairs. Retrieved January 1, 2011, from http://www.ptsd.va.gov/

National Collaborating Centre for Mental Health. (2005). *The management of post traumatic stress disorder in primary and secondary care.* London, UK: National Institute for Clinical Excellence.

National Resource Directory. (2010). Retrieved February 1, 2011, from http://www.nationalresourcedirectory.gov/

Norman, S. B., Wilkins, K. C., Tapert, S. F., Lang, A. J., & Najavits, L. M. (2010). A pilot study of seeking safety therapy with OEF/OIF veterans. *Journal of Psychoactive Drugs, 42*, 83–87.

Pietrzak, R. H., Goldstein, M. B., Malley, J. C., Johnson, D. C., & Southwick, S. M. (2009). Subsyndromal posttraumatic stress disorder is associated with health and psychosocial difficulties in veterans of operations enduring freedom and Iraqi freedom. *Depression and Anxiety, 26*, 739–744.

Pietrzak, R. H., Goldstein, M. B., Malley, J. C., Rivers, A. J., Johnson, D. C., & Southwick, S. M. (2010). Risk and protective factors associated with suicidal ideation in veterans of operations enduring freedom and Iraqi freedom. *Journal of Affective Disorders, 123*, 102–107.

Ramchand, R., Schell, T. L., Karney, B. R., Osilla, K. C., Burns, R. M., & Caldarone, L. B. (2010). Disparate prevalence estimates of PTSD among service members who served in Iraq and Afghanistan: Possible explanations. *Journal of Traumatic Stress, 23*, 59–68.

Reeves, R. R. (2007). Diagnosis and management of posttraumatic stress disorder in returning veterans. *Journal of the American Osteopathic Association, 107*(5), 181–189.

Resick, P. A., Monson, C. M., & Chard, K. M. (2007). *Cognitive processing therapy: Veteran/military version.* Washington, DC: Department of Veterans Affairs.

Rizzo, A. A., & Kim, G. (2005). A SWOT analysis of the field of virtual rehabilitation and therapy. *Presence: Teleoperators and Virtual Environments, 14*, 1–28.

Rizzo, A. A., Schulteis, M. T., & Kerns, K. (2004). Analysis of assets for virtual reality applications in neuropsychology. *Neuropscholological Rehabilitation, 14*, 207–239.

Rothbaum, B. O., Astin, M. C., & Marsteller, F. (2005). Prolonged exposure versus eye movement desensitization and reprocessing (EMDR) for PTSD rape victims. *Journal of Traumatic Stress, 18*, 607–616.

Rothbaum, B. O., Hodges, L., & Ready, D. (2001). Virtual reality exposure therapy for Vietnam veterans with posttraumatic stress disorder. *Journal of Clinical Psychiatry, 62*, 617–622.

Rothbaum, B. O., Rizzo, A., & Difede, J. (2010). Virtual reality exposure therapy for combat-related posttraumatic stress disorder. *Annals of the New York Academy of Sciences, 1208*, 126–132.

Sayer, N. A., Noorbaloochi, S., Frazier, P., Carlson, K., Grevely, A., & Murdoch, M. (2010). Reintegration problems and treatment interests among Iraq and Afghanistan combat veterans receiving VA medical care. *Psychiatric Services, 61*, 589–597.

Schlenger, W. E., Kulka, R. A., Fairbank, J. A., Hough, R. L., Jordan, B. K., Marmar, C. R., & Weiss, D. S. (1992). The prevalence of post-traumatic stress disorder in the Vietnam generation: A multimethod, multisource assessment of psychiatric disorder. *Journal of Traumatic Stress, 5*, 333–363.

Seal, K. H., Bertenthal, D., Miner, C. R., Sen, S., & Marmar, C. (2007). Bringing the war back home: Mental health disorders among 103,788 US veterans returning from Iraq and Afghanistan seen at Department of Veterans Affairs facilities. *Archives of Internal Medicine, 167*, 476–482.

Sesame Workshop. (2011). *Deployments, homecomings, changes, and grief.* Retrieved February 1, 2011, from http://www.sesameworkshop.org/initiatives/emotion/tlc

Shea, M. T., Vujanovic, A. A., Mansfield, A. K., Sevin, E., & Liu, F. (2010). Posttraumatic stress disorder symptoms and functional impairment among OEF and OIF National Guard and Reserve veterans. *Journal of Traumatic Stress, 23,* 100–107.

Sherman, M. (2003). Updates and five-year evaluation of the S.A.F.E. program: A family psychoeducational program for serious mental illness. *Community Mental Health Journal, 42,* 213–219.

Stein, D. J., Ipset, J.C., & McAnda, B. A. (2009). Pharmacotherapy for posttraumatic stress disorder: A review of meta analysis and treatment guidelines. *CNS Spectrums, 14*(1), 25–31.

Stein, D. J., Ipser, J. C., & Seedat, S. (2006). Pharmacotherapy for posttraumatic stress disorder (PTSD). *Cochrane Database Syst Rev.* (1), CD002795.

Street, A. E., Vogt, D., & Dutra, L. (2009). A new generation of women veterans: Stressors faced by women deployed to Iraq and Afghanistan. *Clinical Psychology Review, 29*(8), 685–694.

Surís, A., & Lind, L. (2008). Military sexual trauma: A review of prevalence and associated health consequences in veterans. *Trauma, violence, and abuse, 9,* 250–269.

Surís, A., & Smith, J. (in press). PTSD related to sexual trauma in the military. In W. Penk & B. Moore (Eds.), *Handbook for the treatment of PTSD in military personnel.* New York: Guilford.

Tanelian, T., Jaycox, L. H., Schell, T. L., Marshal, G. N., Burnam, M. A., Eibner, C., et al. (2008). The Invisible Wounds Study Team. *Invisible wounds of war: Summary and recommendations for addressing psychological and cognitive injuries.* Santa Monica, CA: RAND Center for Health Policy Research. Retrieved February 1, 2011, from http://rand.org/pubs/monographs/2008/RAND_MG720.1.pdf

Tuerk, P. W., Yoder, M., Grubaugh, A., Myrick, H., Hamner, M., & Acierno, R. (2011). Prolonged exposure therapy for combat-related posttraumatic stress disorder: An examination of treatment effectiveness for veterans of the wars in Afghanistan and Iraq. *Journal of Anxiety Disorders, 25,* 397–403.

Ursano, R. J., Bell, C., Eth, S., Friedman, M., Norwood, A., Pfefferbaum, B., et al. (2004). Work Group on ASD and PTSD, Steering Committee on Practice Guidelines. Practice guideline for the treatment of patients with acute stress disorder and posttraumatic stress disorder. *American Journal of Psychiatry, 161,* 3–31.

U.S. Department of Defense. (2011). *DoD casualty reports, 2011.* Retrieved February 1, 2011, from http://www.defense.gov/ news/casualty.pdf

U.S. Department of Veterans Affairs. (2008). VA Uniform mental health services in VA medical centers and clinics. In *Veterans health administration handbook 1160.01.* Washington, DC: Author. Retrieved February 1, 2011, from http://www.va.gov/vhapublications/ViewPublication.asp?pub_ID=1762

U.S. Department of Veterans Affairs and Department of Defense. (2009). *VA/DoD clinical practice guideline for management of concussion/mild traumatic brain injury (mTBI), version 1.0.* Washington, DC: Author. Retrieved July 5, 2011, from http://www.healthquality.va.gov/mtbi/concussion_mtbi_full_1_0.pdf

U.S. Department of Veterans Affairs and Department of Defense. (2010). *VA/DoD clinical practice guideline. Management of post-traumatic stress.* Washington, DC: Author.

Vogt, D. S., Pless, A. P., King, L. A., & King, D. W. (2005). Deployment stressors, gender, and mental health outcomes among Gulf War I veterans. *Journal of Traumatic Stress, 18,* 272–284.

Women in Military Service for America Memorial Foundation. (2010). *Press Kit.* Washington, DC: Author. Retrieved February 1, 2011, from http://www.womensmemorial.org/Press/stats.html

21

Users of Assistive Technology: The Human Component

Martin G. Brodwin, Frances W. Siu, and Elizabeth Cardoso

Assistive technology (AT) has a profound impact on the everyday lives and employment opportunities of individuals with disabilities by providing them with greater independence and enabling them to perform activities not possible in the past. AT is defined in the "Technology-Related Assistance of Individuals with Disabilities Act of 1988" (Tech Act; P. L. 100–407) as "any item, piece of equipment, or product system, whether acquired commercially off the shelf, modified, or customized, that is used to increase, maintain, or improve functional capabilities of individuals with disabilities" (Scherer, 2007, p. 185). AT enhances social functioning, recreational activities, and work opportunities, thus decreasing a consumer's functional limitations and helping to "level the playing field" between people with disabilities and those without disabilities.

When utilizing AT, a consumer's self-worth, sense of belonging, and the attitudes of others play a dynamic role. Therefore, consumer involvement is imperative to the process. Initially, in the assessment/evaluation phase of rehabilitation, the rehabilitation counselor should help the consumer identify the priorities and motivation for requesting AT. These should be in the forefront throughout the entire process as they are key to successful implementation and use of AT. By carefully defining achievement goals with the consumer, the counselor will be able to clearly identify what he or she wants to accomplish by using technology. This involves the activities that motivate a consumer to use AT and is crucial to successful adaptation and use.

Self-esteem, self-efficacy, and motivation are described as central elements in increasing a consumer's confidence and belief in self. Good outcomes and efficacy expectations, as well as strong motivation, help lead to successful adaptation to AT. The purpose of this chapter is to present the human component of technology, the relationship between consumers and technological devices/equipment, and the acceptance and use by consumers. Recommendations are offered to assist rehabilitation professionals in helping consumers with accepting, utilizing, and benefiting from technology.

From "Use of assistive technology: The human component," by M. Brodwin, T. Star, and E. Cardoso, 2003, *Journal of Applied Rehabilitation Counseling,* 34, 23–29. The National Rehabilitation Counseling Association.

TECHNOLOGY ACCEPTANCE AND USE

AT increases functional abilities, independence, and access to mainstream society by individuals with disabilities. Currently, more than 20 million Americans with disabilities are using technology; however, a national survey on AT abandonment found that 29% of devices obtained were discarded later (Riemer-Reiss & Wacker, 2000). These researchers found "those individuals who continued to use their technology had significantly higher mean scores than those who discontinued use of their technology in relation to relative advantage, consumer involvement, and compatibility" (p. 48).

Riemer-Reiss and Wacker (2000) researched technology use and abandonment issues by consumers. Their findings inferred that little documentation existed from the consumer's perspective as to why assistive devices had been abandoned. These authors' goal was to determine factors associated with AT continuance or discontinuance using Rogers's (1995) theory of diffusion, based on a consumer's initial decision to accept a device and later reject it. According to Riemer-Reiss and Wacker, discontinuance happens in two ways: (a) replacement, where one device is discarded for an improved one and (b) user disenchantment or dissatisfaction. The researchers derived the following as crucial factors for consumers' continued use of AT: advantage, compatibility, trialability, and reinvention.

Carroll and Phillips (1993), in a survey on abandonment of AT by 25 new users, concluded that characteristics of relative advantage (effectiveness, reliability, ease of use, comfort, and enhancement of the user's performance) were significantly related to not abandoning technology. Compatibility, a factor related to use, is the extent to which the device is perceived by consumers to meet their needs. Trialability was defined as the degree to which the consumer could experiment with the AT device or equipment before acquisition. Reinvention occurs when a new model replaces an older one. Riemer-Reiss and Wacker (2000) hypothesized that the relationship between continuance/discontinuance involved a combination of compatibility, advantage, support, trialability, consumer involvement, and changes when making decisions or setting goals. These authors concluded that further research is necessary in the areas of evaluation and whether the provision of technology is meeting the needs and desires of the consumer.

NONUSE OR USE OF AT

The degree to which a device is essential for a consumer's desired function includes his or her particular needs and becomes crucial in determining whether the consumer uses or abandons the product (Scherer, 2002, 2007). To avoid nonuse, rehabilitation counseling professionals need to identify and consider matching technology with aspects of the person's personality and temperament, characteristics of the setting, and the material traits of the assistive device itself.

Optimal Use

Scherer (2007) further described optimal characteristics of the setting where the AT will be used to include the following: support from others (family, peers, and employer), realistic expectations of family/employer, and an environment that fully supports and rewards use of technology. Positive consumer personality variables involve motivation (how AT will help the consumer accomplish desired tasks), coping skills, capability to use the device, pride in using technology, patience, and self-discipline. Characteristics of the technology that influence consumer use include the following: compatibility with and enhancement of other technologies that the consumer is using, reliability, ease of use, problem-free and timely maintenance, and desirable transportability.

Benefit Expectations

These expectations involve what the consumer wants to accomplish by using AT—the desired tasks that are most important to the consumer. Aspects of technology that will benefit consumers are influenced by the positive and negative attitudes of others. Other areas that may influence continued use are the following: social support, loneliness, isolation, and cultural identity. Research has shown that individuals who do not have social support have an increased chance of discontinuing use of recently acquired technology (Riemer-Reiss & Wacker, 2000; Scherer, 2007). The characteristics related to consumers' acceptance and use include level of technical comfort, cognitive (intellectual) skills, personality traits, adjustment, and outlook, including pre-existing temperament and ways of coping. In addition, technological characteristics to consider include design factors, such as weight, ease of set-up, compatibility with other devices, as well as the consumer's level of comfort when using AT (Reed & Saladin, 2008).

THE HUMAN COMPONENT

The National Council on Disability performed a study in 1993 on the impact of assistive technologies on individuals with disabilities and found that (a) approximately 76% of children who received AT were able to stay in a regular classroom and about 45% were able to reduce school-related services; (b) around 62% of working-age persons were able to be less reliant on their family members and 58% were able to cut down on paid assistance; (c) roughly 80% of senior citizens were able to increase their independence and about half were able to avoid institutionalization; (d) nearly 92% of working individuals reported that AT helped them to work efficiently and effectively and 83% indicated that they increased their income; and (e) almost 67% reported that AT had helped them to obtain employment (Stumbo, Martin, & Hedrick, 2009).

AT does not merely increase the functional abilities and independence of the end users; utilization of AT has powerful influences on the attitude, self-worth, self-esteem, and motivation of older individuals and those with disabilities.

Attitudes

Attitudes exhibited by professionals are crucial in establishing trust and confidence in the counselor–consumer relationship. When a consumer forms a relationship with a professional involving how to effectively use AT, the consumer takes the position of initiating a help-seeking role. This role requires developing a level of courage toward, and trust and confidence in, the professional relationship. The rehabilitation counselor needs to maintain a focus on the consumer's best interests and have a positive attitude. Any negative attitudes exhibited by the professional could have adverse consequences for the consumer in his or her achievement of desired outcomes. The goal is to approach providing technology services from the consumer's perspective when defining specific objectives, needs, and desires. According to Scherer (2007), "assistive technologies are used when consumers have goals and see the devices as valuable to goal achievement. When users have significant input into selection of the devices, they become more invested in using them successfully" (p. 131).

Self-Worth

Schaller and DeLaGarza (1999) affirmed that the self-concepts of consumers with disabilities are influenced by the social context in which they interact, validating either positively or negatively, self-worth. Supportive relationships for consumers promote a sense of belonging and are necessary for the development of positive self-images and self-acceptance. Positive social support promotes more stability, less emotional stress, and greater psychological well-being by buffering negative life events and easing environmental pressures. Consumers with disabilities usually have knowledge of their needs, but have a difficult time expressing and attaining feelings of belonging. Technology can both heighten feelings of being different (in a negative way) and, at the same time, enhance the ability to interact with others. As noted by Best (2009), children with cerebral palsy who use AT are more capable of interacting with children without disabilities.

Self-Esteem

Behavior and cognition are essential elements that contribute to learning, with an emphasis on learning through observation of others. This is certainly true when consumers are adapting to the use of AT. Self-esteem is highly related to an individual's ability to accomplish tasks and goals. The concepts of self-esteem, self-worth, and self-image are defined as the total dimension of the self, with self-concept relating to a specific area in which individuals evaluate their knowledge, capabilities, and skills (Santrock, 2009).

An ability to cope with a problem rather than avoid it contributes to positive self-evaluative thoughts, which generate self-approval, thus enhancing one's self-esteem. Bandura's (1982) theory of individuals believing that they can master a situation and produce a positive outcome is labeled self-efficacy. It is based on the principle that cognitive events are induced and altered by efforts and persistence demonstrated in a task. Personal experience reinforced by successful performance of a task, including use of AT, enhances an individual's belief that goals attempted can be accomplished (Conyers, Enright, & Strauser, 1998; Cook, Polgar, & Hussey, 2008).

Self-Efficacy Theory

Self-efficacy theory proposes that expectations vary in level of challenge (high or low degree), in strength (ability to persevere), and flexibility of self-efficacy (whether it will transfer from one area to another). The above essential elements affect the level of self-efficacy and the extent to which an individual is able to cope with obstacles, and it is applicable to the use of technology. In the first element, a consumer feels confident in knowing what to do with AT and how to do it. The second element involves a belief that, if tried out, success will be achieved. A belief that the chosen behavior will have an effect on the outcome (adaptation to technology) is the third element. The final element brings successful reinforcement to the consumer as he or she believes that the device or equipment is of importance. Thus, the enhancement of activities and reduction of functional limitations provide adequate incentives for performing the behavior in the future (Cook et al., 2008; Scherer, 2007).

Efficacy Expectations and Outcome Expectations

Self-efficacy beliefs consist of two components: efficacy expectations and outcome expectations (Conyers et al., 1998). Efficacy expectations concern a person's beliefs about the ability to undertake a given task (in this case, learning to use technology), and range from high to low. Outcome expectations involve whether a person knows what to do in a given situation and believes that the outcomes of effort will be beneficial or not and also have a range of high to low. Both efficacy and outcome expectations need to be relatively high for people to attempt and succeed at using technology. Self-efficacy includes four essential elements that can be related to the use of AT (Bandura, 1982; Mitchell & Brodwin, 1995):

1. In a given situation, an individual knows what to do and how to do it. In the case of AT, the consumer needs the knowledge on how to successfully use the device.
2. The person has the confidence that he or she can succeed in the activity. This relates to a consumer being self-assured that, if given sufficient instruction, he or she can successfully learn to use the device or equipment.

3. The individual believes that what he or she does will have an impact on the end result. This element involves a consumer believing that he or she can learn to use the technology and that this will result in a positive outcome, in that the consumer will be able to accomplish the desired tasks with use of technology.
4. The outcome is of sufficient importance for the person to want what the outcome will provide. The consumer believes that what the device or equipment provides in decreasing functional limitations and enhancing capabilities is what he or she desires.

Consequently, the level of self-efficacy a consumer maintains will determine, in part, whether he or she will accept, try out, and continue to use AT in the future. When the levels of these four components are high, the consumer typically demonstrates goal-oriented, self-assured, and persistent behavior when dealing with the technology. The higher the consumer's self-efficacy, the greater the likelihood of successful adaptation to, and use of, AT (Conyers et al., 1998).

Motivation

The term motivation is defined as an inner urge or desire that prompts an individual to perform a behavior; motivation produces a particular action or manifests itself as any influence that promotes positive performance (Scherer, 2007). Self-efficacy provides the foundation for motivation by establishing actions that result in positive, repetitive reinforcement. In the process of delivering technology services to a consumer, motivation may result from any point within the process: the consumer, the activity engaged in, the environment, or the AT system components. As noted by Rubin and Roessler (2008), in dealing with consumers and AT, motivation must always be maintained for there to be a successful end result.

Generally, human behavior may be inspired, intrigued, satisfied, or provide feelings of accomplishment at any point in task engagement that reinforces an intrinsic element expressed as motivation. AT can provide motivation in many ways. Social rewards, such as increased interpersonal interaction, may provide the necessary motivation and desire to use technology. For example, when a student derives pleasure from playing games on a computer, he or she will be more motivated and interested in using the computer for homework. By carefully defining the goals of the potential user, devices can be selected that are meaningful and motivating to the particular consumer.

Achievement Motivation

This kind of motivation is based on the need for achievement and defined by the desire to accomplish some purpose or reach a level of excellence by expending an amount of effort to excel. Achievement-oriented individuals are less likely to have fear of failure; they have stronger hopes for success and are moderate risk takers. To learn to use AT involves taking risks that may result in failure. Factors that influence achievement motivation have been identified as early independence training by parents and interaction within an environment with others engaging in strong social modeling of achievement behavior (Santrock, 2009). One can postulate that consumers with this background will more readily adapt to and persist in using technological devices.

Intrinsic and Extrinsic Motivation

According to Santrock (2009), there are two types of motivation components that have been identified: intrinsic and extrinsic. Intrinsic motivation is defined as confidence in one's ability to be competent and to accomplish something for its own sake. Working hard in school with the goal of a higher paying job is an example of extrinsic motivational behavior.

Learning to operate a computer to do better in school or work is another example. The use of a computer to interact socially, using e-mail, chat rooms, playing games, or listening to music is a third example.

Researchers (Rogers, 1995; Santrock, 2009) have identified the roll of the environment in promoting high intrinsic motivation. Factors that contribute to motivation are the variety of experiences and the extent to which the family or caregiver encourages competence and curiosity. Extrinsic motivation may include those resulting from social outcomes or success-ful completion of an activity. Examples of social outcomes involving AT acquisition include conversational discourse, achievement of a goal (moving to a desired location in a power wheelchair), or reinforcement (getting higher grades in school).

BENEFITS AND EXAMPLES OF AT

AT enables consumers with disabilities to reduce and perhaps minimize functional limita-tions. These devices and equipment may be low-tech (mechanical) or high-tech (electro-mechanical or computerized) and can compensate for sensory and functional losses. AT provides the means to move (e.g., wheelchairs, scooters, lifts), speak (e.g., augmentative and alternative communication devices), read (e.g., Braille input, voice recognition devices), hear (e.g., telecommunication devices for the Deaf [TDD], hearing aids), or manage self-care tasks (e.g., remote environmental control systems, prosthetic and orthotic devices). Technology service is "any service that directly assists an individual with a disability in the selection, acquisition, or use of an assistive technology device" (Scherer, 2002, p. 185). Realistically, technology helps equalize the capacities of those individuals with disabilities compared to those without disabilities (Brodwin, 2010).

Technology has many social and recreational applications that enhance the ability of consumers to participate in meaningful activities. For example, a wheelchair with balloon tires allows a consumer to travel on the beach and traverse other rough, outdoor terrain. Greater independence in daily living, including leisure time activities, becomes enhanced with AT. Remote environmental control allows a consumer to do such tasks as turning on lights, a computer, television or radio, answering a telephone, and unlocking the front door. Through reasonable accommodations, many consumers are able to remain on their jobs, and others can seek employment, if not working (de Jonge, Scherer, & Rodger, 2007). A power chair or scooter at work may allow consumer mobility without the use of excess energy required when walking. An adaptive computer at work may permit a consumer to perform required work functions that were previously time consuming or not possible. Consumers with expressive communication deficits may be capable of performing work or school functions with increased and enhanced use of computer-based communication (Brodwin, Parker, & DeLaGarza, 2010).

Another form of technology, custom-designed prosthetic and orthotic devices, helps consumers with upper extremity limitations. These devices enhance manual dexterity, bilat-eral dexterity, and tasks involving eye–hand coordination. Consumers with upper extrem-ity difficulties may be helped by enlarged keyboards, key guards, miniature keyboards, and various specialized user interface switches (optical head pointers, light beams, touch screens) (Rubin & Roessler, 2008). Prosthetic and orthotic devices help consumers with lower extremity limitations perform activities such as standing and walking.

Accommodations for consumers with visual deficits include both optical and nonopti-cal low-vision devices. Examples of optical devices are magnifiers, specially coated lenses, and telescopes. Nonoptical visual aids include talking clocks, talking calculators, closed-circuit televisions that enlarge print electronically, and personal computers and peripherals with the capability of print magnification, speech output, and optical scanning (Brodwin et al., 2010). In addition, hearing aids, TDD, cochlear implants, electronic ears, amplified telephones, and audio loops are helpful AT devices for consumers who are deaf or hard-of-hearing.

Augmentative and alternative communication, commonly known as AAC is a range of communication tools that allows a person to select symbols, pictures, letters, words, or phrases to generate oral communication. This type of AT is usually employed when working with the population who have autism (especially nonverbal individuals) and with people with speech impediments.

Individuals with learning disabilities often have difficulties with reading, writing, speaking, listening, spelling, reasoning, visual perception, or math. They have trouble taking in information through their senses and processing the information accurately to the brain. Information is scrambled and distorted when communicated to the brain, resulting in confused thinking, disorganization, and avoidance behavior. The person may be able to think logically but not be able to articulate in writing and consequently, may appear "lazy" or even "stupid." AT along with personal effort can make a difference. For example, listening to the taped version of the book or using screen reading software to read scanned reading materials allows the person to bypass the reading problem. This alternative learning style is favored in the community with learning disabilities since it promotes independence, reduces anxiety, and fosters self-esteem.

RECOMMENDATIONS FOR REHABILITATION COUNSELING PROFESSIONALS

1. Consumer involvement, from initial assessment through selection and adaptation, is essential to the success of AT. A consumer-driven model provides a feeling of ownership and responsibility and is directly related to continued use of AT (Riemer-Reiss & Wacker, 2000).

2. By having the consumer identify priorities and desires, he or she wants to accomplish through the use of AT, the rehabilitation counselor learns what is foremost in motivating the consumer to use technology.

3. A careful analysis of costs and benefits of AT from the consumer prior to selection should be made. The advantage a device provides must outweigh the costs of using it or the device will probably not be used (Riemer-Reiss & Wacker, 2000).

4. Basic, minimal (low-tech) cost solutions should be considered before expensive high-tech ones. Simple devices may be as effective as more complex ones.

5. The devices should be durable, reliable, and effective (Rubin & Roessler, 2008).

6. Provisions need to be in place for technical assistance, repairs, and routine maintenance (Rubin & Roessler, 2008).

7. To ensure increased functioning and independence (the ultimate goals of using technology), the correct match between consumer and the AT must occur. If not, the chances of continued consumer use of the device or equipment will be minimized (Reed & Saladin, 2008).

8. When recommending AT, the consumer should be presented with any possible alternative choices.

9. Each consumer has preferences, perspectives, and expectations. The counselor needs to realize that professionals and consumers see things from very different perspectives (Scherer, 2007).

10. The degree to which a technological device is essential for desired functioning, the more likely it will be used (Carroll & Phillips, 1993).

11. The counselor needs to make sure the consumer really does want the device and that it is not just something someone else really wants him or her to have (Scherer, 2007).

12. The consumer needs the skills to use the device; it should be easy to operate and require little assistance from others for everyday use (Scherer, 2002).

A change in a consumers' needs can result in product discontinuance (Cook, 2002; Scherer, 2007). Therefore, follow-up and periodic reassessment of a consumer's desires and abilities are crucial for continued use of AT devices.

CONCLUSION

The goal of AT is to increase functional independence for consumers who have disabilities (Brodwin, 2010; Cook et al., 2008). Therefore, the focus is not on the disability but on the remaining functional (residual) abilities that individuals use to accomplish their chosen objectives and their daily tasks. When technological systems are considered for use, the rehabilitation counselor needs to evaluate the various characteristics of the consumer that will effect successful adaptation. According to Scherer (2007), the single most significant factor associated with technology abandonment is a failure to consider the user's opinions and preferences in device selection—in other words, the device is abandoned because it does not meet the person's needs or expectations. Other reasons that AT may be abandoned include a lack of motivation, insufficient training, ineffective device performance, and accessibility problems (Phillips & Zhao, 1993). There needs to be a close and appropriate fit (match) between technological device and consumer. Therefore, the need for the counselor to actively listen and engage the consumer in the process is essential to the effectiveness and outcome of AT success. The closer the counselor matches the consumer's various characteristics to the appropriate device, the greater the chance it will continue to be used. Additionally, the consumer needs to be knowledgeable and trained in the specific device for it to be used efficiently and effectively.

REFERENCES

Bandura, A. (1982). Self-efficacy mechanism in human agency. *American Psychologist, 37*, 122–147.

Best, S. J. (2009). Cerebral palsy. In M. G. Brodwin, F. W. Siu, J. Howard, & E. R. Brodwin (Eds.), *Medical, psychosocial, and vocational aspects of disability* (3rd ed., pp. 305–318). Athens, GA: Elliott & Fitzpatrick.

Brodwin, M. G. (2010). Assistive technology. In I. B. Weiner & W. E. Craighead (Eds.), *Corsini encyclopedia of psychology* (Vol. 1, 4th ed., pp. 158–160). Hoboken, NJ: John Wiley and Sons.

Brodwin, M. G., Parker, R. M., & DeLaGarza, D. (2010). Disability and reasonable accommodation. In E. M. Szymanski & R. M. Parker (Eds.), *Work and disability: Context, issues, and strategies for enhancing employment outcomes for people with disabilities* (3rd ed., pp. 281–323). Austin, TX: Pro-Ed.

Carroll, M., & Phillips, B. (1993). *Survey on assistive technology abandonment by new users* (Cooperative Agreement No. H133E0016). Washington, DC: National Institute on Disability and Rehabilitation Research.

Conyers, L. M., Enright, M. S., & Strauser, D. R. (1998). Applying self-efficacy theory to counseling college students with disabilities. *Journal of Applied Rehabilitation Counseling, 29*(1), 25–30.

Cook, A. M. (2002). Future directions in assistive technology. In M. J. Scherer (Ed.), *Assistive technology: Matching device and consumer for successful rehabilitation* (pp. 269–280). Washington, DC: American Psychological Association.

Cook, A. M., Polgar, J. M., & Hussey, S. M. (2008). *Cook and Hussey's assistive technologies: Principles and practice* (3rd ed.). St. Louis, MO: Mosby Elsevier.

de Jonge, D., Scherer, M. J., & Rodger, S. (2007). *Assistive technology in the workplace*. St. Louis, MO: Mosby.

Mitchell, L. K., & Brodwin, M. G. (1995). Self-efficacy and rehabilitation counseling. *Directions in Rehabilitation Counseling, 6,* 1–4.

Phillips, B., & Zhao, H. (1993). Predictors of assistive technology abandonment. *Assistive Technology, 5*(1), 36–45.

Reed, B. J., & Saladin, S. P. (2008). Assistive technology. In J. D. Andrew & C. W. Faubion (Eds.), *Rehabilitation services: An introduction for the human services professional* (pp. 188–227). Linn Creek, MO: Aspen Professional Services.

Riemer-Reiss, M. L., & Wacker, R. R. (2000). Factors associated with assistive technology discontinuance among individuals with disabilities. *Journal of Rehabilitation, 66*(3), 44–50.

Rogers, E. M. (1995). *Diffusion of innovations* (4th ed.). New York: Free Press.

Rubin, S. E., & Roessler, R. T. (2008). *Foundations of the vocational rehabilitation process* (6th ed.). Austin, TX: Pro-Ed.

Santrock, J. W. (2009). *Life-span development* (12th ed.). New York: McGraw Hill.

Schaller, J., & DeLaGarza, D. (1999): "It's about relationships": Perspectives of people with cerebral palsy on belonging in their families, schools, and rehabilitation counseling. *Journal of Applied Rehabilitation Counseling, 30*(2), 7–18.

Scherer, M. J. (Ed.) (2002). *Assistive technology: Matching devices and consumers for successful rehabilitation.* Washington, DC: American Psychological Association.

Scherer, M. J. (2007). *Living in the state of stuck: How technology impacts the lives of people with disabilities* (4th ed.). Cambridge, MA: Brookline Books.

Stumbo, N. J., Martin, J. K., & Hedrick, B. N. (2009). Assistive technology: Impact on education, employment, and independence of individuals with physical disabilities. *Journal of Vocational Rehabilitation, 30*(2), 99–110.

22

Dance of Disability and Spirituality

BONI BOSWELL, MICHAEL HAMER, SHARON KNIGHT, MARY GLACOFF,
AND JON MCCHESNEY

During the past decade, the scope of literature concerning spirituality has expanded into a wide range of health care contexts (Koenig, 2001; Meraviglia, 2004; Post, Puchalski, & Larson, 2000; Smith & McSherry, 2004). Spirituality issues have been included in areas of research such as oncology (Flannelly, Flannelly, & Weaver, 2002; Meraviglia, 2004), medical psychology (McEwen. 1998; Hill & Pargament, 2003), and cardiac care (Harris et al., 1999). In the field of rehabilitation, the role of spirituality in the lives of individuals with disabilities has become a major topic of study related to coping with severe, chronic suffering and losses (McColl et al., 2000a, 2000b).

Although deemed an important topic by people with disabilities (Chally & Carlson, 2004), there continues to be inadequate information and contrasting perspectives related to people with disabilities in the growing body of spirituality literature. Treloar (2002) reported that spiritual beliefs enabled people with disabilities and family members to establish meaning for disability and to cope with the challenges of losses associated with disability. These results may appear to be encouraging in regard to the potential benefits of spiritual beliefs for individuals with disabilities, but the study included participants affiliated only with evangelical Christian churches. Participants with disabilities from diverse faiths who do not hold similar religious and/or spiritual beliefs may respond quite differently when asked to address the role of spirituality in their lives.

Numerous authors have characterized the experience of disability as a succession of losses, and as such, may create a context for spiritual changes (McColl et al., 2000a; Selway & Ashman, 1998). Disability-associated challenges may prompt one to question traditional concepts about a higher being, as well as to question the purpose of his/her own life, and indeed, the purpose of life in general. Although reflection on these questions may provide the impetus for personal and spiritual development, authors such as Ross (1995) have noted that the increased isolation that often accompanies the experience of disability may make a spiritual quest more difficult. Whether the experience of disability encourages or limits spiritual growth is not fully understood. These notions and the concern that spirituality is "an underused resource in the rehabilitation process" (Underwood-Gordon, Peters, Bijur, & Fuhrer, 1997, p. 225) underscore the need to focus on understanding how spirituality may benefit individuals in long-term rehabilitation.

Many authors have recommended clarifying the meaning of the terms "spirituality" and "religiousness" (Anandarajah, 2001; Koenig, George, Titus, & Meador, 2004). Although related, these terms are not used synonymously. Religiousness is associated with specific

From *Journal of Rehabilitation,* 73(4), 33–40, 2007. Reprinted with permission from the National Rehabiliation Association.

rituals and a doctrine that is shared with a group (Koenig et al., 2004), while spirituality is viewed as one's inner beliefs or worldview about the meaning and purpose of life and/or the quest for understanding these concepts (Thomas, 2000). In this sense, even without religious affiliation, individuals may consider themselves to be strongly spiritual.

Despite clarification of the difference in meaning between spirituality and religion, there continues to be a lack of consensus concerning the definition of spirituality (Bash, 2004; Henery, 2003; MacLaren, 2003; Narayanasamy, 2002; Smith & McSherry, 2004). Howard and Howard (1996) stressed that spirituality refers to a person's "subjective perception and experience of something or someone greater than him/herself" (p. 18). In this view, spirituality is defined as an individual's personal beliefs about the forces that influence his or her life and the transcendent aspects of life. Other authors such as Taylor (2001) have emphasized that spirituality is a cultural phenomenon that should be considered within a cultural context and therefore subjective to a society, with no universal definition. While some researchers have expressed concern over the absence of a universal definition of spirituality, others have stressed the importance of addressing the broad components that are commonly used to characterize spirituality. Concept analyses of spirituality by Meraviglia (1999) and Tanyi (2002) have identified attributes most often used to define spirituality. These attributes include a person's views about what is meaningful, connectedness with self, significant others, nature, and/or higher power.

McColl et al. (2000a) analyzed the commonalities of spiritual characteristics but with a slightly different perspective. They focused on the types of relationships consistently found in the definitions of spirituality, highlighting three types of relationships: self, others, and larger than or beyond the world. The relationship types served as the foundation of their attempt to develop a theoretical base for exploring spiritual disability issues. They used a simple matrix to analyze spiritual issues identified as important by individuals with disabilities in light of these relationships. The authors concluded that the framework offered a meaningful structure for conceptualizing spirituality in relation to individuals with disabilities. While offering an organizational structure for reviewing spiritual issues, this conceptual framework appears to shed little light on understanding the complex role spirituality plays in the lives of people with disability.

Even though a universal definition of spirituality remains elusive, perhaps most authors can agree with Anandarajah's (2001) description of spirituality as "a complex and multidimensional part of the human experience" (p. 82). He continues to elaborate that spirituality is a broad term that includes cognitive and philosophic aspects, namely, "the search for meaning, purpose and truth in life and the beliefs and values by which an individual lives" (p. 83). For the purposes of this study, spirituality was defined broadly as a person's views of the world, particularly, how a person explains the world and the forces that impact her or his life.

The primary goal of the current study was to describe the emerging themes that characterized the role of spirituality in the lives of men and women with severe disabilities. The current study expanded the findings of an earlier study involving women with disabilities (Boswell, Knight, McChesney, & Hamer, 2001), by adding the perspectives of male participants with disabilities to explore spiritual issues discussed by the combined group.

METHODS

This study was conducted using qualitative methods implemented by an interdisciplinary team of five researchers representing areas of expertise that included exercise and sport science, health education and promotion, recreation and leisure, and English. Adults with severe disabilities were recruited for the study through purposive sampling. Face-to-face, individual, in-depth interviews were conducted with each of the 13 participants by one the researchers who has a physical disability. All interviews were audiotaped with the consent of the participants and transcribed verbatim. Each participant received a copy of his or her transcribed interview and verified the accuracy of the transcript before data analysis.

The analysis of data in this study involved the application of the Consensual Qualitative Research Model (Hill, Thompson, & Williams, 1997). The process of consensual qualitative research is based on the assumption that multiple perspectives are more likely to be free of bias (Marshall & Rossman, 1989). This process values collaboration among researchers "to construct a shared understanding of the phenomenon" (Hill et al., 1997, p. 522). Data analysis proceeded in two phases. In the first phase, analysis of the data using this consensual process initially involved three research team members, referred to as the primary team, independently reviewing the data. These three researchers proceeded to participate in group discussions that included reaching consensus concerning domain development, coding, and the construction of core ideas. The fourth researcher served as auditor, a role that entailed checking and challenging the work of the primary team. In response to the auditor's review and challenge of the domains and core ideas, the primary team undertook revisions and subsequent development of categories to describe consistencies and inconsistencies across cases. In the second phase, the fifth member of the research team along with the auditor and one primary team member reviewed coded data in relation to themes. Using the consensual process, these three team members proceeded to identify major themes.

All research team members believed strongly in the basic philosophical premise that disability research should be a collaborative endeavor in which persons with disabilities are an integral part. One of the researchers who has a physical disability served as both interviewer and auditor. Serving in both capacities, this researcher allowed the team as a whole to address two aspects of the methodology that have been identified previously as potential problems. One concern voiced by researchers and practitioners in the area of disability is that nondisabled persons hold sociohistorical perceptions of people with disability that set them apart and marginalize them (Asch, 1998; Fitzgerald, 1997). This view has been characterized as a perception of the disabled as "other than the rest of humanity" (Fitzgerald, 1997, p. 408). The second potential problem noted by disability scholars is that nondisabled researchers of disability are potentially vulnerable to issues that arise from personal anxiety about becoming disabled (Fine, 1994; Fitzgerald, 1997). The full participation of a researcher with a disability as both interviewer and auditor thus served as an important means of addressing not only the quality of the rapport established with the participants during the interviews but also the possible unrecognized biases held by the other members of the research team during the analysis process. As interviewer, this team member facilitated rapport building and enhanced the possibility of creating a climate in which participants living with disability could comfortably and openly explore the issues associated with the focus of the study (Moustakas, 1994).

PARTICIPANTS

Participants ranged in age from 35 to 55 years. These 7 men and 6 women, 11 of whom were Caucasian and 2 of whom were African American, lived with severe disability that included spastic cerebral palsy, quadriplegia, paraplegia, post-polio syndrome, congenital glaucoma, and retinopathy of prematurity. All participants had lived with disability for a minimum of 10 years when interviewed. Each participant experienced an evolution of religious affiliation that stemmed from an upbringing involving Jewish, Catholic, Episcopalian, and Baptist religions and no religious affiliation.

RESULTS

Overall, analysis of the combined data of male and female participants indicated that they described disability and spirituality as essential interactive dimensions of their lives. Despite individual differences such as age of onset of disability, type of disability, religious affiliation, or gender, all but one participant expressed strong beliefs related to a higher being and all participants stressed the influence of these beliefs on their lives as a person with disability. The one participant expressing agnostic views concerning the existence of a higher being described a world view that clearly interacted with his perspective of his disability and the coping strategies he employed. Therefore, the male participants, as the female participants described previously (Boswell et al., 2001), portrayed a complex, reciprocal interaction between the experience of disability and their spiritual or world view. This interaction unfolded in their lives much like that of a dance performed by two partners moving together in rhythm across the floor. This process was characterized by five major themes: purpose, awareness, connections, creativity, and acceptance.

PURPOSE

These participants spoke of their disability and their spiritual views as integral to the purpose and meaning in their lives. Almost all of the nine participants with adult onset of disability explained that their perceptions of the purpose or meaning of their lives changed significantly after their accidents. Only one participant with adult onset stressed that there was no change in the purpose or passion of his life after the onset of disability, but there was a dramatic change related to the paths available to pursue his passions. This participant emphasized his belief that, as Picasso considered, "all art is working with limitations," and he viewed disability as working with a new set of limitations to pursue meaning in his life.

Often, these participants appeared unable to articulate exactly what this life purpose was, but they expressed a strong belief that it was there and that it related to their disability and was rooted in their spiritual views. As voiced by one participant,

> ...this is probably just not a freak accident that I became a quadriplegic. But that has some purpose for the world I live in, and that I am not just here living out the lift of a quad because of fate, but there's some reason,...or some purpose that God intended to fulfill through a disability.

One of the most expressive voices reflecting a struggle to come to grips with the meaning of life came from a male who had begun to think of disability as a gift that enabled him to develop his life career. As an adolescent, his life had been filled with high-risk behaviors involving drugs, alcohol, and fast cars. Stressing that if his accident had resulted in paraplegia as opposed to his "high-level quad" injury, he believed that a continuing ability to drive would have resulted in death. Disability precipitated his relocation away from his hometown into an environment with "new" associations who challenged his beliefs and ultimately invited him to think differently about spirituality and his purpose in life. This participant explained

> In the last few years I have thought of disability as a gift because part of me feels like I'd be dead if I weren't [this] disabled. There is no doubt. There's no way I could be as spiritual, not religious, as spiritual as I am today, at one with myself, my life, my circumstances...I believe that God...in the big sense, not a crucified god or TV evangelist god [after my accident] put people in my life who have shown me a path, and that way I've been able to walk free from a lot of old stuff and walk into a new kind of world.

Several other participants spoke specifically of God or a "higher power" when they discussed the purpose of their lives after onset of their disabilities. Some of these participants suggested that God had sent them a message or intervened because their lives had been "out of control." Two of these participants suggested that disability was a direct consequence of inappropriate behavior and stressed that the turning point in their lives was "being saved." As expressed by one participant, "Just to sum it up, if I had done what I was supposed to have done twenty years ago then there's a possibility that I would not be in the chair." Both these participants continued to abuse drugs and alcohol after their accidents, "to cope with being in a wheelchair everyday" until "being saved." As explained by one participant, "And actually when I got saved, I didn't look at the things that I couldn't do. I thank God for what I could do in the wheelchair." These two participants repeatedly underscored the importance of the event of *being saved* and of *staying saved* to fulfill the purpose in their lives, which they professed to be related to "spreading the teachings of Jesus" to others.

The four participants with congenital disabilities described a different type of struggle to gain and maintain meaning and purpose in their lives compared with participants with adult onset. Without a moment or single event in their lives when the whole world shifted, these participants described a life-long series of both losses and gains of abilities. Although all four wrestled in one way or another to find purpose and meaning in their lives, one of these participants approached the meaning and purpose of his life through an agnostic world view that included great emphasis on individualism. A powerful source of meaning in his life was achieved through attaining a sense of himself, "as an individual first, and secondly as a person with disabilities." His life reflected periods of affiliation with other people with disabilities, but he stressed that his focus was as an individual, "different from all other people," with or without disabilities. The three other participants with congenital disabilities described various periods of questioning and at times great difficulties in their lives, but stressed that they experienced purpose and meaning in life through helping others. Each had chosen to pursue a helping profession that had deepened their sense of purpose as they aged. Through great determination, each had completed advanced educational degrees, and each appeared strongly motivated by a desire to serve others, especially people with disabilities. This aspect of their lives was highlighted in the following response:

> I realized that something was missing for me. I wanted to be able to reach people at a deeper level. I wanted to be able to reach people and help them change their lives and their perspectives. So, that's what made me decide to go back and get a PhD.

AWARENESS

Awareness of self, the environment, and nature was a topic emphasized frequently by these participants and was closely related to the theme of connections. Although linked with connections, many responses about awareness, especially in terms of self-awareness, presented a unique or distinctive quality. This quality related to a sense of realization or discovery that was less apparent in responses about connections. The greatest overlap of awareness and connections was found in comments concerning "others," such as family and friends. Comments related to others were organized under the theme of connections.

An awareness of self was linked to the expression of spirituality as illustrated by the following response:

> I think whatever we use to express it, our spirituality defines some of our self, if not most of it, in what our rituals are, in how we set up our lives, we have to have some sense of involvement with that, in order to know that we are unique.

When addressing the process of becoming aware of self as a person with disabilities, one participant replied, "listen from the heart,...not from the outward appearance of things, [but] what's on the inside of you."

Awareness of self in respect to inner strength for coping and adapting was repeatedly voiced by these participants and often strongly related to spirituality. As described by one participant, "Spirituality means one's capacity to draw on inner strength, one's inner strength to find direction, purpose." She continued by explaining that disability had required her to "draw from inner strength" and that she had realized that the experience had compelled her to question herself and "caused me to look deep in myself."

Participants highlighted the awareness of the details of life such as noticing things in the environment from a different perspective, as described in the following response, "Since becoming a wheelchair user, it has put me in a position to look at the world differently and I think that is where a lot of my spirituality lies. Because when I look around, when I listen...and I see everything that goes on, I find myself paying attention more than I used to."

One participant explained that her experience of disability resulted in a surprising change in her level of awareness and appreciation of nature.

> I think, believe it or not, although most people would think that it's made it less, I think that it's actually made it more....Because every time I go out into nature I always think to myself is this the last time I am going to see this? So, I always have a real intense appreciation of it whenever I am there and so I think in that regard it's made me not take things for granted I guess (that) would be a good way to say it. So it's made my appreciation more.

CONNECTIONS

Strongly associated with awareness, connections to other people and to the community, including the faith community, as well as to the larger world and a higher power, were emphasized in numerous ways and in reference to different dimensions of life, such as the following view:

> I think the fact that you are wounded connects you. It really does. Now, I'm not belittling the fact that disability can isolate the hell out of you...but I think hearing the story of a person who lost a child at childbirth or father who had Alzheimer's, I don't care what the story is, if you're paying attention and you're willing to realize you are not the only person in the universe that has got problems, then you can be enriched and strengthened by other people's stories.

Participants often mentioned that they were aware of or connected to others in a general sense, offering comments such as people with disabilities, "build bridges between people," or comments noting appreciation of others' advice, "I think the important word in all of this is listening....Not only to Christ, but also listen to those around you because they have something to offer." More frequently participants noted the importance of connections with specific family and friends. Comments such as, "I love connecting with other people. I am a social being," and "I know [name] loves me more than life itself. I thank god for that," illustrate the importance of family and friends.

Also, participants expressed frequently the tremendous impact of caretakers, especially paid caretakers. These relationships were discussed often as connections colored by dependency and included the challenges of coping with insensitivities. As expressed by one participant, "a lot of the time when my day's not going well, it's because of attendants, maybe my attendant is a couple of hours late....Almost nothing helps those days."

Connections to community were cited as essential to spirituality by several participants, especially by female participants. Yet, achieving a sense of community in a formalized church setting often posed challenges. The challenges included not only the ability to physically join the worship service but also to feel genuine acceptance. One participant stressed, "Sometimes my disability limits my ability to nurture my spirituality through community. Well, most obvious, transportation. Second most obvious is finding those communities where I do truly feel accepted." She further explained, "… it's really hard to find a church that you really do feel a sense of community. … It's not just that you go to church every Sunday, but that there is a sense of community. There are people there to support you and you are there to support other people". Not only were some churches portrayed as lacking in acceptance but were often described as places of limited understanding of disability. As one participant explained,

> There are some real interesting views on disabilities in the different religions. If you look at the Bible, there are references to God healing people with disabilities and so some people think that if you are a person with a disability, then you must not be saved. … I can't tell you the number of times I've had people want to heal me and I've come to a point in my life where I look at them and say that means you don't accept me for who I am. I used not to be able to understand that enough to be able to say it to people, but now I do, I don't need to be healed, I'm okay.

Closely related to connections and to acceptance of people with disabilities into churches, one participant remarked,

> I don't think the organized church has done the disabled community any favors, and so, I guess it's a bit unnerving to be in such a system. As I look at the statistics, 95% of the disabled world does not see itself as religious, maybe spiritual, but I haven't heard a whole lot about that. I think there is a large void in our disabled community, a void in connecting to our spirituality. Community may be a piece of that, we need some way of expressing and understanding our spirituality. But, that doesn't happen for many, especially the more disabled.

On the other hand, one participant recalled a very different connection with people of a congregation. He recounted, "as my disease progressed they accommodated to that and did an enormous number of helpful things, … so I would say that was a spiritual experience for me to see the lengths people will go to be helpful to another human being."

Feelings of more abstract connections with the world at large were expressed repeatedly as illustrated by the following response, "there's a definite connectiveness you know that I feel now, than before I broke my neck." Connections with a sense of a higher power were often associated with nature, as represented in the following response, "And, a lot of my spirituality I think comes from nature and … there's a force of love or … I don't know exactly how to describe that force, but certainly a force that's bigger than we are." Another participant stated, "Nature, that's where I find my connectedness to a larger sense of being."

CREATIVITY

Several participants stressed the significance of creativity both as it relates to creating art and as it relates to problem solving. Male participants stressed frequently that engaging in the creative process through writing, music, or poetry offered opportunities to transcend the pain and suffering. One male participant emphasized that "Meaning in life can be transformed by the creative process." This participant perceived that living with disability required creativity. Learning to work with limitations was inherent in the creative process and learning to live with disability. On this broad abstract level, creativity was exemplified by the following response, "Creativity is important in adapting to disability and transforming negative experiences into something acceptable." Another participant stated, "I'd say it has played a central role [in my life], I mean more than relationships. There's something really important about creativity."

Overall, the female participants spoke of creativity differently compared with the male participants. Women in this study characterized creativity as essential, but in a more practical, problem-solving manner. This was exemplified by the following response:

> We have to be creative in finding help and in day-to-day survival. I often say to people, just getting up and getting through a day is a full-time job. It demands quite a bit of it (creativity) actually, and especially on the days that things don't work very smoothly.

ACCEPTANCE

All these participants spoke about the necessity of accepting themselves as they are and moving forward in their lives. Several participants expressed a deep and abiding wish to impart strategies for self-acceptance to others with disabilities. Comments from participants were similar to the following statement: "The part of spirituality that I want to bring home to them (others with disabilities) is that you are okay how you are. You are not a freak, you're not weird. You're okay. And that would be the piece that I want to bring to them."

Participants with adult onset described initial periods of resisting and struggling against what had happened as, "going against the grain instead of acceptance," but most of these participants appeared to have progressed to a state of acceptance in the context of disability. Understanding that acceptance was a process in the context of disability was reflected in the following response, "It was a progression because the first couple of years I was still trying to live the lift I used to live and I hadn't accepted all these new limitations with my life and that I have to essentially redefine what life is for me."

Acceptance of physical limitations and ability to "let go" of the need to control life were described as necessary steps toward discovering meaning and growing spiritually. As explained by one participant, "In order to ever get to some stage of acceptance, we must identify and appreciate things that provide happiness and meaning in a redefined life." This participant also explained, "When I think of spirituality myself, it is important to try to accept life for what it is."

All participants described acceptance in society as inconsistent, and at times, self-serving. One participant viewed society's acceptance as a "facade of yes, we want you here, but we wish you had come when we wanted you to, not when you wanted to." One participant remarked,

> You find that some people are accepting and some people are little more curious and some people are just a bit standoffish. We need communities to allow us to grieve, allow us to be pissed, and maybe that's what we have to offer is that we can't cover up our pain. We can't hide. There's no makeup for this.

She believed that acceptance of people with disability by society was difficult because "people have just unloaded because of seeing my disability. I reflect a sense of vulnerability that most people aren't comfortable showing."

DISCUSSION

The results of this study indicated that these participants with disabilities spoke with clarity and candor about the essential interactive role of spirituality in their lives. As explained by one participant, "Spirituality is intimately connected to surviving disability and coping with the deep suffering associated with that experience." All but one of these participants voiced a strong and on-going belief in a higher being and stressed the ongoing development of their spiritual views. Although one specific participant expressed skepticism in relation to a higher being, he revealed a philosophy or worldview that while stressing the importance of individual responsibility, acknowledged the need for social support and acceptance for all people. These views shaped his perspective of disability and his life in general.

Five themes characterized the ongoing interactive process of disability and spirituality: purpose, awareness, connections, creativity, and acceptance. When reviewing these themes, one cannot help but recognize that often these themes interact and overlap with each other. Sometimes, a participant's comments fell clearly into one theme, but at other times, a topic or an event described by a participant cut across themes, indicating a compound or multidimensional relationship between themes. For example, participants spoke about the importance of connections with communities and about strategies that they used to become part of a group, along with the necessity of acceptance of self as a person with a disability for becoming a contributing part of a community.

Most of these participants characterized their disability as contributing to the major purpose and meaning to their lives. Similar to findings in other studies (Lindsey, 1996), these participants expressed positive attitudes about life and about feeling that their lives included purpose. For most of these participants, purpose in life and acceptance of disability strongly influenced coping behaviors. Studies such as McColl et al. (2000a) and Treloar (2002) indicated the importance of both purpose and acceptance. Meraviglia (2004) found that individuals reporting high levels of meaning in life also earned high psychological well-being scores and that as the level of meaning in life increased, symptoms of distress from disease decreased.

Numerous authors have discussed the significance of finding purpose or meaning in life. Lindsey (1966) stressed the importance of meaning in the lives of people with disabilities through application of the ideas of Frankl (1984) formulated from accounts of life in concentration camps. Ross (1995) discussed purpose in terms of its relation with a sense of self. She stressed that finding purpose in life was a natural accompaniment to development of a strong sense of self for most people.

Awareness and connections were less frequently cited in the literature compared with purpose, but were stressed by these participants and were noted by other authors such as McColl et al. (2000a, 2000b) as significant, especially in regard to family and friends. It must be noted that in many of their attempts to express the significance of awareness, these participants spoke of connections. Within the theme of awareness, these participants conveyed a deep sense of appreciation of self. Awareness of self was related especially to inner strength that arose for coping and adapting to the challenges associated with disability.

Female participants emphasized connection with communities as a significant resource of social support more frequently than male participants. Within the theme of connections with communities, experiences with organized religions were described often as sources of frustration. These responses were similar to others found in the literature, such as Fitzgerald (1997) who cautioned that religions may serve as "forms of oppression that limit the spiritual expression of people with disabilities" (p. 407).

Creativity emerged frequently as a significant aspect in the lives of these participants. Creativity as problem solving was portrayed as an essential tool in issues of daily life in the current study and repeatedly emerged in the literature (Lindsey, 1996; Narayansamy, 2002) as important. Effective problem-solving skills have been linked with constructive coping and stress reduction (Treloar, 2002) and positive self-image (Chally & Carlson, 2004). Use of creativity in music, writing, and/or in other arts was stressed particularly by the male participants in the current study as effective means for transforming the negativity of disability into positive experiences. Similar comments about use of the arts as a path to spirituality have been mentioned by Anandarajah (2001).

Acceptance of disability and its influence on identity and self-image appeared to be significant factors in the lives of these participants. These participants repeatedly referred to acceptance of disability as an essential step leading to spiritual progress. Ross (1995) referred to giving up control over life as a motivator for searching for the answer to "who is in control" of our lives, thus creating an impetus for reflection.

IMPLICATIONS

These findings offer convincing support that spirituality was a meaningful and salient part of the lives of these participants with disabilities. For church leaders and congregations, application of these findings can be drawn regarding increasing support and understanding of people with disabilities. Also, in conjunction with the recommendations of Treloar (2002), these findings suggest that church leaders review their teachings in regard to beliefs about disability and sin and about healing practices.

For professionals in the field of rehabilitation, these findings suggest that efforts be increased to ensure that spiritual needs of people with disabilities are addressed. Collaboration with chaplain/pastoral staff and counselors trained to work effectively with people with disabilities can offer help to individuals with disabilities who are struggling with spiritual issues. Sharing resources may include identification of churches that have demonstrated understanding of disabilities and acceptance of people with disabilities. Rehabilitation centers may also wish to recruit people with disabilities from the community who have successfully grappled with spiritual issues to provide consultation not only for the rehabilitation center but also for various congregations.

CONCLUSION

The interaction of spirituality and disability unfolded in the lives of these participants as a dance in which both partners influenced the direction and rhythm of the steps. This interaction was characterized by five major themes: purpose, awareness, connections, creativity, and acceptance. In light of the potential importance of these overlapping themes associated with spirituality, further inquiry is recommended concerning the effectiveness of interventions to promote identification of purpose in life and examination of how purpose in life influences acceptance in the context of disability. A review of strategies for identifying inner strengths may point to a need to develop more effective ways to increase self-awareness. Also, evaluation of interventions that include avenues for creative expression may indicate that these programs promote not only the ability to adapt to the lifelong challenges of living with disabilities, but also as one participant emphasized provide opportunities for, "transforming negative experiences into something acceptable." Lastly, building a sense of connection with family and friends and with the community and the larger world appeared to hold tremendous potential for renewal of the spirit for these participants. Strategies directed at developing these kinds of connections may be an essential component of coping with the overwhelming obstructions and losses associated with disabilities.

REFERENCES

Anandarajah, G. (2001). Spirituality and medical practice: Using the HOPE questions as a practical tool for spiritual assessment. *American Family Physician, 63*(1), 81–89.

Asch, A. (1998). Distracted by disability. *Cambridge Quarterly of Health Care Ethics, 7,* 77–87.

Bash, A. (2004). Spirituality: The emperor's new clothes? *Journal of Clinical Nursing, 13,* 11–16.

Boswell, B., Knight, S., McChesney, J., & Hamer, M. (2001). Disability and spirituality: A reciprocal relationship with implications for the rehabilitation process. *Journal of Rehabilitation, 67,* 20–25.

Chally, P. S., & Carlson, J. M. (2004). Spirituality, rehabilitation, and aging: A literature review. *Archives of Physical Medicine & Rehabilitation, 85*(Suppl 3), S60–S65.

Fine, M. (1994). Working the hyphens: Reinventing self and other in qualitative research. In N. K. Denzin & Y. S. Lincoln (Eds.), *Handbook of qualitative research* (pp. 70–82). Thousand Oaks, CA: Sage.

Fitzgerald, J. (1997). Reclaiming the whole: Self, spirit, and society. *Disability and Rehabilitation, 19*(10), 407–413.

Flannelly, L., Flannelly, K., & Weaver, A. (2002). Religion and spiritual variables in three major oncology nursing journals: *Oncology Nursing Forum, 29,* 679–685.

Frankl, V. E. (1984). *Man's search for meaning.* New York: Washington Square Press.

Harris, W. S., Gowda, M., Kolb, J. W., Strychacz, C.P. Vacek, J. L., Jones, P. G., et al. (1999). A randomized, controlled trial of the effects of remote, intercessory prayer on outcomes in patients admitted to the coronary care unit. *Archives of Internal Medicine, 159,* 2273–2278.

Henery, N. (2003). Constructions of spirituality in contemporary nursing theory. *Journal of Advanced Nursing, 42*(6), 550–557.

Hill, C. E., Thompson, B. J., & Williams, E. N. (1997). A guide to conducting consensual qualitative research. *The Counseling Psychologist, 25,* 517–572.

Hill, P., & Pargament, K. (2003). Advances in the conceptualization and measurement of religion and spirituality and health: Implications for physical and mental health research. *American Psychologist, 58,* 64–74.

Howard, B. S., & Howard, J. R. (1996). Occupation as spiritual activity. *The American Journal of Occupational Therapy, 51,* 181–185.

Koenig, H., George, L., Titus, P., & Meador, K. (2004). Religion, spirituality, and acute hospitalization and long-term care use by older patients. *Archives of Internal Medicine, 164,* 1579–1585.

Koenig, H. G. (2001). Spiritual assessment in medical practice. *American Family Physician, 63*(1), 30–32.

Lindsey, E. (1996). Health within illness: Experiences of chronologically ill/disabled people. *Journal of Advanced Nursing 24,* 465–472.

MacLaren, J. A. (2003). A kaleidoscope of understandings: Spiritual nursing in a multifaith society. *Journal of Advanced Nursing, 45*(5), 457–464.

Marshall, C., & Rossman, G. B. (1989). *Designing qualitative research.* Newbury Park, CA: Sage.

McColl, M. A., Bickenbach, J., Johnson, J., Nishihama, S., Schumaker, M., Smith, K., et al. (2000a). Changes in spiritual beliefs after traumatic disability. *Archives of Physical Medicine and Rehabilitation, 81*(6), 817–823.

McColl, M. A., Bickenbach, J., Johnson, J., Nishihama, S., Schumaker, M., Smith, K., et al. B. (2000b). Spiritual issues associated with traumatic onset disability. *Disability and Rehabilitation, 22,* 555–564.

McEwen, B. S. (1998). Protective and damaging effects of stress mediators. *New England Journal of Medicine, 228,* 171–179.

Meraviglia, M. G. (1999). Critical analysis of spirituality and its empirical indicators, prayer and meaning in life. *Journal of Holistic Nursing, 17,* 18–33.

Meraviglia, M. G. (2004). The effects of spirituality on well-being of people with cancer. *Oncology Nursing Forum, 31,* 89–94.

Moustakas, C. (1994). *Phenomenological research methods.* Thousand Oaks, CA: Sage.

Narayanasamy, A. (2002). Spiritual coping mechanisms in chronically ill patients. *British Journal of Nursing, 11*(22), 1461–1470.

Post, S. G., Puchalski, C., & Larson, D. B. (2000). Physicians and patient spirituality: Professional boundaries, competency, and ethics. *Annals of Internal Medicine. 132*(7), 578–583.

Ross, L. (1995). The spiritual dilemma: Its importance to patient's health, well being, quality of life and its implications for nursing practice. *International Journal of Nursing Studies, 32,* 457–468.

Selway, D., & Ashman, A. F. (1998). Disability, religion and health: A literature review in search of the spiritual dimensions of disability. *Disability and Society, 13,* 429–439.

Smith, J., & McSherry, W. (2004). Spirituality and child development: A concept analysis. *Journal of Advanced Nursing, 45*(3), 307–315.

Tanyi, R. A. (2002). Toward clarification of the meaning of spirituality. *Journal of Advanced Nursing, 39,* 500–509.

Taylor, E. J. (2001). Spirituality, culture, and cancer care. *Seminars in Oncology Nursing, 17,* 197–205.

Thomas, O. C. (2000). Interiority and Christian spirituality. *The Journal of Religion, 80*, 41–60.

Treloar, L. L. (2002). Disability, spiritual beliefs and the church: The experiences of adults with disabilities and family members. *Journal of Advanced Nursing, 40*(5), 594–603.

Underwood-Gordon, L., Peters, D. J., Bijur, P., & Fuhrer, M. (1997). Roles of religiousness and spirituality and the lives of persons with disabilities: A commentary. *American Journal of Physical Medicine and Rehabilitation, 76*, 255–257.

23

Rehabilitation Professionals and Abuse of Women Consumers

MARTIN G. BRODWIN AND FRANCES W. SIU

*I*n American society, men and women with disabilities have been treated stereotypically with disdain and discrimination. Traditional efforts to promote protection of the "weak and disabled" (a societal stereotype) have inadvertently kept individuals with disabilities from accessing resources and education for protection and advancement (Smart & Smart, 2007). One form of discrimination is manifest through the prevalence of abusive behaviors. Powers and Oschwald (2005) reported that abuse is a serious problem for people who have disabilities. Violence is more prevalent among women with disabilities as compared with those without disabilities and with men with disabilities (Nosek, Hughes, Taylor, & Taylor, 2006).

Rehabilitation counselors can begin to assist women with issues of abuse by acknowledging that advocacy and protection from abusive behavior is a priority for many women with disabilities (Chan, 2010). By routinely asking about abuse and addressing issues of safety and control during rehabilitation planning, counselors can provide valuable information, resources, and support that may help prevent abuse from occurring and assist women for whom abuse has occurred (Glover-Graf & Reed, 2006; Powers et al., 2009). Although information pertinent to this area is being disseminated, a network of resources within the community helpful to all parties involved in abuse issues is necessary. Professional referral to psychologists, psychiatric social workers, and vocational training centers can help provide holistic support for consumers. Because of the vulnerability and highly dependent nature of women with disabilities, they rarely complain or voice anger and humiliation. Advocating for these consumers can be a significant part of rehabilitation counselors' job responsibilities.

ABUSE AND VIOLENCE

Abuse is a serious and underreported problem that is prevalent among women with disabilities in the United States. Studies show that the percentage of women with disabilities who have been abused is 62% to 67%; these women experience all kinds of abuse for significantly longer periods of time than those without disabilities (Nosek et al., 2006; Thomas, Joshi, Wittenberg, & McCloskey, 2008). Violence against women cuts across geographic lines and penetrates all socioeconomic levels. Women of all religious, ethnic, economic, and educational backgrounds and of varying ages, physical abilities, and lifestyles are affected by gender-based mistreatment. The phenomenon of violence against women is a complex social, health, criminal justice, and human rights problem occurring throughout the world (Alhabib, Nur, & Jones, 2010).

INTIMATE PARTNER ABUSE

The most common context of violent abuse of women is between intimate partners. A crime commonly referred to as domestic violence, intimate partner violence, spousal abuse, or wife abuse. Females constitute the vast majority of victims, whereas males comprise the majority of perpetrators (U.S. Department of Justice, 2006; World Health Organization, 2001). Each year, approximately 5.3 million incidents of intimate partner violence occur in the United States. On average between 1993 and 2004, approximately 85% of incidents of victimization by intimate partners involved women; about 15% occurred to men (U.S. Department of Justice, 2006). One in four women in America will experience violence in an intimate relationship, and for 24% to 30% of these women, the abuse will be regular and ongoing. The highest rate of domestic violence occurs among young women between 16 and 24 years of age (National Coalition Against Domestic Violence [NCAD], 2007). As a result, two million people are injured and 1,300 killed annually. Intimate partner violence costs this country over $4 billion in medical expenses and $1.8 billion in loss of productivity; eight million days of paid work is lost, equivalent to the loss of 32,000 full-time jobs each year. An estimated 48% of "victimized" women in the United States do not report their abuse to law enforcement agencies (Centers for Disease Control [CDC], 2006).

The genesis of intimate partner violence occurs when a perpetrator exerts power to take control of the victim. As identified by many domestic abuse survivors, a vicious cycle of abuse proceeds in three stages (Hassouneh-Phillips, McNeff, Powers, & Curry, 2005). Stage 1 is the *Tension Building,* where the abuser is edgy, moody, unpredictable, easily agitated, and there is an air of heightened anxiety causing the victim emotional distress; Stage 2 is the *Explosion,* the abuser becomes intensely emotional, angry, explosive, violent, and abusive in various ways; and Stage 3 is the *Honeymoon Period,* the abuser appears to be regretful, apologizes for abusive actions, and returns to being a loving individual, as if nothing had happened. Over the course of the cycle, the victim experiences many feelings, from anger to love to confusion.

A woman is at increased risk of being stalked and even killed after leaving her abusive relationship, because the victim's choice to leave her abuser is likely to be perceived as a challenge to the perpetrator's ability to maintain power and control (Kopala & Keitel, 2003). As a result, considerations of safety should dictate where, when, and how an abused woman decides to leave that relationship. Even if an abused woman eventually leaves her home, the abuse often continues after separation, frequently characterized by different forms of behavior, increased repetitions, and tragically, increased severity (NCAD, 2003).

Types of Abuse

Domestic violence commonly occurs in the forms of physical, emotional, and sexual abuse, which are often concurrent (CDC, 2006). NCAD (2007) estimated that 1.3 million women are physically assaulted by their intimate partners annually, with over 80% being stalked by a current or former intimate partner. Nearly 7.8 million women have been sexually assaulted by an intimate partner at some point in their lives; 31% of women who are stalked by a current or former intimate partner are also sexually assaulted by the same person. Approximately, one-third of women who report abuse to the police are later killed by their spouses or boyfriends. Physical violence and emotional abuse occurring simultaneously is part of a systematic pattern of abusers exercising their need for power and control.

Emotional abuse was characterized as "soul murder" in the Surgeon General's Report on Women's Mental Health (U.S. Department of Health and Human Services

[HHS], 2005), which is an apt definition of a crime in which a woman's spirits are significantly diminished. The report addressed serious concerns about the effects of emotional abuse, which negates a woman's existence and is as damaging as physical and sexual abuse. A pattern of emotional abuse is likely to destabilize a woman's perceptions of herself and her reality (Schaller & Fieberg, 1998). For many physically battered women, emotional abuse is an ongoing backdrop against which physical abuse occurs. As a result, a battered woman's symptoms may reflect the stress of dealing with repetitive verbal abuse, threats, and segregation from society (Dutton, Haywood, & El-Bayoumi, 2000).

ABUSERS

Within an abusive relationship, there is a victim and an abuser. The abuser who exerts power to take control of the victim is often referred to as the perpetrator or batterer. These individuals are likely to be men who are known to the victim, including friends, neighbors, husbands, boyfriends, and extended-family members (NCAD, 2007). Bancroft (2002) found the following five principal behaviors to be characteristic of abusers: (a) exerting power to take control, (b) blaming the "victim" for their problems, so as to have someone to take their frustrations out on, (c) enjoying being the center of attention with priority given to their needs, (d) taking complete financial control of the abused woman, and (e) having a history of being abused. Often, abusive individuals project pleasant and charming images, appearing in public to be unusually fun and loving.

Peterman and Dixon (2001) described a batterer as someone who uses all types of abuse and other behaviors to gain control of what they consider "their" women. Most batterers involved in intimate partner violence do not have criminal records and are rarely violent with anyone except their partners. They frequently have low self-esteem, fear being abandoned by separation and divorce, suspect infidelity or pregnancy, and often choose violence rather than looking for other solutions to perceived problems.

There are three types of batterers: typical batterers, sociopathic batterers, and antisocial batterers.

Typical Batterers

They are the most common type of abuser and usually not diagnosed to have mental illness or a personality disorder, nor are they violent to people outside the family. Typically, they lack criminal records.

Sociopathic Batterers

These individuals may have been diagnosed with personality disorders, accept violence as a way to deal with problems, are more violent than the typical batterer, and too frequently use weapons to hurt their victims. These individuals are very unlikely to have criminal records, although they may be substance abusers and use power and control both inside and outside the family environment.

Antisocial Batterers

These people constitute a very small percentage of the population. They are usually diagnosed with mental illnesses or personality disorders compounded by drug addiction. Their violent acts are far more severe and frequent, with the result that they often have criminal records.

VULNERABILITY TO ABUSE

In addition to experiencing all forms of abuse that happen to women without disabilities, such as physical, emotional, and sexual abuse, women with disabilities also experience abuse unique to their disabilities and which persists for significantly longer periods of time (Nosek et al., 2006; Schaller & Fieberg, 1998), including neglect, coercion, control/restraint, theft of property, arbitrary deprivation of liberty, concealment of medication, restriction of mobility, and the threat of such acts. Not only do women with disabilities experience intimate partner abuse, they also suffer institutional abuse, because they are more likely to be institutionalized and encounter abusive service providers outside their homes (Sobsey, 1994).

Nosek, Howland, Rintala, Young, and Chanpong (2001b) suggested why women with disabilities are more vulnerable to abuse, reporting eight reasons from an analysis by Andrews and Veronen.

- Increased dependence on others for long-term care
- Denial of human rights resulting in perceptions of powerlessness
- Less risk of discovery in the perception of the perpetrator
- Difficulty some survivors have in being believed
- Less education about appropriate and inappropriate sexuality
- Social isolation and increased risk of manipulation
- Physical helplessness and vulnerability in public places
- Attitudes within the field of disabilities valuing mainstreaming and integration, without consideration of each individual's capacity for self-protection

Perpetrators of abuse of women with disabilities include intimate partners, caregivers who are friends, family members, hired personal attendants, and service providers such as health care or independent living personnel in public and private settings (Glover-Graf & Reed, 2006). Moreover, when people with disabilities report abuse, they are often met with skepticism, blunting opportunities to escape further abuse (Powers et al., 2009).

SOCIAL AND PSYCHOLOGICAL ISSUES

Compared with women without disabilities, women with disabilities are more vulnerable and have notably lower self-esteem (Alhabib et al., 2010; Sobsey, 1994). Historically, women with disabilities display defining characteristics: they are (a) more dependent on others, (b) typically socialized to be passive before other people's wishes and demands, (c) short on self-esteem due to frequent rejections, (d) afraid of being placed in an institutional environment, (e) more accepting of abuse as normal behavior because of the habitual effect, (f) socially isolated, (g) perceived as powerless, (h) less believable by others, (i) naïve about sexuality, and (j) directed to mainstream living without resources for self-protection (Glover-Graf & Reed, 2006).

Learned helplessness is a common result of being a victim in an abusive relationship, resulting in beliefs that one cannot leave, fight back, or do anything to control the situation (Deaton & Hetica, 2001). A perception of powerlessness becomes paramount in an individual's thoughts and behavior.

Abuse affects all aspects of a person's life. Many abused individuals' basic survival needs are challenged; a form of abuse peculiar to women with disabilities is deprivation of food, medicine, assistive devices, and mobility (Glover-Graf & Reed, 2006; Hassouneh-Phillips & Curry, 2002). The feeling of safety of such women is threatened by the constant fear and hostility they live with daily. As suggested by Maslow's hierarchy theory of needs, it is difficult and often impossible for these individuals to satisfy higher-level needs such as love, self-esteem, and self-actualization without first satisfying lower-level needs for food, clothing, shelter, and safety. Many abused women acquire multiple disabilities. Approximately, 40% have acquired disabilities because of the abuse and 60% of women seeking help from the Domestic Violence Initiative for Women With Disabilities had disabilities prior to being abused. Others were homicidal or suicidal because of the violence in their lives (Glover-Graf & Reed, 2006).

ABUSE AND EMPLOYMENT

The U.S. Census Bureau (Rubin & Roessler, 2008) estimated that 10% of women between ages 16 and 64 have work disabilities. Among these women, only 14% work full time, compared to 52% of women without disabilities and 22% of men with disabilities. Of those between ages 25 and 64, 9% have college degrees as compared with 26% of women without disabilities and 13% of men with disabilities. Census research has shown that even when women with disabilities have higher levels of education, they are less likely to be employed.

Because of psychosocial debilitating factors, women with disabilities feel that they must work twice as hard as women without disabilities to gain recognition from their employers. Women with disabilities believe that it is vital to first prove that their disabilities do not hinder their competence and reliability. Only then will they feel that employers appropriately value the work they produce. Several additional factors contribute to employment inequalities for women with disabilities (Doren & Benz, 1998).

- Women are less likely than men to receive occupational or vocational training in secondary school.
- Women with disabilities underuse vocational rehabilitation services in comparison to men with disabilities.
- Due to the ramifications of the earning gap, occupational stereotypes, and gender division in the labor market, women with disabilities are less likely to be employed and more likely to be underemployed.
- Employers may be reluctant to promote an employee with a disability because of the fear that added responsibility or extra workload could worsen the disability. Employers may also believe that women with disabilities are sick and, therefore, fragile.
- Women with disabilities are often literally hidden from sight and kept away from customers because they do not fit the stereotypical female image. In addition, co-workers with preconceived notions about women with disabilities may lack understanding.

Regardless of improvement in employment opportunities for women since the working women's movement in the 1970s, women with disabilities have fewer employment opportunities than women without disabilities and men with disabilities. Women with disabilities are more likely to experience poor post-school employment outcomes, lower earnings, negative employment experiences, and little or no support or accommodation. Doren and Benz (1998) suggested that women with disabilities are doubly disadvantaged in the labor market, experiencing dual discrimination because of prejudice toward both gender and disability. Sociologists suggest that minority women with disabilities may experience "triple jeopardy" because they are non-White, "disabled," females. Thus, it stands to reason that abused women with disabilities are very likely to experience "quadruple discrimination."

Even as the economic impact of disability on employment, earnings, and education is more devastating for women than for men (Rubin & Roessler, 2008). Violence in women's lives is yet another significant barrier to employment, which impacts job search and job retention behaviors due to increased mental and physical health hazards (Coulter, 2004). Wettersten et al. (2004) reported that domestic abuse has a profound impact on the prospects of female survivors gaining meaningful employment, possibly as a result of a diminished vocational history and general self-concept that may decrease the ability to work. This group of women have difficulty retaining their jobs and receiving promotions, often turning to welfare and returning to their abusive relationships.

Abuse is a serious health, economic, and human rights issue associated with numerous social problems (U.S. Department of Justice, 2006). Poor health related to chronic illness and sexually transmitted diseases such as HIV/AIDS are abuse-related health hazards within our society. Although intimate partner abuse involving people with disabilities occurs at all socioeconomic levels, it arises frequently among persons with low incomes (James, Johnson, & Raghavan, 2004). Acts of violence have been found to harm the economy, relating directly to decreased productivity, reduced tax proceeds, and poverty. Other social problems related to domestic abuse include homelessness, drug and alcohol abuse, criminal activity, child abuse, teen pregnancy, unwanted pregnancy, prostitution, trafficking, and gang activities (NCAD, 2007).

REHABILITATION SERVICES

Due to widespread violence against women with disabilities, it is likely that rehabilitation professionals will serve clients who have experienced abuse or who are in abusive relationships (Brodwin & Siu, 2007; Siu, 2005). Rehabilitation counselors may be the only individuals who are available and trustworthy with whom to discuss these issues. Vocational rehabilitation can provide hope for such women. Rehabilitation services that include job training, vocational programs, and employment opportunities provide battered women with immediate income to support themselves and their children after leaving their abusers. Securing financial resources through employment is a significant motivator to assist abused women in leaving these relationships and becoming independent (Chronister & McWhirter, 2003).

The philosophy of rehabilitation counseling is to use a holistic approach, integrating programs to empower rehabilitation consumers to achieve fulfilling, socially meaningful, and functionally effective interaction within society (Brodwin & Brodwin, 2009; Patterson, Szymanski, & Parker, 2005). Bitter (quoted in Patterson et al., 2005) stated that equality of opportunity affirming the holistic nature and uniqueness of individuals must provide the philosophical foundation for the practice of rehabilitation.

STRATEGIES TO COMBAT VIOLENCE

Cooperative efforts across disciplines, organizations, and individuals are essential to producing positive influences among people dealing with abuse issues in their lives. To reduce violence against people with disabilities in a meaningful way, greater collaboration among professionals is needed for three principal reasons (Sobsey, 1994). First, most abuse-related programs are developed without consideration of addressing limited accessibility and making reasonable accommodation to meet the needs of people with disabilities. Second, most helping professionals deny responsibility for providing special care unique to people with disabilities. Third, multiple-discipline support team members must incorporate a focus on violence and abuse prevention as part of their operations.

The number one goal when structuring abuse prevention and intervention teams should be to prioritize representation by all relevant disciplines to produce effective interdisciplinary teamwork that inspires reputable working relationships and sensible communication among all team members. Due to the needs of people with disabilities, abuse prevention and intervention team members need to discuss cases with experienced consultants within the social service systems. Psychologists, social workers, and other counselors have primary responsibility for designing and implementing programs to help survivors of abuse overcome the negative effects of their experiences.

Rehabilitation counselors can assist other team members to work together and promote the recovery of any individual who has been abused (Glover-Graf & Reed, 2006). Rehabilitation professionals, especially rehabilitation counselors, must consider casting themselves as prominent representatives, striving to provide a better quality of life for abused individuals by providing rehabilitation services with sensitivity, caring, and cultural understanding.

Consistent with the objectives of developing rehabilitation plans "with" (not for) consumers with disabilities is the essence of respecting their autonomy. Sobsey (1994) suggested that people with disabilities should be included in meaningful ways in every aspect of violence and abuse prevention. The extent and nature of their involvement should be based on a woman's unique situation. Personnel who care for women must understand that safety is the most essential and valuable need, not only for the women at risk but also for everyone in their families. It is important that direct service providers take an active role in prevention and intervention. The most effective approach is to assemble a violence prevention support team or task force made up of disability specialists, medical experts, and other helping professionals who can share experiences and information, support each other's rights to be free of harassment if there is a report of abuse, and create a formalized violence-related support network (Thomas et al., 2008).

Service planners may play a role by developing services with sensitivity to the safety of consumers with abuse issues. Service administrators may help by implementing and coordinating services with the safety of abused consumers in mind. One major contribution is to take initiatives to involve other individuals, such as researchers, consultants, family members, persons with disabilities, members of law enforcement, and child protection specialists, to determine how to provide services that empower and protect this population of consumers (Alhabib et al., 2010; Sobsey, 1994).

Advocates have an important role to play in working to ensure the availability of enhanced services, often through legislation, to prevent abuse of people with disabilities, and to provide accessible treatment for those who have experienced abuse. Advocacy to meet the needs and improve the lives of abused individuals with disabilities is essential. Rehabilitation professionals who specialize in advocating for people with disabilities can serve as expert resources.

Rehabilitation counselors can begin to assist women with issues of abuse by acknowledging that advocacy and protection from abuse is a priority and necessity for many women with disabilities. By routinely asking about abuse and addressing issues of safety and control during rehabilitation planning, counselors can provide information, resources, and support that may help prevent abuse from occurring and assist women for whom abuse has occurred. Although information pertinent to this area is being disseminated, a network of resources within the community helpful to all parties involved in abusive relationships is needed. Professional referral to psychologists, social workers, professional counselors, and vocational training centers provides holistic support for consumers. Because of the vulnerability and highly dependent nature of women with disabilities, these persons rarely complain or voice anger and humiliation (Siu, 2005). Advocating for such clients who have abuse issues can be an important part of the rehabilitation counselor's job responsibilities.

The recovery process for abused women with disabilities has two vital goals: (a) establishing safety and (b) restoring control over their lives (Powers et al., 2009). Establishing safety often begins by focusing on control of the body and then moving outward toward control of the environment. Body control focuses on regulating functions consisting of eating, sleeping, and managing symptoms such as anxiety, depression, flashbacks, and states of dissociation. Rehabilitation counselors can assist women in establishing safety and control over their lives by several means. This includes fostering women with disabilities in a self-image as income-generating workers; providing them information about and assisting in connecting with agencies and resources; supporting them as they establish those connections; empathizing with them about their frustrations, fears, and stress during the process; and acknowledging their successes, even seemingly minor ones. As a result, efforts to aid recovery from abuse have implications for rehabilitation in the areas of health care, transportation services, attendant care, and vocational/career counseling (Schaller & Fieberg, 1998).

As providers of human services, rehabilitation counselors and service providers must understand that although they are responsible to report suspicion of abuse, they are not responsible for proving its occurrence. Counselors' training should include attention to the principle that when in doubt, contacting domestic violence hotlines for guidance is a viable option.

INCLUSION OF STUDY OF ABUSE IN REHABILITATION EDUCATION CURRICULA

The idea of including the study of abuse in rehabilitation curricula has been echoed in multiple studies (Glover-Graf & Reed, 2006; Hassouneh-Phillips & Curry, 2002; Schaller & Fieberg, 1998). The consistent recommendation has been to include topics addressing abuse in rehabilitation curricula for both pre-service and in-service training programs, with the goal of better preparing rehabilitation professionals to deal with consumers' abuse issues that often surface in crisis situations. The sound judgment of rehabilitation professionals could make a difference in the lives and well-being of abused women; discussing issues related to influencing their decision to stay, leave, or return to an abusive relationship. Such judgment may play a significant role in how post-separation battered women manage their safety while re-entering mainstream society. Glover-Graf and Reed (2006) suggested that integrating the content related to the abuse of women with disabilities in rehabilitation counselor training programs is a matter of ethical practice.

Young, Nosek, Walter, and Howland (1998) suggested that to combat violence against women with disabilities, all rehabilitation service providers must (a) take responsibility to be knowledgeable about domestic violence and abuse issues, (b) cultivate a network of resources in the community for helping abuse survivors, and (c) include screening for abuse in routine intake and follow-up procedures. For pre-service education, specific content areas on abuse could be added to the curriculum required by Council on Rehabilitation Education accredited master's degree programs in rehabilitation counseling. Additionally, supervised practicum and internship experiences should include opportunities to work with women who have experienced abuse.

Intimate partner violence has a powerful and harmful impact on women with disabilities. Rehabilitation counselors, as primary service providers for people with disabilities, are likely to have opportunities to help these individuals. To better prepare professionals to provide appropriate rehabilitation services with sensitivity rehabilitation educators must be involved in the design of pre-service and in-service training curricula that include issues of domestic violence and disability. Counselors would benefit from additional training to be able to empower domestic violence survivors to take control and improve their quality of life.

RECOMMENDATIONS FOR REHABILITATION PROFESSIONALS

To address abuse issues of rehabilitation, consumers rehabilitation professionals have several responsibilities to: (a) learn about violence by using available training related to abuse of people with disabilities; (b) to employ universal screening as a routine client-intake procedure; (c) volunteer information, resources, and referrals to clients who are in danger or at risk of an abusive situation; (d) facilitate collaboration with domestic violence shelters to supply personal care services and replace medications and assistive devices left behind in an emergency situation (Hassouneh-Phillips & Curry, 2002); (e) accumulate domestic violence resources to enhance abuse-related services for abuse survivors with disabilities (Hassouneh-Phillips et al., 2005); and (f) raise awareness and offer educational activities to reduce the vulnerability of women with disabilities and increase their ability to protect themselves (Nosek, Foley, Hughes, & Howland, 2001a).

REFERENCES

Alhabib, S., Nur, U., & Jones, R. (2010). Domestic violence against women: Systematic review of prevalence studies. *Journal of Family Violence, 25*, 369–382.

Bancroft, L. (2002). *Why does he do that? Inside the minds of angry and controlling men*. New York: Berkley.

Brodwin, M. G., & Brodwin, S. K. (2009). A case study approach, rehabilitation intervention, and assistive technology. In M. G. Brodwin, F. W. Siu, J. Howard, & E. R. Brodwin (Eds.), *Medical, psychosocial, and vocational aspects of disability* (3rd ed., pp. 1–16). Athens, GA: Elliott & Fitzpatrick.

Brodwin, M. G., & Siu, F. W. (2007). Domestic violence against women who have disabilities: What educators need to know. *Education, 127*(4), 548–551.

Centers for Disease Control. (2006). *National Center for Injury Prevention and Control: Intimate partner violence: Fact sheet*. Retrieved January 15, 2007, from http://www.cdc.gov/ncipc/factsheets/ipv-facts.htm

Chan, J. (2010). Combating violence and abuse of people with disabilities: A call to action. *Journal of Intellectual and Developmental Disabilities, 35*(1), 48–49.

Chronister, K. M., & McWhirter, E. H. (2003). Applying social cognitive career theory to the empowerment of battered women. *Journal of Counseling and Development, 81*, 418–425.

Coulter, M. (2004). *The impact of domestic violence on the employment of women on welfare* (Award Number: 1998-WT-VX-0020. Document No.: 205294). Retrieved November 11, 2006, from http://www.ncjrs.org/pdffiles1/nij/grants/ 205294.pdf

Deaton, W. S., & Hetica, M. (2001). *A therapist's guide to growing free—A manual for survivors of domestic violence*. Binghamton, NY: Haworth.

Doren, B., & Benz, M. R. (1998). Employment inequality revisited: Predictors of better employment outcomes for young women with disabilities. *Journal of Special Education, 31*(4), 425–443.

Dutton, M. A., Haywood, Y., & El-Bayoumi, G. (2000). Impact of violence on women's health. In S. J. Gallant, G. P. Keita, & R. Royak-Schalder (Eds.), *Health care for women* (pp. 41–56). Washington, DC: American Psychological Association.

Glover-Graf, N., & Reed, B. J. (2006). Abuse against women with disabilities. *Rehabilitation Education, 20*(1), 43–56.

Hassouneh-Phillips, D., & Curry, M. A. (2002). Abuse of women with disabilities: State of the science. *Rehabilitation Counseling Bulletin, 45*(2), 96–104.

Hassouneh-Phillips, D., McNeff, E., Powers, L., & Curry, M. A. (2005). Invalidation: A central process underlying maltreatment of women with disabilities. *Journal of Women & Health, 41*(1), 33–50.

James, S. E., Johnson, J., & Raghavan, C. (2004). "I couldn't go anywhere"—Contextualizing violence and drug abuse: A social network study. *Violence Against Women, 10*(9), 991–1014.

Kopala, M., & Keitel, M. A. (Eds.). (2003). *Handbook of counseling women*. Thousand Oaks, CA: Sage.

National Coalition Against Domestic Violence. (2003). *2003 domestic violence statistics-Domestic violence facts*. Retrieved December 20, 2005, from http://www.ncadv.org/files/DV_Facts.pdf

National Coalition Against Domestic Violence. (2007). *2007 domestic violence statistics-Domestic violence facts*. Retrieved August 20, 2007, from http://www.ncadv.org/files/domesticviolencefacts.pdf

Nosek, M. A., Foley, C. C., Hughes, R. B., & Howland, C. A. (2001a). Vulnerabilities for abuse among women with disabilities. *Sexuality and Disability, 19*(3), 177–189.

Nosek, M. A., Howland, C., Rintala, D. H., Young, M. E., & Chanpong, G. F. (2001b). National study of women with physical disabilities: Final report. *Sexuality and Disability, 19*(1), 5–39.

Nosek, M. A., Hughes, R. B., Taylor, H. B., & Taylor, P. (2006). Disability, psychosocial, and demographic characteristics of abused women with physical disabilities. *Violence Against Women, 12*(9), 838–850.

Patterson, J. B., Szymanski, E. M., & Parker, R. M. (2005). Rehabilitation counseling: The profession. In R. M. Parker, E. M. Szymanski, & J. B. Patterson (Eds.), *Rehabilitation counseling: Basics and beyond* (4th ed., pp. 1–26). Austin, TX: Pro-Ed.

Peterman, L. M., & Dixon, C. G. (2001). Assessment and evaluation of men who batter women. *Journal of Rehabilitation, 67*(4), 38–42.

Powers, L. E., & Oschwald, M. (2005). *Violence and abuse against people with disabilities: Experiences, barriers, and prevention strategies.* Retrieved September 24, 2005, from Oregon Health & Science University, Oregon Institute on Disability and Development, Center on Self-Determination Web site: http://www.directcareclearing house.org/download/AbuseandViolenceBrief%203-7-04.pdf

Powers, L. E., Renker, P., Robinson-Whelen, S., Oschwald, M., Hughes, R., Swank, P., et al. (2009). Interpersonal violence and women with disabilities: Analysis of safety promoting behaviors. *Violence Against Women, 15*(9), 1040–1069.

Rubin, S. E., & Roessler, R. T. (2008). *Foundations of the vocational rehabilitation process* (6th ed.). Austin, TX: Pro-Ed.

Schaller, J., & Fieberg, J. L. (1998). Issues of abuse for women with disabilities and implications for rehabilitation counseling. *Journal of Applied Rehabilitation Counseling, 29*(2), 9–17.

Siu, F. W. (2005). Rehabilitation counselors: What we should know about domestic violence. *The Rehabilitation Professional (International Association of Rehabilitation Professionals Journal), 13*(2), 43–47.

Smart, J. F., & Smart, D. W. (2007). Models of disability: Implications for the counseling profession. In A. E. Dell Orto & P. W. Power (Eds.), *The psychological and social impact of illness and disability* (5th ed., pp. 75–100). New York: Springer.

Sobsey, D. (1994). Abuse, neglect, violence, and disability. In D. Sobsey (Ed.), *Violence and abuse in the lives of people with disabilities: The end of silent acceptance* (pp. 13–50). Baltimore: Brooks.

Thomas, K. A., Joshi, M., Wittenberg, E., & McCloskey, L. (2008). Intersections of harm and health: A qualitative study of intimate partner violence in women's lives. *Violence Against Women, 14*(11), 1252–1273.

U.S. Department of Health and Human Services. (HHS, 2005). Social stress factors and stigma. In *Surgeon General's workshop on women's mental health, November 30–December 1, 2005, Denver, Colorado workshop report.* Retrieved December 1, 2007, from http://www.surgeongeneral.gov/topics/womensmentalhealth/ mentalhlth_rpt.pdf

U.S. Department of Justice. (2006, December). *Bureau of Justice Statistics: Intimate partner violence in the U.S.—Offender characteristics.* Retrieved January 15, 2007, from http://www.ojp.usdoj.gov/bjs/intimate/offender.htm

Wettersten, K. B., Rudolph, S. E., Faul, K., Gallagher, K., Trangsrud, H. B., Adams, K., et al. (2004). Freedom through self-sufficiency: A qualitative examination of the impact of domestic violence on the working lives of women in shelters. *Journal of Counseling Psychology, 51*(4), 447–462.

World Health Organization. (2001, June). *WHO fact sheet No 239–Violence against women.* Retrieved December 20, 2006, from http://www.who.int/mipfiles/2269/ 239-ViolenceAgainstWomenforMIP.pdf

Young, M. F., Nosek, M. A., Walter, L., & Howland, C. (1998). *A survey of rehabilitation service providers' perceived knowledge and confidence in dealing with abuse of women with disabilities.* Unpublished manuscript.

IV

Interventions and Resources: Conclusion

DISCUSSION QUESTIONS

1. The chapter on substance abuse counseling provides a distinction between use, abuse, and addiction. What are the criteria that differentiate abuse from addiction?
2. Over the past few decades, there have been efforts to legalize marijuana. This effort has been promoted by an increased use of this drug by HIV/AIDS patients. Medical researchers have shown the benefits of marijuana use as a drug because it decreases the side effects of pharmaceutical products and eases chronic pain, as well as other major benefits. Discuss how the medical use and legalization of marijuana would benefit patients who have chronic and life-threatening illnesses. Also, provide an argument for how the legalization of marijuana both with and without a physician's prescription would benefit people who live with chronic illnesses and disabilities.
3. The ongoing conflicts in Iraq and Afghanistan are resulting in large numbers of returning combat veterans. Discuss specific psychological, emotional, and social factors that challenge this particular group of active-duty military as they transition from military life to home.
4. The ongoing conflicts in Iraq and Afghanistan also have created persons with medical and physical disabilities. Discuss the specific medical and physical needs that active-duty military would benefit from as they transition from military life to home.
5. Women make up a larger percentage of deployed forces than ever before comprising 14% of all deployed personnel. Discuss how the armed forces experience may be different for women than men.
6. Discuss some psychosocial supports and resources that should be offered specifically to women as they transition from active duty to civilian life.
7. Assistive technology (AT) has a profound impact on the lives and opportunities of individuals with disabilities. What is the employment and vocational impact of AT on the lives of people with disabilities? Discuss specifically how AT provides greater independence for people with disabilities while performing activities related to daily living.
8. Why would the individual's self-worth, self-esteem, and self-efficacy improve with the use of AT?
9. Abuse and violence are serious and underreported problems that are prevalent among women with disabilities. Discuss the specific psychosocial factors that are unique to women with disabilities who are abused.
10. The most common form of violence and abuse of women is between intimate partners. How would abusive relationships between partners be both the same and different for women with physical disabilities?

11. Describe the role that religion and spirituality plays in the lives of persons with disabilities. What specific aspects of religiosity and spirituality increase personal coping and resiliency?

12. Discuss some myths and attitudes related to people with disabilities and their religious/spiritual practices.

PERSONAL PERSPECTIVE

The value of tapping into one's spiritual beliefs is engagingly illustrated in Dr. Herbert's essay on his personal journey in recovering from open-heart surgery. The concepts and intervention strategies presented in the different chapters of Part IV assume an everyday impact and understanding when someone is confronted with life-and-death issues. The story of Dr. Herbert's recovery experience is not necessarily told for inspiration but for its teaching and other intervention values. He provides a refreshing perspective on how to cope with the daily hassles of life postsurgery and how to gain a renewed appreciation of the ordinary and unexpected. The lessons emanating from his recovery experience resonate with all of us who are vulnerable to the uncertain effects of the unexpected.

RECOVERY AND THE REHABILITATION PROCESS: A PERSONAL JOURNEY

James T. Herbert

On Thursday, November 7, 2002, I underwent quintuple by-pass, open-heart surgery, or as my cardiac surgeon and new best friend characterized, the "grand slam of heart surgery." I am not sure if he is a baseball fan, but since this procedure was my first surgical experience, I had nothing to compare it with. Given that he was the surgeon and I was the reluctant "designated hitter," I took him at his word. While I am happy to report that my initial and subsequent recovery continues to go well, this experience provided me with an opportunity to conduct a serious inventory of my life and decide whether some changes were in order. This inventory led me to assess life lessons that I either failed to embrace or simply ignored altogether.

I thought this forum might provide the opportunity for me to share some of these lessons as they relate to being a rehabilitation counselor educator. Frankly, I am not sure whether anything that I write on this topic will have the intended impact but, at the very least, I hope what I share provides the opportunity for each of us to stop for a moment and take quick inventory of our professional lives. For some, I suppose, what I share will already be obvious. For others what I share may be dismissed quickly as personal ramblings that have no application to their lives. With apologies to educators in both groups, I am directing my thoughts to the rehabilitation counselor educator who fits somewhere in between.

CALLING ON GOD—WHERE ARE YOU?

One consequence of facing life-threatening or life-altering surgery is that it provides an opportunity to reflect on your life. For the first time, I began to think of my mortality and,

---

From "Recovery and the rehabilitation process: A personal journey," by J. T. Herbert. *Rehabilitation Education, 17*(2), 125–132. Reprinted with permission of *Rehabilitation Education*.

I want to thank the reviewers and co-editors for their helpful comments on the initial draft of this chapter.

in particular, my personal relationship with God. As a rehabilitation counselor educator, I do not talk about God with my students. For reasons of political correctness, religious freedom, personal insecurity, and lack of informed opinion, I have purposely stayed away from any serious engagement on this topic with students. Other than the anecdotal comment that "discussing client spirituality is an important aspect of the rehabilitation process," in retrospect, I provided no clear idea of what this statement involved, how to do it, or why it may be true.

Concerning my own rehabilitation, I realize now that having a personal relationship with God was an important aspect in preparing for surgery and the recovery process. This renewed relationship started with prayer. By prayer, I am not referring to the recital of the "Lord's Prayer" and then waiting for some divine intervention to occur. Certainly, this tried and true approach works for many, but in my case, I had to find a different prayer. More often my prayers were associated with fears and doubts regarding what I was about to face, facing it, and then trying to enhance my spiritual relationship with God. There were times throughout my rehabilitation that prayer provided an important comfort to me and helped me to deal with the emotional, physical, and social aspects of illness. I would ask for comfort and peace and somehow through prayer I found it. There were other times, however, that my prayers did not provide comfort. My intentions were the same as before, but I did not achieve the same results. It was as if I was having a one-way conversation with the "Big Spirit in the Sky." I would pray for spiritual guidance and then I would wait for something—some indication for me to do something. Maybe a voice in the wind would provide a divine response ("Hey God—was that you whispering something to me?" No, it was just our two cats scratching the furniture). Maybe my "inner voice" would say something profound, but often it seemed the voice was simply me having a conversation with me ("Hey God—was that you talking to me or me talking to me?").

Listening to my inner voice was never easy given that I was always unsure who was talking and on whose authority the comments were being made. Still, if I believe that I am made in God's image, then I guess it was God talking to me. (Okay, I recognize this statement reflects my personal religious belief, so we can agree to disagree on its validity.) During particularly difficult times when I would get despondent (most men do not like to use the word depressed), I would sometimes wait for a sign from God that would hopefully help. A multicolored, flashing neon sign dropping from the sky that read, "Jim, I am pleased with you—keep up the good work" would provide clear indication that God was with me. However, even this proof might be asking a bit too much from God. Lowering my expectations of divine intervention, I was willing to settle for a ceiling light flickering off and on when I asked for evidence that God did care about me. Although neither electrical communication method has occurred, I am gradually recognizing how God communicates to me by being more open to spiritual opportunities in my everyday dealings with others. My interactions to share or not share love with others, to take time and acknowledge blessings, to recognize the limits of things I cannot control, and to forgive myself and others were all opportunities to experience a spiritual connection with God. It is not my intention to confuse the issue of religious versus spiritual beliefs and impose my personal beliefs of whom and what God means in this narrative (earlier exception noted). History is replete with examples of personal and social tragedies with each side believing that "God is with us."

On a smaller scale and having direct relevance to my work as a rehabilitation counselor educator, my recent personal experience with illness provided me with new spiritual insights and how I might incorporate them when working with students. For instance, in my supervised clinical practicum, I plan to ask questions that, up to now, were left unexplored. Examples of questions include:

1. What are your views about a higher spiritual power? Have they remained the same over your life? If they have changed, what events have impacted on them?
2. How do your spiritual views impact your daily interactions with people you work with and the people you plan to serve during your professional careers?
3. Are there situations where it is appropriate or inappropriate to discuss your personal spiritual beliefs with your clients or have them discuss their views with you?
4. What aspects are uncomfortable when discussing spiritual beliefs with others?

As I have not addressed these questions in prior supervision experiences, I have no idea what might follow. At the very least, I hope that asking such questions will lead to a better understanding of how spiritual beliefs are as fundamental as inquiring about other personal, social, medical, and vocational aspects of disability and illness. Regardless of one's spiritual or religious beliefs, it is an area that can have tremendous importance to individuals we work with and, if rehabilitation counselors are willing to open the door on the topic, it offers promise for helping others.

TIME KEEPS ON TICKING

Exploring one's spiritual beliefs eventually leads to the issue of mortality, a difficult topic to address with colleagues, family, and friends when facing serious illness. Each of us recognizes that we have finite time to be here, yet there is an undeniably irrational aspect that suggests the contrary. Just like the old Timex watch commercial, we assume that we will just "keep on ticking." Suspending the belief of reincarnation for a moment, if one assumes that the present lifetime is your one and only chance to "get it right," I started considering questions such as "Why did I get this illness and what happens if things do not work out as planned?" "What kind of life have I made for myself and the people I love?" "What did I value throughout my life and how did I recognize its importance?" "Who loves me and how have I loved them in return?" "What kinds of changes do I want to make and what obstacles stand in the way of making beneficial changes?" and "How will I find ways to overcome these obstacles?"

To the extent you have supportive family and friends and your willingness to examine these questions provides you with an opportunity for sobering answers. Some of the rediscovered answers made me realize that I spent too much time and energy on things I could not control. I found that I worried too much and too often about small matters that caused a great deal of personal and professional angst. I allowed work to comprise too much of my personal identity and account for too much of my life activities. Having a healthy career is one thing, but when the hospital social worker asks how you spend your free time and you can't come up with a single avocational activity that provides personal joy, it may be time to reconsider your life balance.

An important step in reevaluating my professional identity and the effort to achieve and maintain it started with the recognition that I do not have all the time in the world: When you start thinking about your life clock and accept the notion that you have limited control on life longevity, you tend to approach the future differently. For a start, you question whether, in fact, there will be a future and, if so, how long? Since none of us knows the answer to this question, the simple recognition that "life goes on without you" is hard to comprehend. Having a serious illness, however, gets you started thinking about the future. In my case, although a positive surgical outcome was expected, there was no guarantee and, in addition, I had to prepare as best I could that more serious injury or death could result from having the surgery. Discussing these possibilities, while unpleasant, sometimes results in people reminding you that your chances of having a successful outcome far exceed that of less successful outcomes. Usually, if I would discuss any doubts about negative surgical outcomes, I would be reminded, "Look, you have a 95% chance that everything is going to work out fine." When I heard this attempt to calm my fears, I sometimes felt like responding, "Suppose I asked you to choose one of 20 playing cards and that one of the cards, if selected, would kill you. Do you still want to play?" When I first learned of my illness, I could not imagine anything more frightening and, like Woody Allen, my thoughts on the whole matter could be summed by saying, "It's not that I'm afraid to die, I just don't want to be there when it happens." Eventually, I came to recognize that while death or more serious injury (heart attack, stroke) was an unlikely outcome, I must be prepared (as best I could) to meet either outcome whether it occurred now or sometime later. Although this obvious realization sounds very rational, the process in getting to this point involved a great deal of emotional expression and spiritual effort.

Perhaps in our discussions regarding death and dying with students, there are academic exercises intended to bring into consciousness the realization of the seemingly short time that all of us share on this planet and intended life contributions each of us wants to make. We might ask our students to imagine what information would their tombstone epitaphs contain, what would be written in their obituaries, what families and friends would say about them publicly and privately after their deaths, and/or if they had one week to live—how would they spend their time? Such discussions provide insight as to how students perceive themselves, what they value, and what may be missing in their current lives. Although I did not complete any written narratives to address these questions, I often initiated internal dialogues when imagining these scenarios. By doing so, I found the experience provided me with a better appreciation of the ordinary. This realization is not cognitively profound but, on an emotional and spiritual level, it reminded me that basic, ordinary appreciation of life is a difficult concept to implement each day. As my medical condition improves with each month, I find that it is a lesson that needs constant reminding.

EVENTUAL APPRECIATION OF THE ORDINARY AND UNEXPECTED

There is a litany of metaphors and sayings that address the essential point of appreciating the everyday things in life including the unexpected occurrences that arise. The familiar phrase "Take time to smell the roses" comes to mind. Prior to my surgery, my approach to life could be described more in keeping with, "So, this is a rose. It sure is pretty. Hey, what about those daisies over there—could they use a little mulch?" It is hard to appreciate roses when you are more concerned about tending to the entire garden. During my recovery, I could think of many missed opportunities where I failed to slow down, observe what was around me and appreciate the ordinary but simple pleasures that life offers. As my recuperation progressed, the ordinary activities such as taking a hot shower, walking in the woods, playing checkers with my son, and talking with my wife were experiences that I appreciated more than ever before. In order to help me appreciate the mundane and miraculous, I take a few brief moments throughout each day to conduct a short and simple prayer of thanks. It allows me to be more present in the moment and gain a better appreciation of life. Taking this time accomplishes what singer/song writer Paul Simon referred to when he wrote, "Slowdown. You move too fast. You've got to make the moments last." Making moments last—I guess if a film company could turn this phrase into a successful advertising campaign then it should be good enough for me.

Although I failed to recognize that having a serious illness could be a gift in disguise, like any adaptation process, time changes perspectives. When I first learned the extent of my illness, my prayers were directed at hoping that I would undergo "no more than an angioplasty with a stent or two." I thought if I could get by with this medical procedure then it would be sufficient in not only improving my physical health but also my spiritual well being. In essence, I was asking God that if you let me get out of this medical jam with limited complications and easy recovery; I would promise to become better spiritually. Anyone recognize some "bargaining" here? Although I had no clear idea of what becoming better spiritually meant, at the time, it seemed sincere if not misguided.

When learning that this procedure was not viable, and that more invasive surgery was in order, my reality went through another adjustment phase. The usual fears and resolution to having the surgery were quickly forgotten when I successfully emerged from the operation. A deep sense of gratitude of having a second chance at life was the central theme. Gradually, this feeling dissipated when I returned home. The physical pain, dependence on others, lack of energy, and, to my amazement, an internal debate about the merits of my surgical outcome contributed to depression. As my physical condition continued to improve, along with continued family support and prayer, I have gradually recognized the benefits of having bypass surgery. I firmly believe that I would not have devoted any serious efforts in making the kinds of life changes that I needed to make without having by-pass surgery. My attempts to develop a greater spiritual presence each day, to think more carefully about life choices I make, and to put forth effort to achieve a more satisfying life all occurred because of this experience. For now, the major task at hand is to retain this perspective as my recovery continues.

REMEMBERING REHABILITATION LESSONS

At this point of my rehabilitation, I have finished my cardiac outpatient program and I am completing the wellness program that follows. I am participating in Weight Watchers and learning that the dietary changes I need to make are lifelong. I also purposefully sought and I am working with a counselor who emphasizes spiritual growth (which, from his perspective, includes everything). You would think with all of these support systems in place that it affords me the opportunity to institute some healthier life changes. It does. Taking time to work on yourself sounds like an opportunity of a lifetime. It is. Still, the greatest challenge for me as I am now seven months postsurgery is to remember the life lessons gained from this experience.

Holding on and building upon these gains is the current challenge at hand. Already I realize that it is very easy to slip into some earlier practices that contributed to coronary artery disease. One maladaptive practice is a lack of patience that I have for myself. For example, several months ago, I engaged in physical activity that my cardiologist reprimanded me for when I shared the fact that "I shoveled snow for several hours but I took my time." When shoveling, I distinctly remember thinking how wonderful it was to be able to perform this type of physical activity without experiencing profuse sweating, shortness of breath, and pain down my left arm. I also thanked God for allowing me to engage in this activity. Despite my attempt to connect physical and spiritual well being, my cardiac professionals saw things a bit differently. Apparently, my body tended to agree with them as I paid for my physical/spiritual experience over the next several days. As an additional reminder of not hurrying the healing process, the next day's lead chapter in the local newspaper contained a story concerning several persons with cardiac problems who died while shoveling snow. OK, so I remain a little slow on the uptake, but I think my recent indiscretion was because I wanted to reclaim an earlier lifestyle. I am relearning that while this reclamation can be beneficial in certain instances; in this case, it was not the best idea.

IMPLICATIONS FOR MY CAREER AS A REHABILITATION COUNSELOR EDUCATOR

When I return to work next academic year, I want to avoid making the same mistakes that contributed to an unhealthy lifestyle. As it pertains to work, it is my intention to remember past lessons that I have learned as a result of illness and recovery. Those lessons have to do with feeling more comfortable about asking for help, developing a greater connection with a higher spiritual power, and placing less emphasis on my career in order to have a more balanced life.

Most of the hassles associated with being an academic are related to obtaining appropriate program resources, negotiating faculty issues within the department, addressing student concerns, fulfilling professional and administrative responsibilities, and balancing teaching, research, and professional service commitments. How well I met those challenges was often associated with how well I was able to effectively use the skills and talents of colleagues. Although I recognize this interdependence, it remains a concept that is sometimes difficult to practice, especially as it concerns the issue of asking for help from colleagues. I found it interesting that asking for help, as it was related to my accomplishing individual rehabilitation goals, was much easier than asking for help at work. Given the conversations that I have with colleagues at other university settings, it seems that my predicament is not unique.

Part of the difficulty in asking for help is associated with the work climate that we perpetuate as academics—one that stresses individual achievement and independence (Herbert, 2001). In this type of setting, asking for help is viewed as a sign of weakness or incompetence, and by doing so, we are admitting that we are vulnerable (human)—an aspect that we try very hard to avoid. Being vulnerable necessitates sharing our thoughts and feelings with our colleagues. It requires us to get closer to one another even when there are obstacles that make it difficult. As I wrote in an earlier editorial (Herbert, 1984), this task would seem fairly easy given our academic training. Yet, how many times have we experienced faculty and student conflicts where we did not employ the same effective listening skills we taught in our counseling skills classes? Sometimes I ask myself, "How come I can demonstrate listening skills within a difficult client–counselor roleplay exercise to my students but I cannot apply the same conditions with a work colleague who is stressed about a particular issue?"

Whether it is a fear of offending someone, an inability to see beyond my own perspective, or some other reason, my recent experience has reminded me that the only person I can change is me. Yes, I know that statement is an espoused mantra that we communicate to our students, but in trying to apply it to my future work, I need to remind myself of the obvious. Further, in situations where I start to feel overwhelmed, I want to validate that it is OK to ask for and receive help. A simple declaration such as "I would like some help with. Can you help me?" is the first step. It took an illness to remind me that it is necessary to repeat it more often when I return to work.

Another outcome that resulted from this life-altering experience was the realization that there was great potential for me to have a stronger connection to God while I am working. Prior to my recent medical excursion, I cannot recall a single incident where I invoked prayer to help me in addressing a work problem. Certainly, there were plenty of opportunities to ask for help in being more patient with my students, more receptive to dissenting views, and more forgiving about personal shortcomings that manifest themselves at work. What seems so obvious now was completely missing in my daily work interactions. For me, God was an occasional afterthought who would only be considered in times of crises. Fortunately, while work can be trying, there was never any time during my academic life that represented a crisis or, atleast, one that I would recognize as such. Besides, why would

God care about my work problems? As a result, I did not ask for any spiritual help as I saw that aspect as totally disconnected to my work life. Sure, I could recite a prayer at the family dinner table or right before I went to sleep but asking for God's help at work?

Given my recent experience, however, I anticipate that there will be many occasions when I will ask or share some simple prayer at work. I anticipate that my prayers will ask God to help me listen better, forgive my own as well as others' shortcomings, and demonstrate patience in handling everyday work stress. I also anticipate giving prayers of thanks for the people I come in contact with each day that bring joy in my life. Through prayer, meditation, or reflection, we have an untapped resource that is always available. As a rehabilitation counselor educator, it is my intention when I return next academic year to take a few moments each day to ask for that help. If nothing else, taking a few moments to collect your thoughts and declare honorable intentions to deal with the work conflicts and demands usually produces a calming effect. We all need a little more peace in our lives.

As I noted earlier, an important impact of my recent experience has resulted in rethinking the importance that work has played in my life. At this point, I need to reevaluate and question roles and responsibilities I have taken on at program, department, college, university, and professional levels. For starters, I made the decision to resign as professor-in-charge of the rehabilitation programs. This decision was both easy and difficult. Easy in the sense of acknowledging that it is time to tone down the importance that work has played in my life; difficult in the sense of letting go and having someone else assume a professional role that I have performed for nearly 13 years. "Passing the torch" signifies a time to let go that requires me to lead in a supportive rather than a proactive role. I expect that giving up perceived administrative control for a program will be difficult during those first several faculty meetings as I believe there will be a natural tendency for me to think, "How would I have handled that situation or that problem?" I imagine there is a natural tendency for most of us who assume administrative roles to believe that we are the best ones to perform these duties. With the successful transition from starting as a pretenured assistant professor to achieving subsequent tenure and promotion to associate and then full professor usually comes with increasing administrative responsibilities. Whether the same requirements to successfully negotiate this career path are the identical ones that make an outstanding administrator is questionable.

Working as an effective rehabilitation counselor educator does not guarantee that one also performs equally well as a program administrator. Certainly, I made my share of mistakes in trying to do what I thought was best for the rehabilitation program. The current task for me, it seems, will be to have patience and show support for my colleague who most likely will experience a similar growth curve.

FINAL THOUGHT

I would like to finish this chapter with a brief story that reminds me of the work that lies ahead. Before my surgery, I was trying to tell my 6-year-old son what was about to happen. I did not want to worry him, yet I also wanted to explain in terms that he could understand why Dad needed surgery. I used a metaphor of how water from the kitchen faucet is decreased when debris gets clogged in the filter screen. I told him that the water pipes represented my heart arteries and that the water symbolized my blood. I also told him that my doctor was "kind of like a plumber who was going to clean and fix Dad's heart pipes." I thought I had reached him with this analogy and, after a few moments, I asked him if he understood. He understood in more ways than I anticipated. As he was sitting next to me, he placed his small hand on my heart and said, "Yes, Daddy's heart is blossoming. Just like a flower in a garden." Tears came to my eyes. He sure was right. Dad's heart continues to blossom.

REFERENCES

Herbert, J. T. (1984). From attitudes to academe: Can they change? [Editorial]. *Rehabilitation Education, 8,* 101–102.

Herbert, J. T. (2001). Thoughts on becoming a rehabilitation counselor educator [Gray Matter]. *Rehabilitation Education, 15,* 307–315.

V

New Directions: Issues and Perspectives: Introduction

*T*he final section of this text contains a number of contemporary issues facing persons with disabilities, counselors, and Americans in general. With obesity, poverty, suicide, constant threat of terrorism, and depression on the rise in the United States, these issues become a necessity to address. At one end of the spectrum, there are individuals, including those with disabilities, who thrive and excel in life, sometimes against tremendous odds. Conversely, there are individuals who are fraught with mental and physical health problems, who struggle through school and/or experience subsequent chronic unemployment difficulties. There is no one single reason for such disparities, but there is a complex myriad ranging from personal traits such as intelligence, resilience, and locus of control, to external variables such as socioeconomic status, social classism, and discrimination.

Chapter 24 by Marini and Chacon is an updated exploration on positive psychology, wellness, and post-traumatic growth. Researchers have focused far too long on the problem issues most individuals face without looking at the traits and characteristics of those who thrive and do exceedingly well in life. Specifically, what is it about successful and healthy individuals that we can learn from and feasibly instill into our own lives and the lives of our clients. The authors discuss research on subjective well-being, hope, optimism, resiliency, happiness, faith, flow, and altruism among other factors found to be important in living well and thriving.

In Chapter 25 by Minkler and Fadem discuss successful aging with a disability rather than giving us yet another discussion about the pathological aspects of aging. The tenor of this chapter is similar to that of Marini and Chacon with regards to characteristics of those who age well, despite ongoing societal marginalization and stigmatization that aging with a disability typically brings. The authors explore the balancing act between diminishing mental and physical abilities with needs for assistance and accommodation, noting once again that societal and environmental barriers can be more disabling than the disability itself. The authors advocate for rehabilitation professionals to consider a more ecological approach to working with older individuals with disabilities.

Chapter 26 is a new addition by David Peterson whose book and numerous publications regarding the International Classification of Functioning Disability and Health (ICF) outline contemporary thinking on disability. In attempting to move away from the narrow pathological classifications of mental and physical disabilities found in the *Diagnostic Statistical Manual* and the *International Classification of Diseases,* the ICF takes a more holistic approach in considering not only the diagnosed disability but also the psychological, social, and environmental factors that may exacerbate a condition. Peterson explores various models of disability, the classifications of the ICF, future research directions and implications. All educators and counselors need to familiarize and begin working with this authoritative text in order to truly consider a holistic approach to working with clients.

Chapter 27 is also a new addition by coeditor Mark Stebnicki, who also "wrote the book" on empathy fatigue. Stebnicki's research and clinical experience in crisis intervention discovered years ago that counselors of all disciplines can be emotionally drained by empathizing with their clients, yet not recognize their own gradual burnout.

Chapter 28 by Romero and Marini is also a new addition that addresses the epidemics of obesity in America and their medical, psychosocial, and vocational implications. It is estimated that the incidence of obesity and obesity-related complications such as Type II diabetes, heart disease, and musculoskeletal problems will cost the U.S. health care system over $3 trillion by 2050 if a radical change in people's lives is not made. People who are overweight and obese are often subjected to ridicule and discrimination both in their personal and professional lives as addressed by the authors reviewing societal attitudes and employment discrimination with this population. Knowing the issues and working with obese persons will continue to become more commonplace in the United States and abroad.

Chapter 29 by Zanskas and Coduti is an updated and ongoing controversial topic on eugenics, euthanasia, and physician-assisted suicide (PAS). The authors summarize the eugenics movement dating back to Charles Darwin and address the catchphrase "survival of the fittest" concept. Then this slippery slope takes the reader through the genocide of Nazi Germany during World War II to exterminate German citizens with disabilities who were viewed as less than human and not qualified to be part of the superior race. Persons with disabilities were called "useless eaters." Zanskas and Coduti flash forward to the present day debate regarding genetic testing, aborting unborn fetuses that may carry a disabling gene, and PAS on the back end of life of individuals with chronic illness and disease who may believe life is no longer worth living. The authors poignantly address humanity going down this path and the implications of who gets to decide what quality of life is and who lives or dies when that quality of life is perceived to be gone.

Chapter 30 by Surís and North is a new and timely chapter pertaining to mental health preparedness for terrorist incidents. The authors outline the reality of the world we now live in post-9/11, noting the various threats to American citizens, and then focus on the psychological repercussions regarding the uncertainty and uncontrollability of such events. As such, they explore the psychological sequelae such as post-traumatic stress disorder (PTSD), psychiatric illness, and disaster stigma. A predominant part of the chapter, however, addresses specific evidence-based interventions, including cognitive behavior therapy, cognitive therapy, psychological first aid, risk communication, building community resilience, and preparedness, in working with survivors of traumatic terrorist incidents. The vast majority of references for this chapter are less than 10 years old, and therefore provide the reader with the most current information on the topic.

Chapter 31 by Bruyère, Harley, Kampfe, and Wadsworth regarding key concepts in employment counseling with aging workers is a new chapter, which again is timely considering the 2008 recession that ultimately left millions of workers with drastically reduced or no 401(k) retirement savings. Considering the economic downturn and the fact that unemployment is still not stabilized in 2011, the reality for many of those retired or near-retired persons in having to return to the workforce is imperative in many cases. As such, the authors specifically address some of the health implications of older workers as well as mental health and employment counseling for this ever-growing population.

Finally, Marini and Stebnicki write a compelling and provocative Chapter 32 in two parts, reflecting each of their opinions and considerations for rehabilitation professionals in the 20th century. Marini provides an overview of where America is in 2011 by highlighting specific events and social issues in American history that have been discussed throughout the book. He then hypothesizes an inconvenient and potentially frightening future for Americans, particularly those of lower socioeconomic status, many of whom are persons and minorities with disabilities. The ramifications of social class and classism are explored, where social injustice perpetuates and exacerbates classism. Marini calls upon rehabilitation counselors and related helping professionals to take a more active and advocacy role beyond their traditional narrow-focused job duties of working almost exclusively with the client to adapt and survive in an able-bodied world. In Part B, Stebnicki discusses how traditional counseling and psychotherapeutic approaches can be integrated into more indigenous and culturally sensitive healing practices. His own beginning and intermediate training in shamanism and his experiences as a Reiki master challenge current practitioners to be respectful and nonjudgmental in examining culturally sensitive approaches to treating chronic illness and disability.

24

Positive Psychology, Wellness, and Post-Traumatic Growth Implications for Rehabilitation Counselor Education

IRMO MARINI AND MITKA CHACON

The impact of a congenital or adventitious disability on an individual and his or her family poses many challenges regarding psychosocial adjustment, vocational options, and independent living functioning. In situations where a disability is relatively stable (e.g., spinal cord injury, amputation), planning for the future may not be as ambiguous or anxiety provoking as it may be for persons with unstable or uncertain diagnoses (e.g., multiple sclerosis, Alzheimer's disease). However, there are many instances where persons with stable disabilities succumb to secondary complications on a regular basis, whereas others with similar disabilities experience few, if any, further health-related problems throughout the remainder of their lives (Antonovsky, 1987).

Antonovsky (1987) distinguished between those individuals who regularly become ill (i.e., a pathological orientation) and those who remain basically healthy despite a severe disability (i.e., a salutogenic orientation). In treating persons with disabilities, a pathological orientation has traditionally been the focus for medical and mental health professionals (Trieschmann, 1981). Stereotypical beliefs and attitudes toward persons with disabilities as being sick, incapable, and dependent have likely facilitated this approach to treatment, likely stemming from the medical model of disability (Marini, 1994).

Rehabilitation counselor practice and education originated from the medical model, or a pathological orientation (Olkin, 1999; Trieschmann, 1981; Vash, 1981). The public vocational rehabilitation program's philosophy of assisting persons with disabilities to reach their maximum potential is a noble ideology, but the program has never really been mandated to explore which factors are indicative of clients with disabilities who not only succeed but also excel in all areas of their lives. This phenomenon of thriving despite having a disability was previously described by Vash (1981) as "transcendence" and Wright (1983) who discussed a strength-based approach, focusing on positive attributes as opposed to negative. More recently, Tedeschi and Calhoun (1988, 1995, 1996) have further explored this concept called post-traumatic growth (PTG).

In exploring factors related to disability and wellness, many of the debilitating primary disabling conditions as well as their secondary complications found today can actually be minimized or even eliminated if individuals with disabilities were to adopt a wellness lifestyle (Pelletier, 1994; Schafer, 1996). Conditions such as high blood pressure, heart

From "The implications of positive psychology and wellness for rehabilitation counselor education," by I. Marini and M. Chacon, 2002, *Rehabilitation Education, 6*(2), 149–164. Reprinted with permission.

377

disease, coronary artery disease, rheumatoid arthritis, gastrointestinal disorders, alcohol and substance abuse, anxiety disorders, and stroke all carry self-induced aspects with them (Pelletier). Pelletier described the field of psychoneuroimmunology as the study of the mind–body connection and how what we think can directly and indirectly affect our physical health status.

This chapter addresses some of the key research findings related to positive psychology, wellness, and PTG by exploring significant factors of healthy individuals and their interaction with the environment. Specifically, what individual traits and practices appear to be related to mental and physical well-being, and what environmental conditions are necessary to nurture wellness in individuals? Research findings in these areas are then discussed with respect to potentially new and emerging areas of disability-related research for rehabilitation educators and areas of practice for rehabilitation counselors.

POSITIVE PSYCHOLOGY AND WELLNESS

The January 2000 issue of *American Psychologist* was devoted to the concept of happiness, excellence, and optimal human functioning. In that issue, American Psychological Association President Martin Seligman and Mihaly Csikszentmihalyi defined the field of positive psychology as being "about valued subjective experiences; well-being, contentment and satisfaction (in the past); hope and optimism (for the future); and flow and happiness (in the present)" (2000, p. 5). At the individual level, positive personal traits such as subjective well-being (SWB), optimism, happiness, perseverance, and self-determination are contributing factors to wellness (Csikszentmihalyi, 1990, 1999; Peterson, 1998; Peterson, Seligman, & Vaillant, 1988; Ryan & Deci, 2000; Seligman & Csikszentmihalyi, 2000; Weisse, 1992). On the environmental level, social support, a sense of belonging, faith in a higher power, having basic financial needs met, and perceived mastery or harmony with one's environment are main external factors contributing to wellness (Arglye, 1986; Dohrenwend et al., 1982; Koenig, 1997; Matthews & Larson, 1997; Pavot, Diener, & Fujita, 1990).

Wellness is defined as "living well—mentally, spiritually and physically—with illness, whether temporary or chronic" (Schafer, 1996, p. 37). Schafer further described a wellness lifestyle as one that includes taking care of the environment; effectively managing emotional problems; thinking critically; maintaining a stable emotional state; spiritual wellness, as in having meaning or purpose; physical habits, including exercise and nutrition; social habits, as in sharing intimacy and establishing good friendships; and time-management habits, such as maintaining a stable work place and developing control over one's time and choices.

This section explores some of the major findings and concepts related to the three levels of analysis for positive psychology described by Seligman and Csikszentmihalyi (2000): the subjective level, the individual level, and the group level. Where relevant, research findings regarding persons with disabilities are integrated with the concept being discussed. The central issue here pertains to how rehabilitation professionals can begin to conceptualize counseling, researching/teaching about disability, and adopt a salutogenic orientation.

SUBJECTIVE LEVEL

Subjective Well-Being

The concept of SWB relates to individuals' cognitive and affective evaluations of their lives (Diener, 2000). It is not the nature of events themselves that elicit well-being, but rather our interpretation of these events. According to Diener, three key concepts imbued in SWB are adaptation, goals, and temperament. Regarding adaptation, Diener stated that we are on a hedonic treadmill where, once we have obtained a possession or accomplishment, we quickly habituate to this level and it no longer makes us happy. Conversely, when people experience misfortune, they also soon adapt emotionally (Brickman & Campbell, 1971). Silver (1982) found that persons with spinal cord injuries reported to be very unhappy immediately following their injuries; but then began to return to a baseline level of adaptation within 8 weeks.

Striving for realistic goals and movement toward obtaining one's goals is also important to SWB, as well as feelings of competence and self-esteem (Cantor & Sanderson, 1999; Diener, 2000). Bandura (1997) described self-efficacy in relation to how individuals feel about their ability or skills to achieve certain goals (efficacy expectations), in relation to the perceived rewards for putting forth the effort to obtain these goals (outcome expectations). If the perceived rewards are not worth the effort, an individual's motivation to pursue the goal is diminished. Marini and Stebnicki (1999) found support for this theory, noting that Social Security Disability Income beneficiaries often report that it is not financially worth the effort to leave disability rolls for minimum wage work and the risk of reinjury as well as the potential loss of health benefits.

One's temperament also appears to be related to SWB. Schafer (1996) cited a number of traits correlated with wellness, such as Type B behavior pattern (an absence of time urgency and hostility), trust in others, hardiness (liking a challenge, strong sense of commitment, and a sense of control), a survivor personality (having grown stronger from some personal crisis), a sense of humor with the ability to laugh at oneself, and self-actualization.

Optimism

Optimism has been defined by Tiger (1979) as "a mood or attitude associated with an expectation about the social or material future—one which the evaluator regards as socially desirable, to his or her advantage, or for his or her pleasure" (p. 18). Peterson (1988, 2000) stated that optimism has been correlated with positive mood, effective problem solving, good health, longer life, and occupational and academic success. Conversely, pessimism has been correlated with passivity, failure, morbidity and mortality, anxiety, and depression.

Buchanan and Seligman (1995) described optimism in terms of an individual's characteristic explanatory style or how he or she attributes the causes of undesirable or poor outcome events. Optimists typically describe such undesirable events as having an external influence with specific causes, whereas pessimists describe undesirable events as being due to something internal and having a global cause. If an individual's response is unrelated to the outcome, this leads to learned helplessness. Seligman's (1991) research has led him to conclude that optimists respond to adversity by asserting internal control whenever feasible, become depressed less often, maintain better health habits, have a stronger immune system, and are healthier. Seligman further concluded that individuals can learn and unlearn to be optimistic or pessimistic.

Taylor (1983) formulated "cognitive adaptation theory," which evolved from interviewing women with breast cancer. Taylor found that those who had "unrealistic" positive beliefs about controlling their prognosis were not negatively affected when learning otherwise. Taylor and Brown (1988) noted that humans have three positive illusions—self-enhancement, unrealistic optimism, and an exaggerated perception of personal control—which have a positive psychological effect. Positive beliefs have additionally been associated with a stronger immune system whereby the type of belief (if positive) affects our emotional state and impacts our neuroendocrine system by eliminating bodily viruses or disease (Stone, Cox, Valdimarsdottir, Jandorf, & Neale, 1987).

The concept of unrealistic optimism is an interesting one, because it fundamentally refutes past strategies of therapeutic treatment whereby clients are counseled to accept their disabilities. Freud (1928) believed that optimism was illusory and came with the cost of denying one's reality. According to Akhtar (1996), one of the defining features of a healthy individual is for him or her to be exposed to the reality of the situation no matter how painful. Current research regarding wellness, however, suggests otherwise (Peterson, 2000). Lazarus (1983) described positive denial as being a factor related to wellness in the presence of adversity. It appears that being overly optimistic about one's future (e.g., health, career) may contribute to a healthy immune system.

Conversely, some researchers believe that unrealistic optimism may have adverse effects on wellness (Oettingen, 1996). Oettingen stated that overly optimistic persons who believe that they will not become ill may postpone or neglect visiting a doctor when they experience symptoms. Cigarette smokers, for example, may ignore or discount the harmful effects of smoking by adopting a bias or creating cognitive dissonance that they are not susceptible to the risks associated with smoking (Gibbons, Eggleston, & Benthin, 1997).

Self-Determination Theory

Self-determination theory is a widely researched and written-about approach to human motivation and personality (Ryan & Deci, 2000). It is the investigation of individuals' inherent growth tendencies and innate psychological needs that provide the basis for self-motivation and personality integration. Ryan and Deci defined three psychological needs: autonomy, competence, and relatedness as concepts of self-determination. When these needs are met, an individual is self-motivated and mentally healthy. Environmental factors, however, can impede personal growth, well-being, and self-motivation (Ryan & Deci, 2000). For example, accessibility barriers and negative societal attitudes toward disability may thwart the growth and motivation of a person with a disability.

Autonomy in this context does not equate to independence but rather to the feeling of mastery one feels when completing a task without assistance. Competence refers to the feelings derived from performing something well, doing it with ease, and being recognized for the work (Harter, 1978). Relatedness refers to perceived support and security from significant others (Ryan & Grolnick, 1986). When we believe there is support available to assist if needed, we feel more secure in pursuing certain goals (Frodi, Bridges, & Grolnick, 1985).

Deci and Ryan (2000) postulated cognitive evaluation theory (CET) as a subtheory to self-determination theory. CET relates to social and environmental factors that facilitate or undermine an individual's intrinsic motivation. The conditions for well-being are more conducive when people are intrinsically motivated toward some goal as opposed to being extrinsically motivated. Intrinsic motivation is facilitated when autonomy, relatedness, and competence are present. Ryan and Deci (2000) stated that positive feedback and rewards can enhance competence and intrinsic motivation. Kasser and Ryan (1993, 1996) found that individuals who placed great importance on intrinsic aspirations were more likely to exhibit indicators related to well-being, self-esteem, and self-actualization. The same study showed a negative relationship between a low-importance rating of intrinsic aspirations and higher levels of anxiety and depression.

Ryan and Deci (2000) noted, however, that in many instances people are driven by extrinsic motivating factors such as threats, coercion, deadlines, and externally imposed goals. Individuals who are driven or externally motivated by environmental factors will, as a consequence, be inhibited in developing a sense of competence, autonomy, or well-being (deCharms, 1968).

Hope

Hope theory (Snyder, 2000) is described as a goal-directed human behavior. Snyder (1994) described hope as a cognitive process of setting goals and developing strategies to accomplish them, known as pathway thinking. Agency thinking is the method used to stay on course and remain motivated to accomplish one's goals. Snyder and Lopez (2002) theorized that successfully moving toward and attaining one's goals brings about positive emotions, whereas failing or being blocked from accomplishing goals result in negative emotions (e.g., depression, low self-esteem). In terms of blocked hope, persons with disabilities sometimes must endure both environmental and attitudinal barriers regarding physical access and/or discriminatory employer attitudes (DiTomasso & Spinner, 1997; Graf, Marini, & Blankenship, 2009; Li & Moore, 1998). Peterson, Maier, and Seligman (1995) described how some individuals may succumb or give up when their goals are blocked and perceived as out of their control, potentially leading to feelings of hopelessness and ultimately learned helplessness (Marini & Stebnicki, 1999). Research regarding the correlates of hope includes possessing an internal locus of control, optimism, the spiritual belief that one will be okay, high self-efficacy to accomplish goals, and strong coping skills (Moore & Stambrook, 1995; Puchalski, 1999; Shnek et al., 1997; Stanton, Danoff-Burg, & Huggins, 2002). Marini and Graf (2011) found that persons with spinal cord injury should never be denied the hope for recovery so long as they continue to move forward in their rehabilitation program and their lives.

Happiness

The pursuit of happiness and what makes individuals happy has received considerable research attention and empirical support over the past decade (Ben-Shahar, 2007; Chapin & Boykin, 2010; Diener, Lucas, & Scollon, 2006; Diener & Seligman, 2002; Lucas, 2007; Marinnic & Brkljacic, 2008; Ryan & Deci, 2000, 2001; Seligman, 2002). The pursuit of happiness can be explored by reviewing three of its theories.

Temporary or fleeting happiness known as *hedonic happiness* relates to engaging in pleasurable activities that gratify us such as buying material goods (e.g., new clothes, car, electronics), socializing with friends, sexual activities, and vacations (Lucas, 2007; Ryan & Deci, 2001). Lucas describes how these daily pleasurable activities are necessary for us to ward off stress; however, that the novelty wears off, we adapt, and we return to an emotional set point shortly after. New clothes have to be replaced with more new clothes, old partners with new ones, etc. This is also described by Lucas as the hedonic treadmill; where something novel initially, becomes adapted or used to, and must be replaced with something novel again to maintain the gratification.

Eudiamonic happiness (Ryan & Deci, 2000) represents the gratification one obtains pursuing self-development activities such as obtaining a degree, mastering a musical instrument, becoming a successful athlete, etc. The sense of accomplishment and mastery is believed to lead to long-term happiness. The sense of self-esteem, self-concept, and self-efficacy can be enhanced as individuals feel more competent and in control of their environment (Bandura, 1997; Ryan & Deci, 2000; Seligman, 2002).

Authentic happiness (Seligman, 2002) is described as a combination of hedonic and eudiamonic happiness at work simultaneously and in moderation. Seligman describes how individuals require both types of happiness activities to lead a good and meaningful life. As individuals work hard to pursue their long-term goals, it becomes prudent in dealing with daily stresses to periodically engage in hedonic activities. Ben-Shahar (2007) suggests that all activities require moderation. For example, being able to choose to go on an exotic vacation for 1 week is likely an activity that most people would look forward to; however, if individuals were somehow forced to remain in the same vacation spot for 1 year, this pleasurable activity would likely lose its novelty and become boring. Conversely, students who do nothing but study all the time or employed persons who work all the time may succumb to a stress-related illness from not taking pleasurable breaks along the way.

Flow

Csikszentmihalyi (1975, 1978) described the concept of "flow" as optimal experiences characterized by high involvement, deep concentration, intrinsic motivation and perception, and difficult challenges matched by an individual's requisite skills. Somewhere between being overwhelmed or stressed and the apathy of being underwhelmed and bored lies the zone Csikszentmihalyi terms flow. Optimal experience promotes individual development and growth as one successfully matches his or her skills to activities and challenges in the environment. Examples of activities that may create flow include sports, work, hobbies, and social interactions. These activities must be appropriately challenging and intrinsically motivating so that the individual perceives personal growth and derives a sense of competence and self-esteem from engaging in them. Activities that are contrary to flow include repetitive and simple tasks and being in an underemployed job. Massimini and Delle Fave (2000) argued that current social and work contexts do not always provide for growth opportunities. As such, more people are turning to leisure activities such as hiking, rock climbing, and high-risk sports for optimal experience. Delle Fave and Bassi (1998) stated that personal growth develops from a focused level of concentration, alertness, active participation, and the perceived importance of the activity.

Research has suggested that persons with disabilities can experience flow (Delle Fave, 1996; Delle Fave & Maletto, 1992). Delle Fave (1996) found that persons who became blind or sustained a spinal cord injury later in life developed a strategy called "transformation of flow. "Transformation relates to situations in which a person with an adventitious disability continues to cultivate former flow activities (e.g., returning to a challenging job). If this is not possible, some individuals seek new sources of concentration and challenge unrelated to their previous experiences.

Massimini and Delle Fave (2000) noted that behavioral flexibility is a crucial feature for adapting to a continually changing environment. Wright (1983) differentiated between coping or adapting to a disability and succumbing to it as well as the environmental barriers imposed by having a disability.

Adaptive Mental Mechanisms

Vaillant (2000) described adaptive mental mechanisms as another internal factor related to positive psychology. Vaillant has identified five adaptive coping mechanisms found at the mature end of the Defensive Function Scale of the *Diagnostic and Statistical Manual of Mental Disorders-IV* (American Psychiatric Association, 1994). Lazurus and Folkman (1984) noted that individuals intentionally use conscious cognitive strategies to make the best of a bad situation. In addition, there are involuntary mental mechanisms that distort our perception of reality to reduce subjective distress.

The five adaptive defense mechanisms that Vaillant (2000) discussed are anticipation, altruism, humor, sublimation, and suppression. Vaillant indicated that adaptive defenses and healthy denial are synonymous. These defenses are independent of social class, education, and intelligence, and they become more salient as we move from adolescence into midlife (Vaillant, 1977). Altruism refers to deriving pleasure from giving to or helping others. Sublimation is defined as a way of indirectly resolving a conflict without adverse consequences or loss of pleasure. Vaillant (2000) described how Beethoven, at the age of 31, contemplated suicide but instead turned this energy into his famous "Ode to Joy"—Ninth Symphony. Suppression involves a semiconscious decision to postpone paying attention to a conflict or emotional pain. Anticipation as a defense mechanism allows us to emotionally deal with some future conflict in small steps and involves both thinking and feeling about the future. Finally, humor can be an expression of emotion without individual discomfort. It can allow us to reframe and view some conflict from a different perspective.

INDIVIDUAL LEVEL

Spirituality

The role of religion and spirituality has gained considerable attention in the counseling field over the last decade (Levin, 2001; Marini & Graf, 2011; Vash & Crewe, 2004). The role of spirituality in positive psychology is with individuals' beliefs and the safe feelings from such beliefs that God or a higher power is watching over them. Levin (2001) summarized the findings of hundreds of epidemiological studies, noting consistent correlational differences between believers and nonbelievers. Findings suggest that those who believe and practice (e.g., pray, go to church, fellowship) have lower divorce, suicide, depression, risky behavior, and substance abuse rates as well as an average 7-year longer life expectancy than nonbelievers. Myers (2000) further found that those who report being close to God indicate being happier.

With regards to persons with disabilities, there is also a growing body of literature suggesting that belief in God or a spiritual power provides many individuals with a sense of meaning and purpose, happiness, and psychological well-being (deRoon-Cassini, de St. Aubin, Valvano, Hastings, & Horn, 2009; Graf, Marini, Baker, & Buck, 2007; Marini & Graf, 2011). Tedeschi and Calhoun (1995), in theorizing the concept of PTG to an adverse event, describes how persons who have thrived postinjury express a new sense of spiritual purpose and meaning in their lives.

Hardiness

Kobasa (1979) postulated the concept of hardiness as a personality trait comprised of three related tendencies: commitment, challenge, and control. In defining these concepts, *commitment* refers to our perceived values and beliefs in striving toward accomplishing goals. Similar to Bandura's (1997) self-efficacy theory, hardy individuals believe they have what it takes to accomplish whatever desirable goals they set out for themselves. And once again, the phenomenon of developing meaning and purpose becomes relevant as individuals and derive these feelings by pursuing their goals. *Challenge* relates to individuals who perceive change as an opportunity to grow and learn, as opposed to something to fear and avoid. Hardy individuals look forward to a new challenge and take moderate risks in pursuing them. *Control* refers to the need hardy individuals have in mastering or controlling their environment, and the sense of self-concept and satisfaction that comes from perceptions of mastery (de Roone-Cassini et al., 2009). Kendall and Buys (1998) described how persons with an acquired disability initially have difficulty adjusting to their situation, and one of the key factors in reestablishing a new sense of self is to reclaim, control, and master their environment as a person with a disability. Person's who believe they have no control over their circumstances and may otherwise feel victimized may succumb to learn helplessness, whereby they simply let others make decisions for them (Marini & Stebnicki, 1999; Peterson et al., 1995).

Resilience

Closely related to the concept of PTG described later, resiliency theory (Kumpfer, 1999; Todd & Worell, 2000) requires two major occurrences to establish whether an individual is resilient: the first is that the individual must have been exposed to some extraordinarily adverse event (e.g., spinal cord injury, amputation) and the second component being despite such trauma, the individual is able to bounce back and thrive beyond anyone's expectations (Yates, Egeland & Sroufe, 2003). Resiliency theory also stresses the interaction between the individual, his or her environment, and situational factors regarding the disability (Kumpfer, 1999; Trieschmann, 1988; Wright, 1983). This complex interdependency and interaction between individual and environment was originally postulated by Lewin (1935) termed somatopsychology. It was not until some 50 years later that Wright (1983) added the variable of disability and factors related to it, as also determining how individuals' adjust or respond to their circumstances.

In Kumpfer's (1999) resiliency theory model, an adverse event or trauma creates disequilibrium for the individual and his or her sense of homeostasis. The individual's personality traits including problem-solving skills, self-efficacy, high self-esteem, among others, is part of the equation in adapting (Masten, Best, & Garmezy, 1990). But the individual's interaction with their environment plays an equally important role in the process of reestablishing equilibrium or adjusting to the disability. Specifically, if the individual is surrounded by dysfunctional significant others, treated negatively, discriminated against, or otherwise devalued by members of the community, he or she will experience difficulty maintaining self-esteem. Conversely, strong family support and community members who treat individuals with dignity and respect serve as the emotional and physical support one needs to adapt positively.

GROUP-LEVEL INDICATORS

Group-level indicators all represent an outward focus by the individual, becoming more concerned with the welfare of others, rather than focusing on one's own problems. This can include taking care of one's family, grandchildren, and friends, as well as assisting others less fortunate in the community by volunteering or making charitable donations. The psychological benefits from such acts are well documented. In helping others less fortunate, researchers describe a *downward social comparison,* particularly for those with disabilities or who have experienced some other traumatic event (e.g., hurricane survivors). Specifically, those who have suffered a trauma generally view their own personal circumstances in a less-severe light when helping other trauma survivors (Klein, 1997; Tedeschi, Park, & Calhoun, 1998; Willis, 1991). In cases of disability, assisting someone with a more severe disability can be particularly rewarding and will develop a more positive affect that their situation could have been much worse in comparison.

The concept of altruism and volunteering has also been extensively studied (see Penner, 2004; Piliavin & Charng, 1990; Wilson, 2000). Volunteering enhances one's feelings of SWB, self-efficacy, and empathy toward others (Penner, 2004; Piliavin & Charng, 1990; Wilson, 2000). It also appears to enhance perceived subjective quality of life from the satisfying feelings derived (Matheis, Tulsky, & Matheis, 2006). Seligman and Csikszentmihalyi (2000) cite one's capacity to love, civility, citizenship, and altruism as important variables for positive well-being. Realtruism specifically, Vollhardt (2009) discusses altruism born of suffering (coined by Staub, 2003) referring specifically to the reasons why some persons who have suffered a trauma or disability, become motivated to help others less fortunate. Janoff-Bulman (1992) suggests that when formerly traumatized individuals help others, it serves to help them rebuild the shattered assumptions about the world and find new meaning or purpose in life, ultimately making them stronger (p. 329). Tedeschi et al. (1998) in describing PTG cite altruism, empathy, and finding meaning or purpose as three significant indicators in the ability to thrive postinjury.

EXTERNAL FACTORS

External or environmental factors relate to dynamics outside of "individual" experience that can either inhibit or enhance wellness. Myers (2000) discussed SWB in terms of who is happy. Self-reports of happiness tend to be reasonably reliable over time despite changing life circumstances (Diener, 1994). Numerous studies provide inconsistent findings as to the current state of peoples' reported happiness. Although some studies indicate people are happy overall, other studies showed that people are becoming increasingly more depressed (Diener & Diener, 1996; Lykken, 1999; Myers & Diener, 1996; Wholey, 1986). Pertinent to many of these studies is the impact that external factors appear to have (e.g., pollution, crime, poverty) on overall well-being.

Income Status

Research regarding wealth and well-being suggests that once people have their basic needs met (i.e., food and drink, safety and security of a home), there is relatively little difference in reported well-being between the poor and the wealthy (Diener, Horwitz, & Emmons, 1985; Inglehart, 1990; Lykken, 1999). Arglye (1986) noted that lottery winners gain only temporary joy from their winnings. Relatedly, persons whose incomes have doubled in the past decade are no happier than those whose incomes have not increased (Diener, Sandvik, Seidlitz, & Diener, 1993). Myers (2000) further noted that Americans' self-reports of being "very happy" over the last 40 years has slightly declined from 35% to 33%, citing the fact that we are twice as rich and no happier. In addition, teen suicide has tripled, divorce has doubled, and depression rates have soared among teens and young adults. These findings present an interesting argument against modern materialism.

Relationships

Along with modern materialism in America is the European American ideal of individualism and autonomy. Although individualism enhances one's identity and self-expression, it may come at a great price. Myers (2000) noted how we spend billions of dollars on cosmetics, diets, and clothes in order to be accepted by others. We also fear loneliness and rejection so much that many people remain in abusive relationships for fear of being alone. In relation to well-being, Pennebaker (1990) found that close, intact relationships and friendships predict health. Studies show that people with leukemia or heart disease have higher survival rates if they have extensive social support (Case, Moss, Case, McDermott, & Eberly, 1992). When a spouse dies or people experience a job loss or divorce, researchers have found that immune defenses appear to weaken for varying periods of time and rates of death and disease increase (Dohrenwend et al., 1982; National Academy of Sciences, 1984).

In exploring findings regarding intimate relationships like marriage, Myers (2000) cited National Opinion Research Center statistics from 1972 and 1996 that indicated married people report being more satisfied with life than divorced or unmarried persons. They are also at less risk for depression. Persons in unhappy marriages, however, are less satisfied with life than unmarried or divorced persons. Further, Veenhoven (1988) found that happy people tend to be more appealing as marriage partners than unhappy persons.

Schafer (1996) described what happens to individuals who experience a loss of social attachments by citing five types of alienation that occur. People essentially may feel powerless (belief that one has little control over a situation), self-estrangement (sense of being separated from the fruit of one's labor), isolation (being detached from others), meaninglessness (life has little meaning or purpose), and normlessness (able to engage in socially unapproved behaviors—not working).

OTHER FACTORS RELATED TO WELLNESS

Goldberger (1982) discussed the concept of sensory deprivation regarding laboratory experiments concerning over- and understimulation. Too little stimulation or deprivational stress results when individuals are involved in boring, isolated jobs (e.g., assembly work); placed in institutions for prolonged periods, or isolated in their homes as is the case of many Medicare homebound patients (Blackwell, Marini, & Chacon, 2001). Goldberger (1982) stated that, after a time, sensory-deprived individuals begin to experience disorientation, anxiety, and depression. Schafer (1996) noted the positive impact of giving nursing home residents a plant to care for, which gives them a sense of control and purpose. For the approximate two thirds of Americans with disabilities who are chronically unemployed, having some other sense of purpose and stimulation becomes important to well-being (Olkin, 1999).

Pelletier (1994), in his book *Sound Mind, Sound Body,* outlined various emotions related to health and wellness versus illness. Wellness emotions include love, faith, will to live, determination, purpose, festivity, and laughter. Distress emotions include anxiety, depression, fear (of isolation and rejection), anger, shame, frustration, and guilt. Livneh (1991), in describing the stages of adjustment to disability, stated that although most persons with disabilities transition through stages of adjustment and subsequently experience many of these distress emotions for a short period, some persons may become "stuck" and never reach an adaptive state. In support of the stage model regarding the "getting stuck" concept, it is known that injured workers who have been off work for an extended period of time often report feelings of depression, anxiety, pessimism about their future, and worry about financially caring for their family (Power & Dell Orto, 1995). Arguing against the stage model, Kendall and Buys (1998) indicated that persons with disabilities go through lifelong periods of occasional sorrow related to their disabilities where many of these distress emotions are experienced on a periodic basis. This assertion is contrary to the findings of other research noted earlier, that persons with spinal cord injury return to an adaptive baseline state of SWB typically within 8 weeks following their injuries (Brickman & Campbell, 1971; Silver, 1982). Seligman (1990) summarized his findings on learned pessimism by stating that it promotes depression and anxiety and that it can become a self-fulfilling prophecy.

Having outlined a number of concepts and research findings related to the psychology of wellness, what aspects of this knowledge is useful in studying disability issues and working with clients with disabilities? What areas of research are fruitful for rehabilitation educators to pursue related to wellness and disability? Finally, how can rehabilitation counselors improve their skills and approaches to counseling with this information?

Post-Traumatic Growth

The concept of PTG (Tedeschi & Calhoun, 1995, 1996) is a fairly recently described concept, pertaining primarily to individuals with disabilities who have essentially become stronger and thrived because of their trauma. Five main areas of positive change postinjury include the following: a greater sense of personal strength, a closer relationship with others, greater overall appreciation of life, spiritual change, and new opportunities and possibilities (Tedeschi & Calhoun, 1996). Calhoun and Tedeschi (2004) noted additional key elements to PTG such as having a strong social support network and the ability to develop new cognitive schema and reframe their situation in a more positive light (Janoff-Bulman, 1992; Kendall & Buys, 1998; Kobasa et al., 1982). Vash and Crewe (2004) noted that "before disability can be transcended, it must first be acknowledged at the three designated levels: recognition of the facts, acceptance of the implications, and embracing the experience." (p. 154). Vash (1981) earlier on described transcendence as the ability to rise above imposed physical limitations and body by exploring one's spiritual growth. Marini and Graf (2010) found persons with spinal cord injury related their spiritual connectedness to happiness, giving new meaning to their lives, and deriving greater strength to deal with future crises through their relationship with God or a spiritual power.

Empirical support for PG is growing, and Tedeschi and Calhoun's (1996) Post-Traumatic Growth Inventory (PTGI) has been used in a number of studies concerning persons with various disabling conditions (Morrill et al., 2008; Pollard & Kennedy, 2007; Steel, Gamblin, & Carr, 2008). Morrill et al. (2008) tested and interviewed 161 women previously treated for breast cancer using the PTGI, a quality-of-life scale, a depression scale, and a post-traumatic stress symptoms scale. Results indicated that the women who scored higher on the PTGI reported a better quality of life, less depression, and less post-traumatic stress. These results are similar to other cancer studies investigating PTG (Stanton, Bower, & Low, 2006).

Pollard and Kennedy (2007) tested 87 persons with spinal cord injury (SCI) at 12 weeks postinjury and were able to follow-up 10 years later with 37 participants. Measures used were the PTGI, a coping strategies inventory, a depression scale, an anxiety inventory, social support scale, and functional independence measure. Findings showed that individuals who initially reported rates of depression and anxiety at 12 weeks postinjury continued to do so at 10 years. Authors found a strong positive relationship between psychological distress and PTG, supporting Tedeschi and Calhoun's (1995) assertion that PTG can be experienced simultaneously with the stress resulting in a paradoxical effect. Znoj (1999) surmised this paradoxical effect by suggesting that although individuals can sustain a trauma and experience the sadness, anxiety, and fear from it, that some also simultaneously grow and become stronger over time which appears to be a survival mechanism that can minimize the impact from the trauma.

SUGGESTED DIRECTIONS FOR FUTURE REHABILITATION RESEARCH

Perhaps the most significant research area derived from the wellness literature concerns not only how this information applies to persons with disabilities but which individual traits and environmental factors enhance the perceived success and wellness of a person with a disability. Vash (1981) cited a number of factors related to disability itself (e.g., time of onset, type of onset, severity, visibility) as well as cultural and environmental variables. However, Vash's factors are anecdotal and do not consider the wellness concepts discussed here. Wright (1983) also addressed concepts such as "as if" behavior (an individual with a disability behaves as if he or she doesn't have a disability) and a coping versus succumbing attitude (individuals either learn to cope and problem solve or give in and become dependent and learn to be helpless) as well as environmental stressors, such as requirement of mourning (an individual with a disability must feel badly and mourn his or her loss of function) and a "just world" phenomena (you deserve what you get), but again doesn't address factors related to those who excel. As such, specific research questions related to wellness and disability follow.

SUGGESTED RESEARCH QUESTIONS

How do persons with various types of disabilities perceive their situations and their futures? Do persons with various disabilities experience flow? Is there a longitudinal difference in self-perceptions and objective measures of health (including secondary complications) between unrealistic optimists and realists and/or pessimists? Are persons with disabilities who practice wellness behaviors (e.g., regular medical checkups, exercise, nutrition, no smoking or abusing substances, relaxation, positive thinking, adequate rest, social connectedness) less ill, less often, compared to those who do not practice wellness behaviors? Do those who practice wellness behaviors experience fewer secondary complications compared with those who do not practice wellness behaviors? What are the ethnic differences in wellness behavior, with specific focus on individualism versus collectivism ideologies? How do demographic variables such as marital status, socioeconomic status, number of close relationships, gender, employment, age, and ethnicity factor in? How do personality variables such as sense of humor, perseverance, locus of control, self-determination, extraversion, and self-concept impact overall wellness and perceived success? These are some intriguing questions for researchers that take us outside of the box regarding what typically has been researched and instead deals with disability holistically.

IMPLICATIONS FOR REHABILITATION COUNSELORS

What can practitioners gain from understanding those individual and environmental elements that enhance a client's lifelong subjective well-being? The educational paradigm dictates that practitioners should teach or empower clients to do for themselves. Although employment and career aspirations have traditionally been a focus for rehabilitation counselors, the reality of secondary complications can often prohibit clients with disabilities from pursuing full-time or ongoing work. For example, persons with mental illness often have cyclical down periods, those with spinal cord injuries succumb to decubitus ulcers which requires bed rest and treatment for weeks or months at a time, and those with diabetes may experience a variety of complications, which could partially be controlled with regular exercise.

The wellness literature translates into a number of counseling strategies for practitioners. An initial technique in educating/encouraging wellness among clients would be to create a bibliography of readings and prescribe bibliotherapy homework for discussion in sessions. Topics on nutrition, exercise, faith, relaxation, positive thinking, and disability-specific complication prevention strategies would be beneficial. This education becomes particularly important due to managed care constraints and shorter lengths of stay for hospitalization as well as diagnostic-related group limitations. Patients are simply not receiving the education needed (i.e., diabetes education) to remain healthy once they leave the hospital.

Behavioral approaches are also relevant in facilitating a client's wellness lifestyle. A behavioral contract and assessment component could be established for a nutrition and exercise program as well as to control and monitor any substance use and abuse. Behavioral homework exercises could be used to build self-confidence by "doing" feared activities rather than simply talking about change. Making sure that clients follow through with stated goals is also possible in this way.

Finally, cognitive approaches could be employed to facilitate client wellness (Beck, 1995). Much of the positive psychology and wellness literature deals with cognitions or having a certain mindset. Subjective well-being, optimism, self-determination, self-efficacy, flow, and adaptive and defense mechanisms are some of the major concepts discussed to this point in this chapter. Correcting irrational belief systems is a hallmark of Albert Ellis' (1977, as cited in Beck, 1995) rational emotive therapy. Cognitive reframing or restructuring is also an excellent technique in assisting clients to think and behave more positively. Seligman (1990) claimed it is possible to unlearn pessimistic ways of thinking in favor of a more optimistic outlook. Not to be overlooked, however, is the reality of environmental factors such as negative societal attitudes. Soliciting from clients what their perceptions are of the world around them becomes important in dispelling irrational beliefs or in acknowledging the accuracy of clients' beliefs.

CONCLUSION

Shorter lengths of hospital stays and reliance on the medical model approach of not dealing with the person "holistically" have rarely allowed acute medical personnel the time to educate patients on wellness or prevention of secondary complications of disability. Because rehabilitation counselors are often involved with clients postrecovery, it behooves researchers, educators, and counselors to not simply pay lip service to the concept of a holistic approach and begin exploring clients' all-around well-being. This involves exploring the wellness behaviors of persons with disabilities, informing students of these findings, and subsequently teaching students counseling skills that promote client wellness. With this truly holistic approach to counseling, clients may experience not only a longer work-life expectancy, but an enhanced state of SWB and perceived quality of life.

REFERENCES

Akhtar, S. (1996). "Someday . . ." and "if only . . ." fantasies: Pathological optimism and inordinate nostalgia as related forms of idealization. *Journal of American Psycholoanalytic Association, 44,* 723–753.

American Psychiatric Association. (1994). *Diagnostic and statistical manual of mental disorders* (4th ed.). Washington, DC: Author.

Antonovsky, A. (1987). *Unraveling the mystery of health: How people manage stress and stay well.* San Francisco, CA: Jossey-Bass.

Arglye, M. (1986). *The psychology of happiness.* London: Methuen.

Bandura, A. (1997). *Self-efficacy. The exercise of control.* New York: Freeman.

Batson, C. D., Schoenrade, P. A., & Ventis, W. L. (1993). *Religion and the individual: A social psychological perspective.* New York: Oxford University Press.

Beck, J. S. (1995). *Cognitive therapy: Basics and beyond.* New York: Guilford Press.

Ben-Shahar, T. (2007). *Happier.* New York: McGraw Hill.

Blackwell, T. L., Marini, I., & Chacon, M. (2001). The impact of the Americans with Disabilities Act on independent living. *Rehabilitation Education, 15,* 395–408.

Brickman, P., & Campbell, D. T. (1971). Hedonic relativism and planning the good society. In M. H. Appley (Ed.), *Adaptation-level theory* (pp. 287–305). New York: Academic Press.

Buchanan, G. M., & Seligman, M. E. P. (1995). *Explanatory style.* Hillsdale, NJ: Erlbaum.

Cantor, N., & Sanderson, C. A. (1999). Life task participation and well-being: The importance of taking part in daily life. In D. Kahneman, E. Diener, & N. Schwarz (Eds.), *Well-being: The foundations of hedonic psychology* (pp. 230–243). New York: Russell Sage Foundation.

Case, R. B., Moss, A. J., Case, N., McDermott, M., & Eberly, S. (1992). Living alone after myocardial infarction: Impact on prognosis. *Journal of the American Medical Association, 267,* 515–519.

Chapin, M. H., & Boykim, R. B. (2010). Integrating positive psychology techniques into rehabilitation counselor education. *Rehabilitation Education, 24*(1), 25–34.

Csikszentmihalyi, M. (1975). *Beyond boredom and anxiety.* San Francisco, CA: Jossey-Bass.

Csikszentmihalyi, M. (1978). Attention and the holistic approach to behavior. In K. S. Pope, & J. L. Singer (Eds.), *The stream of consciousness* (pp. 335–358). New York: Plenum.

Csikszentmihalyi, M. (1990). *Flow: The psychology of optimal experience.* New York: Harper & Row Publishers, Inc.

Csikszentmihalyi, M. (1999). If we are so rich, why aren't we happy? *American Psychologist, 54,* 821–827.

deCharms, R. (1968). *Personal causation.* New York: Academic Press.

deRoon-Cassini, T. A., de St. Aubin, E., Valvano, A., Hastings, J., & Horn, P. (2009). Psychological well-being after spinal cord injury: Perception of loss and meaning making. *Rehabilitation Psychology, 54*(3), 306–314.

Delle Fave, A. (1996). Il processo di 'trasformazione di Flow' in un campione di soggetti medullolesi [The process of flow transformation in a sample of subjects with spinal cord injuries]. In F. Massimini, P. Inghilleri, & A. Delledr Fave (Eds.), *La selezione psicologica umana* (pp. 615–634). Milan: Cooperativa Libraria IULM.

Delle Fave, A., & Bassi, M. (1998, June). *Optimal experience and apathy: The meaning of experience fluctuation in adolescents.* Paper presented at the VI Biennial EARA Conference, Budapest, Hungary.

Delle Fave, A., & Maletto, C. (1992). Processi di attenzione e qualita dell'esperienza soggettiva [Attention processes and the quality of subjective experience]. In D. Galati (Ed), *La psicologia dei non vedenti* (pp. 321–353). Milan: Franco Angeli.

Diener, E. (1994). Assessing subjective well-being: Progress and opportunities. *Social Indicators Research, 31*, 103–157.

Diener, E. (2000). Subjective well-being: The science of happiness and a proposal for a national index. *American Psychologist, 55*, 34–43.

Diener, E., & Diener, C. (1996). Most people are happy. *Psychological Science, 7*, 181–185.

Diener, E., Horwitz, J., & Emmons, R. A. (1985). Happiness of the very wealthy. *Social Indicators, 16*, 262–274.

Diener, E., Lucas, R. E., & Scollon, C. (2006). Beyond the hedonic treadmill: Revising the adaptation theory of well-being. *American Psychologist, 61*, 305–314.

Diener, E., Sandvik, E., Seidlitz, L., & Diener, M. (1993). The relationship between income and subjective well-being: Relative or absolute? *Social Indicators Research, 28*, 195–223.

Diener, E., & Seligman, M. (2002). Very happy people. *Psychological Science, 13*, 81–84.

DiTomasso, E., & Spinner, B. (1997). Social and emotional loneliness: A re-examination of Weiss' typology of loneliness. *Personality and Individual Differences, 22*, 417–427.

Dohrenwend, B., Pearlin, L., Clayton, P., Hamburg, B., Dohrenwend, B. P., Riley, M., & Rose, R. (1982). Report on stress and life events. In G. R. Elliott & C. Eisdorfer (Eds.), *Stress and human health: Analysis and implications of research* (pp. 19–37). New York: Springer.

Freud, S. (1928). *The future of an illusion.* London: Hogarth.

Frodi, A., Bridges, L., & Grolnick, W. S. (1985). Correlates of mastery-related behavior: A short-term longitudinal study of infants in their second year. *Child Development, 56*, 1291–1298.

Gibbons, F. X., Eggleston, T. J., & Benthin, A. C. (1997). Cognitive reactions to smoking relapse: The reciprocal relation between dissonance and self-esteem. *Journal of Personality and Social Psychology, 72*, 184–195.

Goldberger, L. (1982). Sensory deprivation and overload. In L. Goldberger & S. Breznitz (Eds.), *Handbook on stress: Theoretical and clinical aspects* (pp. 410–418). New York: Free Press.

Graf, N. M., Marini, I., Baker, J., & Buck, T. (2007). The perceived impact of religious and spiritual beliefs for persons with chronic pain. *Rehabilitation Counseling Bulletin, 51*(1), 21–33.

Graf, N. M., Marini, I., & Blankenship, C. (2009). 100 words about disability. *Journal of Rehabilitation, 75*(2), 25–34.

Harter, S. (1978). Effectance motivation reconsidered: Toward a developmental model. *Human Development, 1*, 661–669.

Inglehart, R. (1990). *Modernization and postmodernization: Cultural, economic, and political change in societies.* Princeton, NJ: Princeton University Press.

Janoff-Bulman, R. (1992). *Shattered assumptions: Towards a new psychology of trauma.* New York: Free Press.

Kasser, T., & Ryan, R. M. (1993). A dark side of the American dream: Correlates of financial success as a life aspiration. *Journal of Personality and Social Psychology, 65*, 410–422.

Kasser, T., & Ryan, R. (1996). Further examining the American dream: Differential correlates of intrinsic and extrinsic goals. *Personality and Social Psychology Bulletin, 22*, 280–287.

Kendall, E., & Buys, N. (1998). An integrated model of psychosocial adjustment following acquired disability. *Journal of Rehabilitation, 64*(3), 16–20.

Klein, W. M. (1997). Objective standards are not enough: Affective, self-evaluative, and behavioral responses to social comparison information. *Journal of Personality and Social Psychology, 72*, 763–774.

Kobasa, S. C. (1979). Stressful life events, personality, and health: An inquiry into hardiness. *Journal of Personality and Social Psychology, 37*, 1–11.

Kobasa, S. C., Maddi, S. R., & Kahn, S. (1982). Hardiness and health: A prospective study. *Journal of Personality and Social Psychology, 42*, 168–177.

Koenig, H. G. (1997). *Is religion good for your health? The effects of religion on physical and mental health.* Binghamton, NY: Haworth Press.

Kumpfer, K. (1999). Factors and processes contributing to resilience: The resilience framework. In M. D. Glantz, & J. L. Johnson (Eds.), *Resilience and development: Positive life adaptations* (pp. 179–224). New York: Kluwer Academic/Plenum Publishers.

Lazurus, R. S. (1983). The costs and benefits of denial. In S. Benitz (Ed.), *Denial of stress* (pp. 1–30). New York: International Universities Press.

Lazurus, R., & Folkman, S. (1984). *Stress, appraisal and coping.* New York: Springer.

Levin, J. (2001). *God, faith, and health.* New York: Wiley.

Lewin, K. (1935). *A dynamic theory of personality.* New York: McGraw Hill.

Li, L., & Moore, D., 1998. Acceptance of disability and its correlates. *Journal of Social Psychology, 138*(1), 13–25.

Livneh, H. (1991). A unified approach to existing models of adaptation to disability: A model of adaptation. In R. P. Marinelli & A. E. Dell Orto (Eds.), *The psychological and social impact of disability* (3rd. ed., pp. 111–138). New York: Springer.

Lucas, R. E. (2007). Adaptation and the set-point model of subjective well-being: Does happiness change after major life events? *Current Directions in Psychological Science, 16,* 75–79.

Lykken, D. (1999). *Happiness.* New York: Golden Books.

Marini, I. (1994). Attitudes toward disability and the psychosocial implications for persons with SCI. *SCI: Psychosocial Process, 7,* 147–152.

Marini, I., & Graf, N. M. (2011). Religiosity and spirituality among persons with spinal cord injury: Attitudes, beliefs, and practices. *Rehabilitation Counseling Bulletin, 54,* 82–92.

Marini, I., & Stebnicki, M. (1999). Social security's alternative provider program: What can rehabilitation administrators expect. *Journal of Rehabilitation Administration, 23*(1), 31–41.

Marinnic, M., & Brkljacic, T. (2008). Love over gold-the correlation of happiness level with some life satisfaction factors between persons with and without physical disability. *Journal of Development and Physical Disability, 20,* 527–540.

Massimini, F., & Delle Faye, A. (2000). Individual development in a bio-cultural perspective. *American Psychologist, 55,* 24–33.

Masten, A. S., Best, K. M., & Garmezy, N. (1990). Resilience and development: Contributions from the study of children who overcame adversity. *Development and Psychopathology, 2,* 425–444.

Matheis, E. N., Tulsky, D. S., & Matheis, R. J. (2006). The relation between spirituality and quality of life among individuals with spinal cord injury. *Rehabilitation Psychology, 51,* 265–271.

Matthews, D. A., & Larson, D. B. (1997). *The faith factor: An annotated bibliography of clinical research on spiritual subjects* (Vols. I–IV). Rockville, MD: National Institute for Healthcare Research and Georgetown University Press.

Moore, A. D., & Stambrook, M. (1995). Cognitive moderators of outcome following a traumatic brain injury: A conceptual model and implications for rehabilitation. *Brain Injury, 9*(2), 109–130.

Morrill, E. F., Brewer, N. T., O'Neill, S. C., Lillie, S. E., Dees, E. L., Carey, L. A., & Rimer, B. K. (2008). The interaction of post-traumatic growth and post-traumatic stress symptoms in predicting depressive symptoms and quality of life. *Psychooncology, 17,* 948–953.

Myers, D. G. (2000). The funds, friends, and faith of happy people. *American Psychologist, 55,* 56–67.

Myers, D. G., & Diener, E. (1996). The pursuit of happiness. *Scientific American, 274,* 54–56.

National Academy of Sciences. (1984). *Bereavement: Reactions, consequences, and care.* Washington, DC: National Academy Press.

Oettingen, G. (1996). Positive fantasy and motivation. In P. M. Gollwitzer, & J. Bargh (Eds.), *The psychology of action: Linking cognition and motivation to behavior* (pp. 236–259). New York: Guilford Press.

Olkin, R. (1999). *What psychotherapists should know about disability.* New York: Guilford Press.

Pavot, W., Diener, E., & Fujita, F. (1990). Extraversion and happiness. *Personality and Individual Differences, 11,* 1299–1306.

Pelletier, K. R. (1994). *Sound mind, sound body.* New York: Simon & Schuster.

Pennebaker, J. (1990). *Opening up: The healing power of confiding in others.* New York: Morrow.

Penner, L. A. (2004). Volunteerism and social problems: Making things better or worse? *Journal of Social Issues, 60*(3), 645–666.

Peterson, C. (1988). Explanatory style as a risk factor for illness. *Cognitive Therapy Research, 12,* 119–132.

Peterson, C. (2000). The future of optimism. *American Psychologist, 55,* 44–55.

Peterson, C., Maier, S. F., & Seligman, M. E. (1995). *Learned helplessness: A theory for the age of personal control.* Oxford: Oxford University Press.

Peterson, C., Seligman, M. E. P., & Vaillant, G. E. (1988). Pessimistic explanatory style is a risk factor for physical illness: A thirty-five year longitudinal study. *Journal of Personality and Social Psychology, 55,* 23–37.

Piliavin, J. A., & Charng, H. W. (1990). Altruism: A review of recent theory and research. *Annual Review of Sociology, 16,* 27–65.

Pollard, C., & Kennedy, P. (2007). A longitudinal analysis of emotional impact, coping strategies and post-traumatic psychological growth following spinal cord injury: A 10-year review. *British Journal of Health Psychology, 12,* 347–362.

Power, P. W., & Dell Orto, A. E. (1995). Disability management: A family perspective. In D. E. Shrey, & M. Lacerte (Eds.), *Principles and practices of disability management in industry* (pp. 411–432). Winter Park, FL: GR Press.

Puchalski, C. M. (1999). Touching the spirit: The essence of healing. In *Spiritual life.* Washington, DC: Discalced Carmelite Friars of the Washington Province.

Ryan, R. M., & Deci, E. L. (2000). Self-determination theory and the facilitation of intrinsic motivation, social development, and well-being. *American Psychologist, 55,* 68–78.

Ryan, R. M., & Deci, E. L. (2001). On happiness and human potentials: A review of research on hedonic and eudaimonic well-being. *Annual Review of Psychology, 52,* 141–166.

Ryan, R. M., & Grolnick, W. S. (1986). Origins and pawns in the classroom: Self-report and projective assessments of individual differences in children's perceptions. *Journal of Personality and Social Psychology, 50*, 550–558.

Schafer, W. (1996). *Stress management for wellness.* Orlando, FL: Harcourt Brace.

Seligman, M. E. P. (1990). *Learned optimism: The skills to overcome lift's obstacles.* New York: Pocket Books.

Seligman, M. E. P. (1991). *Learned optimism.* New York: Knopf.

Seligman, M. E. P. (2002). *Authentic happiness: Using the new positive psychology to realize your potential for lasting fulfillment.* New York: Free Press.

Seligman, M. E. P., & Csikszentmihalyi, M. (2000). Positive psychology: An introduction. *American Psychologist, SS*, 5–14.

Shnek, Z. M., Foley, F. W., LaRocca, N. G., Gordon, W. A., DeLuca, J., Schwartzman, H. G.,...& Irvine, J. (1997)., Helplessness, self-efficacy, cognitive distortions, and depression in multiple sclerosis and spinal cord injury. *Annals of Behavioral Medicine, 19*(3), 287–294.

Silver, R. L. (1982). *Coping with an undesirable life event: A study of early reactions to physical disability* (Unpublished doctoral dissertation). Northwestern University, Evanston, IL.

Snyder, C. R. (1994). *The psychology of hope.* New York: The Free Press.

Snyder, C. R. (Ed.). (2000). *Handbook of hope: Theory, measures, and applications.* San Diego, CA: Academic Press.

Snyder, C. R., & Lopez, S. J. (2002). The future of positive psychology: A declaration of independence. In C. R. Snyder, & S. J. Lopez (Eds.), *Handbook of positive psychology* (pp. 751–767). London: Oxford University Press.

Stanton, A. L., Bower, J. E., & Low, C. A. (2006). Post-traumatic growth after cancer. In L. G. Calhoun, & R. G. Tedeschi (Eds.), *Handbook of post-traumatic growth* (pp. 138–175). Mahwah, NJ: Lawrence Erlbaum Associates, Inc.

Stanton, A. L., Danoff-Burg, S., & Huggins, M. E. (2002). The first year after breast cancer, diagnosis: Hope and coping strategies as predictors of adjustment. *Psychooncology, 11*, 93–102.

Staub, E. (2003). *The psychology of good and evil: Why children, adults, and groups help harm others.* Cambridge: Cambridge University Press.

Steel, J. L., Gamblin, T. C., & Carr, B. I. (2008). Measuring post-traumatic growth in people diagnosed with hepatobiliary cancer: Directions for future research. *Oncology Nursing Forum, 35*(4), 643–650.

Stone, A. A., Cox, D. X., Valdimarsdottir, H., Jandorf, L., & Neale, J. M. (1987). Evidence that secretory IgA antibody is associated with daily mood. *Journal of Personality and Social Psychology, 52*, 988–993.

Taylor, S. E. (1983). Adjustment to threatening events: A theory of cognitive adaptation. *American Psychologist, 38*, 1161–1173.

Taylor, S. E., & Brown, J. D. (1988). Illusion and well-being: A social psychological perspective on mental health. *Psychological Bulletin, 110*, 193–210.

Tedeschi, R. G., & Calhoun, L. G. (1988). *Perceived benefits in coping with physical handicaps.* Paper presented at the meeting of the American Psychological Association. Atlanta, GA.

Tedeschi, R. G., & Calhoun, L. G. (1995). *Trauma and transformation: Growing in the aftermath of suffering.* Thousand Oaks, CA: Sage.

Tedeschi, R. G., & Calhoun, L. G. (1996). The posttraumatic growth inventory: Measuring the positive legacy of trauma. *Journal of Traumatic Stress, 9*, 455–471.

Tedeschi, R.G., Park, C. L., & Calhoun, L.G. (1998). *Posttraumatic growth: Positive changes in the aftermath of crisis.* Mahwah, NJ: Lawrence Erlbaum Associates Publishers.

Tiger, L. (1979). *Optimism: The biology of hope.* New York: Simon & Schuster.

Todd, J. L., & Worell, J. (2000). Resilience in low-income, employed, African American women. *Psychology of Women Quarterly, 24*, 119–128.

Trieschmann, R. (1981). *Spinal cord injuries: Psychological, social and vocational adjustment.* New York: Pergamon.

Trieschmann, R. (1988). *Spinal cord injuries: Psychological, social, and vocational rehabilitation* (2nd ed.). New York: Demos.

Vaillant, G. E. (1977). *Adaptation to life.* Boston: Little, Brown.

Vaillant, G. E. (2000). Adaptive mental mechanisms: Their role in a positive psychology. *American Psychologist, 55*, 89–98.

Vash, C. (1981). *Psychology of disability.* New York: Springfield.

Vash, C. L., & Crewe, N. M. (2004). *Psychology of disability* (pp. 288–299). New York: Springer.

Veenhoven, R. (1988). The utility of happiness. *Social Indicators Research, 20*, 333–354.

Vollhardt, J. R. (2009). Altruism born of suffering and prosocial behavior following adverse life events: A review and conceptualization. *Social Justice Research, 22*, 53–97.

Weisse, C. S. (1992). Depression and incompetence: A review of the literature. *Psychological Bulletin, 111*, 475–489.

Wholey, D. (1986). *Are you happy?* Boston: Houghton Mifflin.

Wills, T. A. (1991). Similarity and self-esteem in downward social comparison. In J. M. Suls & T. A. Wills (Eds.), *Social comparison* (pp. 51–78). Hillsdale, NJ: Lawrence Erlbaum Associates Publishers.

Wilson, J. (2000). Volunteering. *Annual Review of Sociology, 26,* 215–240.

Wright, B. A. (1983). *Physical disability: A psychological approach* (2nd ed.). New York: Harper & Row.

Yates, T. M., Egeland, B., & Sroufe, L. A. (2003). Rethinking restlience: A developmental process perspective. In S. A. Luthar (Ed.), *Resilience and vulnerability: Adaptation in the context of childhood adversities* (pp. 243–266). New York: Cambridge University Press.

Znoj, H. J. (1999, August). *European and American perspectives on post-traumatic growth: A model of personal growth: Life challenges and transformation following loss and physical handicap.* Paper presented at the Annual Convention of the American Psychological Association, Boston, MA.

25

Successful Aging: A Disability Perspective

MEREDITH MINKLER AND PAMELA FADEM

For much of its short history, gerontology both reflected and reinforced a "decline and loss" paradigm. A heavy accent was placed on notions of aging as a series of decrements or losses in the individual, to which both elders and society needed to adapt or adjust (Phillipson, 1998).

The last 20 years have witnessed the emergence of several alternative perspectives that provide a sharp contrast to this negative view, key among them Rowe and Kahn's (1987, 1997, 1998) conceptualization of "successful aging." This popular perspective holds that many of the health and related problems associated with "normal aging" are in fact not normal at all but, rather, are the result of lifestyle and other factors that put people at high risk for disease and disability in later life.

The concept of successful aging has been helpful in focusing renewed attention on health promotion and disease and injury prevention as means of adding life to years and not merely years to life. Multiple well-designed studies of successful aging similarly have made a real contribution to clarifying the many health-promotion and disease-prevention strategies that can help ensure a healthier old age (Rowe & Kahn, 1998; Seeman, 1994).

Yet, the new emphasis on successful aging is problematic, as well. The concept has been criticized for paying insufficient attention to (a) aging over the life course; (b) race, class, and gender inequities; and (c) the realities and importance of losses and gains in later life (Baltes & Carstensen, 1996; Riley, 1998; Scheidt, Humphreys, & Yorgason, 1999; Schulz & Heckhausen, 1996). Many of these criticisms are highly relevant to the issues and concerns of people with disabilities. To date, however, none of the extant critiques have focused specifically on the limitations of the successful-aging paradigm when applied to this population.

The present chapter attempts to address this gap. We begin with a brief overview of Rowe and Kahn's successful-aging paradigm and its three components— low probability of disease and disease-related disability, high cognitive and physical functioning, and active engagement with life. We then examine each of these characteristics specifically as they relate to the lives of older adults with substantial physical disabilities.[1] We suggest that although the concept of successful aging has moved the field forward in some important new ways, both the term itself and some of its specific dimensions and meanings may serve to further stigmatize and marginalize people who are aging with severe disabilities and who may not meet the criteria for aging successfully. We conclude by making a case for the use of alternative conceptualizations that emphasize the environmental conditions needed to optimize the aging experience for both individuals with disabilities and those without.

SUCCESSFUL AGING: AN OVERVIEW

Although the term *successful aging* was coined more than half a century ago, its use in gerontology today is primarily in reference to Rowe and Kahn's (1987, 1997, 1998) paradigm. As suggested earlier, these investigators made a clear distinction between "successful aging" and "usual aging," with the latter referring to the large proportion of elders who function well but are at substantial risk for disease or disability.

Rowe and Kahn (1987) first described successful aging solely in reference to the avoidance of disease and disability. Aided by the MacArthur Study of Successful Aging—a $10 million, 10-year effort by dozens of scientists to develop a conceptual basis for a "new gerontology" based on an appreciation of the positive aspects of aging (Rowe & Kahn, 1998)—the model subsequently was broadened. Successful aging, thus, was seen as encompassing two additional components: maintenance of high physical and cognitive functional capacity and active engagement in life. Briefly, the avoidance of disability involves increased, rather than decreased, attention to preventive health care and health promotion in the later years, in part to "compress" morbidity (Fries, 1980), so that illness and disability comprise a much smaller portion of the last years of life (Rowe & Kahn, 1998). Maintaining physical and mental function also involves an accent on both prevention and health promotion. This component of the successful-aging paradigm presupposes that (a) fears of loss of function are often greatly exaggerated, (b) much functional loss can indeed be prevented, and (c) many functional losses can be regained.

Finally, the third aspect of successful aging—active engagement with life—was put forward as a direct counter to the earlier (and now largely discredited) "disengagement theory" (Cumming & Henry, 1961). That theory had conceptualized late life as a time of mutual withdrawal and letting go, during which individuals gradually relinquished roles and responsibilities while society prepared to replace its older members. In contrast to disengagement theory, the third prong in Rowe and Kahn's (1998) conceptualization of successful aging suggests that "maintaining close relationships with others, and remaining involved in activities that are meaningful and purposeful, are important for well-being throughout the life course" (p. 46).

These three components were seen as hierarchically ordered such that

the absence of disease and disability makes it easier to maintain mental and physical function. And maintenance of mental and physical function in turn enables (but does not guarantee) active engagement with life. It is the combination of all three—avoidance of disease and disability, maintenance of cognitive and physical function and sustained engagement with life—that represents the concept of successful aging most fully. (Rowe & Kahn, 1998, p. 39)

Each of these conceptual components has particular salience and meaning when viewed from a disability perspective.

LOW PROBABILITY OF DISEASE AND DISEASE-RELATED DISABILITY

Proponents of the successful-aging paradigm are careful to acknowledge that "vulnerability to disease and disability is not wholly under our control, nor is it likely to become so" (Rowe & Kahn, 1998, p. 40). At the same time, they argue that many of the losses associated with usual aging are in fact caused primarily by extrinsic factors (e.g., diet and exercise) and therefore are subject to alteration. Rowe and Kahn indeed go further to suggest that "successful aging is dependent upon individual choices and behaviors. *It can be attained through individual choice and effort*" [italics added] (p. 37).

On the one hand, of course, few would argue that the high incidence of conditions such as diabetes and hypertension in the elderly reflect, to a considerable degree, earlier lifestyle and environmental factors, rather than normal, age-related changes. On the other hand, however, an overemphasis on the role of individual choices and behaviors in determining the probability of disease and disease-related disability is problematic. As Riley (1998) argued, such equations do not pay adequate attention to the fact that "changes in lives and changes in social structures are fundamentally interdependent" (p. 15). Such factors as the "structural opportunities in schools, offices, nursing homes, families, communities … and society at large" (Riley, 1998, p. 151), in short, have a heavy impact on one's prospects for aging successfully.

The situation of people with disabilities represents a striking case in point. Data from the *Survey of Income and Program Participation* (SIPP), thus, showed an employment rate of just 32.2% in 1994; in 1995, men and women with disabilities earned, respectively, just 72.1% and 72.7% of the income earned by their counterparts without disabilities. For men, moreover, this income gap represents a substantial increase over recent years (Kaye, 1998). People with disabilities living in the community are also twice as likely as people without disabilities to live alone (19.6% vs. 8.4%; Kaye, 1998)—a factor that, like low income, is associated with poorer diet and exercise patterns and other risk factors (Seeman, 2000).

Although a 1994 Harris poll of Americans with disabilities had almost two thirds of the respondents reporting an improved quality of life over the preceding 4 years (Leitman, Cooner, & Risher, 1994), and although the 1990 Americans with Disabilities Act has substantially increased awareness of the need for environmental changes and accommodations, "statistical evidence for real improvements in the lives of those with disabilities—more opportunities for employment and improved economic status, greater freedom of movement and ease of access, and increased levels of social integration—has been slow to materialize" (Kaye, 1998, p. 1). Without concomitant action to substantially improve the "responseability" of people with disabilities, including access to programs and policies that ensure a decent standard of living, and opportunities to build on strengths and participate fully in society, calls for greater personal responsibility for health are likely to have limited appeal (Minkler, 1996). Furthermore, an overemphasis on the resources and motivations of elders themselves also risks the implication of blame for elders who fail to meet the criteria for minimizing their risk of disease or disability (Cassell & Neugarten, 1991; Kennedy & Minkler, 1998; Minkler, 1990; Scheidt et al., 1999; Tornstam, 1992). Indeed, as Scheidt et al. pointed out, it is ironic that the successful-aging model's emphasis on the critical role of intrinsic factors, such as individual choice concerning smoking, diet, and exercise, is not supplemented by an equal emphasis on the role of extrinsic factors. The latter would include factors such as poverty and inaccessibility and in other ways deleterious environments.

With regard to physical fitness and exercise, for example, which Rowe and Kahn (1998) identified as the crux of successful aging, recent analyses of Behavioral Risk Factor Surveillance System (http://www.cdc.gov/nccdphp/brfss) data, which were stratified by gender and controlled for education and race, are instructive. These analyses revealed that persons 65 and older who live in unsafe neighborhoods are significantly less likely to engage in regular exercise than those in safe neighborhoods (Weinstein, Feigley, & Pullen, 1999). For elders with disabilities, the difficulties of engaging in regular exercise in high-crime neighborhoods are likely to be further compounded by heightened concerns about physical vulnerability and lack of environmental access.

MAINTENANCE OF HIGH PHYSICAL AND COGNITIVE FUNCTION

Characterizations of successful aging as closely related to the maintenance of high physical and cognitive function are also problematic, particularly when used in relation to people who enter old age with significant (and often lifelong) disabilities. As Scheidt et al. (1999) noted, "The term *successful* as used to describe older individuals who age with no or minimal loss of function ... connotes a fixed standard" (p. 279) and the achievement of static end points. As an example, they highlight Rowe and Kahn's (1997) argument that older persons can indeed move "*in and out* of success over time," with those who are most resilient being able to "return to meeting the criteria of success" (p. 439).

As Fadem (1999) has argued, people who have lived a substantial portion of their lives relying on others for assistance with activities of daily living long ago redefined for themselves what independence and effective functioning are about. Furthermore, they "are likely to repeat this process of redefinition many times as their level of physical functioning [changes] and slowly (or quickly) deteriorate[s]" (Fadem, 1999, p. 4). The difference here is subtle but important: People with progressive disabilities, and those for whom a "stable" disability becomes more limiting later in life, often continue to see themselves as functioning effectively and having a good quality of life, while acknowledging the need for increasing assistance and accommodations. Rather than viewing themselves as moving "out of success over time," they frequently view their functional ability as increasingly dependent on the success with which their *environments* can adapt and change to accommodate their changing bodies and personal needs.

This perspective is complemented by Fried et al.'s (1991) emphasis on "compensatory strategies," or manipulations of the environment that prevent an impairment from becoming disabling or restricting in terms of the individual's ability to perform particular tasks or functions. In the case of people who are already disabled, the level of financial and other resources available, which can determine the possibility of home modifications and other compensatory strategies, often is the key factor in determining whether effective adaptation (and successful aging) can be achieved.

As suggested below, the inclusion of "active engagement with life" as a component of successful aging in Rowe and Kahn's model was designed, in part, to make conceptual room for people such as physicist Stephen Hawking, who was highly successful and engaged with life despite being severely disabled by amyotrophic lateral sclerosis, or Lou Gehrig's disease. Yet, when "high physical and cognitive function" is named as a necessary component of successful aging, a different and contradictory message may be sent. Indeed, in the foreword to their book *Successful Aging*, which reports on the results of the MacArthur Study, Rowe and Kahn state that "in sum, we were trying to pinpoint the many factors that conspire to put one octogenarian on cross-county skis and another in a wheelchair" (p. xii).

Statements such as this one may serve to reinforce both handicappism and what Cohen (1988) called "the elderly mystique," which refers to the phenomenon of prejudice against the old in general being replaced with a more specific prejudice against elders who are or become disabled. This perspective frequently is internalized by elders themselves, who conclude that "when disability arrives, hope about continued growth, self realization and full participation in family and society must be abandoned so that all energy can he directed toward the ultimate defeat which is not death but institutionalization" (Cohen, 1988, p. 25). By substantially lowering the bar of dreams and expectations for and by elders with disabilities, this new variant of ageism ironically can mitigate against the very proactive health-promotion and health-maintenance activities advocated by proponents of successful aging (Minkler, 1996).

Taking a cue from Cohen (1998), we argue that considering "high mental and physical function" to be a necessary component of successful aging may serve to reinforce the fears and negative images that both elders themselves and society at large hold about aging with a substantial disability. The focus on personal responsibility, moreover, risks ignoring the environmental and policy contexts that can facilitate or severely limit an individual's ability to achieve and sustain high functioning in society.

ACTIVE ENGAGEMENT WITH LIFE

Rowe and Kahn's (1998) third and final component of successful aging—active engagement with life—was defined as having two dimensions: relating to and being connected with others through social relationships and continuing productive activities. The first of these dimensions was used to underscore the plethora of evidence on the importance of social networks, and the social support given and received through those networks, for health and well-being in both earlier and later life (Cohen & Syme, 1985; Seeman, 2000). The second dimension stresses the importance of productive behavior, defined broadly as "all activities, paid or unpaid, that create goods or services of value" (Rowe & Kahn, 1997, p. 47). As noted earlier, the addition of this social dimension to a model that previously had focused solely on disease and disease-related disability has been hailed as an important step forward (Riley, 1998). Rowe and Kahn (1998) did make a special effort to argue that even individuals with the most severe disabilities can remain actively engaged with others and make "heroic achievements" (p. 38) and contributions despite their functional limitations.

Fadem (1999) underscored this point, providing telling examples of individuals with severe disabilities who "effectively mobilized both consumer rights and political campaigns" (p. 5) and provided "seasoned peer mentorship" (p. 5) by telephone to scores of younger people with disabilities while never leaving home. Such constructive engagement is mirrored as well in the birth and evolution of one of the significant social movements of the latter part of the twentieth century.

Traditional measures of social connection and productive engagement, however, may not fully capture the reality of the lives of older people with disabilities (Carstensen, 1991; Fadem, 1999; Holstein, 1998; Pennix et al., 1998). Pennix et al.'s (1998) study of emotional vitality among older women with disabilities, for example, revealed that with respect to social relations, the primary element valued was not "availability or frequency of contacts but perceiving enough warmth and understanding to meet an individual's needs" (p. 814). Similarly, as Carstensen has pointed out, selective *reduction* in the frequency of social interactions may help some individuals achieve a more satisfying and adaptive old age. Viewed from this perspective, efforts to either measure or enhance the social-relationship dimension of successful aging by simplistic, across-the-board approaches to what constitutes healthy social engagement may well miss the mark.

Furthermore, as Holstein (1998) has argued, although the concept of productive aging has been expanded to include voluntarism, informal caregiving, and other unpaid and often invisible activities, "productivity, understood culturally, is closely linked to paid work, a link that will be difficult to sever" (p. 363). She goes on to note, "A work-oriented definition of productivity can obscure diversity, establish new standards for an acceptable old age, and support someone else's vision of social and economic needs" (p. 366). For older people with disabilities, older women, older people of color, and low-income elders, whose relationship to the labor market often has been one of marginalization, viewing productive aging narrowly in terms of paid work is particularly dangerous.

Finally, beyond this very real concern lies the fact that a paid or unpaid "goods and services" approach to productive aging may leave little room for constructive engagement with questions of the meaning and significance of aging and old age. As Cole (1988) argued, the renewed emphasis on successful aging is part of a historical pattern based on dichotomizing old age into positive and negative poles and emphasizing one of those poles, rather than appreciating the essential unity and dialectic that aging ultimately represents. The latter, more complex perspective respects the diversity of aging and its place as part of a natural and unified lifetime (Cole, 1988). The vision of aging as a dialectic involving losses and gains holds particular relevance if we are to more fully value the lives and contributions of people who are aging with substantial disabilities. It also provides an important alternative to what Cole (1992) described as our culture's "relentless hostility to physical decline and its tendency to regard health"—and, we would add, the absence of disability—"as a form of secular salvation" (p. 239). He went on to note, "By transforming health as a means of living well into an end unto itself, 'successful aging' reveals its bankruptcy as an ideal" (p. 239), one that fails to make room for the realities of physical disability, decline, and death.

IMPLICATIONS

Successful aging has become a central theoretical paradigm within the fields of geriatrics and gerontology. Summarizing a large body of theoretical and empirical research on this paradigm, Seeman (1994) argued that

> the concept of successful aging provides for a critical refocusing of attention on the substantial heterogeneity in patterns of aging among older persons, particularly the existence of more positive trajectories of aging that avoid many, if not all, of the common age-related diseases and disabilities. (p. 61)

We agree with Seeman that a more positive view of aging can play a critical role in helping individuals achieve and maintain higher levels of function as they grow older. We would argue, however, that from a disability perspective neither the semantics nor the theoretical conceptualization of successful aging constitutes the best approach to achieving this goal, for "disability, or more accurately the disablement process, is a dynamic social phenomenon that has as much to do with cultural norms and socioeconomic status as it does with individual physiological conditions" (Kennedy & Minkler, 1998, p. 92). Bearing this in mind, and building on the arguments presented in this chapter, we underscore the need for further research involving the development and testing of broader ecological approaches to successful aging with a disability. As defined by Bronfenbrenner (1992), such approaches consider and attend to the individual, the immediate settings in which he or she lives, the larger contexts in which these settings are embedded, and the interactions among all of these levels.

An early and promising model in this regard was put forward by Baltes and Baltes (1990), who replaced the term *successful aging* with *optimal aging* in reference to "a kind of utopia, namely, aging under development-enhancing and age-friendly environmental conditions" (p. 8). As Marsiske, Lang, Baltes, and Baltes (1995) have suggested, the focus in such a model is on "how individuals and life environments can manage opportunities for, and limits on, resources at all ages" (p. 6). Such a perspective implicitly recognizes that social/physical environmental changes are critical if optimal aging—with or without a disability—is to be achieved (see also Kaplan & Strawbridge, 1993; Satariano, 1997; Verbrugge & Jette, 1994).

The continued development and refining of conceptual approaches to research that stress optimal aging is consistent with the "new paradigm of disability," which holds that a person with a disability "should no longer be viewed as someone who cannot function because of an impairment, but rather as someone who needs an accommodation in order to function" (Bleecker, 2000, p. 1). When this approach is taken, disability research and research-driven program and policy interventions stress changing the physical and social environments within which both aging and the disablement process take place.

Research also is needed into optimal aging for those who are growing older with developmental disabilities. Although organizations such as ARC have produced excellent material on aging with a developmental disability (Brown & Murphy, 1999), this topic has received scant attention in the academic literature (see LeBlanc & Matson, 1997; Walz, Harper, & Wilson, 1986). Many of the issues and concerns discussed in the present chapter with regard to successful aging and physical disability can and should also be raised with respect to aging and developmental disabilities. To better explore this area, further studies, including qualitative research into the lived experience of people aging with developmental disabilities, should be undertaken.

Finally, further research is needed into the development of theoretical approaches that move beyond dichotomous notions of successful/unsuccessful or healthy/unhealthy aging and old age. By acknowledging that losses and gains, and limits and potentials, are a critical part of the aging process (Baltes & Carstensen, 1996; Scheidt et al., 1999), these newer perspectives make room for questions about the meaning and significance of aging and old age. They help us move beyond what Moody (1988) described as the ever-more technical and "instrumental" orientation of academic gerontology, within which "the problems of later life are treated with scientific and managerial efficiency, but with no grasp of their larger political or existential significance. The last stage of life is progressively drained of meaning" (p. 82).

Continuing efforts to move beyond the confines of the successful-aging paradigm can build in part upon the foundations laid by feminist research. As Harper (1997) has pointed out, for example, feminist scholarship concerning new reproductive technologies and the control of women's bodies may hold special relevance for research into "the medicalization and control of the *ageing* body" (p. 167) and the associated development of successful-aging norms and ideals. Similarly, and building on Moody's (1988) concerns just noted, scholarship is needed that continues to question whether the narrow successful-aging paradigm is ultimately simply a logical extension of our continuing quest to fulfill scientific and biotechnological imperatives (Cassel & Neugarten, 1991).

From the perspective of practice, as Satariano (1997) has suggested, the conceptual framework provided by the "new paradigm of disability" suggests the importance of having public health professionals collaborate with architects, city planners, transportation experts, and engineers in the design of both indoor and outdoor environments that truly accommodate elders of diverse abilities and functional limitations. Taking a cue from the World Institute on Disability (WID), attending to the broader environments within which aging takes place also would have us explore the critical dimension of consumer control over personal assistance services (PAS) and other needed resources. WID's finding that publicly funded PAS programs around the nation often fail to provide services around the clock and/or 7 days a week is an example of the need for changing both current practices and policies that "represent a substantial barrier to full participation" (Bleecker, 2000, p. 3).

Finally, from a policy perspective, broader conceptualizations of optimal aging would have us work for legislation that supports, rather than hinders, the capacity of people aging with disabilities to participate fully in society, in part through the provision of adequate resources. Such policy-level change would include, for example, additional mandates and funding for responsive and affordable transportation services and adequate personal assistance (including assistance outside the home) to enable people with disabilities to remain engaged in their communities.

In the conclusion to *Successful Aging*, Rowe and Kahn (1998) call for better allocation of paid employment, education, and training throughout the life course, as well as better integration of work, education, parenting, leisure, and other activities to "make successful aging more attainable for all of us" (p. 206). These recommendations are laudable and important; however, without far greater attention to the substantial and growing disparities among the old and the future old (Kaye, 1998), and similarly, heightened attention to the ways in which a concept like successful aging can inadvertently hurt those who are already devalued and marginalized in our society, such prescriptions are unlikely to be realized. As we attempt to design research, programs, and policies that can help maintain and promote health and well-being across the life course, we must ensure that those studies and interventions are in fact broadly inclusive. They should reflect the strengths, as well as the needs and concerns, of the "quiet revolution" represented by the greatest diversity of elders ever witnessed (Burton, Dilworth-Anderson, & Bengston, 1992, p. 129). Current and future elders with disabilities represent a critical part of this revolution, and one whose individual and collective voices concerning concepts such as successful aging must be sought out and heard.

NOTE

1. Due mainly to space limitations, we have intentionally focused this chapter primarily on aging with physical disabilities. It should be noted, however, that many of the same arguments and issues discussed here can and should be raised with respect to successful aging and developmental and other mental disabilities. Although there is a relative paucity of work on aging and developmental disabilities in academia, this topic is well examined in the nonacademic literature, and the reader is referred to the June 1999 *Arc Newsletter* for excellent recent coverage of this topic (Brown & Murphy, 1999).

ACKNOWLEDGMENT

Support for this project was provided by the University of California (UC) at Berkeley's Committee on Research. The authors also gratefully acknowledge the helpful comments received from Dr. Martha Holstein, Dr. Jae Kennedy, and members of UC Berkeley's Working Group of Aging. Thanks, finally, are also due to Lisa Butler and Laura Spautz for the research assistance and clerical support they provided.

REFERENCES

Baltes, M., & Carstensen, L. (1996). The process of successful aging. *Ageing and Society, 16,* 397–422.

Baltes, P. B., & Baltes, M. M. (1990). Psychological perspectives on successful aging: The model of selective optimization with compensation. In P. B. Baltes & M. M. Baltes (Eds.), *Successful aging: Perspectives from the behavioral sciences* (pp. 1–34). Cambridge, UK: Cambridge University Press.

Bleecker, T. (2000). The new paradigm of disability: Implications for research and policy. *Consumer Choice, 4,* 1–3.

Bronfenbrenner, U. (1992). Ecological systems theory. In R. Vasta (Ed.), *Annals of child development. Six theories of child development: Revised formulations and current issues* (pp. 187–249). London: Jessica Kingsley.

Brown, A., & Murphy, L. (1999, June). Aging with developmental disabilities: Women's health issues. *ARC Newsletter.*

Burton, L., Dilworth-Anderson, P., & Bengston, V. (1992). Creating culturally relevant ways of thinking about aging and diversity: Theoretical challenges for the 21st century. In E. P. Stanford & F. M. Tores-Gil (Eds.), *Diversity: New approaches to ethnic minority aging* (pp. 129–140). New York: Baywood.

Carstensen, L. (1991). Selectivity theory: Social activity. In K. W. Schaie & M. P. Lawton (Eds.), *Annual review of gerontology and geriatrics* (pp. 195–217). New York: Springer.

Cassel, C. K., & Neugarten, B. (1991). The goals of medicine in an aging society. In R. Binstock & S. Post (Eds.), *Too old for health care?* (pp.75–91). Baltimore: Johns Hopkins.

Cohen, E. (1988). The elderly mystique: Constraints on the autonomy of the elderly with disabilities. *The Gerontologist, 28*(Suppl.), 24–31.

Cohen, S., & Syme, S. L. (Eds.). (1985). *Social support and health.* New York: Academic Press.

Cole, T. (1988). The specter of old age: History, politics and culture in America. *Tikkun, 3,* 14–18, 93–95.

Cole, T. (1992). *The journey of life: A cultural history of aging in America.* Cambridge, UK: Cambridge University Press.

Cumming, E., & Henry, W. E. (1961). *Growing old: The process of disengagement.* New York: Basic Books.

Fadem, P. S. (1999, November). *Long-term disability and successful aging.* Paper presented at the annual meeting of the Gerontological Society of America, San Francisco, CA.

Fried, L. P., Herdman, S. J., Kuhn, K. E., Rubin, G., & Turano, K. (1991). Pre-clinical disability. *Journal of Aging and Health, 3,* 285–300.

Fries, J. F. (1980). Aging, natural death, and the compression of morbidity. *The New England Journal of Medicine, 303*(3), 130–135.

Harper, S. (1997). Constructing later life/constructing the body: Some thoughts from feminist theory. In A. Jamieson, S. Harper, & C. Victor (Eds.), *Critical approaches to ageing and later life* (pp. 160–172). Buckingham: Open University Press.

Holstein, M. (1998). Women and aging: Troubling implications. In M. Miner & C. L. Estes (Eds.), *Critical gerontology* (pp. 359–373). Amityville, NY: Haywood.

Kaplan, G. A., & Strawbridge, W. I. (1993). Behavioral and social factors in healthy aging. In R. A. Ables., H. C. Gift, & M. G. Ory (Eds.), *Aging and quality of life.* New York: Springer.

Kaye, H. S. (1998). Is the status of people with disabilities improving? *Disability Statistics Abstract, 21,* 1–4.

Kennedy, J., & Minkler, M. (1998). Disability theory and public policy: Implications for critical gerontology. In M. Minkler & C. L. Estes (Eds.), *Critical gerontology.* Amityville, NY: Baywood.

LeBlanc, L. A., & Matson, J. L. (1997). Aging in the developmentally disabled: Assessment and treatment. *Journal of Clinical Geropsychology, 3*(1), 37–55.

Leitman, R., Conner, E., & Risher, P. (1994). *N.O.D. Harris survey of Americans with disabilities.* New York: Louis Harris and Associates. Inc., N.O.D.

Marsiske, M., Lang, F. R., Baltes, P. B., & Baltes, M. M. (1995). Selective optimization and compensation: Life-span perspectives on successful human development. In R. A. Dixon & L. Blackman (Eds.), *Psychological compensation: Managing losses and promoting gains* (pp. 35–79). Hillsdale, NJ: Erlbaum.

Minkler, M. (1990). Aging and disability: Behind and beyond the stereotypes. *Journal of Aging Studies, 4,* 245–260.

Minkler, M. (1996). Critical perspectives on ageing: New challenges for gerontology. *Ageing and Society, 16,* 467–487.

Moody, H. (1988). *Abundance of life: Human development policies for an aging society.* New York: Columbia University Press.

Pennix, B., Guralinik, J. M., Simonsick, E. M., Kasper, J. D., Ferrucci, L., & Fried, L. P. (1998). Emotional vitality among disabled older women: The women's health and aging study. *Journal of the American Geriatrics Society, 46,* 807–815.

Phillipson, C. (1998). *Reconstructing old age: New agendas in social theory and practice.* London: Sage.

Riley, M. W. (1998). Letter to the editor. *The Gerontologist, 38,* 151.

Rowe, J., & Kahn, R. (1987). Human aging: Usual and successful. *Science, 137,* 143–149.

Rowe, J., & Kahn, R. (1997). Successful aging. *The Gerontologist, 37,* 433–440.

Rowe, J., & Kahn, R. (1998). *Successful aging.* New York: Random House.

Satariano, W. (1997). The disabilities of aging: Looking to the physical environment. *American Journal of Public Health, 87,* 331–332.

Scheidt, R. L., Humphreys, D. R., & Yorgason, J. B. (1999). Successful aging: What's not to like? *The Journal of Applied Gerontology, 18,* 277–282.

Schulz, R., & Heckhausen, J. (1996). A life span model of successful aging. *The American Psychologist, 51,* 702–714.

Seeman, T. E. (1994). Successful aging: Reconceptualizing the aging process from a more positive perspective. In B. Vellas & J. Albarede (Eds.), *Facts and research in gerontology* (pp. 61–73). New York: Springer.

Seeman, T. E. (2000). Health promoting effects of friends and family on health outcomes in older adults. *American Journal of Health Promotion, 14,* 362–370.

Tornstam, L. (1992). The Quo Tad is of gerontology: On the scientific paradigm of gerontology. *The Gerontologist, 32,* 318–326.

Verbrugge, L., & Jette, A. (1994). The disablement process. *Social Science and Medicine, 38,* 1–14.

Weinstein, A., Feigley, P., & Pullen, P. (1999). Neighborhood safety and the prevalence of physical inactivity—selected states, 1996. *Morbidity and Mortality Weekly Report, 48,* 143–146.

26

An International Conceptualization of Disability: The International Classification of Functioning, Disability, and Health

DAVID B. PETERSON

*T*he International Classification of Functioning, Disability, and Health (ICF; World Health Organization [WHO], 2001), and its predecessors—the International Classification of Impairments, Disabilities and Handicaps (ICIDH and ICIDH-2; WHO, 1980, 1999)—have been influential in the conceptualization of the construct of disability in the United States and internationally for more than three decades. Any discussion of the psychological and social impact of illness and disability would be incomplete with considering the ICF's influences on this social discourse.

We will begin with a brief overview of the history of classification of health and illness, and the role that different conceptualizations of disability have played along the way. We will then review the development of the ICF within the context of these conceptualizations, introduce its key concepts, conceptual framework, and a brief orientation to its use. We will conclude with consideration of the current and future impact of the ICF on conceptualizing psychological and social aspects of illness and disability.

In a chapter that reviews the ICF, it is difficult to avoid being redundant with other similar publications. A variety of reviews have discussed and critiqued the ICF (see volume 50 of *Rehabilitation Psychology*, 2005; volume 19 of *Rehabilitation Education*, 2005; and volume 25 of *Disability & Rehabilitation*, 2003). Several book chapters have been written for seminal handbooks in the counseling and psychology professions (Peterson, 2009; Peterson & Elliott, 2008; Peterson, Mpofu, & Oakland, 2010;), and most recently a text focusing on the psychological aspects of functioning, disability, and health (Peterson, 2011). These publications not withstanding any explanation of the ICF can and should be referenced back to the ICF itself (WHO, 2001).

CONCEPTUALIZATIONS OF DISABILITY: ICD, ICIDH, ICF

The concept of disability has manifested itself in various ways across stakeholders in our health care system. An awareness of the prevailing perspectives on disability can inform intervention targeting and the evaluation of health care intervention outcomes, and is therefore very informative in conceptualizing clinical work with people with disabilities. At the same time, a concise review of the medical, social, and biopsychosocial models of disability illustrates the development of the ICF and its predecessors.

Several texts have compared and contrasted various models of disability, including a chapter in the present volume. Previous iterations of this text (Dell Orto & Powers, 2007) provide detailed reviews of how disability has been defined and conceptualized in the literature. *The Handbook of Counseling Psychology* (Brown & Lent, 2008) includes a chapter discussing advancements in conceptualizing disability (Peterson & Elliott, 2008). More recently, the text *Psychological Aspects of Functioning, Disability and Health* (Peterson, 2011) provides a review of models of disability as they relate to the ICF. A concise review of the medical, social, and biopsychosocial models of disability highlights perspectives held by various stakeholders in the health care system, which may inform our collaboration with multiple disciplines in today's health care environment.

Origins of Classifications of Health

International classification of population health began with a focus on the prevalence of medical diagnoses and causes of death with the *International Statistical Classification of Diseases and Related Health Problems* (ICD, now in its 10th revision, WHO, 1992). A brief review of the ICD is important to understanding the conceptual development of the construct of disability, as well as knowing that the ICD serves as the sister classification for the ICF; more on that in a moment. The ICD provides an etiological classification of health conditions (e.g., diseases, disorders, injuries) related to mortality (death) and morbidity (illness). The ICD was first formalized in 1893 as the Bertillon Classification or the International List of Causes of Death; the ICD acronym persists till date.

The United States uses the clinical modification of the ICD-9, even though the ICD-10 was approved by the World Health Assembly in 1992; it is scheduled to use the ICD-10 in 2013. Neighboring Canada has been using the ICD-10 for some time now. The WHO is in the process of updating the ICD-10 in order to make it a better tool to diagnose and treat disease; the ICD-11 is due for publication in 2015. It promises to be a global, multilingual, multidisciplinary system of classification, and its development transparent and free from commercial input. The system's context will allow for interactive information sharing using modern technology and integrated into health informatics systems worldwide. The new system is intended for daily clinical use with simpler diagnostic criteria (Martin, 2009).

Although various stakeholders in the health care system hold varying and opposing views on how to conceptualize disability, making consensus difficult to achieve, it is important to define disability so that those who are disadvantaged by their experience of disability can be identified, their life experiences compared with those who are not disabled, and disparities in life experiences can be noted so that inequalities can be observed, measured, and ultimately remedied (Leonardi, Bickenbach, Üstün, Kostanjsek, & Chatterji, 2006).

Medical Model

The medical model has been the dominant force in health care service provision, focusing on the diagnosis of a disease, disorder, or injury (Wright, 1980). The medical model can be described as a treatment process that first identifies a pathogen or cause of injury or other disease process (often classified by the ICD), and then selects an appropriate treatment protocol for the condition identified (Reed et al., 2008). Within the United States, a classification of procedures associated with treatment of illness or injury employed in this treatment process is the Current Procedural Terminology or CPT codes (American Medical Association [AMA], 2007).

The medical model has neither focused on contextual factors (e.g., social and environmental factors) nor on the subjective experiences of individuals with disabilities. Disability within this context tends to be conceptualized as a personal problem that requires treatment by a medical professional (WHO, 2001). More contemporary perspectives on disability have posited that behavioral and social factors affect the course of chronic disease and disability over the life span, moving the focus from the individual to one's context.

The medical model and related diagnostic information have limited utility for assessment and treatment due to the lack of focus on important contextual factors in health and functioning. Historical evidence suggests that diagnostic information alone, without functional data, may not adequately reflect an individual's health condition (see Peterson, 2005; Reed et al., 2005). Disease or impairment may manifest differently across individuals; similar functioning does not imply similar health conditions. Diagnoses alone have not sufficiently predicted length (McCrone & Phelan, 1994) or outcome of hospitalization (Rabinowitz, Modai, & Inbar-Saban, 1994), level of necessary care (Burns, 1991), service needs (National Advisory Mental Health Council, 1993), work performance (Gatchel, Polatin, Mayer, & Garcy, 1994), receipt of disability benefits (Bassett, Chase, Folstein, & Regier, 1998; Massel, Liberman, Mintz, & Jacobs, 1990; Segal & Choi, 1991), or social integration (Ormel, Oldehinkel, Brilman, & vanden Brink, 1993).

For instance, someone with the diagnosis of major depressive disorder, according to the *Diagnostic and Statistical Manual of Mental Disorders* (*DSM-IV-TR*; American Psychological Association [APA], 2000), must experience at least five of the nine possible characteristic symptoms in order to qualify for the diagnosis. These symptoms can range from an inability to concentrate to weight gain or loss. The functional implications of any of the nine symptoms may be quite disparate, and the possible combinations of the five symptoms required for the diagnosis will have varying clinical presentations. When one considers the possible combinations of presentations, it becomes clear that diagnostic information alone is limited without clear descriptions of function that inform the diagnosis.

Notwithstanding the limitations of the medical model, it is very important to note that it has not been without utility. The medical model contributed to advances in science that helped researchers to better describe disease processes and related etiology, and so allowed more rapid and effective response to the acute needs of persons with physical disabilities and other chronic health conditions. The medical model also informed early initiatives to address issues of improved care, survival, and quality of life. Medical definitions of disability provide the cornerstone for determining disability for legal and occupational purposes, and for determining eligibility for financial assistance (Peterson & Elliott, 2008). Although it continues to be influential, limitations of the medical model and the focus on the civil rights–related and disability activism helped to develop the opposing *social model* of disability.

Social Model

The medical model was challenged by the civil rights era and related disability advocacy efforts, encouraging a movement away from the medical model of disability and functioning toward a social model that considered the role of environmental barriers in health and functioning (Peterson & Elliott, 2008; Rusk, 1977; Smart, 2005; Wright, 1980, 1983). As just reviewed, diagnostic information alone, without functional data, may not adequately reflect an individual's health condition (see Peterson, 2005, 2011; Reed et al., 2005). Disease or impairment may manifest differently across individuals; similar functioning does not imply similar health conditions.

Beyond the variety of presentations of diagnoses and potential functional limitations that may or may not present in an individual, Leonardi et al. (2006) wrote that the quality of life experience of a person dealing with health issues is an important focus of clinical attention. It was their position that it is important to distinguish between objective descriptions of the "disability experience" and an individual's satisfaction with that experience: "... data about quality of life, well-being, and personal satisfaction with life are useful for health and policy planning; but these data are not necessarily predicted by the presence or extent of disability" (p. 1220).

In contrast to the medical model, the social model of disability highlights the importance of a person's subjective experience as it relates to facilitators and barriers that the environment may present, their impact on health and functioning and ultimately an individual's quality of life (Elliott, Kurylo, & Rivera, 2002; Hurst, 2003; Smart, 2005; Ueda & Okawa, 2003). In the social model of disability, disability is no longer a simple personal attribute, but a complex social construct reflecting the interaction between the individual and his or her environment (WHO, 2001, p. 20).

The social paradigm focuses on the barriers and facilitators to functioning, such as daily activities, life skills, social relations, life satisfaction, and participation in society. This model suggests that any problem related to disability is influenced by, if not due in large part to, societal attitudes and barriers in the environment. Within the social model paradigm, the individual is seen as the organizing core, but impairments are defined by the environment (Olkin, 1999; Olkin & Pledger, 2003). The environment is typically construed as the "... major determinant of individual functioning" (Pledger, 2003, p. 281). The social model highlights the need for increased access and opportunities for people with disabilities, and it has historically been favored by advocates for the civil rights of persons with disability, who historically have disapproved of the medical model in general.

Limitations associated with the social model of disability include that it has neither clearly distinguished who qualifies as a person with a disability nor how disability is measured or determined. Further, researchers in this area have not established a distinct body of scholarship that systematically posits empirically testable and potentially falsifiable hypotheses (Peterson & Elliott, 2008). Perhaps, this is due to the fact that some supporters of the social model of disability regard psychological theory and scholarship as part and parcel to the medical model where disability is equated with person-based pathology, largely independent of environmental and social factors (see Olkin & Pledger, 2003).

Biopsychosocial Model

The origins of the biopsychosocial framework can be traced back to an article from the 1970s arguing for a new medical model for biomedicine (see Engel, 1977). The biopsychosocial model of disability integrates useful aspects of both the medical and social models of disability, addressing biological, individual, and societal perspectives on health. Planning treatments and documenting outcomes of interventions from the body, individual and societal perspectives can improve the quality of health care service provision and consequently the quality of life of people with disabilities, as well as increase the participation of individuals with disabilities in society (Peterson & Threats, 2005). The biopsychosocial perspective defines health care in the broadest sense by using a universal, culturally sensitive, integrative, and interactive model of health and disability that is sensitive to social and environmental aspects of functioning (Peterson, 2005, 2011).

The ICF integrates the medical and social models of disability, addressing biological, individual, and societal perspectives on health in a biopsychosocial approach (Peterson, 2005; WHO, 2001). Ultimately, the biopsychosocial model integrates all that is useful in both the medical and social models of disability. Next, we turn to a discussion about the evolution of the ICF and its influence on the international discourse on functioning, disability, and health.

ICD, ICIDH to the ICF

The development of the ICF began in 1974, when two separate classifications were developed, the first addressing impairments related to changes in health and the second handicaps that considered the role of the environment in disability and functioning. Discussions generated from work since 1972 were formally submitted for consideration at the October

1975 International Conference for the Ninth Revision of the International Classification of Diseases (ICD). In May 1976, the 29th World Health Assembly adopted a resolution that approved the trial publication of the supplementary classification of impairments and handicaps as a complement to the ICD. The first edition of the ICIDH, the ICF's predecessor, was published in 1980 for trial purposes. This trial edition of the ICIDH presented the origins of a more holistic model of disability, stressing the role of environmental determinants in the performance of day-to-day activities and fulfillment of social roles by persons with disabilities (Brandsma, Lakerveld-Heyl, & Van Ravensberg, 1995; De Kleijn-De Vrankrijker, 2003).

The ICIDH was instrumental in defining key concepts within the Americans with Disabilities Act (ADA). Two critical terms, impairments and disability, were defined parallel to those employed in the ICIDH. Brown (1993) argued for advantages of linking the ICIDH with the ADA such as the creation of a uniform framework for discussion and a standardized measurement tool for data collection. For a succinct overview of contributions of the ICIDH in the development of the ADA definitions and implementation, see Nieuwenhuijsen (1995).

The revision of the ICIDH began with its reprinting in 1993, which ultimately led to the provisionally titled ICIDH-2. It was referred to and incorporated in the Standard Rules on the Equalization of Opportunities for Persons with Disabilities (United Nations Department of Public Information [UNDPI], 1993), which was adopted by the United Nations General Assembly at its 48th session in December 1993. The ICIDH-2 was accepted as one of the United Nations' social classifications, subsequently affecting international human rights mandates as well as national legislation.

At a 1996 meeting in Geneva, work from various collaborating centers was collated and an alpha draft was produced, which was pilot tested from May 1996 through February 1997. Comments and suggestions were compiled at WHO headquarters, and primary issues were identified and circulated to contribute to the ongoing revision process. The primary principle held that the classification should contain a culturally meaningful order of categories relying on consensus from potential stakeholders, including professionals in health care service provision, insurance, social security, and other entitlement programs; labor; education; economics; social policy development; and allied corporate entities. Another guiding principle for the ICIDH-2 revisions was respect for the different languages represented in the international community. They maintained that the ICF should be attractive to its users and should appeal to managers and policymakers who would support its use and that it needed to have continuity with previous classification systems in order to complement systems already in place (WHO, 2001).

Feedback obtained during testing of the alpha draft of the ICIDH-2 was used to develop a beta-1 draft that was tested from June 1997 through December 1998. These results were used to inform development of a beta-2 draft, which underwent testing from July 1999 through September 2000, which is when the writer became involved with the ICIDH-2 development efforts.

Feasibility and reliability studies of case evaluations were conducted during the beta-2 field trials that involved 24 countries, 1,884 case evaluations, and 3,216 evaluations of case summaries. Focus groups and various other studies contributed to the beta-1 and -2 revision processes. The revisions formulated for the beta-2 draft of the ICIDH-2 signified the shift from a focus on impairment and disorder to a focus on health. These revisions were designed to reflect changes in disability policy development and reforms of health care systems internationally and also mirror the medical, social, and biopsychosocial perspectives on disability just reviewed, and their development over time.

International field testing occurred in over 50 countries (WHO, 2001) at various centers and nongovernmental and intergovernmental organizations affiliated with the United

Nations through the efforts of more than 1,800 scientists, clinicians, persons with disabilities, and other experts. Results of the studies led to several conclusions including that the ICIDH-2 was a useful and meaningful public health tool. It was agreed that training was needed in the implementation of the system, particularly in the application of its conceptual framework.

After preliminary review of the systematic beta-2 field trial data, the prefinal draft was completed in October 2000 and presented at a revision meeting the following month. Suggestions from the meeting were incorporated into the version submitted to the WHO Executive Board in January 2001. The final draft was presented at the 54th World Health Assembly in May 2001. The Assembly voted for the adoption of the ICIDH-2 and elected to rename the system from the second edition of the ICIDH (ICIDH-2) to the International Classification of Functioning, Disability and Health, or the ICF. A summary of the ICIDH/ICF revision process can be found in the seventh annex of the ICF (WHO, 2001).

Prior to its most current form as the ICF in 2001, Hurst (2003) challenged the ICIDH development efforts by saying that it perpetuated the medical model, countered the social model of disability, and presented barriers to the understanding of issues related to social justice and disability among health care providers. In response to this criticism, WHO made a concerted effort to involve people with disabilities and disability rights advocates in the ICIDH revision process that produced the ICF. Such criticism had great influence on the evolution of the ICF and its increased focus on contextual factors, and ongoing participation of international stakeholders will continue to shape the ICF in its future iterations.

From a disability-rights activist perspective, the interactive model informing the ICF's conceptual framework is complementary to the social model of disability (disability being an interaction between impairment, functioning, and environment). The social model of disability is very helpful in describing how environmental factors are key to understanding disability and how advocacy occurs through social change (Hurst, 2003). The name was changed from the ICIDH to the ICF to reflect the paradigm shift away from a focus on consequences of disease as found in the 1980 version toward a focus on the components of health found in the current version (WHO, 2001). Rather than an emphasis on "impairment, disability, and handicap" exclusively, the revised classification incorporated the terms activity and participation to denote positive experiences related to function and health. In the current version of the classification, the term *impairment* is defined as a problem with a body function or structure and the term *handicap* has been replaced with the term participation restriction, meaning a problem an individual may experience in life situations.

The evolution of the ICIDH to the current iteration of the ICF reflects the international zeitgeist to embrace a biopsychosocial model of disability rather than a medical or social model exclusively. We now have at our disposal an etiologically neutral framework and classification that was created through global consensus building to identify all aspects of a person's health experience at the individual and contextual levels (Stucki et al., 2005).

INTERNATIONAL CLASSIFICATION OF FUNCTIONING DISABILITY AND HEALTH

The ICF(WHO, 2001) was published in 2001 as the latest addition to the WHO family of classifications, as a new taxonomy of health and functioning that promotes the use of universal classifications of function that are complementary to the use of diagnostic information in health care service provision. A sister classification to the ICD defined earlier, the two systems are used together to classify a holistic conceptualization of health and functioning.

The ICF embraces a biopsychosocial approach for conceptualizing and classifying mental and physical health functioning (body functions and structures), disability (activity limitations and participation restrictions), environmental barriers, and facilitators; collaborating with the person being assessed in determining these factors (personal factors), targeting interventions, and evaluating treatment efficacy. These terms are further defined in the next section.

The ICF is a significant development in health care, as it can be used as a standard for defining concepts, building constructs, hypothesizing relationships, and proposing new theories that will further research and practice in counseling (Bruyère & Peterson, 2005; Bruyère, Van Looy, & Peterson, 2005). Detailed classification of functioning requires reading the ICF and receiving training in its use, so an overview of its details is outside the scope of this chapter. However, the reader is referred to various published references to become familiar with the full classification system, and oriented to its use (Peterson, 2005, 2011; Peterson & Paul, 2009; WHO, 2001).

ICF Conceptual Framework

For our purposes, the ICF conceptual framework is reviewed here as a potential template to inform health care professionals working with people with disabilities. The ICF is based on a universal, culturally sensitive, integrative, and interactive model of health and functioning that provides sensitivity to psychosocial and environmental aspects of health and disability (Simeonsson et al., 2003; Üstün, Chaterji, Bickenbach, Kostanjsek, & Schneider, 2003). The ICF conceptual framework portrays health as a dynamic interaction between a person's functioning and disability within a given context (see Figure 26.1).

The conceptual framework of the ICF consists of two parts: *Functioning and Disability* and *Contextual Factors*. Each part contains two components; within the first part, the *Body* component consists of two parallel classifications, *Body Functions* and *Body Structures*. The second component, *Activities and Participation*, covers domains of functioning from an individual and a societal perspective. For health care professionals conceptualizing a case, they can use this framework to first explore biological bases of behavior (body functions and body structures). Once the physical and mental health and functioning of an individual are clarified at the individual level, then how that person functions in his or her environment can be explored with respect to potential (activity) versus actual ability to participate within a social context (participation). The discrepancy between identified potential (activity) and actual participation can serve as the focus of clinical attention for intervention targeting.

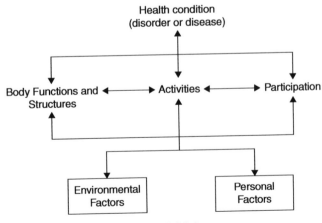

FIGURE 26.1

Interactions between the components of ICF.

The second part of the ICF classification addresses *Contextual Factors* through two components, the first is *Environmental Factors*, or factors in the physical, social, or attitudinal world ranging from the immediate to more general environment. The biopsychosocial model has supported the utility of considering facilitators and barriers present in the environment when planning treatment interventions for people with disabilities. The second component is *Personal Factors*, calling attention to the need to consider unique factors such as gender, race, age, fitness, religion, lifestyle, habits, upbringing, coping styles, social background, education, profession, past and current experience, overall behavior pattern and character, individual psychological assets, and other health conditions (WHO, 2001).

Key Concepts

Within the ICF, the term *health* refers to components of health that are a focus of health care professionals (e.g., hearing, learning, remembering, seeing, speaking, walking) as well as health-related components of well-being that are not typically a focus of health care systems (e.g., education, labor, social interactions, transportation). As reviewed above, the literature suggests that attending to contextual factors that are not typically a focus of health care systems can lead to improved treatment outcomes. The ICF conceptual framework can help clinicians account for various contextual factors that may be influencing someone's health and functioning as impacted by *disorder* or *disease*, including factors that may escape the focus of many health care providers.

Functioning within the ICF conceptual framework is defined as all body functions, activities, and participation in society. *Disability* refers to any impairments, activity limitations, or participation restrictions, or "the outcome or result of a complex relationship between an individual's health condition and personal factors, and of the external factors that represent the circumstances in which the individual lives" (WHO, 2001, p. 17). Note that the terms used in the ICF are capitalized to distinguish them from their lay uses (Threats & Worrall, 2004).

APPLYING THE ICF CONCEPTUAL FRAMEWORK

The following scenario will help illustrate the utility of the biopsychosocial framework and the ICF for case conceptualization. Consider a 22-year-old man who due to a head trauma has a cognitive disorder not otherwise specified, and a co-occurring diagnosis of major depressive disorder, single episode, severe. We will use this scenario to illustrate several points.

A clinician may encounter a variety of perspective across and within health care agencies. Understanding these perspective can help to identify allies and inform strategies to address barriers in the system. For instance, if a clinician is encountering a health care entity focused on the medical model of service provision, the clinician's advocacy efforts can focus on social and contextual factors to encourage a holistic program of health care.

In our example, treating hospital may be focused on medical presentations of impairment related to his head trauma and the degree of depressive symptomology and related risks. The ICF's conceptual framework addresses these foci through body functions and body structures (which do include the brain). In addition, the biopsychosocial approach embraced within the ICF's conceptual framework will take into careful account contextual issues such as the client's family system, social circles, and greater community. Further, through a consideration of activities and participation, the client's potential based on his functioning and impairments can be compared with how his current context facilitates or hinders his functioning.

Clinicians may find that some health care systems are more open to the biopsychosocial approach than others. It is important to capitalize upon the strengths inherent in a given system and to carefully suggest ideas that may enhance treatment based on a framework like that proposed within the ICF. They can in turn use the ICF conceptual framework to highlight the role of contextual factors in facilitating or hindering healthy functioning.

CLASSIFYING WITH THE ICF

The size and scope of the ICF, with just under 1,500 categories of classification, may make it appear difficult to use at first. It is important to review the ICF in its entirety and participate in available training opportunities in order to become proficient with the ICF. For the purpose of introduction, a general overview of using the ICF is available in a journal article by Peterson (2005), and specific application to working with psychological impairments is available in a text by Peterson (2011).

To provide some encouragement and perspective on the ICF, one could compare its use with that of any comprehensive reference; it is not necessary or practical to read most reference material from cover to cover in a brief time period, rather, one searches for specific information according to a specific need. Once familiar with the basic structure of the ICF, the user can search purposefully for information related to health and functioning with some facility.

There are two versions of the ICF: the full version that provides all four levels of classification detail and the short version that provides two levels of classification. In either case, units of classification are qualified with numeric codes that specify the magnitude or extent of disability or function in a given category as well as the extent to which an environmental factor is a facilitator or a barrier. To allow quick and easy classification, the WHO has created an electronic version of the ICF that is searchable through the ICF Browser or CD-ROM (WHO, 2001). An alphabetical index is also available in the hardcopy version of the ICF.

One-Level Classification

The categories of function for a given domain begin at a general level of detail and expand to levels of greater detail. The one-level classification of the ICF expands on the core structure as follows: (1) the body functions component contains eight chapters that address "physiological functions of body systems (including psychological functions)" (WHO, 2001, p. 12); (2) the body structures component contains eight chapters that parallel the body functions component and deal with "anatomical parts of the body such as organs, limbs, and their components" (p. 12); (3) the activities and participation component contains nine chapters, with activities addressing "the execution of a task or action by an individual" and participation addressing "involvement in a life situation" (p. 14); and (4) the environmental factors component contains five chapters focusing on "the physical, social, and attitudinal environment in which people live and conduct their lives" (p. 171), organized from the immediate to more general environment. The maximum number of codes available at the one-digit level of classification is 34.

Two-Level Classification

The two-level classification is the first branching level of the ICF, comprising specific chapter headings. Alphanumeric codes begin with a letter (b for body functions, s for body structures, d for activities and participation, and e for environmental factors) and a three-digit numeric classification indicating chapter and specific categories within each chapter. For example, the classification associated with the psychological function of emotion is found in the first chapter of body functions (its code begins with "b") under the specific mental function section, called emotional functions, or alphanumeric code b152. The two-level items total 362 distinct, three-digit codes.

Detailed Classification

The detailed classification with definitions lists all categories within the ICF along with their definitions, inclusions, and exclusions, providing greater levels of detail using four- and five-digit numeric codes. The level of classification used depends on the clinical context. Examining emotional functions, examples of level of detail include appropriateness of emotion (b1520), regulation of emotion (b1521), and range of emotion (b1522). Code groups also offer an other specified (e.g., b1528) and unspecified (e.g., b1529) codes for functions not detailed in the current classification.

Codes at the detailed level of classification number up to 1,424 items. However, the ICF suggests that typical use of the system in a health or health-related setting for surveys and clinical outcome evaluation will generate a set of 3–18 codes to describe a case with two-level (three-digit) precision. The more precise four-level codes would be used for more specialized services (rehabilitation outcomes, geriatrics, and mental health) and research.

Hierarchical, Mutually Exclusive Code Example

Within components, as units of classification become more detailed, there is the assumption that more detailed units share the attributes of the broader units in the hierarchy order in which they fall. For example, range of emotion b1522 shares the attributes of the higher level of classification emotional functions b152. It is worth mentioning again that categories within the same level are designed to be mutually exclusive. More than one category may be used to accurately classify specific functioning as warranted.

Turning to an example within the ICF from the mental functions chapter, page 49, the orientation functions (b114) section of global mental functions (b110–139), which are second-level codes. Orientation functions can be classified more precisely to address orientation to person (b1142, a third-level code) and even more precisely as orientation to others (b11421), a five-digit code. This represents the pathway from a two-level code in mental functions to a more detailed classification.

Qualifiers

Qualifiers provide inherent meaning to the ICF codes, reflect the magnitude of the issue classified, and appear as one, two, or three digits after the decimal point that follows the ICF code. Students of the ICF will benefit from a review of the second annex of the ICF (pp. 219–233) that provides coding guidelines, including an overview of the ICF organization and structure and general and specific coding rules. Annex Four of the ICF (pp. 238–241) provides specific case examples for applying the ICF. However, there is work to be done with respect to the consistent clinical implementation of the ICF.

CLINICAL IMPLEMENTATION OF THE ICF

Manual

Although the ICF was adopted as the complement to the ICD-10, the 191 member states that are encouraged by the WHO to use it must generate their own resources to guide its clinical implementation. These efforts have not been consistent or well coordinated across the member states. In order to facilitate implementation of the ICF in clinical settings in the United States, the APA and WHO formed a series of interdisciplinary teams of experts to develop *The Procedural Manual and Guide for the Standardized Application of the ICF: A Manual for Health Professionals* (Reed et al., 2005).

Reed et al. (2005), some of whom were members of the alpha drafting team for the joint-manual effort, including the author, detailed the initial template development that led to work completed thus far on the implementation manual. The manual development effort proved challenging and is still ongoing. The size of the manual has grown over time and generated discussion regarding the utility of a paper manual versus an electronic computerized matching system approach to implementing the ICF. The manual is currently undergoing a multidisciplinary editing process.

Once the manual is published, studies will need to be conducted that evaluate the clarity of the manual, the utility of the manual in clinical practice, and ultimately the application of the ICF given the new implementation guidelines. Training needs to be developed to promote consistent coding of guidelines from the WHO and its collaborating centers (Reed et al., 2008). Clinical judgment, assessment biases, and interactional dynamics between rater and participants are further areas of complexity to address in standard use of the ICF, so much work lies ahead. A thorough review of the APA's collaboration with the WHO in the development of a clinical implementation manual can be found in Reed et al. (2005, 2008).

Ethical Use of the ICF

The ICF incorporates a set of ethical provisions that when applied responsibly and used with consumer participation in a collaborative and informational process, assures ethical use of the ICF. The ICF is not something that is done to someone, rather, it is *done with* or in collaboration with a person (Peterson & Threats, 2005; Threats & Worrall, 2004). The 11 ethical provisions are actually a part of the ICF's classification system. In order to maintain the spirit of its intended use, it is important for ICF users to be informed by the ethical provisions when applying the ICF to practice.

The 11 ethical provisions were established in the sixth annex of the ICF to reduce the risk of disrespectful or harmful use of the classification system. The provisions address three general areas: (1) respect and confidentiality, (2) clinical use of the ICF, and (3) social use of ICF information (WHO, 2001a, pp. 244–245). The sixth annex of the ICF prefaces the ethical guidelines for the use of ICF as follows:

> Every scientific tool can be misused and abused. It would be naïve to believe that a classification system such as ICF will never be used in ways that are harmful to people. As explained in Appendix 5, the process of the revision of ICIDH has included persons with disabilities and their advocacy organizations from the beginning. Their input has lead to substantive changes in the terminology, content and structure of ICF. This annex sets out some basic guidelines for the ethical use of ICF. It is obvious that no set of guidelines can anticipate all forms of misuse of a classification or other scientific tool, or for that matter, that guidelines alone can prevent misuse. This document is no exception. It is hoped that attention to the provisions that follow will reduce the risk that ICF will be used in ways that are disrespectful and harmful to people with disabilities. (WHO, 2001a, p. 244)

The 11 provisions are listed here according to three broad themes.

Respect and Confidentiality

1. ICF should always be used so as to respect the inherent value and autonomy of individual persons.
2. ICF should never be used to label people or otherwise identify them solely in terms of one or more disability categories.

3. In clinical settings, ICF should always be used with the full knowledge, cooperation, and consent of the persons whose levels of functioning are being classified. If limitations of an individual's cognitive capacity preclude this involvement, the individual's advocate should be an active participant.
4. The information coded using ICF should be viewed as personal information and subject to recognized rules of confidentiality appropriate for the manner in which the data will be used.

Clinical Use of ICF

5. Wherever possible, the clinician should explain to the individual or the individual's advocate the purpose of the use of ICF and invite questions about the appropriateness of using it to classify the person's levels of functioning.
6. Wherever possible, the person whose level of functioning is being classified (or the person's advocate) should have the opportunity to participate and in particular to challenge or affirm the appropriateness of the category being used and the assessment assigned.
7. Because the deficit being classified is a result of both a person's health condition and the physical and social context in which the person lives, ICF should be used holistically.

Social Use of ICF Information

8. ICF information should be used, to the greatest extent feasible, with the collaboration of individuals to enhance their choices and their control over their lives.
9. ICF information should be used toward the development of social policy and political change that seeks to enhance and support the participation of individuals.
10. ICF, and all information derived from its use, should not be employed to deny established rights or otherwise restrict legitimate entitlements to benefits for individuals or groups.
11. Individuals classed together under ICF may still differ in many ways. Laws and regulations that refer to ICF classifications should not assume more homogeneity than intended and should ensure that those whose levels of functioning are being classified are considered as individuals (WHO, 2001a, pp. 244–245).

FUTURE DIRECTIONS FOR THE ICF

WHO wrote in the eighth annex of the ICF that the ICF is owned by all its users. There is much left to be done by the international community owners of this important but developing system. WHO suggested the following foci for future work with the ICF:

1. Promote the use of the ICF at the country level for development of national databases.
2. Establish an international dataset and the framework to permit international comparisons.
3. Identify algorithms for eligibility for social benefits and pensions.
4. Study disability and functioning of family members (e.g., a study of third-party disability due to the health condition of significant others).
5. Develop the personal factors component.
6. Develop precise operational definitions of categories for research purposes.
7. Develop assessment instruments for identification and measurement.
8. Provide practical applications by means of computerization and case recording forms.

9. Establish links with quality-of-life concepts and the measurement of subjective well-being.
10. Research into treatment or intervention matching.
11. Promote use in scientific studies for comparison between different health conditions.
12. Develop training materials on the use of ICF.
13. Create ICF training and reference centers worldwide.
14. Research environmental factors to provide the necessary detail for use in describing the standardized and current environment (WHO, 2001a, pp. 251–252).

The literature reviewed in this chapter suggests that considerable progress has been made in meeting the goals suggested by WHO. It is an exciting time to be involved with the development of the ICF as its owners take responsibility for making the system the best it can be for society. We conclude this chapter with a review of important future developments for the ICF.

Mental Health Parity

The ICF was designed to be etiologically neutral, addressing health and function regardless of diagnosis. Consequently, the ICF promotes parity between physical and mental health care service provision. For example, difficulties in attention are classified the same regardless of whether they are caused by problems with physical pain, the effects of medication, or depression. When functioning becomes the focus of describing health, the differences between physical and mental impairments are not a focus of attention, supporting aspirations for mental health parity (Peterson & Threats, 2005).

Unfortunately, mental health–related services are often relegated to mental health carve out resources that are not as well resourced as services for physical medicine. While mental health care parity legislation was passed recently in the United States, it has yet to effectively challenge the lack of parity with respect to third-party resources provided for the treatment of physical versus mental disabilities. The ICF has brought international attention to this dilemma through the associated Mental Health Task Force (see Kennedy, 2003).

If health care classification becomes more etiologically neutral and focuses on functioning (what a person does, what he or she can do given the opportunity), the rationale for mental health parity becomes more salient. Hopefully, the ICF will continue to play an important role in achieving mental health parity and in treating people with mental disorders comparably to people dealing with physical disorders. For a thorough review of the important work of the Mental Health Task Force described in our historical development discussion of the ICF, see the study by Kennedy (2003).

Social Justice and Disability Advocacy

While the original ICIDH (WHO, 1980) was developed in close circles of rehabilitation professionals who did not systematically consult with people with disabilities, efforts began in 1993 to revise the classification system with input sought from the disability community, including individuals with disabilities and related organizations. Disabled Peoples' International contributed its time and energies to the revision process, and the ICF reflects their important input (Duggan, Albright, & LeQuerica, 2008; Hurst, 2003; WHO, 2001a, p. 242). Subsequently, the United Nations recognized the ICIDH's value and endorsed its use "as a basis for human rights advocacy around the world" (Üstün et al., 2003, p. 569). Future efforts to revise the ICF will present an international opportunity for those interested in social justice to meaningfully contribute to the ICF's ongoing development.

Advocacy is an ethical responsibility of all health care professionals. The ethical provisions of the ICF encourage health care professionals to use the ICF to facilitate the empowerment and inclusion of persons with disabilities in society. One way to advocate social justice for those who may be marginalized by society is to include them in the development of practical solutions, as was done in the development of the ICF (Peterson & Threats, 2005). The ICF greatly benefited from significant input from all of its stakeholders, an example of social justice in action.

The disability community was also involved in and had an important impact on the identification of key constructs within the classification during latter phases of the development of the ICF (see Hurst, 2003; Üstün et al., 2003). For example, the term *handicap* was eliminated from the classification because of its pejorative connotations in English. Disability was purposefully avoided as a name of any component of the ICF and is used as an umbrella term that is operationalized as activity limitations or participation restrictions (see definitions described previously).

Another important outcome of the disability community's involvement was the establishment of the Environmental Task Force (ETF), one of the three task forces created for the recent revision process. ETF was funded by the Centers for Disease Control and chaired by Rachel Hurst, a disability rights activist (Hurst, 2003). People with disabilities were the majority of the members of the ETF, representing WHO-based geographic regions and expertise in environmental factors and disability. The work of the ETF resulted in the development of the environmental factors component of the ICF, which encouraged consideration of the influence of interactions between an individual and his or her environment rather than focusing on the person's impairment exclusively (Schneidert, Hurst, Miller, & Üstün, 2003).

The contextual factors (environmental and personal factors) developed in collaboration with the disability community provided a more holistic picture of health and functioning. Classifying health and functioning in light of contextual factors facilitates more effective health care service provision for people with disabilities and greater social justice. Social policy developers can consider contextual factors and related databases when establishing legislation, services, and interventions for people with disabilities (Hurst, 2003; Schneidert et al., 2003).

Future Research

Recent reviews of the literature generated by ICF stakeholders suggest a number of areas of ongoing research on the ICF (Peterson, 2005; Peterson & Rosenthal, 2005; Peterson et al., 2010). Validity studies are necessary to provide evidence to support the model of disability and functioning proposed by WHO. Further operationalization and quantification of ICF codes and qualifiers are necessary. Researchers must collect data on the various constructs presented, explore associations, and hypothesize and confirm causal links. ICF core sets have been and continue to be developed in order to assemble useful collections of disability-specific codes sets. As research progresses on more specific applications of the ICF, evidences for validity of specific applications will become apparent (Peterson & Paul, 2009).

Chute (2005) proposed that the evolving knowledge base of medical information has outgrown our ability to consume it effectively. Systems like the ICF and its sister classification, the ICD, in electronic and searchable formats, can help construct shared semantics, vocabularies, and terminologies that are accessible and clinically useful in a way that helps us to use medical knowledge effectively for treating people in health care settings. Medical informatics is a very complex area of research. Aspects of health and functioning are important metrics of wellbeing and so are important to include in this evolving research area (Chute, 2005).

The ICF contributes to an increasingly unified global discourse about the health and well-being of groups including people with disabilities. Researchers involved in clinical practice and in using the ICF need to continue developing international and interdisciplinary collaborations to facilitate this discourse (Martin, 2009). Ongoing clinical implementation efforts will help us understand the ICF's utility in conceptualizing functioning, disability, and health within this international and multidisciplinary paradigm.

Some believe that the ICF is still missing important aspects of life and living currently summarized under the personal component of contextual factors. Ueda and Okawa (2003) suggest that the entire "subjective dimension" or "experience" is missing from the ICF entirely. They define the "subjective experience of disability" as

> a set of cognitive, emotional and motivational states of mind of any person, but particularly of a person with health condition and/or disability. … It is a unique combination of, on one hand, a disability experience, i.e. a reflection (influence) of existing health conditions, impairments, activity limitations, participation restrictions and negative environmental factors (obstacles) into the person's mind (negative subjective experience), and on the other hand an experience of a positive nature, which includes, among other things, the psychological coping skills developed, often unconsciously, in order to overcome these negative influences (positive subjective experience). (p. 599)

It is reasonable to propose that there may be considerable overlap between subjective experience and personal factors, which are currently undefined within the contextual part of the ICF. To the ICF's credit, developing this component is prioritized as important future work for the ICF (WHO, 2001a, p. 251).

CONCLUSION

The ICF promises to inform our international health efforts by providing a unified language of health and functioning that will facilitate the exchange of information worldwide. Future assessment, treatment, and research efforts using the ICF can revolutionize the way we think about physical and psychological functioning, disability, and health; improve the quality of care for individuals internationally; generate and disseminate universal research data on disability and functioning; and ultimately influence culturally sensitive global health policy.

Those who want to learn more about the ICF should consult the ICF itself for more precise coding guidelines, paying close attention to annexes at the end of the document, specifically, Annexes 2, 3, and 4, seek training from WHO affiliates knowledgeable in the ICF, and read more of the seminal references noted in this chapter. Ultimately, we can anticipate the release of the manual from the APA/WHO (see Reed et al., 2008), and the related training that will undoubtedly develop as a result.

REFERENCES

American Medical Association. (2007). *Current procedural terminology.* Washington, DC: Author.

American Psychiatric Association. (2000). *Diagnostic and statistical manual of mental disorders* (4th ed., text rev.) Washington, DC: Author.

Bassett, S. S., Chase, G. A., Folstein, M. F., & Regier, D. A. (1998). Disability and psychiatric disorders in an urban community: Measurement, prevalence and outcomes. *Psychological Medicine, 28*, 509–517.

Brandsma, J. W., Lakerveld-Heyl, K., & Van Ravensberg, C. D. (1995). Reflection on the definition of impairment and disability as defined by the World Health Organization [Special issue: The International Classification of Impairments, Disabilities, and Handicaps (ICDH): Perspectives and developments, 119–127.]. *Disability & Rehabilitation: An International Multidisciplinary Journal, 17*(3–4), 119–127.

Brown, S. C. (1993). Revitalizing "handicap" disability research. *Journal of Disability Policy Studies, 4*, 55–73.

Brown, S., & Lent, R. (Eds.). (2008). *Handbook of counseling psychology* (4th ed.). Hoboken, NJ: John Wiley & Sons.

Bruyère, S. M., & Peterson, D. B. (2005). Introduction to the special section on the International Classification of Functioning, Disability and Health (ICF): Implications for rehabilitation psychology. *Rehabilitation Psychology, 50,* 103–104.

Bruyère, S. M., Van Looy, S. A., & Peterson, D. B. (2005). The International Classification of Functioning, Disability and Health (ICF): Contemporary literature review. *Rehabilitation Psychology, 50,* 113–121.

Burns, C. (1991). Parallels between research and diagnosis: The reliability and validity issues of clinical practice. *The Nurse Practitioner, 16*(10), 42–45, 49–50.

Chute, C. G. (2005, June). *The spectrum of clinical data representation: A context for functional status.* Symposium conducted at the meeting of the World Health Organization's North American Collaborating Center, Mayo Clinic, Rochester, MN.

De Kleijn-De Vrankrijker, M. W. (2003). The long way from the International Classification of Impairments, Disabilities and Handicaps (ICIDH) to the International Classification of Functioning, Disability and Health (ICF). *Disability and Rehabilitation, 25,* 561–564.

Dell Orto, A. E., & Power, P. W. (Eds.). (2007). *The psychological and social impact of illness and disability.* New York: Springer.

Duggan, C. H., Albright, K. J., & LeQuerica, A. (2008). Using the ICF to code and analyse women's disability narratives. *Disability and Rehabilitation, 30,* 978–990.

Elliott, T., Kurylo, M., & Rivera, P. (2002). Positive growth following an acquired physical disability. In C. R. Snyder & S. Lopez (Eds.), *Handbook of positive psychology* (pp. 687–699). New York: Oxford University Press.

Engel, G. L. (1977). The need for a new medical model: A challenge for biomedicine. *Science, 196,* 129–136.

Gatchel, R. J., Polatin, P. B., Mayer, T. G., & Garcy, P. D. (1994). Psychopathology and the rehabilitation of patients with chronic low back pain disability. *Archives of Physical Medicine and Rehabilitation, 75,* 666–670.

Hurst, R. (2003). The international disability rights movement and the ICF. *Disability and Rehabilitation, 25,* 572–576.

Kennedy, C. (2003). Functioning and disability associated with mental disorders: The evolution since ICIDH. *Disability & Rehabilitation, 25,* 611–619.

Leonardi, M., Bickenbach, J., Üstün, T. B., Kostanjsek, N., & Chatterji, S. (2006). Comment: The definition of disability: What is in a name? *Lancet, 368,* 1219–1221.

Martin, S. (2009). Improving diagnosis worldwide. *Monitor on Psychology, 40*(9), 62–65.

Massel, H. K., Liberman, R. P., Mintz, J., Jacobs, H. E. (1990). Evaluating the capacity to work of the mentally ill. *Psychiatry: Journal for the Study of Interpersonal Processes, 53,* 31–43.

McCrone, P., & Phelan, M. (1994). Diagnosis and length of psychiatric in-patient stay. *Psychological Medicine, 24,* 1025–1030.

National Advisory Mental Health Council. (1993). Health care reform for Americans with severe mental illness: Report of the National Advisory Mental Health Council. *American Journal of Psychiatry, 150,* 1447–1465.

Nieuwenhuijsen, E. R. (1995). The ICIDH in the USA: Applications and relevance to ADA goals. *Disability and Rehabilitation, 17,* 154–158.

Olkin, R. (1999). *What psychotherapists should know about disability.* New York: Guilford Press.

Olkin, R., & Pledger, C. (2003). Can disability studies and psychology join hands? *American Psychologist, 58,* 296–304.

Ormel, J., Oldehinkel, T., Brilman, E., & vanden Brink, W. (1993). Outcome of depression and anxiety in primary care: A three wave 3 1/2 year study of psychopathology and disability. *Archives of General Psychiatry, 50,* 759–766.

Peterson, D. B. (2005). International Classification of Functioning, Disability and Health (ICF): An introduction for rehabilitation psychologists. *Rehabilitation Psychology, 50,* 105–112.

Peterson, D. B. (2009). The International Classification of Functioning, Disability & Health: Application to professional counseling. In M. A. Stebnicki & I. Marini (Eds.), *The professional counselor's desk reference* (pp. 529–542). New York: Springer Publishing.

Peterson, D. B. (2011). *Psychological aspects of functioning, disability and health.* New York: Springer Publishing.

Peterson, D. B. & Elliott, T. R. (2008). Advances in conceptualizing and studying disability. In S. Brown and R. W. Lent (Eds.), *Handbook of counseling psychology* (4th ed., pp. 212–230). Hoboken, NJ: Wiley & Sons.

Peterson, D. B., Mpofu, E., & Oakland, T. D. (2010). Concepts and models in disability, functioning, and health. In E. Mpofu & T. Oakland (Eds.), *Rehabilitation and health assessment: Applying ICF guidelines* (pp. 3–26). New York: Springer Publishing.

Peterson, D. B., & Paul, H. (2009). Using the International Classification of Functioning, Disability and Health (ICF) to conceptualize disability functioning in psychological injury and law. *Psychological Injury and Law, 2*(3–4), 205–214.

Peterson, D.B., & Rosenthal, D. (2005). The international classification of functioning, disability and health: A primer for rehabilitation educators. *Rehabilitation Education, 19,* 81–94.

Peterson, D. B., & Threats, T. T. (2005). Ethical and clinical implications of the International Classification of Functioning, Disability and Health (ICF) in rehabilitation education. *Rehabilitation Education, 19,* 129–138.

Pledger, C. (2003). Discourse on disability and rehabilitation issues: Opportunities for psychology. *American Psychologist, 58,* 279–284.

Rabinowitz, J., Modai, I., & Inbar-Saban, N. (1994). Understanding who improves after psychiatric hospitalization. *Acta Psychiatrica Scandidavica, 89,* 152–158.

Reed, G. M., Dilfer, K., Bufka, L. F., Scherer, M. J., Kotzé, P., Tshivhase, M.,et al. (2008). Three model curricula for teaching clinicians to use the ICF. *Disability and Rehabilitation, 30,* 927–941.

Reed, G. M., Lux, J. B., Jacobson, J. W., Stark, S., Threats, T. T., Peterson, D. B., et al. (2005). Operationalizing the International Classification of Functioning, Disability and Health (ICF) in clinical settings. *Rehabilitation Psychology, 50,* 122–131.

Rock, M. (2005, June). *Welcome WHO/ICF NACC to Mayo clinic.* Symposium conducted at the meeting of the World Health Organization's North American Collaborating Center, Mayo Clinic, Rochester, MN.

Rusk, H. A. (1977). *Rehabilitation medicine* (4th ed.). St. Louis, MO: Mosby.

Schneidert, M., Hurst, R., Miller, J., & Üstün, B. (2003). The role of environment in the International Classification of Functioning, Disability and Health (ICF). *Disability and Rehabilitation, 25,* 588–595.

Segal, S. P., & Choi, N. G. (1991). Factors affecting SSI support for sheltered care residents with serious mental illness. *Hospital and Community Psychiatry, 42,* 1132–1137.

Simeonsson, R. J., Leonardi, M., Lollar, D., Bjorck-Akesson, E., Hollenweger, J., & Martinuzzi, A. (2003). Applying the International Classification of Functioning, Disability and Health (ICF) to measure childhood disability. *Disability and Rehabilitation, 25,* 602–610.

Smart, J. (2005). The promise of the International Classification of Functioning, Disability & Health (ICF). *Rehabilitation Education, 19,* 191–199.

Stucki, G., Üstün, T. B., & Melvin, J. (2005). Applying the ICF for the acute hospital and early post-acute rehabilitation facilities. *Disability and Rehabilitation, 27,* 349–352.

Threats, T. T., & Worrall, L. (2004). Classifying communication disability using the ICF. *Advances in Speech-Language Pathology, 6,* 53–62.

Ueda, S., & Okawa, Y. (2003). The subjective dimension of functioning and disability: What is it and what is it for? *Disability and Rehabilitation, 25,* 596–601.

Üstün T. B., Chatterji S., Bickenbach, J., Kostanjsek, N., & Schneider M. (2003). International classification of functioning, disability and health: A new tool for understanding disability and health. *Disability and Rehabilitation, 25,* 565–571.

United Nations Department of Public Information (UNDPI). (1993). *The standard rules on the equalization of opportunities for persons with disabilities.* Adopted by the United Nations General Assembly, 48th session, resolution 48/96, annex, of 20 December, 1993.

World Health Organization. (1980). *International Classification of Impairments, Disabilities, and Handicaps* (ICIDH). Geneva, Switzerland: Author.

World Health Organization. (1992). *International statistical classification of diseases and related health problems, tenth revision* (ICD-10). Geneva, Switzerland: Author.

World Health Organization. (1999). *ICIDH-2: International Classification System of Functioning and Disability: Beta-2 draft, Short Version.* Geneva, Switzerland: Author.

World Health Organization. (2001). *International Classification of Functioning, Disability and Health: ICF.* Geneva, Switzerland: Author.

Wright, G. N. (1980). *Total rehabilitation.* Boston, MA: Little, Brown and Company.

Wright, B. A. (1983). *Physical disability: A psychosocial approach* (2nd ed.). New York: Harper & Row.

27

Psychosocial Impact of Empathy Fatigue on Professional Helpers

MARK A. STEBNICKI

*I*n traditional Native American beliefs, each time you heal someone you give away a piece of yourself. The medicine man or woman understands that the healer at some point in time will become wounded; thus he or she will require healing (Tafoya & Kouris, 2003). Nouwen (1972) speaks to this type of experience from his concept of the *wounded healer*. He suggests that paradoxically we withdraw into ourselves, thus creating a sacred space for no other person to enter. Many in the helping professions have a wounded healer type of experience also. I refer to this phenomenon as empathy fatigue. A word I coined, that results from a state of psychological, emotional, mental, physical, spiritual, and occupational exhaustion that occurs as the counselors' own wounds are continually revisited by their clients' life stories of chronic illness, disability, trauma, grief, and loss (Stebnicki, 1999, 2000, 2001, 2007, 2008, 2009a, 2009b). Thus, it is of paramount importance that counselor educators, supervisors, and professional helpers know how to recognize and cultivate resiliency and self-care practices.

The wounded healer experience or counselor impairment and fatigue syndromes have been recognized by nurses, psychologists, counselors, and other mental health professionals. For example, compassion fatigue, first introduced in the nursing literature by Joinson (1992) and then expanded by Figley (1995), Stamm (1995), and others in psychology, suggests that therapists who deal with survivors of extraordinarily stressful and traumatic events are more prone to compassion fatigue or a secondary traumatic stress type of reaction as a result of feeling compassion and empathy toward others' pain and suffering. McCann and Perlman (1989) refer to this experience as "vicarious traumatization" where the therapist becomes deeply emotionally affected by the client's traumatic stories. Other professional counselors experience a special type of burnout (Maslach, 1982, 2003) where there is an organizational–environmental impact on the person who feels emotionally and physically exhausted, depleted, and has reached the point of depersonalization with their professional colleagues.

Empathy fatigue, as opposed to other fatigue syndromes and counselor impairments, is experienced by professional counselors who primarily use person-centered and empathy-focused interactions to build rapport with their clients so they can achieve a therapeutic working relationship. Indeed, many counselors spend a tremendous amount of time and energy acting in compassionate and empathic ways searching for the meaning of their client's mind, body, and spirit that has been lost to trauma, incest, addictions, and other stressors that prompt questions concerning the meaning of their lives. As a consequence, professional counselors become affected by the same persistent or transient physical, emotional, and psychological symptoms as their clients. This phenomenon affects the whole self; mind, body, and spirit.

Clearly, the search for personal meaning in one's chronic illness, disability, or traumatic experience is an existential and spiritual pursuit (Stebnicki, 2006). In many cultures, the most significant and meaningful questions relate to where we came from before birth and where we will transcend at the time of our death (Pedersen, 2000). The wounded healer searches for existential meaning in the significance of his or her chosen occupation as a professional helper. Such questions as *How could life and death, joy and suffering, love, self-acceptance, and healing exist all within the same day in the lives of my clients?* are disorienting and call on a divine source to acquire a deeper level of understanding.

This chapter provides a description of the empathy fatigue experience from a mind, body, and spiritual growth perspective. Further, I offer a functional risk factor assessment, the Global Assessment of Empathy Fatigue (GAEF) Functioning (Stebnicki, 2009b) as a guideline or screening measure for professional counselors who experience counselor impairments and professional fatigue syndromes such as empathy fatigue. Also, the broader meaning of the phenomenon of empathy fatigue will be explored within a sociocultural context.

EMPATHY AS A THERAPEUTIC APPROACH

Throughout the history of the helping professions, the most fundamental approach to helping others has been rooted in compassion and empathy. Empathy has a rich history of being at the core of most humanistic theoretical orientations within counselor education and training programs. The skills of empathy are a prerequisite for becoming a competent helper and are integral to person-centered approaches that practitioners use to facilitate interpersonal effectiveness and enhance client outcomes (Corey & Corey, 2003; Egan, 1998; Ivey & Ivey, 1999; Truax & Carkhuff, 1967). Empathy has been discussed in the counseling and psychology literature as a skill that can be both developed and learned if facilitated properly in therapeutic interactions (Barone et al., 2005). Many suggest that empathy-focused interactions are qualitatively distinct from other therapeutic approaches. This is because there are multiple variables that mediate the therapeutic relationships. Oftentimes, perceptions of empathy are dependent upon who is measuring or rating this experience; the professional helper, the client, or the counselor educator/supervisor. If facilitated competently by the therapist, empathy can (1) increase client self-awareness, (2) be a motivation for personal growth and change, and (3) cultivate new ways of thinking, feeling, and acting to achieve optimal levels of mind, body, and spiritual wellness.

Rogers (1980) talked passionately about empathy and empathic listening as a "way of being" with a client. Rogers (1957) hypothesized that clients who perceive their therapist as facilitating positive regard, empathy, and congruence during a session demonstrate a more positive outcome with their client. He appeared to have an understanding of counselor fatigue syndromes also, as he observed a significant need for therapists to rebalance their minds, bodies, and spirits after spending countless hours in psychotherapy sessions. However, there is an emotional and physical cost to entering the private perceptual world of the client because the counselor may be a "sponge" for their client's emotional and physical pain. Overall, the conscious and unconscious absorption of the client's emotional, physical, spiritual, and existential issues is a natural artifact of helping others at intense levels of service.

Professional helpers are in a "high touch" profession and are at the epicenter of their client's life stories. Many client stories contain themes of extraordinary stressful and traumatic events, pain, and suffering and result in client transference and negative countertransference of toxic energy during the session. Accordingly, there is a shadow side to facilitating empathic approaches during day-to-day counseling interactions. Indeed, professional helpers must be present at a much higher level of listening, attending, and empathic responding; perhaps more so than professionals who perform medical, psychological, or vocational assessments. Overall, the limited use of empathy-focused therapeutic interactions, by professionally distancing or personally detaching oneself from such engagements, may in fact be a coping mechanism for some, whereby avoiding the experience of empathy fatigue.

EMPATHY FROM A SOCIOCULTURAL PERSPECTIVE

The conceptual roots of empathy can be traced back long before its modern application in Western research and practice as described by Rogers (1902–1987), who published his seminal work, *Client Centered Therapy* in 1951. According to Katz (1963), the term empathy was first used in nonclinical terms and conceptualized in 1897 by Theodore Lipps (1851–1914). His concept, originally termed *Einfuhlung* in German, referred to the process of becoming totally absorbed in an external object (art form) or projecting oneself into an aesthetic form of art. It was not until Sigmund Freud referred to Lipps's concept of *Einfuhlung* in relation to a person's feelings. Freud suggested that *Einfuhlung* (empathy) may produce a specific psychological state that could potentially be projected from oneself into the psychological state of another person. Although Freud's use of empathy was discussed in nonclinical terms, the conceptual underpinnings can be traced back to non-western theorists over 100 years ago.

Counselors who work in traditional mental health practice settings and those who facilitate western-style empathy-focused therapeutic interactions may experience a higher degree of empathy fatigue than persons who work in other occupations. The research strongly supports that counselor impairment and burnout are real among professionals who work with clients who have some of the following experiences: (a) loss (i.e., grief, divorce, extramarital affairs), (b) substance abuse issues (i.e., mental health concerns, family issues, legal problems, career issues), (c) career development issues (i.e., company downsizing, work-related job stress, career transitions), (d) chronic health conditions (i.e., cancer, HIV/AIDS), (e) trauma (e.g., acute and post-traumatic stress issues), and (f) issues of generalized anxiety, depression, and other general stress conditions (Stebnicki, 2008).

The majority of counselor education programs incorporate humanistic and person-centered approaches in their training and supervision of pre-professional counselors. However, it is important to recognize that there are unique cultural differences in the use of empathy. The skills of empathy are integrated into many of the theories in counseling and psychology that have been developed by early European and 20th century psychoanalytic theorists and practitioners (e.g., Freud, Jung, Rogers). Accordingly, empathy-focused therapeutic interactions among counselors and psychologist appear to be a natural occurrence but may have limited use with specific cultural groups. If the skills of empathy are not facilitated in a culturally sensitive manner (e.g., expecting a client to disclose multiple feelings/emotions during session) then the counselor may not be working in a culturally competent and ethical manner.

It is critical to understand the "fourth force" of counseling as proposed in the multicultural counseling literature that views the construct of empathy somewhat differently. Some multicultural theorists see empathy as a skill that is pancultural or universal (Ponterotto & Bensesch, 1988; Ridley, 1995). For example, the scale of ethnocultural empathy (Wang et al., 2003) measures cultural-specific empathy. Wang et al. hypothesized that ethnocultural empathy is composed of the following counselor traits: (a) intellectual empathy (e.g., the ability to understand a culturally different person's thinking and feelings); (b) empathic emotions (e.g., the attention that one gives to the other's feelings and emotions); and (c) communication or expression of ethnoculturally empathic thoughts and feelings toward culturally different individuals and groups. Theoretically, ethnocultural empathic skills can be developed by the counselor over time much like the western use of empathy. Training culturally skilled and competent counselors utilizes models that assist in developing counselors' knowledge, awareness, and understanding of another person's unique cultural experiences as it relates to their feelings and emotions. Others in the muliticultural counseling literature (see Ibrahim, 1991; Ridley & Lingle, 1996) also confirm that cultural empathy is a skill that can be developed and learned by the counselor.

The transition from traditional use of empathy to a more culturally centered practice can be a difficult yet enriching experience. West (2005) suggests that if we truly want to experience the richness of each client's cultural healing system, then we may want to be immersed through understanding and integrating indigenous health and healing practices. Understanding the differences in how culturally different clients think, feel, and act in terms of psychosocial response to chronic illnesses and disabilities may be an indicator of how well the professional helper can facilitate therapeutic interactions in a culturally competent and ethical manner.

WHAT IS EMPATHY FATIGUE?

This author hypothesizes that empathy fatigue may be different from other types of counselor impairment and fatigue syndromes (Stebnicki, 2008). This is primarily because empathy fatigue (1) is viewed as a counselor impairment that can occur early on in one's career due to an interaction of variables that include, but are not limited to, personality traits, general coping resources, age and developmental related factors, opportunities to build resiliency, organizational and other environmental supports, and the interrelationship between the person's mind, body, and spiritual development (Stebnicki, 2000); (2) many times goes unrecognized by the individual and the professional counseling setting or environment because of its subtle characteristics; (3) may be experienced as both an acute and a cumulative type of emotional, physical, and spiritual stressor that does not follow a predictable linear path to total burnout or fatigue; and (4) is a highly individualized experience for most individuals, because the counselor's perception toward the client's story and life events differs depending on the issues presented during session.

In view of this hypothesis, professional counselors who experience empathy fatigue appear to have a diminished capacity to listen and respond empathically to their client's stories that contain various themes of acute and cumulative psychosocial stress, not necessarily stories of acute and posttraumatic stress. Consequently, the professional counselor acquires feelings of grief, loss, detachment, anxiety, depression, and a type of professional burnout, in which he or she feels like his or her therapeutic interactions with others have very little meaning and purpose in the client's overall life.

Client stories that have themes such as addictions, physical or sexual abuse, and psychological trauma can adversely affect the mind, body, and spirit of the counselor. Remembering emotions related to such painful or traumatic events and recreating an internal "emotional scrapbook" can be extremely painful and difficult for clients as well as counselors. This is especially relevant for new professional counselors who have not had the opportunity to cultivate self-care strategies for professional wellness.

THE NEUROSCIENCE OF EMPATHY FATIGUE

Kabat-Zinn (1990; see Berger, 2006) indicates that empathy fatigue can be scientifically measured in the brain because there are specific neurological pathways to empathetic responses. The complexities of studying how emotions affect our mind, body, and spirit require studying such problems from a multidisciplinary perspective that includes the fields of psychology, neurology, immunology, and biology. The discipline of psychoneuroimmunolgy (PNI) has provided a model by which researchers can study emotions and the brain. The task of PNI researchers is a difficult one because as Sapolsky (1998) suggests, our emotions, particularly the stress response, have their own unique physiological arousal patterns of magnitude, frequency, and intensity.

New studies on the mind–body connection report that the shared emotions and physiological arousal experienced between client and therapist can contribute to our knowledge of how empathic connections are developed during counseling sessions. For example, Marci, Ham, Moran, and Orr (2007) studied clients being treated for mood and anxiety disorders using 20 client–therapist pairs. These researchers specifically focused on the therapeutic relationships that were formed during psychotherapy sessions. They took physiological reaction measures of both client and therapist and as well as the client's perceived level of their therapist's empathy. They found that when high positive emotions and empathy were experienced by the client and therapist, then similar physiological responses were experienced as measured by electrical skin conductance recordings, heart rate, voice dynamics, and body movement. Thus, the therapist at some level may be experiencing both same and similar emotions as the individuals they serve.

From a purely dynamic physiological state, emotions involve different body systems and are measured much differently by neuroscientists than experimental psychologists. In the study of emotions and the brain, it is hypothesized that there are discrete, basic, and universal emotions that persons react to on a mind, body, and spiritual dimension (Bar-On & Parker, 2000; Mayne & Bonanno, 2001). Despite that many individuals express universal emotions (e.g., anger, love, happiness, sadness) with varying levels of experience and intensity, Mayne and Ramsey (2001) indicate that this only constitutes a measure of personal experience and a self-report of emotional expression.

Our individual perception of critical events determines how our parasympathetic and sympathetic nervous system is activated during times of an actual or anticipated stressful event. This is because people differ in how they turn-on their stress mechanism and other emotional responses in the brain. After prolonged periods of physiological stress such as seen by professionals who work with the traumatized, it is evident that chronic activation of the stress response has both a physiological and emotional cost. Consequently, professionals who work at such intense levels of service may experience anxiety and depressive disorders. This may account for some aspects of the emotional and physical fatigue experienced by those who report counselor fatigue syndromes such as empathy fatigue. As Sapolsky (1998) notes, if we are constantly trying to mobilize energy, we never have the opportunity to store it; especially when we need it later to achieve calm and relaxed states of consciousness. Accordingly, there is a physical and emotional cost to persistent sympathetic arousal because of the heavy secretion of glucocorticoids released in the body that are markers for depression and anxiety disorders.

Brothers (1989) points to the amygdale–cortical pathway in the brain as part of the key neural circuitry that underlies the emotions associated with the empathy response. The amygdale appears to be the specific structure of the brain that orchestrates the most intense electrical activation when reading, interpreting, or trying to understand the emotions of others. Over time, the counselor's inability to express a healthy and facilitative emotional response (such as empathy) based on the client's expression of such feelings as stress, grief, or trauma appears to have a bio-psycho-social-spiritual cost to the counselor. In other words, the chronic and cumulative activation of the emotional brain and habitual repression of emotions can compromise our immune system, which increases our resistance to infections, chronic illness, and diseases (Pert, Dreher, & Ruff, 2005; Sapolsky, 1998; Weil, 1995).

Overall, it appears that a much stronger working alliance or social–emotional attachment is formed in therapy than once perceived. Because of the empathetic psychophysiological connection that forms between client and therapist, there appears to be potential for some degree of emotional, mental, physical, and spiritual exhaustion experienced by intense, cumulative, and regular therapeutic interactions.

EMPATHY FATIGUE FROM A GLOBAL PERSPECTIVE

More recently, the experience of empathy fatigue has been extended to other cultures. This author's previous work *Empathy Fatigue: Healing the Mind, Body, and Spirit of Professional Counselors* (see Stebnicki, 2010) interestingly has been translated into Korean, which suggests that this phenomenon may be experienced by professional helpers from other cultures. Journalists who cover stories from around the globe also report being affected by empathy fatigue. Many journalists are at the epicenter of natural disasters and human-made atrocities. They report experiencing some degree of empathy fatigue during and after covering such stories related to tsunamis, tornadoes, hurricanes, floods, and conflicts in Iraq, Afghanistan, and other parts of the world (Thompson, 2011; Zaki, 2009). In fact, in the last several years alone we have seen unprecedented number of naturally occurring disasters and human-made atrocities in Pakistan, Libya, Japan, Haiti, Gulf of Mexico, and many other places around the globe.

The use of the term *empathy fatigue* has been used frequently in the social online media where it is suggested that scientists and journalists should work together to stop human rights abuses because empathy is the primary human quality that fuels our instincts of protecting others (Decolonizing Solidarity, 2011; Phillips, 2011; Zaki, 2009). Dean (2003) suggests that there is a danger to constant exposure to gruesome images of suffering as seen in various media outlets, which could in fact desensitize us to such suffering. As a result, some online journalists and social media outlets describe a type of acute stress response; an actual physical, emotional, mental, spiritual, and occupational exhaustion. Perhaps we are all suffering from soul loss, which according to Native American shamanism is a major cause of mental, physical, and spiritual illness (Ingerman, 1991), thus, we may all need a "soul retrieval" to get us back to balance globally.

MEASURING THE EMPATHY FATIGUE RESPONSE

The GAEF (see Table 27.1) rating scale is a theoretical measure of the experience of empathy fatigue (Stebnicki, 2009b). The intent and purpose of the GAEF in its early stage of development is to provide a holistic means of viewing the overall level of functioning as the professional helper reports the experience of empathy fatigue within the last 2 weeks. This measure was developed through an extensive review of the literature in

TABLE 27.1 Global Assessment of Empathy Fatigue Rating Scale (GAEF)

	Level V	Level IV	Level III	Level II	Level I
Cognitive	Diminished concentration; preoccupied; disorganized thoughts; detachment from client	Diminished concentration; preoccupied; slightly disorganized thoughts; detachment; possible irrational thinking	Exhibit some diminished concentration; somewhat preoccupied; thought organization loose; fair focus on therapeutic process; quiet attending of counselor to internal thoughts and feelings; having an "off day"	Slight problems in concentration; occasionally preoccupied; need to continually refocus; good focus on therapeutic process; some response to internal thoughts and feelings; thoughts of hopefulness	Slight problems in concentration and thought organization; more preoccupied than usual; responding to internal thoughts and feelings more than usual, but therapeutic process good
Behavioral	Impatience; irritability; aggression; cynical with client; hypervigilance; poor eye contact; strained, erratic, slow, or fast-paced speech	Impatient; irritable; competitive; very cautious; eye contact fair; somewhat strained, erratic, slow, or fast-paced speech; somewhat cynical with clients	Exhibit signs of restlessness or impatience; slightly inattentive eye contact; slightly strained vocal tone and pace of speech	Physical signs of being restless or impatient, but controls behaviour; eye contact good; occasionally strained vocal quality and pace of speech	Exhibit physical signs of restlessness or impatience, but controls behaviour; eye contact good; vocal quality and pace of speech good, but sometimes strained
Spiritual	Detached from spiritual support; lack meaning and purpose in faith or spiritual beliefs; communication of these deficits	Lack some meaning and purpose with regard to faith or spiritual beliefs; some detachment of spiritual support; communication of lack of meaning and purpose spiritually	Confusion regarding meaning and purpose with regard to faith or spiritual beliefs; separation from spiritual support	Sense of awareness of refocusing on meaning and purpose with regard to faith or spiritual beliefs; attempts to remain connected spiritually; makes attempts to become reconnected to spiritual support	Sense of connectedness to faith restored after self-reassurance; attempts to become reconnected to spiritual support
Process skills	Lack of rapport with client; strained working alliance; nonexistent attending and listening; no genuine empathetic responses; resistant; apprehensive; hypersensitive; high degree of countertransference;	Rapport difficult to establish; no working alliance; poor attending and listening; gather information in session vs. processing client story; superficial empathic responses; some degree of countertransference;	Longer time to establish rapport; working alliance achieved more slowly; listening and attending to clients fair to good; empathetic responses more genuine; session involves gathering basic information;	Working alliance takes longer to achieve but remains stable; empathic response more genuine, deeper, more frequent; session goes beyond data gathering; nonverbal incongruencies in session; avoids dealing	Rapport takes slightly longer to establish; working alliance takes somewhat longer to achieve, but work with client remains intact and stable; attending and listening is appropriate; integration of client content,

(continued)

TABLE 27.1 Global Assessment of Empathy Fatigue Rating Scale (GAEF) (continued)

	Level V	Level IV	Level III	Level II	Level I
	lack of open-ended questioning; lack of solution-focused probes; diminished use of brainstorming techniques; basic information gathering sessions vs. processing client story; misses opportunities to integrate client content, experience, and affect	little use of open-ended questioning; little use of solution-focused probes; little use of brainstorming techniques with clients; somewhat resistant or apprehensive during session; show little nonverbal interest during testing	some missed opportunities in therapeutic interactions; responses have only basic empathy; somewhat resistant or apprehensive; little nonverbal interest during session; some degree of countertransference; little use of open-ended questioning; little use of solution-focused probes; little use of brainstorming techniques	with countertransference; uses some open-ended questioning, solution-focused probes, or brainstorming techniques; rapport takes longer to establish, but eventually is good; working alliance takes longer to achieve; ongoing therapeutic work with client remains intact and stable; attending and listening is good	experience, and affect better; few missed therapeutic opportunities; empathic responses somewhat deeper; somewhat hesitant to explore new areas of client support and resources; some nonverbal incongruencies; increased interest in understanding countertransference; open-ended questioning, solution-focused probes, and brainstorming techniques used
Emotional	Diminished affective state; moodiness; sadness; tearfulness; negative; pessimistic; clear high and low emotions; depleted; exhausted	Somewhat diminished affective state; moodiness; slight mood swings; moderate level of sadness; emotionally fatigued; negative; Pessimistic	Affective state fair; slight moodiness; dysthymic; appears emotionally tired; negative; pessimistic	Affective state good; sense of dysthymic mood; slightly emotionally tired; feeling negative or pessimistic	Affective state could be better; sense of a slightly "down" mood; somewhat emotionally tired; slightly negative; pessimistic, but initiates self-correction
Physical	Shallow breathing; sweating; fatigue; discomfort while sitting; dizziness; nausea; disturbance in visual acuity; facial grimace of pain; muscle tremors or twitches; severe headache	Shallow breathing; slight sweating; fatigue; facial grimacing; feelings of wooziness; lack of appetite due to upset stomach; occasional muscle tremors or twitches; moderate degree of headache; disturbance in visual acuity	Exhibit tiredness; sighs of frustration with breath; facial grimacing; lack of appetite; occasional muscle twitches; slight sense of headache; dry eyes	Exhibits slight tiredness but takes steps to avoid fatigue. Occasional signs of frustration; use internal dialogue to relax while sitting; Some discomfort appetite and eating habits somewhat irregular; muscles slightly tense; needs constant reminder to rebalance physical wellness	Slight tiredness. Takes steps to avoid fatigue. Occasional sighs of frustration. Uses internal dialogue to relax; appetite and eating habits somewhat irregular; muscles feel slightly tense; constant reminder to rebalance wellness

Occupational				
Missing at least one day of work per week; cancelling sessions; not showing up for sessions; avoids meetings; avoids colleague at work; Leaves work early every day	Missing 2–3 days of work per month	Missing 1–2 days of work per month	May feel the need to take off 1–2 days of work per month	May feel the need to take off 1–2 days of work per month
Sick or cynical sense of humor	Rescheduling client appointments	Some avoidance of starting session on time	Has thoughts of client "no shows"	Thoughts of client "no shows"
Poor coping skills	Avoids meetings	Hope for client "no shows"	Occasionally makes excuses for leaving meetings early	Conducts sessions on time and for usual duration
Shows little resiliency	Avoids colleagues at work	Cuts session shorter than usual	Minimal contact with colleagues at work	Will make excuses for leaving meetings early
Difficulty separating professional and personal life	Leaves work early on average	Makes excuses to try and leave meetings and work early	Has difficulties transitioning to social self	Contact with colleagues less than usual
	Consistently cuts sessions short	Superficial contact with colleagues at work	Some difficulties separating professional and personal life	Exhibits usual sense of humor
	Exhibits cynical sense of humor	Exhibits inappropriate sense of humor	Better coping abilities and resiliencies	Difficulties transitioning to social self
	Difficulties separating professional and personal life	Some difficulties separating professional and personal life		Some difficulties separating professional and personal life
	Struggling	Some difficulties with coping abilities and resiliency		Better coping skills and resiliency
	Exhibiting decreased coping abilities and resiliency			

Source: Reprinted with permission from M. A. Stebnicki (2009b). Empathy fatigue: Assessing risk factors and cultivating self-care. In I. Marini, & M. A. Stebnicki (Eds.) *The professional counselor's desk reference* (pp. 813–830). New York: Springer Publishing.

counseling, psychology, mental health, and the biopsychosocial research in nursing and medicine.

This measure includes five levels of empathy fatigue experience. Level V indicates the highest level and Level I the lowest level of empathy fatigue. It is hypothesized that professional helpers may experience and project this unique professional fatigue experience in seven distinct areas: (1) cognitively, (2) behaviorally, (3) spiritually, (4) through process/counseling skills, (5) emotionally, (6) physically, and (7) occupationally. The GAEF may be used as a (1) self-rating measure by the professional helper, (2) rating measure by the therapists' clients, (3) rating measure used by the therapists' clinical supervisor or independent observer, and/or (4) ratings by other objective persons (e.g., peers). Accordingly, the rater would utilize the I–V rating scale within each of the content areas above. Undoubtedly, there will be potential for interaction effects because of the seven discrete areas in which the person may experience the phenomenon of empathy fatigue. Thus, it may be important for ratings to be taken at various times throughout the day, after client sessions, or other time-sampling points throughout the week.

As with all self-report measures, person(s) doing the rating should understand that there are limitations in rater objectivity and bias, as well as subjective rating of the individual's mood, affect, personality traits/states, levels of stress, attitude, motivation, level of satisfaction, and other measures of personal well-being. Overall, in its beginning stages of development, the GAEF may serve as a prevention screening measure for a phenomenon experienced by many professional helpers who work at intense levels with persons who have chronic illnesses and disabilities.

CONCLUSION

The experience of empathy fatigue is both similar and different from other types of counselor impairment or professional fatigue syndromes. Thus, it is hypothesized that the cumulative effects of multiple client sessions throughout the week may lead to a deterioration of the counselor's resiliency or coping abilities. Healing the minds, bodies, and spirits of professional counselors should be a collective responsibility among professional counseling associations, as well as counselor educators, clinical supervisors, and the counselor's work setting. One of the most troubling aspects of counselor impairment and fatigue syndromes is that counselor educators, supervisors, and professional counseling associations have been slow to prepare counselor trainees/supervisees for cultivating self-care approaches. We do a good job of preparing competent and ethical practitioners for diagnosing and treating a variety of mental health conditions and addressing other counseling related issues; however, the role and function of professional counselors have expanded significantly in the last 10 years. Today, many counselors provide mental health and disaster relief services to those involved in a multitude of extraordinary stressful and traumatic events (e.g., hurricanes, fires, floods, school shootings, workplace violence). Consequently, providing the mental health rescue to those at the epicenter of critical incidents profoundly affects the mind, body, and spirit of professional counselors.

Facilitating empathic approaches in the counseling relationship requires that we help our clients unfold the layers of their stress, grief, loss, or traumatic experiences by searching through their emotional scrapbooks. The search for personal meaning and purpose of our client's pain and suffering may contribute to our own spiritual fatigue experience. If counselors are mindful of this experience and view this as an opportunity for nurturing personal growth and development then they may create opportunities for resiliency so that they can replenish their wounded spirits.

REFERENCES

Bar-On, R., & Parker, J. D. (2000). *The handbook of emotional intelligence: Theory, development, assessment, and application at home, school, and in the workplace.* San Francisco: Jossey-Bass.

Barone, D. F., Hutchings, P. S., Kimmel, H. J., Traub, H. L., Cooper, J. T., & Marshal, C. M. (2005). Increasing empathic accuracy through practice and feedback in a clinical interviewing course. *Journal of Social and Clinical Psychology, 24*(2), 156–171.

Berger, R. M. (2006). Prayer: It does a body good. *Sojourners Magazine, 35*(2), 17.

Brothers, L. (1989). A biological perspective on empathy. *American Journal of Psychiatry, 146*(1), 1–16.

Corey, M. S., & Corey, G. (2003). *Becoming a helper* (4th ed.). Pacific Grove, CA: Group/Brooks/Cole.

Dean, C. (2003). Empathy, pornography, and suffering. *A Journal of Feminist Cultural Studies, 14*(1), 88–124.

Decolonizing Solidarity. (2011). *Decolonizing Solidarity.* Retrieved on July 22, 2011, from http://decolonizingsolidarity.blogspot.com/2011/03/solidarity-fatigue.html

Egan, G. (1998). *The skilled helper: A problem-management approach to helping* (6th ed.). Pacific Grove, CA: Brooks/Cole.

Figley, C. R. (1995). *Compassion fatigue: Coping with secondary traumatic stress disorder in those who treat the traumatized.* Bristol, PA: Brunner/Mazel.

Ibrahim, F. (1991). Contribution of cultural world view to generic counseling and development. *Journal of Counseling & Development, 70,* 13–19.

Ingerman, S. (1991). *Soul retrieval: Mending the fragmented self.* San Francisco: Harper San Francisco.

Ivey, A. E., & Ivey, M. B. (1999). *Intentional interviewing and counseling: Facilitating client development in a multicultural society.* Pacific Grove, CA: Brooks/Cole.

Joinson, C. (1992). Coping with compassion fatigue. *Nursing, 22*(4), 116–122.

Kabat-Zinn, J. (1990). *Full catastrophe living: Using the wisdom of your body and mind to face stress, pain, and illness.* New York: Dell.

Katz, R. L. (1963). *Empathy: Its nature and uses.* New York: Free Press.

Marci, C., Ham, J., Moran, E., & Orr, S. (2007). Physiologic correlates of perceived therapist empathy and social-emotional process during psychotherapy. *Journal of Nervous and Mental Disorders, 195,* 103–111.

Maslach, C. (1982). *The burnout: The cost of caring.* Englewood Cliffs, NJ: Prentice-Hall.

Maslach, C. (2003). *Burnout: The cost of caring.* Cambridge, MA: Malor Books.

Mayne, T. J., & Bonanno, G. A. (2001). *Emotions: Current issues and future directions.* New York: Guilford Press.

Mayne, T. J., & Ramsey, J. (2001). The structure of emotion: A nonlinear dynamic systems approach. In T. J. Mayne & G. A. Bonanno (Eds.), *Emotions: Current issues and future directions* (pp. 1–37). New York: Guilford Press.

McCann, L., & Perlman, L. A. (1989). Vicarious traumatization: A framework for understanding the psychological effects of working with victims. *Journal of Traumatic Stress, 3*(1), 131–149.

Nouwen, H. J. M. (1972). *The wounded healer.* New York: An Image Book/Doubleday.

Pedersen, P. (2000). *A handbook for developing multicultural awareness* (3rd ed.). Alexandria, VA: American Counseling Association.

Pert, C. B., Dreher, H. E., & Ruff, M. R. (2005). The psychosomatic network: Foundations of mind-body medicine. In M. Schlitz, T. Amorok, & M. Micozzi (Eds.), *Consciousness and healing: Integral approaches to mind-body medicine* (pp. 61–78). St. Louis, MO: Elsevier, Churchill, & Livingstone.

Phillips, K. (2011). Can social media relieve empathy fatigue? Retrieved July 20, 2011 from http://webcache.googleusercontent.com/search?q=cache:1XmE9w9NPQYJ:www.getlucid.net/blog/2011/03/can-social-media-relieve-empathy-fatigue/+empathy+fatigue&cd=28&hl=en&ct=clnk&gl=us&source=www.google.com

Ponterotto, J. G., & Bensesch, K. F. (1988). An organizational framework for understanding the role of culture in counseling. *Journal of Counseling & Development, 66,* 237–241.

Ridley, C. R. (1995). *Overcoming unintentional racism in counseling and therapy: A practitioner's guide to intentional intervention.* Thousand Oaks, CA: Sage.

Ridley, C. R., & Lingle, D. W. (1996). Cultural empathy in multicultural counseling: A multidimensional process model. In P. B. Pederson & J. G. Draguns (Eds.), *Counseling across cultures* (4th ed., pp. 21–46). Thousand Oaks, CA: Sage.

Rogers, C. R. (1951). *Client-centered therapy: Its current practice, implications, and theory.* Boston: Houghton Mifflin.

Rogers, C. R. (1957). The necessary and sufficient conditions of therapeutic personality change. *Journal of Consulting Psychology, 21,* 95–103.

Rogers, C. R. (1980). *A way of being*. Boston: Houghton Mifflin.

Sapolsky, R. M. (1998). *Why zebras don't get ulcers: An updated guide to stress, stress-related diseases, and coping*. New York: W. H. Freeman.

Stamm, B. H. (1995) *Compassion fatigue: Coping with secondary traumatic stress disorder in those who treat the traumatized*. New York: Brunner-Routledge.

Stebnicki, M. A. (1999, April). *Grief reactions among rehabilitation professionals: Dealing effectively with empathy fatigue*. Presentation made at the NRCA/ARCA Alliance Annual Training Conference, Dallas, TX.

Stebnicki, M. A. (2000). Stress and grief reactions among rehabilitation professionals: Dealing effectively with empathy fatigue. *Journal of Rehabilitation, 6*(1), 23–29.

Stebnicki, M. A. (2001). Psychosocial response to extraordinary stressful and traumatic life events: Principles and practices for rehabilitation counselors. *New Directions in Rehabilitation, 12*(6), 57–71.

Stebnicki, M. A. (2006). Integrating spirituality in rehabilitation counselor supervision. *Rehabilitation Education, 20*(2), 137–159.

Stebnicki, M. A. (2007). Empathy fatigue: Healing the mind, body, and spirit of professional counselors. *Journal of Psychiatric Rehabilitation, 10*(4), 317–338.

Stebnicki, M. A. (2008). *Empathy fatigue: Healing the mind, body, and spirit of professional counselors*. New York: Springer.

Stebnicki, M. A. (2009a). Empathy fatigue in the counseling profession. In I. Marini & M. A. Stebnicki (Eds.), *The professional counselor's desk reference* (pp.802–812). New York: Springer Publishing.

Stebnicki, M. A. (2009b). Empathy fatigue: Assessing risk factors and cultivating self-care. In I. Marini, & M. A. Stebnicki (Eds.), *The professional counselor's desk reference* (pp.813–830). New York: Springer Publishing.

Stebnicki, M. A. (2010). *Empathy fatigue: Healing the mind, body, and spirit of professional counselors*. Korean translation by Hakjisa Publisher, South Korea.

Tafoya, T. & Kouris, N. (2003). Dancing the circle: Native American concepts of healing. In S. G. Mijares (Ed.), *Modern psychology and ancient wisdom: Psychological healing practices from the world's religious traditions* (pp. 125–146). New York: Haworth Integrative Healing Press.

Thompson, A. (2011). *Empathy fatigue 2.0*. Retrieved July 23, 2011, from http://triblocal.com/wheaton/community/stories/2011/05/empathy-fatigue-2-0

Truax, C. B., & Carkhuff, R. R. (1967). *Towards effective counseling and psychotherapy*. Chicago: Aldine.

Wang, Y., Davidson, M. M., Yakushko, O. F., Bielstein Savoy, H., Tan, J. A., & Bleier, J. K. (2003). The scale of ethnocultural empathy: Development, validation, and reliability. *Journal of Counseling Psychology, 50*(2), 221–234.

Weil, A. (1995). *Spontaneous healing*. New York: Ballantine.

West, W. S. (2005). Crossing the line between talking therapies and spiritual healing. In R. Moodley & W. West (Eds.), *Integrating traditional healing practices into counseling and psychotherapy* (pp. 38–49). Thousand Oaks, CA: Sage.

Zaki, J. (2009). *Empathy fatigue and what the press can do about it*. Retrieved July 20, 2011, from http://webcache.googleusercontent.com/search?q=cache:JfvHLhbUUKIJ:www.huffingtonpost.com/jamil-zaki/empathy-fatigue-and-what_b_199361.html+empathy+fatigue&cd=3&hl=en&ct=clnk&gl=us&source=www.google.com

28

Obesity as a Disability: Medical, Psychosocial, and Vocational Implications

Maria G. Romero and Irmo Marini

Until recently, the American social condition of being overweight or obese had not received much attention from researchers or the media. The medical, psychosocial, and vocational implications of obesity have quickly moved to the forefront of study for researchers, counselors, and the medical community. Obesity is now considered the second leading cause of preventable death after cigarette smoking, and it is estimated that over 300,000 people die each year in the United States from obesity-related complications (Fontaine & Bartlett, 1998; Puhl & Brownell, 2001). In much greater numbers, however, are the rapidly growing secondary disabilities associated to obesity, which have direct, indirect, and personal costs to the individual and the community (Seidell, 1999). In the United States, where over $33 billion is spent by consumers each year on weight loss/management remedies and where less than 5% of the population is able to keep the weight off, it seems apparent this epidemic requires a greater understanding and better treatment alternatives (Seidell, 1999; Seligman, 1994).

In this chapter, a range of topics related to obesity including its prevalence, medical aspects, and associated complications are explored. Other relevant areas include the psychosocial factors pertaining to societal attitudes and individual mental health issues, vocational implications concerning work/wage discrimination, Social Security regulations, and Americans with Disabilities Act protections. The implications for rehabilitation counselors regarding vocational and mental health counseling are also discussed.

DEFINING OVERWEIGHT AND OBESITY

Before any issues related to being overweight or obese are discussed, it is important to understand the medical definitions of each. Obesity is determined by using the body mass index (BMI) in which a person's weight in kilograms is divided by height in meters squared. BMI is a measurement tool to determine a person's excess body weight and utilizes the following categories: overweight is a BMI of 25 kg/m² or more, obesity is a BMI of 30 kg/m² or greater, and severe obesity is BMI of 40 kg/m² or more. Consequently, a BMI under 18.5 kg/m² is defined as underweight, and a BMI between 18.5 and 24.9 is considered normal weight (Visscher & Seidell, 2001). BMI identifies persons considered to be at increased risk of weight-related disorders and premature death (Hunter, Reid, & Noble, 1998). Cross-sectional studies have also shown that a large waist circumference, considered to be in excess of 102 cm in men and 88 cm in women, is also associated with increased morbidity (Molarius

From *Journal of Applied Rehabilitation Counseling*, 2006, 37(1), 21-29. http://nrca-net.org/jarc_indices. html. Reprinted with permission from the National Rehabilitation Counseling Association.

& Seidell, 1998). The Metropolitan Life Insurance (MLI) Company tables have established mortality rates based on height and weight ratios. The MLI tables list mild obesity as being 20% to 40% over ideal weight, moderate obesity as 41% to 99% over ideal weight, and morbid obesity at 100% or more over ideal weight (Metropolitan Life, 1996). The MLI tables and BMI calculations can be found at www.halls.md/body-mass-index.

Aside from this mathematical definition, obesity is also defined as an excessively high amount of body fat or adipose tissue in relation to lean body mass (Centers for Disease Control [CDC], 2004). The amount of body fat (or adiposity) includes the distribution of fat throughout the body and the size of the adipose tissue deposits (CDC, 2004).

PREVALENCE

The sudden rise in the number of children and adults who are obese has led researchers to conclude that obesity has become an epidemic in the United States (Peters, Wyatt, Donahoo, & Hill, 2002). Obesity is not only the second leading cause of preventable death in the United States (Fontaine & Bartlett, 1998), its comorbidity with other diseases/disabilities makes it one of the most debilitating and costly disorders of the 21st century (American Obesity Association [AOA], 2004; Crossrow, Jeffery, & McGuire, 2001; Goodman & Whitaker, 2002; Li, et al., 2004; Mustillo et al., 2003). Despite the obvious health problems and severity of obesity and its complications, it is believed that the U.S. medical establishment and government have largely ignored the problem until recently (AOA, 2004; Gordon-Larson, 2001).

The incidence of obese persons has steadily increased during the past 25 years both in the United States and other countries (Puhl & Brownell, 2001). Obesity is described by the AOA (2004) as a disease that affects nearly one-third of the adult American population. In the United States approximately 127 million adults are overweight, 60 million are obese, and 9 million are severely obese.

Gender

In the past 25 years male obesity has increased from 13% to 20%, and female obesity has increased from 15% to 25%. The prevalence of being overweight is reported by the AOA to be higher for men than for women. The prevalence of obesity and severe obesity, however, is higher for women, 34% higher than men with obesity and 6.3% higher than men with severe obesity (AOA, 2004).

Ethnicity

A number of studies suggest that there is a higher prevalence of obesity among middle-aged Hispanic women of low socioeconomic status (Cantero, Richardson, Baezconde-Garbanati, & Marks, 1999; Winkleby, Gardner, & Taylor, 1996). Macdonald (1999) reported that over 66% of African American women, 64% of Mexican American women, and 64% of Mexican American men had a BMI of 25 or more. Neumark-Sztainer (1999), in their analysis of data between 1988 and 1994, noted ethnic differences among female children, finding that non-Hispanic Whites had the lowest incidence of obesity at 11.9%. They further found that 17.9% of African American and 15.8% of Mexican American female children were reportedly obese. Female adolescents had similar disparities, with non-Hispanic Whites at 9.6%, African Americans at 16.3%, and Mexican Americans at 14% during the same time period.

Age

Obesity among younger Americans has increased, especially with findings that obese children have a 79% likelihood of later becoming obese adults (AOA, 2004). Today's youth are considered the most inactive generation in history, in part because of less rigorous physical education programs offered in schools, the sedentary activities of television and video game playing, and the media blitz directed at children for cereals and fast food. The AOA reports that an estimated 30% of children ages 6 to 11 are overweight and 15% are obese, with similar numbers found for adolescents ages 12 to 19. Boys tend to be more overweight than girls, at 32% versus 27% (AOA, 2004).

MEDICAL IMPLICATIONS

The medical community has been reluctant to educate or dictate to patients the impact obesity has on the body (Cleator et al., 2002). In one study, nearly 50% of obese patients indicated that their physician had not recommended any treatment for weight loss and 75% reported that they had little or any faith in their physician to assist them with weight loss (Wadden et al., 2000; Wee, McCarthy, Davis, & Phillips, 1999). Relatedly, physicians have generally reported a negative bias toward overweight patients (Ajzen & Fishbein, 1977; Eagly & Chaiken, 1993; Teachman & Brownell, 2001). Indeed, physicians may not only perceive overweight and obese patients differently but some have also been found to spend less time with heavier patients (approximately 9 minutes) and have less of a desire to help them (Hebl & Xu, 2001). Hebl, Xu, and Mason (2003) found that although male overweight patients did not perceive their quality of care to be lower than that of non-overweight patients, female patients did perceive poorer quality care from their physicians.

Secondary Complications of Obesity

As noted earlier, the health effects of obesity make it the second leading cause of preventable death (Puhl & Brownell, 2001). Independent of this, however, are the tens of millions of persons at risk of developing more serious chronically disabling conditions. The AOA (2004) reports that obesity is associated with more than 30 medical conditions with very strong evidence linked with at least 15 secondary conditions. The highest prevalence ratio is linked with high blood pressure where essentially the heavier one is, the greater the likelihood of having this condition. The AOA reports that over 75% of hypertension cases can be directly attributed to obesity, and the risk of developing hypertension is five to six times greater than that in non-obese individuals between 20 and 45 years of age (AOA, 2004; Diamanti-Kandarakis & Bergiele, 2001). Hypertension related to obesity has been found across all age and ethnic groups, gender, and socioeconomic status. Hypertension is further related to cardiovascular disease due to blood lipid levels (triglycerides or bad cholesterol—low-density lipoproteins) and eventually coronary heart disease across all groups.

The incidence of coronary heart disease follows the same prevalence trajectory as hypertension in that the higher an individual's BMI, the higher the percentage of reported coronary heart disease. For example, the prevalence of coronary heart disease among women with a BMI of 18.5 to 24.9 is 6.87%, whereas the prevalence among women with a BMI of greater than 40 is 19.22% (National Health and Nutrition Examination Survey [NHANES] III, 1988–1994). Other circulatory-related disorders associated with obesity include chronic venous insufficiency, deep vein thrombosis, and stroke.

A third strong risk factor with high prevalence rates related to obesity is type 2 diabetes (NHANES III, 1988–1994). The AOA (2004) projects that as many as 90% of persons with type 2 diabetes are overweight or obese, and this is especially true for certain minority groups such as Hispanics and American Indians. As the BMI index rises in size, there is a proportionate increase in the percentage of persons with diabetes. Obesity has been found to be the strongest environmental influence for type 2 diabetes onset (AOA, 2004). The medical ramifications of obesity with diabetes are that obesity increases insulin resistance thereby making drug treatment less effective.

A fourth major complication of obesity is the effect of excessive weight on the body's musculoskeletal system leading to a higher prevalence of osteoarthritis (NHANES III, 1988–1994). Prevalence percentages for persons with a BMI greater than 40 are 17% for women and 10% for men. Obesity has been correlated with the development of osteoarthritis in the back, knees, hips, and hands. It has also been associated with rheumatoid arthritis, carpal tunnel syndrome, low back pain, joint pain, and heel spurs (AOA, 2004; Onyike, Crum, Lee, Lyketsos, & Eaton, 2003; Visscher & Seidell, 2001).

Finally, there are a host of other complications that have been associated with obesity including mental health issues (primarily depression and anxiety), pancreatitis, sleep apnea, urinary stress incontinence, chronic odor, liver disease, impaired immune response, impaired respiratory function, gallbladder disease, and a variety of cancers including breast cancer, esophagus and gastric cancer, colorectal cancer, endometrial cancer, and renal cell cancer (AOA, 2004; Mustillo et al., 2003; Onyike et al., 2003; Palinkas, Wingard & Barrett-Connor, 1996; Ross, 1994; Visscher & Seidell, 2001).

PSYCHOSOCIAL IMPLICATIONS OF OBESITY

Societal Attitudes

Negative societal attitudes toward persons who are obese begin for those persons at a generally young age. Early research indicated that children as young as age 6 describe obese children as lazy, dirty, stupid, ugly, and cheaters (Staffieri, 1967). Current research on obesity indicates that there remains a "widespread, culturally acceptable stereotype and negative attitude of obese people" (Crossrow, Jeffery, & Mcguire, 2001, p. 208) and that culture determines what is attractive. Other research findings have shown that being obese is associated with negative attitudes such as being aesthetically unpleasant to look at (Wooley & Wooley, 1979), morally and emotionally impaired (Keys, 1955), and alienated from their sexuality (Millman, 1980). The implications of such attitudes can lead to prejudice and discrimination, in part due to a largely held belief that obesity is something that is controllable and that persons who are overweight are lazy and weak willed (Myers & Rosen, 1999; Wadden & Stunkard, 1985). This perception elicits the concept of attribution of blame on the individual and/or the family for not being strong enough to control the problem (Gordon-Larsen, 2001; Neumark-Sztainer, 1999; Puhl & Brownell, 2001). Although there is evidence that obesity is part genetically and part environmentally caused, most laypersons continue to believe obesity to be largely environmentally based (Neumark-Sztainer, 1999). Puhl and Brownell (2003) note how attributional explanations of weight stigma are related to the Protestant work ethic and "just world bias" (p. 216) in blaming the individual. This attitude tends to be more prevalent in cultures that promote individualism and thinness.

Employer Attitudes

Although the implications of employer discrimination toward persons who are obese are discussed later, suffice it to note that employer discrimination against overweight or obese persons is found at virtually all stages of employment including hiring (Klesges, et al., 1990), placement (Bellizzi, Klassen, & Belonax, 1989), compensation (Register & Williams, 1990), promotion (Bordieri, Drehmer, & Taylor, 1997), discipline (Bellizzi & Norvell, 1991), and discharge (Kennedy & Homant, 1984). Klesges et al.'s (1990) laboratory study found that even though qualified overweight candidates were mostly preferred over unqualified normal-weight candidates, overweight candidates were most often assessed with qualities such as lacking self-control and discipline, being depressed, and having an offensive appearance. Other studies have suggested that employers perceive that obese job applicants lack self-discipline, have low supervisory potential, are less ambitious, and lack poor personal hygiene and appearance (Larkin & Pines, 1979; Rothblum, Miller, & Garbutt, 1988).

Mental Health

Although obesity has been associated with physical and chronic medical conditions fairly consistently, the effect that obesity has on severe psychiatric disorders is more contradictory (Onyike, et al., 2003; Wadden & Stunkard, 1985). It has not been shown that overweight persons have any more serious psychological disturbance than the general population (Wadden & Stunkard, 1985). Conversely, Fontaine and Bartlett (1998) indicate that it is well known that obesity has a negative impact on health and has an effect on other important aspects of life. Obesity has been closely associated with depression, eating disorders in children and adults, and behavior problems among children such as oppositional defiant disorder (Burrows & Cooper, 2002; Li et al. 2003; Onyike et al., 2003). Studies have shown both positive and negative correlations between depression and obesity (Crisp, Queenan, Sittampaln, & Harris, 1980; Palinkas et al., 1996; Paykel, 1977). Palinkas et al. (1996), however, discuss the concept of "jolly fat," which proposes that obese people are jolly and not depressed. This hypothesis stems from the theory that the dietary habits of obese persons may protect them against depression, anxiety, and dysphoria.

Since an individual's perception about himself or herself is to a degree influenced by the attitudes of others, overweight individuals "may suffer low self-esteem, have negative self-images, think others dislike them, and thus have high levels of depression" (Ross, 1994, p. 64). Wadden and Stunkard (1985) indicate that although it is believed that being overweight and obese are closely linked to emotional disturbance, recent research has suggested that disturbances among individuals may in some cases be the consequence of obesity and the social prejudice and discrimination that are demonstrated against them (Puhl & Brownell, 2003). Li et al. (2003) indicates, however, that societal attitudes toward obesity and its impact on individuals are culture specific.

Self-Esteem

In Western societies where billions of dollars in advertising are spent annually on the rewards of being thin, the stigmatization of being obese can impact an individual's self-esteem and radically change their behavior in quest for the glorified, yet often unrealistic, perfect body (Carlisle-Duncan & Robinson, 2004; Seligman, 1994). Self-esteem is regarded as a socially derived state, such as when a person who is obese does not measure up to society's view of thinness, which can cost them potential employment and marital opportunities (Klesges et al., 1990; Pingitore, Dugoni, & Tindale, 1994; Sobal, 1984). Although some studies show being obese does not affect one's level of self-esteem (Grilo, Wilfley, Brownell, & Rodin, 1994), other studies suggest that self-esteem is indeed impacted (Burrows & Cooper, 2002; Goodman & Whitaker, 2002; Gordon-Larsen, 2001; Lumeng, Gannon, Cabral, Frank, & Zuckerman, 2003; Miller, Rothblum, Brand, & Felicio, 1995; Mustillo et al., 2003).

Miller and Downey (1999) suggest that gender is the factor that determines how weight affects self-esteem. In the United States, the standards of thinness are more extreme for women than they are for men and self-esteem may be more of an important aspect for women than for men (Grilo et al., 1994). Women are more dissatisfied with their bodies than are men and are more likely to work hard toward achieving the thin ideal (Jambekar, Quinn, & Crocker, 2001). They are also more likely to diet, suffer from eating disorders (Miller & Downey, 1999), and feel poorly about themselves when they cannot achieve the thin ideal (Jambekar et al., 2001).

Socioeconomic Status

There is some evidence to suggest that obesity may be more prevalent among those of lower socioeconomic status and with lower levels of education, factors which tend to be inter-related (Averett & Korenman, 2001; Gordon-Larsen, 2001; Gortmaker, Walker, Weitzman, & Sobol, 1990; Rosmond & Björntorp, 1999). There also appears to be a stronger relationship of obesity among women in comparison to men in relation to socioeconomic status from traditionally being paid less in the workforce. Researchers hypothesize a cycle of low educa-tion associated with lower paying jobs, and lower income is further associated with poorer food and nutritional consumption behavior including the inexpensiveness of the more fatty foods (Averett & Korenman, 2001; Rosmond & Björntorp, 1999). This cycle is further influ-enced by employer discrimination toward persons who are overweight or obese in that if they are not skilled or educated, women more so than men, are hired in lower paying jobs if they are hired at all (Macdonald, 1999; Pagan & Davila, 1997; Roehling, 1999). When ethnicity is considered, there are numerous studies indicating a high prevalence of obesity among middle-aged Hispanic and African American women of low socioeconomic status (Winkleby et al., 1996).

Fat Pride

In 1969, the National Association to Advance Fat Acceptance (NAAFA) was established with the overall objective of improving the quality of life for fat people. Its mission is to eliminate discrimination based on body size, self empower overweight persons, educate its members on nutritional information, and support for improving self-image and being comfortable with one's body size (NAAFA, 1994). NAAFA believes its mission is similar to that of the civil rights movement and other related movements, and although changing attitudes has been slow, business marketing trends are catering more to oversized persons as evident in their magazines and commercials.

VOCATIONAL IMPLICATIONS

The issue of weight discrimination in employment has received greater interest over the past several years due to the growing increase in the incidences of obesity, the greater number of lawsuits based on weight discrimination, and employer concerns about health care–related costs (Johnson & Wilson, 1995; Lippman, 1998; Taussig, 1994; Zablocki, 1998). This section explores existing legislative protections concerning employment discrimina-tion of persons who are obese and existing evidence toward prevalence of employment discrimination.

Legislative Protections

Two relevant areas fall within this purview: protections set forth from the Rehabilitation Act of 1973 (RHA) and protections from Title I of the Americans with Disabilities Act (ADA) of 1990. The Social Security Administration follows the Clinical Guidelines in the classifica-tion of obesity utilizing the BMI described earlier.

Prior to October 1999, obesity was considered an impairment in which applicants for benefits could be awarded solely for being obese (Federal Register, 2002). Subsequent to the October 1999 ruling deleting obesity as a primary disabling condition, the administra-tion added paragraphs to the prefaces of musculoskeletal, respiratory, and cardiovascular body system listings, reminding adjudicators that the effects of obesity secondary to other impairments can have a greater impact on functioning than by considering each impair-ment separately. Despite the ruling, however, obesity can still "equal" (classify as disabled) a listing by itself if it is classified as "severe" in addition to considering an individual's age, education, and past work history (Federal Register, 2002). Unfortunately, as shown by its definition, there is no specific BMI level that differentiates between "severe" and "nonsevere" obesity. As such, Administrative Law Judges have much discretion in deciding what is severe. Generally, there will have to be some other disabling condition such as musculoskeletal, respiratory, or heart condition that significantly limits the individual completing activities of daily living (Roehling, 1999).

Regarding other federal protection under ADA or RHA, both have parallel definitions of disability and neither law specifically mentions obesity is a disability. Instead, both laws define an individual with a disability as someone with a mental or physical impairment that substantially limits one or more major life activities. Legally, the courts have consistently ruled using the Equal Employment Opportunity Commission regulations that coverage of obesity as a disability will be considered a rare occurrence. To establish obesity as a disability, two factors must be met: obesity was caused by a physiological condition and the employee must be morbidly obese or 100% over his ideal body weight (*Cook v. Rhode Island, 1993*). This requirement is, of course, extremely difficult to prove, and statistically less than 1% of Americans are considered morbidly obese (Rodin, 1993). Even when plaintiffs can show a physiological cause for morbid obesity, the Supreme Court has ruled that ADA definitions of disability do not cover conditions that are medically correctable as obesity arguably can be (*Albertson's Inc. v. Kirkingburg, 1999; Murphy v. United Parcel Service, 1999*).

Although there appears to be scant protection for obesity discrimination in employment, there are two additional laws that can be more favorable for those filing employment discrimination lawsuits. The first is "perceived disability," which stems from the ADA and RHA definitions considering an employee who is "regarded as" disabled. In the 1993 *Cook v. Rhode Island* decision, the plaintiff did not have to prove he had a disability, but rather that the employer perceived he had one (i.e., regarded as) and was suffering from a weight condition and assumed he could not perform the functions of the job.

Other protections fall under Title VII of the 1964 Civil Rights Act addressing "disparate treatment and disparate impact" categories of discrimination (*Gerdom v. Continental Airlines, Inc. 1982*). The first refers to cases where an employer treats some employees differently as apparent in the Continental Airlines case where the court determined that the airline's hire/fire policies treated employees differently based on gender due to differences in male versus female flight attendant weight restriction policies. This disparate treatment category also takes into consideration whether the established job requiring characteristic (slender female flight attendants) is a bona fide occupational qualification. If an employer can prove that having heavier female flight attendants will somehow hurt their business, then they are not obligated to hire the individual. The disparate impact discrimination category refers to whether an employer's hiring policies have a disparate impact on a designated group of people based on gender, age, or race. If, for example, an employer wanted to hire exclusively males, however, had no bona fide occupational qualification as to how the business might be negatively impacted by hiring women, the employer would be liable under the disparate impact category of discrimination (Roehling, 1999).

Prevalence of Employment Discrimination

Discrimination against overweight employees occurs in the employment arena as well involving hiring, promotion, termination, and insurance coverage (Bordieri, Drehmer, & Taylor, 1997; Klesges et al., 1990; Register & Williams, 1990). Despite the fact that over 99% of persons who are overweight or obese are not protected or recognized under existing disability legislation, research in this area continues to show a link between employment discrimination and obesity irrespective of court rulings (Roehling, 1999).

Lang (2002) reported that Caucasian women who weighed an average of 65 lbs more earned approximately 7% less than their slimmer coworkers; however, no significant differences existed among minority women. Gortmaker et al. (1993) found that obese women earned approximately $6,700 less than slender women. Haskins and Ransford (1999) studied the relationship between weight and career payoffs among 306 women and found that weight had no effect on income when education, length of service, and age were controlled. It did, however, have an effect on level of career access, with 65% of the thinner women holding professional and managerial positions compared with only 39% of the overweight women. For blue-collar workers, a reverse trend was observed. There are also reported cases where overweight employees must pay higher health-care premiums (Paul & Townsend, 1995), are denied benefits altogether due to their weight, or are terminated because of their weight (Rothblum, Brand, Miller, & Oetjen, 1990).

Evidence also suggests that persons who are overweight or obese are disadvantaged in not only being hired but also the type of position they may be hired for (Puhl & Brownell, 2001). Several studies note when business students or managers are asked to rate identical candidates' resumes, overweight persons are often not selected for the job, or they are hired in less desirable positions (Decker, 1987; Klassen, Jasper, & Harris, 1993; Larkin & Pines, 1979; Rothblum, et al., 1988).

COUNSELING IMPLICATIONS

The implications of working with persons who are obese or overweight may be broken down into mental health counseling and/or vocational counseling. Although each of these is discussed separately, it is important to note that clients may come in for assistance with overlapping concerns.

Mental Health Counseling

Although a relationship between obesity and psychiatric disorders such as depression is not well established, there are several studies that indicate depression to be most consistently correlated with severe obesity in women (Carpenter, Hasin, Allison, & Faith, 2000; Noppa & Hallstrom, 1981; Roberts, Kaplan, Shema, & Strawbridge, 2000). Since, however, other chronic medical conditions related to obesity such as diabetes, arthritis, or musculoskeletal pain often coexist with obesity, it is difficult to distinguish what role obesity itself has with depression (Katon & Ciechanowski; 2002; Katon & Sullivan, 1990). Other possible coexisting contributors that can impact individual's mental health previously discussed include unemployment or underemployment in lower paying jobs (Bordieri, Drehmer, & Taylor, 1997; Pagan & Davila, 1997), lower socioeconomic status (Sobal & Stunkard, 1989), and being discriminated against in employment, by family members, and treating medical professionals (Adams, Hicken, & Salehi, 1988; Crandall, 1995; Price, Desmond, Krol, Snyder, & O'Connell, 1987; Teachman & Brownell, 2001).

In working with the mental health needs of persons who are obese, Olkin (1999) has advocated for disability-affirmative therapy whereby counselors must explore their own biases and beliefs about obesity, recognize and acknowledge the inequity and discrimination directed at those who are obese, and view the counseling process from a social construct approach that does not attribute blame to the individual, but rather stems from negative societal attitudes. It is also important that counselors do not make a client's size the salient issue in counseling. Automatically assuming a client's size is the cause of his/her problems and can not only derail establishing rapport but also offend the client (Rush, 1998). Olkin (1999) recommends directly asking clients whether they perceive their medical condition has an impact as to their seeking counseling. In situations where this is the case, cognitive reframing can be an excellent strategy in changing a client's perspective in placing a lesser value on his/her physique and instead focusing on other positive interpersonal attributes (Leahy, 2001; Wright, 1983).

Additional strategies counselors can use where clients' weight is a precipitating factor in their mental health could include behavior modification, rational emotive therapy, reality therapy, support groups, and bibliotherapy. Behavior modification strategies could focus around establishing a baseline for eating behavior, times of day, diary recording what one's affect is like prior to/after eating (i.e., anxious, stressed, sad), and subsequently replacing eating behaviors for healthier behaviors (Spiegeler & Guevremont, 1998). Rational emotive therapy could be effective in changing clients' perceptions toward building self-esteem; however, they should recognize that many of their beliefs about being discriminated against are likely true and must be validated by the counselor (Ellis & Maclaren, 1998; Wessler & Wessler, 1988). Reality therapy again must be used with caution in that it assumes individual responsibility for one's situation (Glasser, 2000). Support groups or group counseling can be effective in helping clients to validate each others' perceptions regarding discrimination, motivating each other to overcome their difficulties, and providing friendship in situations outside of the group (Jacobs, Masson, & Harvill, 2002). Finally, bibliotherapy can be effective in educating clients across a gambit of areas including weight control, exercise, and eating behaviors.

Vocational Counseling

In vocational counseling where obesity is a factor, counselors again must first acknowledge the fact that employer discrimination does exist and empower clients if relevant with information about legislation involving disparate treatment and disparate impact. As with counseling other persons with disabilities, clients who are obese should be encouraged to focus on what their qualifications are to perform jobs. Counselors and clients must also work together in dispelling myths and misconceptions about overweight employees.

In assessing clients with obesity for vocational opportunities, it is important to know whether there are other secondary disabilities such as respiratory, musculoskeletal, diabetes, or heart disease problems. This would typically be detailed in client medical records and should be verified as to severity with the client regarding functional limitations. With this in mind, counselors have a better understanding of client's physical capabilities in performing work and in conducting a transferable skills analysis. Client education, past work experience, occupational interests, and age play a significant role in successfully placing clients. Typically, higher level of education generally corresponds with work that is less physically demanding. For those clients with lower levels of education (i.e., less than grade 12), counselors should explore the unskilled, sedentary, and light levels of work that are generally less strenuous. Such positions may include video surveillance monitor, parking lot attendant, ticket taker, garment sorter, clothing or other production inspectors, machine operators, assembly workers, and file clerks. Those clients with higher levels of education are generally easier to place in less physically demanding jobs and have been shown in the literature to be less discriminated against by employers when they are qualified (Klesges et al., 1990).

Vocational counseling should also encompass any perceived anxiety clients who are obese may have regarding employment. Although ability to perform the job would generally not be a concern for qualified clients, dealing with negative or stereotypical attitudes of employers and coworkers may carry some trepidation. Clients can be empowered by role-playing mock job interviews by teaching clients to focus on strengths/assets to perform the job, to know their rights, and to convey these in a nonthreatening manner to employers. Being prepared to respond appropriately to possible coworker degradation comments would also be beneficial to practice as well. Similarly, client's self-esteem may be enhanced by refocusing cognitions of self-worth away from physique/physical appearance, and direct cognitions more toward one's abilities to perform the work.

Finally, counselors may benefit from being familiar with the stages of change theory. Some clients may not perceive having a problem and therefore obesity may be viewed as an addictive behavior. Miller and Rollnick (2004) describe the stages from precontemplation (not acknowledging a problem), contemplation (suspecting a problem however being unsure as to wanting to change), determination (making a cognitive decision to change), action (engaging in change behaviors), maintenance/exit, or in some cases relapse. Understanding motivational interviewing can assist counselors in helping clients to move toward recognizing and developing a more healthy lifestyle.

SUMMARY

Obesity and related medical complications have soared to the forefront of medical conditions that lead to premature death, discrimination in employment, compromised quality of life, and negative psychosocial implications. Its prevalence is statistically found across all groups and ages, particularly so among persons of minority and low socioeconomic status. The impact of being obese affects individuals in a number of nonmedical ways as well: being the subject of negative societal attitudes and affecting one's self-esteem, the type of job one obtains, and potentially one's mental health. Counselors who are aware of the medical, psychosocial, and vocational implications of obesity can assist clients in a variety of ways keeping Olkin's (1999) recommendations in mind regarding disability-affirmative therapy. Although legislatively obesity is not recognized for over 99% of its arguable population, research has shown this stigmatized group is nevertheless discriminated against as any other minority group might be. As such, it would benefit rehabilitation counselors to be well prepared to work with this ever-increasing population.

REFERENCES

Adams, G. R., Hicken, M., & Salehi, M. (1988). Socialization of the physical attractiveness stereotype: Parental expectations and verbal behaviors. *International Journal of Psychology, 23*, 137–149.

Ajzen, I., & Fishbein, M. (1977). Attitude-behavior relations: A theoretical analysis and review of empirical research. *Psychological Bulletin, 84*, 888–918.

Albertsons, Inc. v. Kirkingburg, 199 S. Ct. 2162 (1999).

American Obesity Association. (2004, October 13). Retrieved October 30, 2004, from http://www.obesity.org/sub/fastfacts/obesity_US.shiml

Averett, S., & Korenman, S. (2001). The economic reality of the beauty myth. *The Journal of Human Resources, 31*, 304–330.

Bellizzi, J. A., Klassen, M. L., & Belonax, J. J. (1989). Stereotypical beliefs about overweight and smoking and decision making in assignments to sales territories. *Perceptual and Motor Skills, 69*, 419–429.

Bellizzi, J. A., & Norvell, D. W. (1991). Personal characteristics and salesperson's justifications as moderators of supervisory discipline in cases involving unethical sales force behavior. *Journal of the Academy of Marketing Science, 19*, 11–16.

Blouw, E. L., Rudolph, A. D., Narr, B. J., & Sarr, M. G. (2003). The frequency of respiratory failure in patients with morbid obesity undergoing gastric bypass. *American Association of Nurse Anesthetists Journal, 71*(1), 45–50.

Bordieri, J. E., Drehemer, D. E., & Taylor, D. W. (1997). Work life for employees with disabilities: Recommendations for promotion. *Rehabilitation Counseling Bulletin, 40*, 181–191.

Burrows, A., & Cooper, M. (2002). Possible risk factors in the development of eating disorders in overweight pre-adolescent girls. *International Journal of Obesity, 26,* 1268–1273.

Cantero, P. J., Richardson, J. L., Baezconde-Garbanti, L., & Marks, G. (1999). The association between acculturation and health practices among middle-aged and elderly Latinas. *Ethnicity & Disease, 9,* 166–180.

Carlisle-Duncan, M., & Robinson, T. T. (2004). Obesity and body ideals in the media: Health and fitness practices of young African-American women. *Quest, 56,* 77–104.

Carpenter, K. M., Hasin, D. S., Allison, D. B., & Faith, M. S. (2000). Relationships between obesity and DSM-IV major depressive disorder, suicide ideation, and suicide attempts: Results from a general population study. *American Journal of Public Health, 90,* 251–257.

Centers for Disease Control and Prevention. (2004, June 24). Overweight and obesity (n.d.). *Nutrition and Physical Activity.* Retrieved October 29, 2004, from http://www.cdc.gov /nccdphp/dnpa/obesity/index. htm

Cleator, J., Richman, E., Leong, K. S., Mawdsley, L., White, S., & Wilding, J. (2002). Obesity: Under-diagnosed and under-treated in hospital outpatient departments. *International Journal of Obesity, 26,* 581–584.

Cook v. Rhode Island Department of Mental Health, 10F.2d 17, 2AD 1476(1ˢᵗ Cir. 1993).

Crandall, C. S. (1995). Do parents discriminate against their heavy-weight daughters? *Personality and Social Psychology Bulletin, 21,* 724–735.

Crisp, A. H., Queenan, M., Sittampaln, Y., & Harris, G. (1980). "Jolly fat" revisited. *Journal of Psychosomatic Research, 24,* 233–241.

Crossrow, N. H. F., Jeffery, R. W., & McGuire, M. T. (2001). Understanding weight stigmatization: A focus group study. *Journal of Nutrition Education, 33*(4), 208–214.

Decker, W. H. (1987). Attributions based on managers' self-presentation, sex, and weight. *Psychological Reports, 61,* 175–181.

Diamanti-Kandarakis, E., & Bergiele, A. (2001). The influence of obesity on hyperandrogenism and infertility in the female. *Obesity Reviews, 2,* 231–238.

Eagly, A., & Chaiken, S. (1993). *The impact of attitudes on behaviors. The psychology of attitudes.* London: Harcourt Brace.

Ellis, A., & Maclaren, C. (1998). *Rational emotive behavior therapy: A therapist guide.* San Luis Obispo, CA: Impact.

Federal Register. (September 12, 2002). SSR 02–01 p: Policy ruling Titles II and XVI.

Fontaine, K. R., & Bartlett, S. J. (1998). Estimating health-related quality of life in obese individuals. *Disease Management & Health Outcomes, 3*(2), 61–70.

Gerdom v. Continental Airlines, Inc., 692, 30 FEP 235 (9ᵗʰ Cir. 1982; en banc), cert denied, 460 U.S. 1074 (1983).

Glasser, W. (2000). *Reality therapy in action.* New York: HarperCollins.

Goodman, E., & Whitaker, R. C. (2002). A prospective study of the role of depression in the development and persistence of adolescent obesity. *Pediatrics, 109*(3), 497–504.

Gordon-Larsen, P. (2001). Obesity-related knowledge, attitudes, and behaviors in obese and non-obese urban Philadelphia female adolescents. *Obesity Research, 9*(2), 112–118.

Gortmaker, S., Walker, D., Weitzman, M., & Sobol, A. (1990). Chronic conditions, socioeconomic risks, and behavioral problems in children and adolescents. *Pediatrics, 85,* 267–276.

Grilo, C. M., Wilfley, D. E., Brownell, K. D., & Rodin, J. (1994). Teasing, body image, and self-esteem in a clinical sample of obese women. *Addictive Behaviors, 19*(4), 443–450.

Haskins, K. M., & Ransford, H. E. (1999). The relationship between weight and career payoffs among women. *Sociological Forum, 14*(2), 295–318.

Hebl, M., & Xu, J. (2001). Weighing the care: Physicians' reactions to the size of a patient. *International Journal of Obesity Related Metabolic Disorders, 25,* 1246–1252.

Hebl, M., Xu, J., & Mason, M. (2003). Weighing the care: Patients' perceptions of physician are as a function of gender and weight. *International Journal of Obesity, 27,* 269–275.

Hunter, J. D., Reid, C., & Noble, D. (1998). Anesthetic management of the morbidly obese patient. *Hospital Medicine, 59,* 481–483.

Jacobs, E. E., Masson, R. L., & Harvill, R. L. (2002). *Group counseling: Strategies and skills* (4th ed.). Pacific Grove, CA: Brooks/Cole.

Jambekar, S., Quinn, D. M., & Crocker, J. (2001). The effects of weight and achievement messages on the self-esteem of women. *Psychology of Women Quarterly, 25,* 48–56.

Johnson, T., & Wilson, M. C. (1995, April). An analysis of weight-based discrimination: Obesity as a disability. *Labor Law Journal,* 238–244.

Katon, W., & Ciechanowski, P. (2002). Impact of major depression on chronic mental illness. *Journal of Psychosomatic Research, 53,* 859–863.

Katon, W., & Sullivan, M. D. (1990). Depression and chronic medical illness. *Journal of Clinical Psychiatry, 51*(Suppl.), 3–11.

Kennedy, D. B., & Homant, R. J. (1984). Personnel managers and the stigmatized employee. *Journal of Employment Counseling, 21,* 89–94.

Keys, A. (1955). Obesity and heart disease. *Journal of Chronic Diseases, 1,* 456–460.

Klassen, M. L., Jasper, C. R., & Harris, R. J. (1993). The role of physical appearance in managerial decisions. *Journal of Business and Psychology, 8,* 181–198.

Klesges, R. C., Klem, M. L., Hanson, C. L., Eck, L. H., Ernst, J., O'Laughlin, D., et al. (1990). The effects of applicant's health status and qualifications on simulated hiring decisions. *Journal of Obesity, 14,* 527–535.

Larkin, J. C., & Pines, H. A. (1979). No fat persons need apply: Experimental studies of the overweight stereotype and hiring preference. *Sociology of Work Occupations, 6,* 312–327.

Leahy, R. L. (2001). *Overcoming resistance in cognitive therapy.* New York: Guilford Press.

Li, Z. B., Ho, S. Y., Chan, W. M., Ho, K. S., Li, M. P, Leung, G. M., et al. (2004). Obesity and depressive symptoms in Chinese elderly. *International Journal of Geriatric Psychiatry, 19,* 68–74.

Lipman, H. (1998). Courts weigh in on obesity. *Business and Health, 63,* 53–54.

Lumeng, J. C., Gannon, K., Cabral, H. J., Frank, D. A., & Zuckerman, B. (2003). Association between clinically meaningful behavior problems and overweight in children. *Pediatrics, 112*(5), 1138–1145.

Macdonald, S. M. (1999). Obesity: Worldwide prevalence and trend. *Healthy Weight Journal, 13*(6), 84–92.

Metropolitan Life Insurance Company. (1996). *Weigh in!* New York: Author.

Miller, C. T., & Downey, K. T. (1999). A meta-analysis of heavy-weight and self-esteem. *Personality and Social Psychology Review, 3*(1), 68–84.

Miller, C. T., Rothblum, E. D., Brand, P. A., & Felicio, D. M. (1995). Do obese women have poorer relationships than nonobese women? Reports by self, friends, and coworkers. *Journal of Personality, 63*(1), 65–85.

Miller, R. W., & Rollnick, S. (2004). *Motivational interviewing: Preparing people for change.* New York: Guilford Press.

Millman, M. (1980). *Such a pretty face: Being fat in America.* New York: Norton.

Molarius, A., & Seidell, J. C. (1998). Selection of anthropometric indicators for classification of abdominal fatness—A critical review. *International Journal of Obesity, 22,* 719–727.

Murphy v. United Parcel Service, 119 S. Ct. 2133 (1999).

Mustillo, S., Worthman, C., Erkanli, A., Keeler, G., Angold, A, & Costello, E. J. (2003). Obesity and psychiatric disorder: Developmental trajectories. *Pediatrics, 111*(4), 851–859.

Myers, A., & Rosen, J. C. (1999). Obesity stigmatization and coping: Relation to mental health symptoms, body image, and self-esteem. *International Journal of Obesity, 23,* 221–230.

National Association to Advance Fat Acceptance. (1994). *Fighting size discrimination and prejudice.* Sacramento, CA: Author.

National Health and Nutrition Examination Survey (1988–1994). National Center for Health Statistics. Plan and operation of the Third National Health and Nutrition Examination Survey, 1988–1994. Series III: Programs and collection procedures. *Vital Health Stat, 1* 1994:1–407.

Neumark-Sztainer, D. (1999). The weight dilemma: A range of philosophical perspectives. *International Journal of Obesity, 23,* S31–S37.

Noppa, H., & Hallstrom, T. (1981). Weight gain in adulthood in relation to socioeconomic factors, mental illness and personality traits: A prospective study of middle-aged women. *Journal of Psychosomatic Research, 25,* 83–89.

Olkin, R. (1999). *What psychotherapists should know about disability.* New York: Guilford Press.

Onyike, C. U., Crum, R. M., Lee, H. B., Lyketsos, C. G., & Eaton, W. W. (2003). Is obesity associated with major depression? Results from the third national health and nutrition examination survey. *American Journal of Epidemiology, 158*(23), 1139–1147.

Pagan, J. A., & Davila, A. (1997). Obesity, occupational attainment, and earnings. *Social Science Quarterly, 78,* 756–770.

Palinkas, L. A., Wingard, D. L., & Barrett-Connor, E. (1996). Depressive symptoms in overweight and obese older adults: A test of the "jolly fat" hypothesis. *Journal of Psychosomatic Research, 40*(1), 59–66.

Paul, R. J., & Townsend, J. B. (1995). Shape up or ship out? Employment discrimination against the overweight. *Employee Responsibilities Rights Journal, 8,* 133–145.

Paykel, E. S. (1977). Depression and appetite. *Journal of Psychosomatic Research, 21,* 401–407.

Peters, J. C., Wyatt, H. R., Donahoo, W. T., & Hill, J. O. (2002). From instinct to intellect: The challenge of maintaining healthy weight in the modern world. *Obesity Reviews, 3,* 69–74.

Pingitore, R., Dugoni, B. L., & Tindale, R. (1994). Bias against overweight job applicants in a simulated employment interview. *Journal of Applied Psychology, 79,* 909–917.

Price, J. H., Desmond, S. M., Krol, R. A., Snyder, F. F., & O'Connell, J. K. (1987). Family practice physicians' beliefs, attitudes, and practices regarding obesity. *American Journal of Preventive Medicine, 3,* 339–345.

Puhl, R. M., & Brownell, K. D. (2001). Bias, discrimination, and obesity. *Obesity Research, 9,* 788-805.

Puhl, R. M., & Brownell, K. D. (2003). Psychosocial origins of obesity stigma: Toward changing a powerful and pervasive bias. *Obesity Reviews, 4,* 213-227.

Register, C. A., & Williams, D. R. (1990). Wage effects of obesity among young workers. *Social Science Quarterly, 71,* 130-141.

Roberts, R. E., Kaplan, G. A., Shema, S. J., & Strawbridge, W. J. (2000). Are the obese at greater risk for depression? *American Journal of Epidemiology, 152,* 163-170.

Rodin, J. (1993). Cultural and psychosocial determinants of weight concerns. *Annals of Internal Medicine, 119,* 643-650.

Roehling, M. V. (1999). Weight-based discrimination in employment: Psychological and legal aspects [Electronic version]. *Personnel Psychology, 52*(4). Retrieved December 6, 2004, from EBSCO Host database.

Rosmond, R., & Björntorp, P. (1999). Psychosocial and socio-economic factors in women and their relationship to obesity and regional fat distribution. *International Journal of Obesity, 23,* 138-145.

Ross, C. E. (1994). Overweight and depression. *Journal of Health and Social Behavior, 35,* 63-78.

Rothblum, E. D., Brand, P. A., Miller, C. T., & Oetjen, H. A. (1990). The relationship between obesity, employment discrimination, and employment-related victimization. *Journal of Vocational Behavior, 37,* 251-266.

Rothblum, E. D., Miller, C. T., & Garbutt, B. (1988). Stereotypes of obese female job applicants. *International Journal of Eating Disorders, 6,* 277-283.

Rush, L. L. (1998). Affective reactions to multiple social stigmas. *Journal of Social Psychology, 138,* 421-430.

Seidell, J. C. (1999). The burden of obesity and its sequelae. *Disease Management & Health Outcomes, 5*(1), 13-21.

Seligman, M. E. P. (1994). *What you can change & what you can't.* New York: Knopf.

Sobal, J. (1984). Marriage, obesity, and dieting. *Marriage and Family Review, 7,* 115-139.

Sobal, J., & Stunkard, A. J. (1989). Socioeconomic status and obesity: A review of the literature. *Psychological Bulletin, 105,* 260-275.

Spiegeler, M. D., & Guevremont, D. C. (1998). *Contemporary behavior therapy* (3rd ed.). Pacific Grove, CA: Brooks/Cole.

Staffieri, J. R. (1967). A study of social stereotypes of body image in children. *Journal of Personality and Social Psychology, 7,* 101-104.

Taussig, W. C. (1994). Weighing in against discrimination: Cook v. Rhode Island, Department of Mental Health, Retardation, and Hospitals and the recognition of obesity as a disability under the Rehabilitation Act and the Americans With Disabilities Act. *Boston College Law Review, 35,* 927-963.

Teachman, B. A., & Brownell, K. D. (2001). Implicit anti-fat bias among health professionals: Is anyone immune? *International Journal of Obesity, 25,* 1525-1531.

Visscher, T. L. S., & Seidell, J. C. (2001) The public health impact of obesity. *Annual Review Public Health, 22,* 355-375.

Wadden, T. A., Anderson, D. A., Foster, G. D., Bennett, A., Steinberg, C., & Sarwer, D. B. (2000). Obese women's perceptions of their physicians' weight management attitudes and practices. *Archives of Family Medicine, 9,* 854-860.

Wadden, T. A., & Stunkard, A. J. (1985). Social and psychological consequences of obesity. *Annals of Internal Medicine, 103,* 1062-1067.

Wee, C. C., McCarthy, E. P., Davis, R. B., & Philips, R. S. (1999). Physician counseling about exercise. *Journal of American Medical Association, 282,* 1583-1588.

Wessler, R. A., & Wessler, R. L. (1988). *The principles and practice of rational-emotive therapy* (5th ed.). San Francisco: Jossey-Bass.

Winkleby, M. A., Gardner, C. D., & Taylor, C. B. (1996). The influence of gender and socioeconomic factors on Hispanic/White differences in body mass index. *Preventive Medicine, 25,* 203-211.

Wooley, S. C., & Wooley, O. W. (1979). Obesity and women: I. A closer look at the facts. *Women's Studies International Quarterly, 2,* 69-79.

Wright, B. A. (1983). *Physical disability: A psychosocial approach* (2nd ed.). New York: Harper & Row.

Zablocki, E. (1998). Weight and work. *Business and Health, 16,* 20-24.

29

Eugenics, Euthanasia, and Physician-Assisted Suicide: An Overview for Rehabilitation Professionals

STEVE ZANSKAS AND WENDY CODUTI

*E*ugenics, euthanasia, and physician-assisted suicide (PAS) are passionately debated practices. These value-laden topics have polarized opinions across all segments of our society. Advances in the Human Genome Project, increased knowledge of the Nazi atrocities against persons with disabilities, and recent court decisions regarding the right to die have combined to foster the existing controversy. Rehabilitation professionals are noticeably absent from these discussions. Review of the literature reflects that the preponderance of scholarly or popular writing regarding these practices lies outside the field of rehabilitation. This chapter is intended to provide the rehabilitation professional with a primer about eugenics, euthanasia, and PAS. To accomplish this task, the following topics are addressed: definitions and historical context, conceptual models, international experience, social and ethical considerations, economic aspects, implications for practice, and future research.

DEFINITIONS AND HISTORICAL CONTEXT

Eugenics

The concept of improving the human race through selective reproduction is reflected in Plato's *Republic* (Barnett, 2004; Larson, 2002). The Greek word *eugenes* means "well born" (Mahowald, 2003). Eugenics is defined as the study of hereditary improvements of the human race by controlled selective breeding (Smart, 2008). The word was conceived in England by Sir Francis Galton, a naturalist, a statistician, and Charles Darwin's cousin. Sir Galton first used the word he coined in one of his publications in 1883 (Barnett, 2004).

The eugenics movement peaked in the United States between 1900 and 1935 (Lombardo, 2003). Eugenicists adopted two approaches, referred to as positive and negative eugenics, to prevent individuals considered to have disabilities from reproducing. Public education and voluntary abstinence were considered positive eugenics. Compulsory sterilization was considered negative eugenics (Larson, 2002). Anyone the state considered socially undesirable appeared subject to involuntary sterilization, including individuals with hereditary deafness or blindness, those considered to have mental illness or developmental disabilities, and those with epilepsy, criminals, prostitutes, or the poor (Larson, 2002; Lombardo, 2003). Social Darwinism, an outgrowth of Darwinism, proposed that social characteristics were inherited along with biological characteristics. Social Darwinism was used as a justification

---

From "Eugenics, euthanasia, and physician assisted suicide: An overview for rehabilitation professionals," by S. Zanskas and W. Coduti, 2006, *Journal of Rehabilitation*, 72(1), 27–32. National Rehabilitation Association.

to eliminate socially undesirable characteristics through eugenic practices (Mostert, 2002). In the early 1900s, almost every state had at least one institution to segregate individuals with disabilities, and 32 enacted compulsory sterilization laws. Between 1907 and 1945, 40,000 eugenic sterilization procedures were performed in the United States; half were conducted in the state of California (Bachrach, 2004). More than 60,000 people were sterilized under these laws in the United States (Larson, 2002).

The most famous case of involuntary sterilization was that of Carrie Bell, a woman from Virginia, who was alleged to have had mental retardation. Ms. Bell was the first woman in Virginia to undergo compulsory sterilization after the Supreme Court affirmed the state's compulsory sterilization law (Mostert, 2002; Larson, 2002; Lombardo, 2003; Palmer, 2003). The U.S. Supreme Court upheld Virginia's 1924 Involuntary Sterilization Act with its 1927 decision in *Buck v. Bell*. This Supreme Court decision has been repudiated, but it has never been overruled (Palmer, 2003). The state of Virginia repealed its sterilization law in 1974.

Eugenics became associated with the concept of racial hygiene in Europe. In 1926, Denmark, Finland, Norway, and Sweden began institutionalized sterilization programs (Barnett, 2004). Influential social and economic forces in Germany, particularly after World War I, foreshadowed the genocide of people with disabilities (Mostert, 2002; Bachrach, 2004). In 1933, Germany's compulsory sterilization law was drafted (Mostert, 2002; Bachrach, 2004). Through a propaganda effort, individuals with disabilities were characterized as a separate group, perceived as different criminals and of little or no economic value. Approximately 400,000 people considered to have a hereditary sickness were sterilized under the Law for the Prevention for Genetically Diseased Offspring. Officially, another 70,273 adults with disabilities were euthanized through centers created by a program created in 1939 called Aktion T-4 (Mostert, 2002).

Following World War II, public awareness of the Nazi Holocaust discredited the word eugenics, and it essentially disappeared from use. The genomic era of medicine began on April 14, 2003, approximately 50 years following the first description of the structure of DNA, when the Human Genome Project completed the sequencing of the human genome (Guttmacher & Collins, 2003). Conservative estimates suggest that at least 13 million people in the United States are affected by genetic conditions (Koch, 2001). Genetic researchers estimate that every individual carries five to seven lethal recessive genes (Larson, 2002). Ethical debate about the Human Genome Project and genetic testing has fostered a resurgence of interest and debate regarding eugenics and genetic practices (Barnett, 2004).

Euthanasia

Euthanasia is derived from the Greek word *eu,* meaning "well," and *thanatos,* meaning "death," and early on it signified a "good" or "easy" death (Nadeau, 1995). Today euthanasia has come to mean "a deliberate intervention, by act or omission, in the life of a dying person with the intention of putting an end to that person's life and suffering" (Nadeau, 1995, p. 10). Euthanasia is performed by physicians and has been further defined as "active" or "passive." Active euthanasia refers to a physician deliberately acting in a way to end a patient's life. Passive euthanasia pertains to withholding or withdrawing treatment necessary to maintain life (Frileux, Lelievre, Munoz Sastre, Mullet, & Sorum, 2003). Sir Francis Bacon, an English philosopher and statesman, termed the phrase euthanasia early in the 17th century. At that time, euthanasia was used as a way to describe a pain-free, peaceful, and natural death that individuals desired to have (Yount, 2000).

The historical societal perspectives of euthanasia often parallel those of suicide. During ancient times in Greece, individuals could request government assistance with suicide, which was sometimes seen as a noble act (Yount, 2000). However, when Christianity became the dominant religion in the Western world, those beliefs changed. The condemnation of suicide became a part of Christian teachings, and there were even antisuicide laws in place. It wasn't until the 20th century when these laws were reviewed. Society found not only that punishing the family of the person who committed suicide was unfair but also that those who did commit suicide usually were viewed as doing so because of a mental illness (Yount, 2000).

In the United States, the first bill to legalize voluntary euthanasia by a physician was introduced in the Ohio legislature in 1906, but it failed (Yount, 2000). The idea of euthanasia was again brought to the social forefront during World War II in Nazi Germany, when adults and children considered mentally deficient were involuntarily put to death (McKhann, 1999). Currently, in the United States, physician-assisted dying in the form of assisted-suicide is legal in Oregon and Washington (Quill & Battin, 2004; Washington State Department of Health, 2010).

Physician-Assisted Suicide

PAS differs from euthanasia, as euthanasia embodies that the dying person may or may not be aware of what is happening to them, and may or may not have requested to die (Hawkins, 2002). With PAS, the terminal patient wants to die and seeks assistance from a doctor in doing so (Dworkin, Frey, & Bok, 1998). The U.S. Supreme Court ruled on June 26, 1997 that individuals do not have a constitutional right to PAS (Hawkins, 2002). Following this, voters in the state of Washington passed the "Death with Dignity Act" (RCW 70.245) in 2008. The act, which became law in 2009, allows adults with less than 180 days to live due to a terminal illness the right to request lethal doses of medication from their physician. Subsequently, the Montana Supreme Court ruled in a 4–3 decision that PAS was not illegal under Montana state statute or public policy (Arce, 2010).

Euthanasia and PAS are often linked together and intertwined in discussions. PAS is also associated with the right-to-die movement, which gained momentum in the 1970s as medical advances kept individuals living who previously would have died. Living wills were first developed during this time, as individuals wanted the right to refuse life-prolonging medical treatment and have some type of ownership over the quality of their life, especially during the very end stages (Yount, 2000).

During the 1980s, the right-to-die movement gained even more momentum with the advent of durable power of attorney, which directed surrogates in making health care decisions for individuals if they were, or became, incompetent to do so for themselves (Yount, 2000). PAS moved to the forefront in the 1990s, largely in part due to Dr. Jack Kevorkian and his public crusade of practicing and accepting PAS (Yount, 2000). Dr. Kevorkian was incarcerated for practicing PAS.

CONCEPTUAL MODELS

The polarization of opinion regarding eugenics, euthanasia, and PAS is represented by the differences between the medical and minority models of disability. One paradigm favors eugenics, euthanasia, and assisted suicide while the other opposes these practices and advocates social support for persons with disabilities (Koch, 2004). Historically, the field of genetic counseling has relied upon the medical model of health and disease (Patterson & Satz, 2002).

The medical model of disability conceptualizes disability as a negative variation of the physical or cognitive norm, disadvantaging a person's life and his/her quality of life (Koch, 2001). The traditional physical definition of disability used in the medical model portrays a person who cannot independently perform tasks or actions (Koch, 2001).

Autonomy and self-sufficiency have become the defining aspects of the normal human existence. The emphasis upon individual autonomy, self-determination, and independence is compatible with, although not an endorsement of, the practices of eugenics, euthanasia, or assisted suicide (Koch, 2001). Individual models of disability, particularly the medical model, have been criticized as inadequate for explaining the complex phenomena of disability (Reindal, 2000). Adhering to a causal understanding of the interaction between impairment and disability, the medical model of disability promotes value judgments by the professional community regarding the quality of life a person with a disability may lead (Reindal, 2000).

In contrast, the minority or social model of disability attributes the concept of disability to the lack of environmental accommodation and negative societal reaction to individuals with disabilities. The minority model suggests that rather than the limits a condition imposes, it is the lack of understanding about the effects of a disability or a failure to accommodate a physical or cognitive difference that is the source of disability (Olkin, 1999; Smart, 2001; Koch, 2004). Social difference theorists and disability rights advocates insist that a physically dependent or interdependent life is as full and viable as one that is autonomous and independent (Koch, 2004; Parens & Asch, 2003). Personhood is perceived as communal or relational experience rather than an individual experience. Individuals in this paradigm are defined not by their disease or limitations, but by their capacity for having relationships with others. The value of a person is absolute, and it cannot be decreased or withdrawn in this conceptualization. Many authors with disabilities argue that the worst aspect of having a disability is not the disability itself, but the societal prejudice against any deviation from the norm (Chen & Schiffman, 2000). Eugenics, euthanasia, and assisted suicide are not supported by the minority or social perspective of disability (Koch, 2004).

INTERNATIONAL PERSPECTIVES

Eugenics

Internationally, China and the Netherlands continue eugenic practices. China passed the Maternal & Infant Health Care Law in 1994. In that year, China's population reached 1.2 billion. A policy of one child per couple was established in order to achieve a population goal of less than 1.4 billion in 2010 (Mao, 1998). A national survey in China conducted in 1987 revealed that there were 51.64 million people with disabilities. Birth defects and genetic diseases accounted for 35.09% of the population with a disability (Ming & Jixiang, 1993). A survey of Chinese geneticists suggested most Chinese perceived individuals with disabilities as a severe burden to families and society (Mao, 1998). Public education was considered an effective approach to reduce the number of genetic diseases. Social, cultural, and economic differences between China and the West were believed to be the likely causes for differences regarding eugenics (Mao, 1998).

Galjaard's study of gene testing and social acceptance as cited in Mao (1998) revealed that the Netherlands operates seven regional genetics centers providing pre- and postnatal chromosomal analysis, biochemical and DNA diagnosis, and genetic counseling services. The genetics centers are funded by national health insurance. As a result of the combined testing and counseling activities, it is estimated that the births of 800 to 1600 children with severe disabilities are prevented annually. The annual cost of operating the genetic counseling centers is estimated at $50 million. However, the averted cost of care for the medical and psychosocial needs required by the 800 to 1600 children with disabilities prevented each year was calculated as ranging between $500 million and $1 billion during an average 10-year lifespan (Galjaard, 1997; as cited in Mao, 1998).

Euthanasia/PAS

Euthanasia, both active and passive, has been practiced in the Netherlands since 1970s and holds the largest source of data for physicians aiding in end-of-life decisions (Kaplan, Harrow, & Schneiderhan, 2002). In 1990, the Dutch government initiated the Remmelink

Commission to survey the practice of PAS and euthanasia in the Netherlands. They found that at least 25,000 cases annually consisted of the withdrawal of life support (passive euthanasia), and of those, 27% were administered morphine in order to shorten life. About 9% of the deaths in the Netherlands in 1990 were attributed to PAS or euthanasia (Nadeau, 1995).

The Remmelink Report, as it has now become known, found that between 6,000 and 12,000 cases annually were reported by Dutch hospitals where PAS or euthanasia was practiced. In 90% of those cases, it was a question of involuntary euthanasia, even though active euthanasia remains illegal (Gentles, 1995). The Board of Royal Dutch Medicine Association endorses euthanasia for newborns and infants with extreme disabilities (Gentles, 1995).

In the Netherlands study, the reasons for choosing to die included loss of dignity, intolerable pain, and not wanting to have an unworthy death. Wanting to avoid being or becoming dependent on others and feeling tired of life were also cited as reasons in choosing to end one's life (Kaplan et al., 2002). Cases in Australia have been studied as well regarding the choices people make for seeking PAS. In 1995, the Northern Territory of Australia legalized the option of euthanasia for the terminally ill, which is defined as those individuals having less than six months to live. In the first year under this policy, seven individuals with cancer sought to use this law to end their lives. Of those seven, pain did not appear to be a reason for their choosing to end their lives. Among the psychosocial factors listed as reasons for wanting to end one's life were social isolation, depression, anticipatory fear, sense of futility, and loss of dignity (Kaplan et al., 2002).

SOCIAL AND ETHICAL CONSIDERATIONS

Eugenics

The history of the eugenics movement has impacted the current practice of genetic counseling. Genetic counselors are guided by a nondirective standard of practice (Larson, 2003; Parens & Asch, 2003; Patterson & Satz, 2002). The goal of the therapist is to provide clear information in an unbiased manner (Saranji, 2002).

Knowledge and attitude of health care professionals is known to influence patient communication and medical decision-making. In one study, medical students, residents, and genetic counseling students, characterized as having minimal experience with disability or genetics, completed a survey regarding their attitudes about disability and genetic screening (Ormond, Gill, Semcik, & Kirschner, 2003). The results of this study indicated that majority of the participants felt that disability caused significant suffering for the person with the disability and 64% felt that having a disability also caused significant suffering for family members. Perceptions about the quality of life for a person with a disability or their family were based upon cognitive functioning, pain experienced, and level of available social support. Among those surveyed, 62% felt that research should be directed toward preventing genetic disability (Ormond et al., 2003).

Genetic testing can assist individuals with understanding the risk of having a child when a family history of a genetic disorder exists and how to manage personal health decisions when planning for a pregnancy (Bodenhorn & Lawson, 2002). Tests exist for genetic factors associated with more than 400 human conditions (Larson, 2002). Genetic tests fall within three broad categories: predictive gene testing, carrier testing, and prenatal testing (Glannon, 1998; Larson, 2002). However, identifying a genetic basis for a disability does not guarantee that a disabling condition exists or will develop (Larson, 2002).

Despite widespread prenatal testing, limited research has been conducted that addresses the decision-making process during prenatal testing. Available studies are primarily qualitative and suggest that the perceived benefits and emotional factors influence the decision to undergo prenatal testing. Patient knowledge and actual risk factors have not been shown to be strong predictors of test use among those eligible for testing. Review of the literature reflects that deciding to undergo genetic testing is primarily related to subjective risk factors and emotions (Lerman, Croyle, Tercyak, & Hamman, 2002). How a genetic test is offered also appears to influence whether or not a person will elect to undergo genetic testing. Individuals are more likely to undergo testing if it is offered in person and carried out immediately (Marteau & Croyle, 1998).

Research regarding the psychological impact of genetic testing is similarly limited. It does suggest, however, that adverse reactions to test results are uncommon when provided through a program that separates the offer of testing from the testing itself and provides clear information and emotional support before and after testing (Lerman et al., 2002; Marteau & Croyle, 1998). The psychological impact of testing results appears to depend more on pretest expectations, mood, and social support than on the test results themselves (Marteau & Croyle, 1998). As an example, pretest levels of depression and hopelessness were found to be the best predictors of levels of hopelessness following test result disclosure rather than the actual results (Meiser & Dunn, 2000).

The psychological impact of certain disease diagnoses does appear to be influenced by the nature of the diagnosis. Suicide occurs with an incidence of four times greater than the general U.S. population, following a diagnosis of Huntington's disease (Meiser & Dunn, 2000). Stress response syndrome has been predicted to develop in 20% of individuals receiving the results of a genetic risk for a "dire" illness (Horowitz, Sundin, Zanko, & Lauer, 2001). Knowledge about the phases of response, an individual's defensive style, and supportive counseling can assist recently diagnosed individuals with understanding and integrating the implications of their diagnosis (Horowitz et al., 2001).

Family relationships may become strained by the results of genetic testing. Partners of the person undergoing testing may be more affected by the results of genetic testing than the person undergoing testing (Marteau & Croyle, 2001). Compared with noncarrier's partners, the partners of carriers of Huntington's disease had substantially higher levels of distress at 1 week, 6 months, and 3 years after the disclosure of positive test results (Meiser & Dunn, 2000). A case study about a male spouse's experience during the decision to terminate a pregnancy reflects that he did not feel his grieving needs were met or recognized during genetic counseling (Robson, 2002). The increased need for family support is related to the sense of loss of control, feelings of guilt, and personal concerns that may affect others in the family who are not directly involved with the testing (Bodenhorn & Lawson, 2002).

Adults who were interviewed regarding their perception of genetic counseling appreciated the opportunity to receive direct education from experts in the field. Participants in this study indicated that they gained a thorough understanding of the risks and conditions, and they appreciated having control of the decision making process. Positive genetic counseling experiences were associated with appointments longer than the traditional physician appointments, provision of reading material, and the involvement of family members in the process (MacLeod, Crawford, & Booth, 2002).

Women at risk for carrying a fetus with Down syndrome or spina bifida were surveyed regarding their experience with genetic counseling (Roberts, Stough, & Parrish, 2002). The survey reflected that 87% were referred to genetic counseling by their doctor, with the primary concern being their age. Among those surveyed, 65% indicated that they would terminate a pregnancy if a disorder were present in their fetus. Results indicated that as knowledge of the resources available for individuals with disabilities increased, the choice to continue a pregnancy became more likely. However, the vast majority of the participants expressed that they were not encouraged to meet with the parent of a disabled child by either their genetic counselor or other medical personnel, were not provided information regarding future quality of life issues for a child with a disability, and were not provided either the positive or negative aspects of giving birth to a child with a disability (Roberts et al., 2002).

Attitudes of people with physical disabilities toward genetic counseling and prenatal diagnosis have rarely been addressed in the literature. Anticipating that individuals with physical disabilities would parallel the literature and express skeptical or negative attitudes toward genetic counseling, 15 adults with physical disabilities were interviewed regarding their feelings about genetic counseling (Chen & Schiffman, 2000). Results of this study indicated that approximately 78% of the participants did not feel that genetic counseling was eugenic. The majority of the participants did not correlate genetics with eugenics and expressed that they felt genetic advancements could improve the health of individuals. None of those interviewed recognized antidisability perspectives about prenatal diagnosis (Chen & Schiffman, 2000).

Quality of life for persons with disabilities is central to the debate about eugenics, euthanasia, and assisted suicide. Semistructured interviews conducted with 153 people who were described as having moderate to severe disabilities indicated that 54% reported experiencing an excellent or good quality of life (Albrecht & Devlieger, 1999). Analysis of the content of the interviews revealed that the definition of quality of life was dependent upon finding a balance between body, mind, and spirit and maintaining relationships within the person's social context and environment (Albrecht & Devlieger, 1999). Interviews with persons having Huntington's disease or cystic fibrosis indicated that the participants felt that others perceived them as unworthy of living and as unnecessary burdens upon society (Chapman, 2002).

Numerous fundamental, ethical, and value questions are raised throughout the present literature review. Examples of major value questions cited by Bodenhorn and Lawson (2002) include the following: What constitutes a life worth living? Who should make decisions? How should life be valued? Ensuring that the decision maker is provided with balanced and current information to arrive at an informed decision and that each individual has the right to make decisions without external pressure presents additional ethical concerns (Chapman, 2002).

Euthanasia/PAS

Ethical debates about euthanasia and PAS center around the concepts of rational suicide, aid in dying, and hastened death (Werth & Gordon, 1998). Rational suicide describes a decision-making process in which a person with a terminal illness who is experiencing intolerable suffering, choosing to end his or her life without coercion. Aid in dying involves providing the person with the actual means of ending their life. The most comprehensive concept, hastened death, refers to anything done to facilitate the process of dying. Hastened death includes rational suicide, aid in dying, and withdrawing or withholding life support (Werth & Gordon, 1998).

Perhaps the most commonly known practitioner of aid in dying was Dr. Jack Kevorkian. Kaplan et al. (2002) studied 93 of Dr. Kevorkian's cases to understand an individual's choice for PAS. Information was gathered through medical reports, death certificates and from medical examiners themselves. A psychological autopsy was also administered to friends and relatives of 47 of Kevorkian's patients. The psychological autopsy has been widely used to study individuals who have attempted suicide. It allows a reconstruction of the psychological profile of the decedent, garnered through those closest to the person, and is parallel to physical autopsies (Kaplan et al., 2002).

In the 97 cases studied, 87% of individuals chose PAS because of a disability and another 36% were described as depressed. Fear of dependency occurred in 90% of the cases while 31.1% were terminally ill, which was listed as having less than 6 months to live (Kaplan et al., 2002). The gender ratio of general completed suicides in the US was 18.9% women in 1995, but in the Kevorkian study 68% were women and 32% were men (Kaplan et al., 2002). Although 73.6% of the individuals reported having pain, only 42.6% had an anatomical basis for that pain (Kaplan et al., 2002). The average age of the decedents was 58.3 years and the majority were white (Kaplan et al., 2002).

The attitudes toward euthanasia and PAS were investigated using a semistructured interview of 70 individuals with terminal cancer (Wilson, et al., 2000). Among those surveyed, 73% felt that euthanasia or PAS should be legalized and 58% believed that if it was legalized, they would make a request for hastened death (Wilson et al., 2000). Psychological factors were cited as being as at least as important as the physical symptoms of those patients indicating they would request hastened death if it were made legal (Wilson et al., 2000). Previous studies have shown that "younger age, greater education, affluence, and White race are all predictors of patient preference for less aggressive treatment and in favor of physician aid in dying" (Steinberg, & Younger, 1998, p. 3). Treatment choices for patients, families and physicians, are influenced by age, religion, ethnicity, and socioeconomic status (Steinberg & Younger, 1998).

What does the above information tell us about the social implications of PAS? Perhaps most telling are the reasons why an individual chooses PAS. As the data from international studies show, the psychosocial aspects of PAS are less related to physical burdens and more toward personal. Similar to the Kevorkian study, where Kaplan et al. (2002) correlated women choosing PAS due to worries about their marriage breaking up and a deterioration of their economic state, women in Oregon chose PAS due to concerns about being a burden to their spouse.

Ethical considerations for physicians weigh heavily in the literature regarding PAS and euthanasia. The ethical issues focus on patient's choice versus medical responsibility. This debate was carried out in the judicial arena, specifically with the Terri Schiavo case in Florida, which may ultimately change the face of the current movement (Campo-Flores, 2005).

The National Association of Social Workers (NASW, 1994) and the American Psychological Association (APA, 1997) were among the first professional associations to issue policy statements regarding client choice and end-of-life decision-making. Ethical guidance for rehabilitation counselors engaged in counseling clients who have a terminal illness is now available through the American Counseling Association's Code of Ethics (ACA, 2005) and The Commission on Rehabilitation Counselor Certification's Code of Professional Ethics for Professional Rehabilitation Counselors (CRC, 2009). Both ethical codes address quality of care issues, counselor competence, choice, referral, and confidentiality while working with terminally ill clients. None of these professional organizations address end-of-life decision-making for individuals with chronic long-term illness or disabilities that are not life threatening. Nor do they advocate for or against PAS. Rather, each code or policy emphasizes high quality end-of-life care, self-determination, and informed decision-making (ACA, 2005; APA, 1997; CRC, 2009; & NASW, 1994). Regardless of the rehabilitation professional's values, the ethical principles or dilemmas involved rehabilitation professionals are advised to employ an ethical decision-making model to address the complexity of providing services to clients considering euthanasia or PAS (CRC, 2009).

Professional intervention was once the standard of care for individuals with a terminal illness considering rational suicide or hastened death (Bongar, 1991; Werth, 1999; Werth & Holdwick, 2000). However, the majority of state involuntary commitment laws require that a person must be a harm to his/her as a result of mental illness for commitment to proceed (Werth, 1996). A terminally ill client's desire to discuss rational suicide is no longer considered to fall within the "danger–to–self" doctrine. Werth and Holdwick (2000) argue that a terminally ill client's rational exploration of options when he/she has 6 or less months to live is inconsistent with impaired judgment due to a mental illness. Terminal illness is no longer considered synonymous with mental illness.

End-of-life care for terminally ill clients is addressed in Section A.9 of both the ACA and CRC codes of ethics (ACA 2005; CRC, 2009). Both codes offer much needed guidance for the rehabilitation professional working with a terminally ill client who wishes to explore end-of-life decision-making. Rehabilitation professionals are directed to facilitate their clients to obtain holistic and high-quality end-of-life care, maximize their self-determination, afford every opportunity for the client to make informed decisions, and to ensure that their clients receive complete and adequate assessment regarding their ability to make competent decisions (ACA, 2005; CRC, 2009). Acknowledging the importance of the personal values of the rehabilitation professional in the counseling relationship, neither the ACA (2005) nor the CRC (2009) code of ethics require counselors to work with terminally ill clients interested in exploring their end-of-life choices. Recognizing the limits of competence, rehabilitation professionals who feel ill equipped to address end-of-life decision making are advised to provide referral to providers with appropriate experience (ACA, 2005; CRC 2009).

Rehabilitation professionals who provide services to terminally ill clients interested in hastening their own deaths are advised to consider applicable laws and the circumstances of each case before making a decision about breaking or preserving their client's confidentiality (ACA, 2005; CRC, 2009). Professional and legal consultation is also recommended when rehabilitation professional is confronted with the choice of breaking their client's confidentiality. Adding to the complexity of the dilemma about disclosure, rehabilitation professionals providing services to client's exploring hastened death need to consider whether the client's confidentiality is privileged communication, who owns the privilege, and who is responsible for exercising the privilege.

ECONOMIC ASPECTS

Euthanasia/PAS

The argument regarding euthanasia and PAS becomes even more intense when economics is considered. Steinberg and Younger (1998) reported that the increased emphasis on cost savings and managed care will become the basis for decision-making for the terminally ill, whereas prior decisions were primarily clinically based. The business of health care generates the dilemma with which Americans are faced.

Estimates show that about one-third of all families with a terminally ill family member will end up in poverty (Bilchik, 1996). Bilchik (1996) also reported that care for the terminally ill accounts for 10% of the national health care costs and that 27% of all Medicare-spending occurs during the last year of a person's life (40% of the total is for the last month alone). Drugs for assisted suicide cost between $35 and $45 and could ultimately be considered as the less expensive treatment for death (Marker, & Hamlon, 2005).

In Oregon, 83% of doctors stated that financial pressures were a factor in a patient's request to die (Bilchik, 1996). Some fear that a "right to die" may soon become a "duty to die" in order to eliminate families from financial ruin. A report from Harvard University stated that one-half of all bankruptcies in the United States are caused by medical bills. At the time of illness onset, more than three-quarters of those people had health insurance and most were middle class and educated. Considering that 16.4% (46.2 million) of the individuals in the United States are uninsured, the idea of choosing death over bankruptcy of your family may become more appealing.

CONCLUSION

Implications for Practice

Rehabilitation professionals have long been absent from the discussion about eugenics, euthanasia, and assisted suicide. Although recent updates to the ACA (2005) and CRC (2009) ethical codes for counselors have addressed end-of-life decision-making, our historical absence from the debate reflects a large disservice to people with disabilities. Many of the cases discussed in the available research involved individuals who would or could have participated in services provided by rehabilitation professional. Counselors need to be aware of the social, ethical, and economic implications for clients who feel like a burden to their family or lack the medical or economic resources to ensure a reasonable quality of life.

Educating individuals with disabilities about alternatives, options, and available resources may make the decision to live with a disability more manageable. Educating the general public about the resources available to enhance one's quality of life appears equally important as socially- and environmentally imposed handicaps appear to have a greater impact on the decision to undergo PAS or to terminate a pregnancy than the illness or disability itself.

Becoming aware of the ethical and psychosocial aspects of euthanasia and PAS also affect the field of rehabilitation. Factors leading to the decision to live, die, or terminate a pregnancy are entangled with race/ethnicity, age, spirituality, gender, and the legal system. Knowing how all of these factors affect individuals with disabilities and their decisions to live or die should be a primary concern of the rehabilitation field.

Future Research

Areas for future research related to the field of rehabilitation are numerous. Further the majority of the research regarding genetic counseling with people who have a genetic condition or disability is qualitative, exploratory, or limited to opinion pieces. Two of the most critical areas are the psychosocial aspects of patients choosing PAS and the involvement of rehabilitation counselors. Additional studies regarding the attitudes of people with disabilities toward genetic counseling and testing are needed. The role of rehabilitation professionals regarding how and when they could become involved in the decision-making process requires exploration. Issues regarding the economics of health care are another area ripe for research. Studying the relationship between health care costs and decisions related to PAS and/or termination of pregnancy could yield significant information for rehabilitation professionals.

Perhaps the starting point for research in the rehabilitation field should begin with the general knowledge, attitudes, and beliefs rehabilitation professionals possess about the practices discussed in this paper. Developing a strong understanding of the attitudes and values rehabilitation professionals possess about quality-of-life decisions and the implications of eugenics, euthanasia, and PAS could lead to better training of rehabilitation counseling students. Expanded discussion of these topics appears appropriate for inclusion in courses about ethics, multicultural counseling, and psychosocial adjustment to disability. The research ideas mentioned above are starting points for developing a knowledge base specific to rehabilitation. The time has come to align our knowledge and actions as rehabilitation professionals with the needs of people with disabilities relative to eugenics, euthanasia, and PAS.

REFERENCES

Albrecht, G. L., & Devlieger, P. J. (1999). The disability paradox: High quality of life against all odds. *Social Science & Medicine, 48*(8), 977–988.

American Counseling Association. (2005). *ACA code of ethics*. Alexandria, VA: Author. Retrieved July 27, 2010, from http://www.counseling.org/PDFs/ACA_2005_Ethical_Code.pdf

American Psychological Association. (1997). *Terminal illness and hastened death requests: The important role of the mental health professional*. [Brochure]. Washington, DC: Author. (Reprinted as *Professional psychology: Research and practice, 28*, 544–547, by R. K. Farberman, 1997.)

Arce, D. (2010). Montana supreme court rules physician assisted suicide not banned by state law. *Jurist Legal News & Research*. Retrieved October 6, 2010, from http://juristlaw.pitt.edu/paperchase/2010/01/montana-supreme-court

Bachrach, S. (2004). In the name of public health-Nazi racial hygiene. *The New England Journal of Medicine, 351*, 417–420.

Barnett, R. (2004). Keywords in the history of medicine: Eugenics. *The Lancet, 363*, 1742.

Bilchik, G. S. (1996). *Dollars & death*. Hospitals & Health Networks, 70, 18–22.

Bodenhorn, N., & Lawson, G. (2002). Genetic counseling: Implications for community counselors. *Journal of Counseling and Development, 81*, 497–501.

Bongar, B. (1991). *The suicidal patient: Clinical and legal standards of care*. Washington, DC: American Psychological Association.

Buck v. Bell, 274 U.S. 200 (1927).

Campo-Flores, A. (2005). The legacy of Terri Schiavo. *Newsweek, 22–28*.

Chapman, F. (2002). The social and ethical implications of changing medical technologies: The views of people living with genetic conditions. *Journal of Health Psychology, 7*, 195–206.

Chen, E. A., & Schiffman, J. F. (2000). Attitudes toward genetic counseling and prenatal diagnosis among a group of individuals with physical disabilities. *Journal of Genetic Counseling, 9*(2), 137–152.

Commission on Rehabilitation Counselor Certification. (2009). *Code of professional ethics for rehabilitation counselors*. Schaumburg, IL: Author.

Dworkin, G., Frey, R. G., & Bok, S. (1998). *Euthanasia and physician-assisted suicide*. Cambridge, UK: Cambridge University Press.

Frileux, S., Lelievre, C., Munoz Sastre, M. T., Mullet, E., & Sorum, P. C. (2003). When is physician assisted suicide or euthanasia acceptable? *Journal of Medical Ethics, 29*, 330–336.

Galjaard, H. (1997). Gene technology and social acceptance. *Pathologie Biologie, 45*, 250–255.

Glannon, W. (1998). Genes, embryos, and future people. *Bioethics, 12*(3), 187–211.

Guttmacher, A. E., & Collins, F. S. (2003). Welcome to the genomic era. *The New England Journal of Medicine, 349*(10), 996–998.

Hawkins, G. (2002). *Physician assisted suicide*. San Diego, CA: Greehnaven Press.

Horowitz, M., Sundin, E., Zanko, A., & Lauer, R. (2001). Coping with grim news from genetic tests. *Psychosomatics, 42*(2), 100–105.

Kaplan, K. J., Harrow, M., & Schneiderhan, M. (2002). Suicide, physician-assisted suicide and euthanasia in men versus women around the world: The degree of physician control. *Ethics & Medicine, 18*, 33–50.

Koch, T. (2001). Disability and difference: Balancing social and physical constructions. *Journal of Medical Ethics, 27*, 370–376.

Koch, T. (2004). The difference that difference makes: Bioethics and the challenge of "disability." *Journal of Medicine and Philosophy, 29*(6), 697–716.

Larson, E. F. (2002). The meaning of human gene testing for disability rights. *University Of Cincinnati Law Review, 70*, 913–938.

Lerman, C. Croyle, R. T., Tercyak, K. P., & Hamman, H. (2002). Genetic testing: Psychological aspects and implications. *Journal of Consulting and Clinical Psychology, 70*(3), 784–797.

Lombardo, P. (2003). *Eugenics bibliography*. Retrieved January 22, 2005, from www.healthsystemvirginia.edu

Lombardo, P. A. (2003). Taking eugenics seriously: Three generations of ??? are enough? *Florida State Law review, 30*(2), 191–218.

MacLeod, R., Crawford, D., & Booth, K. (2002). Patient's perceptions of what makes genetic counseling effective: An interpretive phenomenological analysis. *Journal of Health psychology, 7*, 145–156.

Mahowald, M. B. (2003). Aren't we all eugenicists? Commentary on Paul Lombardo's "taking eugenics seriously". *Florida State Law Review, 30*(2), 219–235.

Marker, R. L., & Hamlon, K. (2005). *Euthansia and assisted suicide:Frequently asked questions*. International Task Force on Euthanasia and Assisted Suicide. Retrieved January 2, 2005, from http://www.internationaltaskforce.org/faq.htm

Mao, X. (1998). Chinese geneticists' views of ethical issues in genetic testing and screening: Evidence for eugenics in China. *American Journal of Human Genetics, 63*, 688–695.

Marteau, T. M., & Croyle, R. T. (1998). Psychological responses to genetic testing. *British Medical Journal, 316*, 693–696.

McKhann, C. (1999). *A time to die.* London: Yale University Press.

Meiser, B., & Dunn, S. (2000). Psychological impact fo genetic testing for Huntington's disease: An update of the literature. *Journal of Neurology, Neurosurgery, Psychiatry, 69*, 574–578.

Ming, G., & Jixiang, M. (1993). Demography of people with disabilities in China. *International Journal of Rehabilitation Research, 16*, 299–301.

Mostert, M. P. (2002). Useless eaters: Disability as genocidal marker in Nazi Germany. *The Journal of Special Education, 36*, 155–168.

Nadeau, R. (1995). Charting the Legal Trends. In I. Gentles (Ed.), *Euthanasia and assisted suicide: The current debate* (pp. 7–27). Toronto, Canada: Stoddart Publishing Co. Limited.

National Association of Social Workers. (1994). Client self-determination in end-of-life decisions. *Social work speaks* (3rd ed., pp 58–61). Washington, DC: NASW Press.

Olkin, R. (1999). *What psychotherapists should know about disability.* New York: The Guilford Press.

Ormond, K. E., Gill, Semcik, P., & Kirschner, K. L. (2003). Attitudes of health care trainees about genetics and disability: Issues of access, health care communication, and decision making. *Journal of Genetic Counseling, 12*(4), 333–349.

Palmer, L. I. (2003). Genetic health and eugenic precedents: A voice of caution. *Florida State Law Review, 30*(2), 237–264.

Parens, E., & Asch, A. (2003). Disability rights critique of prenatal genetic testing: Reflections and recommendations. *Mental Retardation and Developmental Disabilities and Research Reviews, 9*, 40–47.

Patterson, A. & Satz, M. (2002). Genetic counseling and the disabled: Feminism examines the stance of those who stand at the gate. *Hypatia, 17*(3), 118–142.

Quill, T. E., & Battin, M. P. (2004). *Physician assisted dying.* Baltimore, MD: Johns Hopkins University Press.

Reindal, S. M. (2000). Disability, gene therapy and eugenics-a challenge to John Harris. *Journal of Medical Ethics, 26*, 89–94.

Roberts, C. D., Stough, L. M., & Parrish, L. H. (2002). The role of genetic counseling in the elective termination of pregnancies involving fetuses with disabilities. *The Journal of Special Education, 361*(1), 48–55.

Robson, F. (2002). "Yes!-a chance to tell my side of the story": A case study of a male partner of a woman undergoing termination of pregnancy for fetal abnormality. *Journal of Health Psychology, 7*, 183–193.

Saranji, S. (2002). The language of likelihood in genetic counseling discourse. *Journal of Language and Social Psychology, 21*, 7–31.

Smart, J. (2008). *Disabled, society, and the individual.* (2nd ed.). Austin, TX: Pro-Ed.

Steinberg, M. D., & Younger, S. J. (1998). *End of life decisions.* Washington, DC: American Psychiatric Press, Inc.

Washington State Department of Health (2010). *Executive Summary: 2009 Death with Dignity Act Report.* Retrieved October 1, 2010, from http://www.doh.wa.gov/dwda/forms/DWDA_2009.pdf

Werth, J. L., Jr. (1996). *Rational suicide? Implications for mental health professionals.* Washington, DC: Taylor & Francis.

Werth, J. L., Jr. (1999). Mental health professionals and assisted death: Perceived ethical obligations and proposed guidelines for practice. *Ethics and Behavior, 9*, 159–183.

Werth, J. L., Jr., & Gordon, J. R. (1998). Helping at the end of life: Mental health professionals and hastened death. In L. Vandecreek, S. Knapp, & T. L. Jackson (Eds.). *Innovations in clinical practice: A sourcebook* (pp. 385–398). Sarasota, FL: Professional Resource Press.

Werth, J. L., Jr., & Holdwick, D. J. (2000). A primer on rational suicide and other forms of hastened death. *The Counseling Psychologist, 28*, 511–539.

Wilson, K. G., Scott, J. F., Graham, I. D., Kozak, J. F., Chater, S., Viola, R. A., et al. (2000). Attitudes of terminally ill patients toward euthanasia and physician-assisted suicide. *Archives of Internal Medicine, 160*, 2454–2460.

Yount, L. (2000). *Physician-assisted suicide and euthanasia.* New York: Facts On File, Inc.

30

Mental Health Preparedness for Terrorist Incidents

ALINA M. SURÍS AND CAROL S. NORTH

BACKGROUND

*A*mericans have been warned that it is a matter of "when, not if" (Ackerman & Tamsett, 2009, p. 84) terrorists will attack the United States with weapons of mass destruction (WMD) (Flynn, 2004). On the eve of the April 11, 2010, Nuclear Security Summit in Washington, DC, President Obama remarked:

> The single biggest threat to US security...short term, medium term, and long term, would be the possibility of a terrorist organization obtaining a nuclear weapon....

> ...organizations like al Qaeda are in the process of trying to secure a nuclear weapon...that they have no compunction at using. Unfortunately, we have a situation in which there is a lot of loose nuclear material around the world. (Office of the Press Secretary, 2010)

Nuclear weapons comprise only one type of WMD. In the weeks after the September 11, 2001, terrorist attacks on New York City and Washington, DC, deliveries of weaponized anthrax to several media and US Congressional office targets via the U.S. mail system represented the first bioterrorist attack on American soil (North et al., 2009a). Other forms of WMD are radioactive devices, chemical weapons, and conventional explosives.

There is no single definition of terrorism recognized by researchers or government agencies. For the purposes of this chapter, terrorism will be defined as:

> illegal use or threatened use of force or violence; an intent to coerce societies or governments by inducing fear in their populations; typically with ideological and political motives and justifications, an "extrasocietal" element, either "outside" society in the case of domestic terrorism or "foreign" in the case of international terrorism. (National Research Council, 2002, pp. 14–15)

Terrorism can be conceptually distinguished from other types of violence based on several unique characteristics: (1) it is premeditated, (2) it is designed to create deep and widespread fear, (3) its effects are directed at a wider audience than the immediate physical target, (4) it involves attacks on symbolic targets or random attacks on civilians, (5) it is viewed by society as violating the norms of dispute regulation and dissent, and (6) it is typically used to influence political behavior of governments, communities, or social groups (Schmid & Jongman, 1988; Wilkinson, 1997). The goal of a terrorist attack is thus not simply to injure and kill people but to also disrupt the broader community and diminish the public's sense of safety by terrorizing the entire population. These distinctive characteristics may serve to magnify mental health effects in comparison with other types of disasters.

THE PLACE OF TERRORISM WITHIN THE LARGER
TYPOLOGY OF DISASTER

Terrorism is a specific type of disaster within a broader category of disasters or mass casualty incidents (North & Surís, 2011). The typology of disasters is broadly conceptualized as falling into three major categories of causality: (1) *natural disasters* such as floods, tornados, hurricanes, earthquakes, and volcanic eruptions; (2) *technological accidents* such as mass transportation accidents (e.g., plane crashes), structural collapses, and explosions caused by human error rather than intent; and (3) *willful human-caused incidents of mass violence* such as mass shootings in the workplace or in public, and domestic or international terrorism. Terrorism is a specific type of willful human-caused disaster, differentiated from other acts of intentional mass violence by its ideological and political motives and its operation outside of societal norms.

Disaster mental health sequelae may vary among the three main types of disasters. There is some evidence that, on average, natural disasters have milder mental health effects than technological accidents, and willful human-induced incidents have more severe mental health consequences than either technological accidents or natural disasters (Neria, Nandi, & Galea, 2008; North, 2007), but definitive data to demonstrate that this is the case do not yet exist. Because disasters vary considerably from one to another in scope and magnitude, there is likely to be considerable variation of disaster severity within disaster types. No studies have been done with sufficient numbers and variation on different types of disasters, or adequately sized research samples assessed with uniform methods from study to study to be able to demonstrate these relationships empirically. This is actually such a very difficult task that we should not expect to see the accumulation of sufficiently comprehensive and methodologically sound data to provide definitive answers to this question any time soon. For the time being, however, it will have to be enough to know that most experts consider willful human acts of mass violence to be the potentially most serious type of disaster in terms of mental health consequences. This is intuitive: due to the fact that someone is intentionally inflicting personal harm adds a heinous psychological dimension to the trauma. For additional reasons that will become more apparent as this chapter proceeds, the terrorism subset of the willful human-induced category of disasters has the potential to have particularly serious mental health consequences.

Disaster typology is complicated by the observation that disasters do not fit neatly into these categories. For example, natural disasters are often complicated by human error (e.g., failure of human controls to prevent catastrophic consequences of what nature doles out or inability of human support systems to provide adequate care for disaster victims). Some disasters, such as firestorms, can be caused by nature (lightning), human error (mismanagement of flammable items such as cigarettes), or willful human intent (arson), and the source may be difficult to identify.

Terrorism can be further subclassified according to the specific type of weapon or agents used. The acronym "CBRNE" stands for chemical, biological, radiological, nuclear, and explosive types of incidents, collectively representing the kinds of agents used in WMD. An example of a chemical attack was the incident in the Tokyo subway system in which the deadly gas sarin was released in many subway tunnels, killing several people and injuring many more. The anthrax attacks in the United States in 2001 were an example of a biological attack. A radiological incident could occur if terrorists place sources of radiation in public places (e.g., under a park bench) with the intent of exposing many people. Nuclear bombs are easily recognized as potential WMDs. The bombings of the U.S. Embassies in East Africa are examples of terrorism using conventional explosives. On September 11, 2001, terrorists hijacked commercial airplanes full of people and used them in a novel way to create explosions and cause extensive damage and destruction in key U.S. locations.

Chemical, biological, and radiological terrorism in particular have characteristics of special importance because of their potential to produce mental health consequences of types and magnitudes not experienced with other types of terrorism or in many other types of disasters. These special characteristics are: (1) the exposures may not be perceptible; (2) the exposures are characterized by uncertainty; (3) symptoms of the exposures are easily misinterpreted; and (4) behavior is directed by personal perceptions of the exposure, not necessarily the actual exposure (North, 2007). This combination of uncertainties is destined to lead to untoward emotional, psychological, and behavioral responses within individuals and collectively within populations. Of note, similar characteristics have been well documented in association with infectious epidemics and accidental contamination incidents (Dunn, Taylor, Elliott, & Walter, 1994; Ginzburg, 1993; Koscheyev, Leon, Gourine, & Gourine, 1997; Meredith et al., 2011), which thus share certain effects with chemical, biological, and radiological terrorism. In contrast, conventional weapons such as bombs and other types of disasters such as tornadoes and plane crashes have immediate and visible consequences. These types of disasters leave little doubt about exposure and injury from the outset. It is hypothesized that the invisibility and uncertainty inherent in these forms of terrorism are important components of their psychological permeability among affected populations. It is also established that the mental health effects of a disaster are more severe when the incident occurs without warning, causes precipitous changes to a scene, creates serious injuries and/or fatalities, is of long duration, and disrupts social support systems. These characteristics may apply to terrorist incidents (Meyers, 2001; Rodriguez & Kohn, 2008).

PSYCHOSOCIAL SEQUELAE OF TERRORISM

The understanding that the distinctive characteristics of terrorism and agents of mass destruction can be expected to have different mental health consequences compared with other kinds of disasters and mass violence incidents may help inform not only mental health interventions but also preparedness for terrorist attacks. Because the disruption intended by terrorist incidents is aimed so widely, terrorism can be expected to have especially far-reaching psychosocial consequences that can reverberate through a community, nation, and even the world if the incident is of sufficient magnitude and significance.

Massive terrorist incidents can be expected to divide affected populations into distinct subgroups with different psychosocial and mental health issues based on the group's exposure level. The larger, more severe, widespread, and heinous the event, the farther the mental health repercussions will be felt from the epicenter of the physical impact. Those closest to the direct impact zone can be expected to have the most severe mental health consequences, and their numbers will be relatively small compared with the larger populations outside the direct impact zone. Those outside the impact zone can be expected to have less-severe mental health effects, but the overall impact in terms of numbers of people affected may be much larger because of the size of the population outside the direct impact zone. Because different exposure groups can thus be expected to have very different mental health effects that create different intervention needs, it is imperative to assess them accurately so that appropriate mental health resources can be directed to different groups and individuals based on their needs (North, 2004; North & Pfefferbaum, 2002, 2004).

Only people with qualifying exposures to a terrorist attack (defined by the *Diagnostic and Statistical Manual of Mental Disorders*, 4th Edition, Text Revision [*DSM-IV-TR*]; American Psychiatric Association, 2000)—being directly exposed to physical harm, personally witnessing the attack, or indirectly exposed through the direct exposure of a close associate—can be considered candidates for a diagnosis of post-traumatic stress disorder (PTSD). Those exposed who lack sufficient symptoms and those not exposed (even those who are highly symptomatic) cannot, by definition, have a diagnosis of PTSD; these subgroups may be considered to have psychosocial reactions, including mass fear and anxiety, uncertainty, and psychological distress.

The September 11, 2001 attacks presented new complexities in conceptualization of exposure required to determine candidacy for a diagnosis of PTSD. Published research considered symptomatic people five or more miles away from "Ground Zero" in the Manhattan area to be sufficiently exposed to consider a diagnosis of PTSD (Galea et al., 2002; Hasin, Keyes, Hatzenbuehler, Aharonovich, &Alderson, 2007). Other studies (Schlenger et al., 2002; Schuster et al., 2001; Silver, Holman, McIntosh, Poulin, & Gil-Rivas, 2002) reported prevalence rates of PTSD-related disorders in U.S. population samples outside of the Manhattan area that would not have qualifying exposures required for diagnosis of PTSD. Determining PTSD prevalence and differentiating it from psychological distress and psychosocial reactions is needed to determine numbers of people with PTSD and to plan effective interventions appropriate to the needs of those with PTSD as well as to provide mental health resources appropriate to all exposure groups.

Psychiatric Illness

Postdisaster psychiatric disorders are well documented in the research literature. PTSD is considered the "signature diagnosis" of disasters (North, Hong, & Pfefferbaum, 2008). The most prevalent psychiatric disorder among directly exposed disaster survivors is usually PTSD, but the reported prevalence varies widely across studies, from 0% to 100%, but usually 50% or less (Neria et al., 2008; North, 2007; North et al., 2008; North & Surís, 2011). The most prevalent post-traumatic symptoms after disasters are intrusive thoughts and images and hyperarousal (especially sleep disturbance, difficulty concentrating, and being jumpy or easily startled) (North et al., 1999). These post-traumatic symptoms are so common (experienced by the vast majority) that they may be considered normative reactions to extreme events. Research has further demonstrated that these common symptoms do not by themselves represent psychiatric illness, and thus they may be best conceptualized as emotional or psychological distress (National Academy of Sciences Institute of Medicine, 2003; North et al., 2008; North & Pfefferbaum, 2002, 2004; North & Westerhaus, 2003). Avoidance and numbing symptoms, however, are relatively uncommon, and these symptoms are strongly predictive of PTSD and central to the psychopathology of this disorder (Breslau, 2001; Ehlers, Mayou, & Bryant, 1998; Maes et al., 1998; McMillen, North, & Smith, 2000; North et al, 1999; North, Surís, Davis, & Smith, 2009b).

PTSD does not usually emerge in isolation from other psychopathology after disasters (North, Surís, & Adewuyi, 2011b; North & Surís, 2011). Psychiatric comorbidity with PTSD is typical and should be assessed and treated, because comorbid diagnoses are more severe and are associated with additional disability (North et al., 1999, 2011b). Major depression is usually the second most prevalent disorder in directly exposed disaster survivors (David et al., 1996; Green, Lindy, Grace, & Leonard, 1992; McFarlane & Papay, 1992; North, Smith, & Spitznagel, 1994; North et al., 1999; North, 2007; North & Surís, 2011). Although substance use may increase following disasters (Vlahov et al., 2002), this phenomenon apparently does not translate into new (i.e., incident) substance-use disorders, which do not often first develop in the postdisaster setting (David et al., 1996; Norris et al., 2002b; North et al., 1999, 2008; North, Ringwalt, Downs, Derzon, & Galvin, 2011a; North et al., 2011b; North & Surís, 2011). Despite this collective evidence of psychiatric disorders after disasters, most disaster survivors do not develop psychiatric disorders, reflecting general human resilience (North, 2007; North et al., 2008; North & Surís, 2011).

The collective disaster literature has identified female sex and pre-disaster psychopathology among the most robust predictors of post-disaster PTSD (Norris et al., 2002b; North & Pfefferbaum, 2004). Other less-consistent predictors identified by previous research have included greater disaster exposure, younger age, higher level of education, ethnic minority status, socioeconomic disadvantage, non-married marital status, other life stressors, and lack of social support (Norris et al., 2002b; North, 2007; North & Pfefferbaum, 2004).

PTSD tends to begin very soon after disasters, with symptoms commencing within days (North et al., 1997, 1999). Delayed-onset of PTSD (defined in *DSM-IV-TR* as when the symptoms begin after a period of more than 6 months has passed since the traumatic event; American Psychiatric Association, 2000) is uncommon after disasters (Norris et al., 2002b; North et al., 1999, 2008; North, 2007). PTSD is often chronic (defined by *DSM-IV-TR* as persisting for at least 3 months; American Psychiatric Association, 2000) after disasters, and PTSD can persist for decades (Marcus, 2001; North, McCutcheon, Spitznagel, & Smith, 2002; North et al., 2008; North, Pfefferbaum, Kawasaki, et al., 2010b; North, 2007).

Much less is known, however, about psychiatric disorders such as PTSD specific to terrorist incidents. A 2004 review of research on directly exposed survivors of terrorist incidents identified seven studies reporting prevalence estimates of PTSD in adult terrorism survivors in the first postdisaster months (North & Pfefferbaum, 2004). Most of these incidents were bombings and mass shooting incidents. Estimated PTSD prevalence associated with these terrorist incidents ranged from 18% to 50%. However, some of the studies reported current prevalence, others reported postdisaster prevalence, and some provided estimates based on symptom screener tools, obfuscating potential for comparison of prevalence findings. The most definitive work on postdisaster PTSD prevalence is from a study of the Oklahoma City bombing that found that 34% of this directly exposed sample, fully assessed with *DSM-III-R* criteria (American Psychiatric Association, 1987), developed PTSD in the first 6 months after the bombing (North et al., 1999). A recently published study of evacuees from the World Trade Center towers on September 11 provided a current (1-month) PTSD prevalence estimate (determined by exceeding a symptom scale threshold) in 15% of survivors assessed 2 to 3 years afterward, but postdisaster PTSD prevalence estimates were not provided (DiGrande, Neria, Brackbill, Pulliam, & Galea, 2011). Little is known about other psychiatric disorders arising following terrorist incidents, aside from a comprehensive study by North et al. (1999) of 182 directly exposed survivors of the Oklahoma City bombing diagnostically assessed approximately 6 months after the bombing, which found that 23% had postdisaster major depression, and other postdisaster anxiety disorders and substance-use disorders were each found in less than 10%.

Psychosocial Reactions

Emotional, psychological, behavioral, and social responses after a terrorist attack vary based on the event, the population, and timing relative to the incident. Terrorist attacks of any kind may elicit acute fear and mass flight responses, such as those seen in the familiar images of crowds of people running from the dust and debris cloud emerging with the collapse of the World Trade Center towers. Hollywood movies dramatize disasters with scenes of mass panic with mobs running in the streets screaming and flailing. Despite these popular images, research has failed to support news accounts of widespread frenzied panic following disasters (Becker, 2005). Regardless, in large terrorist events, large numbers of individuals may engage in fear-based behaviors that are counterproductive to the public's safety. For example, 3,300 people were advised to evacuate during the Three Mile Island crisis, but for every one person asked to leave, 45 did so; a mass of 150,000 evacuating citizens clogged the highways, hindering the evacuation of those who were advised to leave (Becker, 2009; Erikson, 1994). This mass exodus likely represents an understandable human response of confusion and alarm in the face of insufficient information, rather than a situation of panic overriding basic safety instructions (Becker, 2009).

Terrorist attacks implemented with nuclear, radiological, chemical, and/or biological agents may be especially frightening, because they are invisible, leaving survivors with persistent uncertainties about their exposure and/or level of exposure (Norwood, Holloway, & Ursano, 2001). Erroneous assumptions about exposure may feed the development of symptoms through interpretation of bodily sensations as indicators of exposure. Alternatively, interpretation of extraneous bodily sensations as symptoms of exposure may lead to erroneous assumptions of exposure. Emotions that may accompany or augment these processes include fear, anxiety, and dread. The response to terrorism is thus disarticulated—or separated—from the actual exposure or injury, being directed by the individual's belief in exposure rather than by the exposure itself (North, 2007; North et al., 2009a; Stuart, Ursano, Fullerton, Norwood, & Murray, 2003). As a result, people's beliefs about their exposure status may predict their health and mental health responses apart from their actual exposures (Stuart et al., 2003). A study found that among unexposed congressional staff after the 2001 anthrax attacks on Capitol Hill, belief in exposure was associated with nearly double the likelihood of receiving antibiotics for anthrax prophylaxis and more than five times the likelihood of receiving a 60-day course of antibiotics (North et al., 2009a). Another study found that among Gulf War veterans, belief in exposure to chemical or biological agents was correlated with mental illness and psychological stress (Stuart et al., 2003; Stuart, Ursano, Fullerton, & Wessely, 2008).

Large numbers of individuals who were not exposed to a disaster agent but interpret their bodily sensations as evidence of exposure may gravitate to medical care centers in large numbers. These mass health care–seeking behaviors create a surge effect, overwhelming the health care systems that are needed to treat those who were injured or became ill through exposure (Fullerton, Ursano, & Norwood, 2004; Roy, 2004). Widespread fear and anxiety invoked by the invisibility and uncertainty of exposure were observed in a radioactive incident with cesium-137 in 1987 in Goiânia, Brazil; although only 250 people were actually contaminated and just 20 developed radiation sickness (four of whom died), more than 100,000 people seeking radiation monitoring overwhelmed local health care capacities. Many of these individuals seeking evaluation presented with classic symptoms of radiation sickness such as vomiting, diarrhea, and rashes, and the fear was so intense that people fainted as they queued up for monitoring (Becker, 2005; Meredith et al., 2011). In the Tokyo sarin gas attacks, more than 5,500 people sought acute medical care but less than 1% suffered serious exposure-related illness or death (Bowman, 1999).

Radiologic incidents are among the most feared of all hazards, and situations involving radioactive contamination and nuclear threat produce especially great apprehension, alarm, and dread (Becker, 2007). Worries over long-term health effects such as birth defects and cancer can be long lasting and may result in persistent psychological ramifications for exposed individuals. Days into the reactor crisis following the major 2011 earthquake and tsunami in Japan, a woman who had evacuated and was interviewed by CNN said, "I'm due to give birth soon....I want to know what's going on at the nuclear plant. I'm scared" (Tuchman et al., 2011). Terrorist incidents involving invisible agents are especially feared. For example, a congressional staff worker who was exposed to the October 2001, anthrax attacks on Capitol Hill said, "Oh my God, I am going to die of anthrax and it's horrible" (North et al., 2005a).

In the post-terrorist attack environment, rumors and misinformation may flourish, and distrust of authorities and institutions may fester and boil (North et al, 2005b, 2009a; North, Pfefferbaum, Hong, et al., 2010a; Weisæth & Tønnessen, 2003). In this environment, at the community level, disruption of infrastructures and systems can engender feelings of helplessness, hopelessness, discouragement, demoralization, disillusionment, and nihilism. Interpersonal dynamics that may play out in the wake of a terrorist incident are anger, blaming scapegoating, and loss of trust for authorities that victims perceive as failing to protect them (Alexander & Klein, 2003). Terrorist attacks can shatter core assumptions and beliefs about the world and one's safety, especially after an unprecedented attack of the magnitude and scope of the 9/11 attacks on the United States (Alexander & Klein, 2003).

Terrorist attacks, which are committed by an "unseen enemy" and are unpredictable, may generate widespread paranoia and a sense of persecution (Alexander & Klein, 2003, p. 493). Collective paranoia may breed conspiracy theories, especially in circumstances where little substantive information is available and people are outraged (Sunstein & Vermeule, 2008), circumstances likely to occur in the wake of a terrorist attack. September 11 conspiracy websites abound, such as the 9/11 Truth Movement comprised of loosely affiliated organizations and individuals who question the accepted account of the 9/11 attacks (BBC Mobile News Magazine, 2008; BBC News, 2010). Polls conducted after the 9/11 attacks found that substantial proportions of the U.S. public believed that the U.S. government was involved either through participation in the attacks or through failure to prevent them (Hargrove & Stempel III, 2006; Zogby International, 2004).

Disaster stigma may complicate disasters involving contamination, infection, or radiation. In such instances, stigma may be directed against those who were exposed or who have evacuated from exposure zones and are assumed to be exposed (Alexander & Klein, 2003; Becker, 2005, 2007). After widespread contamination of the Goiânia, Brazil area by cesium-137 in 1987, agricultural produce would not sell, tourism fell off dramatically, and evacuees were refused hotel accommodations, food service, and passage on airplanes; evacuees driving cars with Goiânia license plates were stoned (Becker, 2004). Terrorist incidents may engender stigma based on assumptions about its perpetrators. Stigma against Muslims and individuals whose ethnicity resembled that of the terrorists was well documented after the 9/11 attacks (Davis & Silver, 2004; Federal Bureau of Investigation, 2001; Hendricks, Ortiz, Sugie, & Miller, 2007; Saad, 2010; Sheridan, 2006; Swahn et al., 2003), reflected in the statistical spike of hate-related violent acts against these groups (Federal Bureau of Investigation, 2001; Swahn et al., 2003; Zogby, 2001). Specific and tragic examples of this stigma were the murders of a turban-wearing Sikh from India who owned a gas station in Arizona, a Christian Egyptian grocer in California, an American citizen who was a Yemen native and a father of four in Detroit, and a Yemini shopkeeper in California, among several others (Lewin, 2001).

INTERVENTIONS

Available disaster mental health interventions were developed for disasters in general, not specifically for terrorist incidents. The most prudent approach to providing interventions post-terrorism is thus to adapt the more general principles of disaster mental health intervention and adapt them to fit the specific needs anticipated for terrorism-exposed populations.

As a general rule, disaster mental health interventions are most effective when they are practical, flexible, empowering, compassionate, and respectful to the needs of the affected individuals as well as to the communities in which they reside (Disaster Mental Health Subcommittee of the National Biodefense Science Board, 2008). Terrorist events, like all disasters, are each unique in terms of population affected (*targeted* in terrorism), type of incident (*agent used* in terrorism), amount of destruction, and psychological effects. Therefore, flexibility in design and implementation is paramount to meeting individual and community needs. The Disaster Mental Health Subcommittee of the National Biodefense Science Board (2008) recommended that the design and implementation of mental health interventions not only take into consideration the ecology of the culture but also the place of the attack and the type of trauma at a systems level in order to optimize the effectiveness of interventions.

The first task for disaster mental health intervention efforts is to subdivide the affected population into those who are psychiatrically ill versus those who are distressed. These groups require different intervention strategies. Inappropriately broad application of psychiatric treatments to the entire population can be counterproductive and ineffective, as interventions needs of people with psychiatric illness are clearly different from those experiencing distress that does not reach diagnostic proportions. If appropriate treatment matching does not occur, people experiencing normative distress can be inappropriately pathologized and exposed to unneeded and potentially harmful interventions, e.g., inappropriate medications (North & Westerhaus, 2003).

Effective disaster mental health response thus begins by identifying individuals with emotional distress and differentiating those who have psychiatric disorders most commonly identified in association with exposure to disaster such as PTSD and major depression. When large populations need assessment, screening procedures can identify those at risk for psychiatric disorders, and high-risk cases identified through screening can be triaged for full psychiatric assessment and treatment, if appropriate. Individuals with known risk factors for psychiatric disorders as described earlier in this chapter may warrant special attention.

Fortunately, the mental health consequences of disasters, including long-term cost and morbidity, can be mitigated by providing services within the first few weeks after the event (Homish, Frazer, McCartan, & Billittier, 2010). However, this requires planning and coordination of mental health interventions with other emergency and medical services to assure rapid mobilization and implementation. Because symptoms and emotional distress begin quickly after disasters, mental health responses also need to start quickly. Even though psychosocial manifestations of disaster exposure most often begin within days of the incident, those affected often delay in seeking treatment or fail to obtain treatment altogether (Weisæth, 2001). The disaster response operation must therefore provide outreach to identify cases and help them connect with appropriate mental health services (Lindy, Grace, & Green, 1981; North & Hong, 2000).

Provision of appropriate mental health interventions needs to be flexible based on the amount of time that has passed since the attack. It takes weeks for new psychiatric disorders such as PTSD and major depressive episodes to fully develop and be diagnosable. Therefore, in the first few days after disaster, diagnosis and treatment of psychiatric disorders will be mostly limited to pre-existing disorders fully established before the disaster that continue or are even exacerbated in the short term after the disaster. Mental health interventions during this period will therefore otherwise be mostly concerned with providing relief for distress and symptoms such as insomnia and anxiety. Psychiatric personnel may therefore be needed in the early postdisaster period to refill prescriptions and assess the status of existing psychiatric illness, and, if needed, provide interventions for more particularly distressing symptoms (e.g., sleep aids for profound insomnia).

The unique characteristics of chemical, biological, and radiological terrorist attacks including imperceptibility and uncertainty of exposures and misinterpretation of symptoms as evidence of exposure present special challenges that may affect intervention needs after this type of disaster (North, 2007). Widespread fear, rumors, and stigmatization of groups of people that may follow terrorist incidents may create special intervention needs to counter these types of problems. Thus, intervention needs may be expected to include not just treatment for psychiatric disorders and measures for relief of distress, but also prevention and management of mass surge behaviors, rumors and misinformation, distrust, and stigmatization.

Treatment of Psychiatric Disorders Following Terrorism

Psychiatric treatment is appropriate for individuals with psychiatric disorders. Traditional pharmacotherapy may be needed for the treatment of disorders such as PTSD, other anxiety disorders, and depressive disorders that may arise in the weeks and months following disasters. Pre-existing disorders such as schizophrenia or bipolar disorder that are endemic in general populations may require re-evaluation and treatment in postdisaster settings.

Psychotherapy may also be a useful intervention for psychiatric disorders arising after terrorist incidents. To our knowledge, there is only one randomized, controlled study of a cognitive-based psychotherapy in a disaster setting (Basoglu, Salcioglu, Livanou, Kalender, & Acar, 2005). Conducting randomized clinical control trials of treatments after terrorist attacks or other disasters has largely been prohibitive due to logistics of chaotic postdisaster settings and the amount of time required to secure cooperation of agencies, research funding, and institutional human studies approvals. Therefore, it should be recognized that recommendations for interventions after disasters have not been subjected to randomized controlled trials, although they are guided by available data. Hobfoll et al. (2007) proposed a set of empirically supported principles to guide interventions particularly in the early to mid-stage periods after disasters and mass violence, with the goals of promoting a sense of safety, calming, a sense of self and collective sense, connectedness, and hope. Many of these elements are the same as those found in traditional therapies for psychiatric disorders such as PTSD.

Cognitive–behavioral psychotherapy is recommended by disaster researchers to reduce the incidence, duration, and severity of acute stress disorder, PTSD, and depression after disasters (Meredith et al., 2011). Cognitive–behavioral approaches to therapy may be particularly useful for addressing specific psychological issues generated by terrorist attacks. Because terrorist incidents are carried out to undermine and destroy the public's sense of safety, psychological effects may include the shaking of people's world views and the shattering of myths of American safety and the government's ability to protect the populace. In contrast to natural disasters and technological accidentals, terrorist attacks are personal attacks with someone "out to get you." The uncertainties characteristic of terrorist attacks, such as not knowing when the immediate danger is over, not knowing the extent of damage or the spread of a chemical, biological, or radiological agent, and not knowing when the next attack will come, may demolish perceptions of safety. In this situation, people may exhibit cognitive distortions such as overgeneralizing and catastrophizing, which may in turn lead to negative emotions.

Cognitive therapy addresses such cognitive distortions by first identifying and challenging them and then replacing them with more accurate and balanced thoughts about the current situation and the future. Cognitive therapy is an established and widely used form of therapy with proven efficacy for treatment of PTSD and other psychiatric disorders (National Academy of Sciences Institute of Medicine, 2007; Nemeroff et al., 2006; Ponniah & Hollon, 2009), and the principles of treatment are applicable for the psychological difficulties of people who have experienced a terrorist attack. Some of the most researched cognitive–behavioral therapies for PTSD are prolonged exposure therapy (Cahill, Foa, Hembree, Marshall, & Nacash, 2006) and cognitive processing therapy (Resick, Monson, & Chard, 2007).

A form of cognitive behavioral therapy has been developed to treat postdisaster distress by targeting a range of common problems in the disaster setting (e.g., anger, anxiety, substance abuse, depression) rather than focusing on a specific disorder (Hamblen, Gibson, Mueser, & Norris, 2006). These techniques would also be appropriate for application in postdisaster settings of terrorist attacks. The therapy is designed to function as an intermediate step between psychological first aid (PFA) and long-term evidence-based treatments.

It is generally recommended that participation in therapy, whether in group or individual sessions, should be voluntary and that providers tailor the pace of the therapy sessions to the progress of the individual, avoiding the probing of long-term problems or issues unrelated to the current disaster situation (Meredith et al., 2011). Readers may find more detailed information on treatment in the general disaster setting in the chapter in this text entitled "Psychiatric and psychological issues in survivors of major disasters."

Other Mental Health Interventions

In general, delivery of mental health interventions in disaster settings should be brief, with the aim of increasing resilience and emotional coping by focusing on problem solving (Meredith et al., 2011).

Psychological First Aid

PFA is mental health assistance that is provided by mental health workers and other disaster-response workers, in the immediate aftermath of disaster and terrorism to reduce initial distress and foster coping and functioning (Terrorism and Disaster Branch of the National Child Traumatic Stress Network and the National Center for PTSD, 2005). This evidence-informed intervention is designed to be delivered in the first few days to weeks after a disaster. It is provided flexibly, depending on the needs of those being served. Offering a wide range of related services (such as helping survivors contact family members and connecting people with local resources) also help reduce distress (Meredith et al., 2011). Readers are directed to http://www.vdh.state.va.us/EPR/pdf/PFA9–6-05Final.pdf for a complete description of PFA with strategies for its application to adults as well as children and adolescents.

Risk Communication

In the post-terrorism environment, effective risk communication is vital to reducing widespread fear and dispelling rumors, and stigma reduction is needed to counter widespread stigmatization. As such, risk communication is a critical component of mental health response to disaster. This practice is applied before, during, and after a terrorist attack.

Risk communication is a process of information exchange that provides guidance to help people respond appropriately and safely to hazardous situations, offers appropriate reassurance, and informs the public of what is being done for them, especially plans to address public safety and recovery (Covello, Peters, Wojteki, & Hyde, 2001). Effective risk communication includes the public as a partner; listens to the concerns of the people; carefully plans and evaluates communication efforts; is honest, frank, and open; speaks with compassion; meets the needs of the media; and involves credible sources to increase the effectiveness of communication (Covello & Allen, 1988). Timely and accurate risk communication can greatly reduce unwarranted fear in the population, mitigate the disaster impact, and reduce excessive demands on the health care system generated by psychosocial responses such as anxiety and fear (Beaton et al., 2007).

Risk communication preparedness depends on the availability of a repertoire of scientifically based messages that have been pretested to assure comprehension by the general public and ready for immediate release if a terrorist attack occurs. Depending on the characteristics of a particular terrorist attack, different key concepts and specific facts must be disseminated to the public. In a radiological/nuclear event, for example, the most important first message to get to the public is that people should stay inside (i.e., "shelter in place") until radiation levels subside to a safe level after several hours. As more information is needed, instruction on how to determine exposure and contamination can be communicated along with specific directions for decontamination (Becker, 2004). Dissemination of this kind of information to the public can substantially reduce morbidity and mortality (Becker, 2007). The Centers for Disease Control and Prevention (CDC) website (http://emergency.cdc.gov) provides specific hazards fact sheets providing detailed information of this type for a variety of chemical, biological, and radiological agents, and what to do if exposed.

In the event of a terrorist attack, information for risk communication can be disseminated through multiple modes of communication. The traditional means of communication in such circumstances is through the media (e.g., newscasts, newspapers, public announcements). Speaking to the media for risk communication purposes is most effective when certain principles are followed, as distilled and summarized by Covello and Allen (1988) and Covello et al. (2001). First, the credibility of the spokesperson in a crisis situation is the key to attaining and maintaining the public trust that is vital for messages to be heeded. Therefore, partnering with credible and trusted sources of information is a key to the success of risk communication. The best approach is to be honest and forthcoming, modeling calmness, confidence, and compassion (Covello, 2001). An excellent example of this strategy was demonstrated by New York City mayor Rudy Giuliani in the aftermath of the September 11, 2001, terrorist attacks on the World Trade Center. Hours after the attacks, when asked about the number of casualties, he simply responded, "More than we can bear." His compassion and his openness about his own emotional pain humanized him and allowed people everywhere to identify with him (Lundgren & McMakin, 2009).

Basic principles of effective risk communication have been established (Covello, 2001; Covello et al., 2001; Norwood et al., 2001). To optimize the effectiveness of dissemination of risk communication messages, it is best if the message can be planned in advance, prepared for a target audience, and directed toward specific desired goals. The communication should have no more than two or three major "take-home" messages ("talking points"), and the content should be clear and succinct. There are several common errors to be avoided. These are communication of mixed or inconsistent messages, inadvertent nonverbal communication of unintended messages, humor (which is inconsistent with the grave emotional climate of crisis situations and likely to be taken as off-putting and even offensive), technical jargon and unfamiliar acronyms, extensive use of language conveying negative connotations (a general rule is to balance one negative with three positives), and giving the appearance of withholding information (e.g., through use of the phrase "no comment"; Covello, 2001). It is best to promise only what can be delivered. It is best to stay with the known situation rather than to indulge invitations to visit imaginary worst-case scenarios. It is also better to admit not knowing a fact rather than guessing, which may quickly destroy one's credibility.

Risk communication can also be disseminated through currently available mass communication technologies such as mobile phones and email and through other technologically efficient means such as the Internet, YouTube, blogs, podcasts, RSS feeds, wikis, Twitter feeds, and social networking sites such as Facebook (Project for Excellence in Journalism, 2011). Most Americans use the internet daily: 48% say they use search engines at least once a day and 69% believe this is the fastest way to get news and health information (MSN-Harris, 2004). During the 2001 anthrax scare, internet news sites were the most common way that internet users accessed information about anthrax: the CDC had more than one half million visits to their website in 1 week, and "Anthrax" was the fifth most often searched term on the Google search engine for the entire year (Bar-Ilan & Echerman, 2005). Risk communicators can take advantage of these powerful and easily accessible modes of communication via media links to provide facts and information about health and safety to wide audiences following terrorist attacks.

The CDC (2010) has developed a three-part strategy for emergency and risk communication through Web-based systems: (1) blend emergency risk communication principles with Web usability principles, (2) seek out and utilize opportunities to educate the public through effective Web link design and email updates, and (3) target internet accessibility for specific audiences through a variety of Web channel technologies. Specific risk communication principles have been delineated for internet dissemination that incorporate and build on traditional risk communication principles (CDC, 2010). These principles are emphasizing the agency's plan and where it can be found, avoiding excessive reassurance, acknowledging public uncertainties and fears, giving people reasonable and specific actions to take in the moment, and providing anticipatory guidance. Adapting traditional risk communication principles for internet use should take into account the fact that users functionally have tunnel vision, impatiently scanning rather than carefully reading web pages, and they will leave pages if they don't quickly find what they are looking for. Therefore, Web-based information must be clearly and succinctly laid out, easily located, and direct and to-the-point in its message to be widely accessed.

BUILDING COMMUNITY RESILIENCE

Along with providing interventions for distressed individuals after terrorism, attention to postdisaster issues at the community level may further benefit the rebuilding of resilience of the community. Norris, Friedman, and Watson (2002a) emphasized the important role of communities in emotional recovery and mental health outcomes of people in the community. A resilient community can provide a buffering and nurturing environment for individuals and families within it.

A resilient community is one that has resources, competencies, and natural support systems that help it and its members withstand major trauma and loss, overcome adversity, and bounce back and rebuild. As soon as possible following a terrorist incident, a careful, but quick community needs assessment should be conducted. Initial population-level psychosocial interventions should be focused on implementation of adaptive coping, restoring a sense of safety, modeling calm and communal and self-efficacy, fostering hope, promoting connectedness, and providing accurate information (Disaster Mental Health Subcommittee of the National Biodefense Science Board, 2008).

Hobfoll et al. (2007) described the role of the resilient community in helping its members after a collective trauma:

> The advantage of a community model over the individual, in this regard, is that the group (e.g., mosque, school, business organization, chamber of commerce, Rotary Club) can develop hope–building interventions, such as helping others clean up and rebuild, making home visits, organizing blood drives, and involving members of the community who feel they cannot act individually because of the magnitude of the problem.

Walsh and McGoldrick (2004) and Saul (2002) have identified four main processes to facilitate healing and resilience after traumatic loss and disaster. The first involves developing an information base to inventory losses, clarifying circumstances and ambiguities, and identifying needs of the people. The second involves sharing in survivorship and loss through memorials and group activities or rituals; sharing of stories, social support, spirituality; and communal emotional and cognitive processing and finding meaning in what has happened. The third process involves planning for the well-being of survivors, taking care of people, and starting to rebuild homes, businesses, social networks, lives, and community. Finally, the fourth process involves moving forward to develop new hopes and aspirations;

revising future plans to accommodate necessary realities after the event; and finding new purpose in life. Saul (2004) observed that the breadth and diversity of the skill sets of the people of a community coming together to work toward a common purpose are its tools to rebuild and move forward in community functioning. A valuable source of community resilience after a disaster may spring from the creativity of its people whose artistic, musical, and spiritual endeavors may provide cultural vehicles for communal processing and finding meaning in what has happened to them and their community.

Walsh (2007) pointed out that healing communities typically exhibit attitudes of tolerance, openness, and attitudes of respect toward differences among the peoples that make up the community. This is a particularly salient issue in the wake of terrorist events, when suspicion, distrust, intolerance, and divisiveness between groups may afflict communities. It is also relevant for terrorist incidents that involve perceptions of contamination and result in stigmatization of disaster victim and evacuee groups. Application of risk communication efforts may be warranted in such situations to help educate members of the community, clarify misunderstandings, correct misinformation, and model positive attitudes. Additionally, community leaders, grassroots organizers, and stakeholders may help communities overcome some of these problems by encouraging activities and discourse that humanize members of diverse groups and bring people together in discourse and activities toward a common goal of rebuilding the community.

In communities attempting to recover from profound terrorist incidents, collective cognitive distortions may arise that may seed the spread of discouragement, promote a communal sense of nihilism, and increase the public's fear. For example, after the 9/11 attacks, there was a sense of collective despair, shock, and loss of the former sense of safety in America; the phrase "Life will never be the same again" was often repeated in the media. On the surface, many people might have agreed that life may never be the same again, but closer examination of what this phrase really states reveals it to be a cognitive distortion that involves inappropriate overgeneralization. It may be true that certain specific things may never be the same again, such as the loss of the Twin Towers on the Manhattan skyline and the new levels of airport security procedures. However, most things have not permanently changed, such as most New Yorkers still live in New York, Broadway shows go on, people buy their groceries in the same stores they always did, people eat turkey at Thanksgiving, students graduate from high school, babies are born, etc. When overgeneralized negative phrases are propagated in the media and by word of mouth, they elicit negative emotions such as despair and fear. Replacement of the distorted statement with more balanced and accurate assessments of the general state of affairs and projection into the future may promote healthier public perceptions and attitudes, ultimately promoting resilience. Public education campaigns such as public service announcements might be able to help members of affected communities develop more realistic and positive attitudes by addressing these distortions.

PREPAREDNESS

The 9/11 attacks increased the American focus of attention toward prevention of terrorism and heightened awareness of the need for preparedness plans. In particular, it is recognized that psychosocial responses must be developed and tested along with medical responses and integrated with the medical response for the nation to be sufficiently prepared for any future terrorist attacks. Mental health preparedness must deal with the current reality that existing mental health resources are already severely strained and could be completely overwhelmed in the days and weeks after a terrorist attack (North & Westerhaus, 2003).

Successful mitigation of the psychosocial consequences of disasters (including acts of terrorism) requires adequate preparedness in three distinct areas: application of appropriate interventions; education and training of providers, leaders, and the public; and enhancement of and targeting communication and messaging (Disaster Mental Health Subcommittee of the National Biodefense Science Board, 2008).

The Department of Homeland Security has outlined a National Response Framework (NRF) that contains the guiding principles for preparation and provision for a unified national response to disasters and emergencies, including terrorist attacks. A link to the website is http://www.fema.gov/NRF/pdf/emergency/nrf/nrf-core.pdf. This guide for the Nation's all-hazards response describes 15 Emergency Support Functions (ESFs) that can be called up as needed and coordinated within an Incident Command System. Each ESF has a coordinator and support functions including several points that are relevant for post-terrorism mental health preparedness functions, especially ESF-8 (Public Health and Medical Services) and ESF-6 (Mass Care, Emergency Assistance, Housing, and Human Services). ESF-6 incorporates mental health preparedness functions and plans. The Federal Emergency Management Agency (FEMA) also outlines 15 national planning scenarios with all but three being directly applicable to terrorist attacks, and these can be accessed through the following link: http://www.fema.gov/pdf/media/factsheets /2009/ npd_natl_plan_scenario.pdf). Although National Level Exercises have been carried out with new ones scheduled on an at least annual basis, mental health preparedness has not been featured prominently in these exercises and plans. A pivotal roundtable meeting was convened by the CDC in December, 2005, with the aim of identifying major gaps in the management of radiological terrorism challenges. The roundtable recommended better integration of psychosocial preparedness into the Nation's planning, training, exercises, and incident management protocols (CDC, 2006). These recommendations are applicable to all types of terrorist events. Based on these recommendations, the Nation can expect to achieve new levels of psychosocial preparedness for terrorist incidents, demonstrated with the availability of new plans and readiness training for mitigating the psychosocial effects of future terrorist incidents.

REFERENCES

Ackerman, G., & Tamsett, J. (2009). Jihadist tactics and targeting. In J. J. F. Forest & S. Salama (Eds.), *Jihadists and weapons of mass destruction* (pp. 83–99). Boca Raton, FL: CRC Press.

Alexander, D. A., & Klein, S. (2003). Biochemical terrorism: Too awful to contemplate, too serious to ignore: Subjective literature review. *British Journal of Psychiatry, 183,* 491–497.

American Psychiatric Association. (1987). *Diagnostic and statistical manual of mental disorders,* 3rd Revised edition. Washington, DC: Author.

American Psychiatric Association. (2000). *Diagnostic and statistical manual of mental disorders,* 4th Edition, Text Revision. Washington, DC: Author.

Bar-Ilan, J., & Echerman, A. (2005). The anthrax scare and the Web. A content analysis of Web pages linking of resources on anthrax. *Scientometrics, 63,* 443–462.

Basoglu, M., Salcioglu, E., Livanou, M., Kalender, D., & Acar, G. (2005). Single-session behavioral treatment of earthquake-related posttraumatic stress disorder: A randomized waiting list controlled trial. *Journal of Traumatic Stress, 18,* 1–11.

BBC Mobile News Magazine. (2008). The evolution of a conspiracy theory. *BBC.* Retrieved March 26, 2001, from http://news.bbc.co.uk/2/hi/uk_news/magazine/7488159.stm.

BBC News. (2010). The conspiracy files. *BBC News.* Retrieved March 26, 2011, from http://news.bbc.co.uk/2/hi/programmes/conspiracy_files/default.stm.

Beaton, R., Stergachis, A., Oberle, M., Bridges, E., Nemuth, M., & Thomas, T. (2007). The sarin gas attacks on the Tokyo subway: 10 years later—Lessons learned. In S. Mahan & P. Griset (Eds.), *Terrorism in perspective* (pp. 296–307). London: Sage.

Becker, S. M. (2004). Emergency communication and information issues in terrorist events involving radioactive materials. *Biosecurity and Bioterrorism, 2,* 195–207.

Becker, S. M. (2005). Addressing the psychosocial and communication challenges posed by radiological/nuclear terrorism: Key developments since NCRP Report No. 138. *Health Physics, 89*, 521–530.

Becker, S. M. (2007). Communicating risk to the public after radiological incidents. *BMJ, 335*, 1106–1107.

Becker, S. M. (2009). Preparing for terrorism involving radioactive materials: Three lessons from recent experience and research. *Journal of Applied Security Research, 4*, 9–20.

Bowman, M. L. (1999). Individual differences in posttraumatic distress: Problems with the DSM-IV model. *Canadian Journal of Psychiatry, 44*, 21–33.

Breslau, N. (2001). The epidemiology of posttraumatic stress disorder: What is the extent of the problem? *Journal of Clinical Psychiatry, 62*, 16–22.

Cahill, S. P., Foa, E. B., Hembree, E. A., Marshall, R. D., & Nacash, N. (2006). Dissemination of exposure therapy in the treatment of posttraumatic stress disorder. *Journal of Traumatic Stress, 19*, 597–610.

Centers for Disease Control and Prevention. (2006). Roundtable on the psychosocial challenges posed by a radiological terrorism incident. A summary report. *Ogilvy Public Relations Worldwide under CDC contract.* Retrieved April 6, 2011, from http://www.bt.cdc.gov/radiation/pdf/rt-psychosocial.pdf.

Centers for Disease Control and Prevention. (2010). Emergency and risk communication on the web. *The Risk Communicator Newsletter.* Retrieved March 28, 2011, from http://www.bt.cdc.gov/ercn/03/rcn01.asp.

Covello, V. T. (October 24, 2001). *Lessons learned from the front lines of risk and crisis communication: 21 guidelines for effective communication by leaders addressing high anxiety, high stress, or threatening situations.* Keynote address, U.S. Conference of Mayors, Emergency, Safety, and Security Summit, Washington, DC.

Covello, V. T., & Allen, F. H. (1988). *Seven cardinal rules of risk communication.* Pamphlet #OPA-87-020. Washington, DC: U.S. Environmental Protection Agency.

Covello, V. T., Peters, R. G., Wojteki, J. G., & Hyde, R. C. (2001). Risk communication, the West Nile virus, and bioterrorism: responding to the challenges posed by the intentional or unintentional release of a pathogen in an urban setting. *Journal of Urban Health, 87*, 382–391.

David, D., Mellman, T. A., Mendoza, L. M., Kulick-Bell, R., Ironson, G., & Schneiderman, N. (1996). Psychiatric morbidity following Hurricane Andrew. *Journal of Traumatic Stress, 9*, 607–612.

Davis, D. W., & Silver, B. D. (2004). Civil liberties vs. security: public opinion in the context of the terrorist attacks on America. *American Journal of Political Science, 48*, 28–46.

DiGrande, L., Neria, Y., Brackbill, R. M., Pulliam, P., & Galea, S. (2011). Long-term posttraumatic stress symptoms among 3,271 civilian survivors of the September 11, 2001, terrorist attacks on the world trade center. *American Journal of Epidemiology, 173*, 271–281.

Disaster Mental Health Subcommittee of the National Biodefense Science Board. (2008). Disaster mental health recommendations: report of the Disaster Mental Health Subcommittee of the National Biodefense Science Board. *National Biodefense Science Board.* Retrieved April 3, 2011, from http://www.phe.gov/Preparedness/legal/boards/nbsb/Documents/nsbs-dmhreport-final.pdf

Dunn, J. R., Taylor, S. M., Elliott, S. J., & Walter, S. D. (1994). Psychosocial effects of PCB contamination and remediation: The case of Smithville, Ontario. *Social Science & Medicine, 39*, 1093–1104.

Ehlers, A., Mayou, R. A., & Bryant, B. (1998). Psychological predictors of chronic posttraumatic stress disorder after motor vehicle accidents. *Journal of Abnormal Psychology, 107*, 508–519.

Erikson, K. (1994). *A new species of trouble: The human experience of modern disasters.* New York: WW Norton.

Federal Bureau of Investigation. (2001). Hate crimes statistics, 2001. *Uniform Crime Reporting System, US Department of Justice.* Retrieved August 13, 2010, from http://www.fbi.gov/ucr/01hate.pdf

Flynn, S. E. (2004). *America the vulnerable: How our government is failing to protect us from terrorism.* New York: HarperCollins.

Fullerton, C. S., Ursano, R. J., & Norwood, A. E. (2004). Planning for the psychological effects of bioterrorism. In R. J. Ursano, A. E. Norwood, & C. S. Fullerton (Eds.), *Bioterrorism: Psychological and public health interventions* (pp. 2–14). Cambridge: Cambridge University Press.

Galea, S., Ahern, J., Resnick, H., Kilpatrick, D., Bucuvalas, M., Gold, J., & Vlahov, D. (2002). Psychological sequelae of the September 11 terrorist attacks in New York City. *New England Journal of Medicine, 346*, 982–987.

Ginzburg, H. M. (1993). The psychological consequences of the chernobyl accident—Findings from the International Atomic Energy Agency Study. *Public Health Report, 108*, 184–192.

Green, B. L., Lindy, J. D., Grace, J. C., & Leonard, A. C. (1992). Chronic posttraumatic stress disorder and diagnostic comorbidity in a disaster sample. *Journal of Nervous and Mental Disease, 180*, 760–766.

Hamblen, J. L., Gibson, L. E., Mueser, K. T., & Norris, F. H. (2006). Cognitive behavioral therapy for prolonged postdisaster distress. *Journal of Clinical Psychology, 62*, 1043–1052.

Hargrove, T, & Stempel, G. H., III (2006). A third of U.S. public believes 9/11 conspiracy theory. *Scripps Howard News Service.* Retrieved January 15, 2008, from http://www.shns.com/shns/g_index2.cfm?action=detail&pk=CONSPIRACY-08-02-06

Hasin, D. S., Keyes, K. M., Hatzenbuehler, M. L., Aharonovich, E. A., & Alderson, D. (2007). Alcohol consumption and posttraumatic stress after exposure to terrorism: Effects of proximity, loss, and psychiatric history. *American Journal of Public Health, 97*, 2268–2275.

Hendricks, N. J., Ortiz, C. W., Sugie, N., & Miller, J. (2007). Beyond the numbers: Hate crimes and cultural trauma within Arab American immigrant communities. *International Review of Victimology, 14*, 95–113.

Hobfoll, S. E., Watson, P., Bell, C. C., Bryant, R. A., Brymer, M. J., Friedman, M. J.,...Ursano, R. J. (2007). Five essential elements of immediate and mid-term mass trauma intervention: Empirical evidence. *Psychiatry, 70*, 283–315.

Homish, G. G., Frazer, B. S., McCartan, D. P., & Billittier, A. J. (2010). Emergency mental health: lessons learned from flight 3407. *Disaster Medicine and. Public Health Preparedness, 4*, 326–331.

Koscheyev, V. S., Leon, G. R., Gourine, A. V., & Gourine, V. N. (1997). The psychosocial aftermath of the Chernobyl disaster in an area of relatively low contamination. *Prehospital and Disaster Medicine, 12*, 41–46.

Lewin, T. (2001). Sikh owner of gas station is fatally shot in rampage. *The New York Times*. Retrieved March 26, 2011, from http://www.nytimes.com/2001/09/17/us/sikh-owner-of-gas-station-is-fatally-shot-in-rampage.html

Lindy, J. D., Grace, M. C., & Green, B. L. (1981). Survivors: Outreach to a reluctant population. *American Journal of Orthopsychiatry, 51*, 468–478.

Lundgren, R. E., & McMakin, A. H. (2009). *Risk communication: A handbook for communicating environmental, safety, and health risks*, 4th edition. Hoboken, NJ: Wiley.

Maes, M., Delmeire, L., Schotte, C., Aleksander, J., Creten, T., Mylle, J.,...Rousseeuw, P. J. (1998). Epidemiologic and phenomenological aspects of post-traumatic stress disorder: DSM-III-R diagnosis and diagnostic criteria not validated. *Psychiatry Research, 81*, 179–193.

Marcus, A. (2001). *Attacks spark rise in substance abuse treatment: Group says stress-related drug, alcohol problems will worsen*. Arlington, VA: The Health Central Network, HealthScoutNews. Retrieved August 31, 2005, from http://healingwellpsych.subportal.com/health/Drugs_Alcohol_Tobacco/Drug_Abuse/505078.html

McFarlane, A. C., & Papay, P. (1992). Multiple diagnoses in posttraumatic stress disorder in the victims of a natural disaster. *Journal of Nervous and Mental Disease, 180*, 498–504.

McMillen, J. C., North, C. S., & Smith, E. M. (2000). What parts of PTSD are normal: Intrusion, avoidance, or arousal? Data from the Northridge, California earthquake. *Journal of Traumatic Stress, 13*, 57–75.

Meredith, L. S., Eisenman, E. P., Tanielian, T., Taylor, S. L., Basurto-Davila, R., Zazzali, J.,...Shields, S. (2011). Prioritizing "psychological' consequences of disaster preparedness and response: a framework for addressing the emotional, behavioral, and cognitive effects of patient surge in large-scale disasters. *Disaster Medicine and Public Health Preparedness, 5*(1), 73–80.

Meyers, D. (2001). Weapons of mass destruction and terrorism: mental health consequences and implications for planning and training. *Weapons of Mass Destruction/Terrorism, Orientation Pilot Program*. Pine Bluff, AR: Clara Barton Center for Domestic Preparedness.

MSN-Harris. (2004). MSN-Harris interactive survey asks: what is America searching for? *Microsoft News Center*. Retrieved March 28, 2011, from http://www.microsoft.com/presspass/press/2004/aug04/08-02searchpollpr.mspx

National Academy of Sciences Institute of Medicine. (2003). *Preparing for the psychological consequences of terrorism: A public health strategy*. Washington, DC: National Academy Press.

National Academy of Sciences Institute of Medicine. (2007). *Treatment of posttraumatic stress disorder: An assessment of the evidence*. Washington, DC: The National Academies Press.

National Research Council, Smelser, N. J., & Mitchell, F. (Eds). (2002). *Terrorism: Perspectives from the behavioral and social sciences*. Washington, DC: The National Academies Press.

Nemeroff, C. B., Bremner, J. D., Foa, E. B., Mayberg, H. S., North, C. S., & Stein, M. B. (2006). Posttraumatic stress disorder: A state-of-the-science review. *Journal of Psychiatry Research, 40*, 1–21.

Neria, Y., Nandi, A., & Galea, S. (2008). Post-traumatic stress disorder following disasters: A systematic review. *Psychological Medicine, 38*, 467–480.

Norris, F. H., Friedman, M. J., & Watson, P. J. (2002). 60,000 disaster victims speak: Part II. Summary and implications of the disaster mental health research. *Psychiatry, 65*, 240–260.

Norris, F. H., Friedman, M. J., Watson, P. J., Byrne, C. M., Diaz, E., & Kaniasty, K. (2002b). 60,000 disaster victims speak: Part I. An empirical review of the empirical literature, 1981–2001. *Psychiatry, 65*, 207–239.

North, C. S. (2004). Approaching disaster mental health research after the 9/11 World Trade Center terrorist attacks. *Psychiatric Clinics of North America, 27*, 589–602.

North, C. S. (2007). Epidemiology of disaster mental health response. In R. J. Ursano, C. S. Fullerton, L. Weisæth, & B. Raphael (Eds.), *Textbook of disaster psychiatry* (pp. 29–47). New York: Cambridge University Press.

North, C. S., & Hong, B. A. (2000). Project C.R.E.S.T.: A new model for mental health intervention after a community disaster. *American Journal of Public Health, 90*, 1-2.

North, C. S., Hong, B. A., & Pfefferbaum, B. (2008). P-FLASH: Development of an empirically-based post-9/11 disaster mental health training program. *Missouri Medicine, 105*, 62-66.

North, C. S., McCutcheon, V., Spitznagel, E. L., & Smith, E. M. (2002). Three-year follow-up of survivors of a mass shooting episode. *Journal of Urban Health, 79*, 383-391.

North, C. S., Nixon, S. J., Shariat, S., Mallonee, S., McMillen, J. C., Spitznagel, E.L., & Smith, E. M. (1999). Psychiatric disorders among survivors of the Oklahoma City bombing. *JAMA, 282*, 755-762.

North, C. S., & Pfefferbaum, B. (2002). Research on the mental health effects of terrorism. *Journal of the American Medical Association, 288*, 633-636.

North, C. S., & Pfefferbaum, B. (2004). The state of research on the mental health effects of terrorism. *Epidemiology and Psichiatry Society, 13*, 4-9.

North, C. S., Pfefferbaum, B., Hong, B. A., Gordon, M. R., Kim, Y. S., Lind, L., & Pollio, D. E. (2010). The business of healing: focus group discussions of readjustment to the post-9/11 work environment among employees of affected agencies. *Journal of Occupational and Environmental Medicine, 52*, 713-718.

North, C. S., Pfefferbaum, B., Kawasaki, A., Lee, S., & Spitznagel, E. L. (2010). Psychosocial adjustment of directly exposed survivors 7 years after the Oklahoma City bombing. *Comprehensive Psychiatry, 52*, 1-8.

North, C. S., Pfefferbaum, B., Vythilingam, M., Martin, G. J., Schorr, J. K., Boudreaux, A. S.,...Hong, B. A. (2009a). Exposure to bioterrorism and mental health response among staff on Capitol Hill. *Biosecurity and Bioterrorism, 7*, 379-388.

North, C. S., Pollio, D. E., Pfefferbaum, B., Megivern, D., Vythilingam, M., Westerhaus, E. T.,...Hong, B. A. (2005a). Capitol Hill staff workers' experiences of bioterrorism: qualitative findings from focus groups. *Journal of Traumatic Stress, 18*, 79-88.

North, C. S., Pollio, D. E., Pfefferbaum, B., Megivern, D., Vythilingam, M., Westerhaus, E. T.,...Hong, B. A. (2005b). Concerns of Capitol Hill staff workers after bioterrorism: Focus group discussions of authorities' response. *Journal of Nervous and Mental Disease, 193*, 523-527.

North, C. S., Ringwalt, C. L., Downs, D., Derzon, J., & Galvin, D. (2011a). Postdisaster course of alcohol use disorders in systematically studied survivors of 10 disasters. *Archives of General Psychiatry, 68*, 173-180.

North, C. S., Smith, E. M., & Spitznagel, E. L. (1994). Posttraumatic stress disorder in survivors of a mass shooting. *American Journal of Psychiatry, 151*, 82-88.

North, C. S., & Surís, A. M. (2011). Psychiatric and psychological issues in survivors of major disasters. In I. Marini & M. Stebnicki (Eds.), *The psychological and social impact of illness and disability*. New York: Springer.

North, C. S., Surís, A. M., & Adewuyi, S. (2011). PTSD and psychiatric comorbidities. In D. Benedek & G. H. Wynne (Eds.), *Clinical manual for the management of posttraumatic stress disorder* (pp. 101-127). Washington, DC: American Psychiatric Press.

North, C. S., Surís, A. M., Davis, M., & Smith, R. P. (2009b). Toward validation of the diagnosis of posttraumatic stress disorder. *American Journal of Psychiatry, 166*, 1-8.

North, C. S., & Westerhaus, E. (2003). Applications from previous disaster research to guide mental health interventions after the September 11 attacks. In R. J. Ursano, C. S. Fullerton, & A. E. Norwood (Eds.), *Terrorism and disaster: Individual and community mental health interventions* (pp. 93-106). Cambridge: Cambridge University Press.

Norwood, A. E., Holloway, H. C., & Ursano, R. J. (2001). Psychological effects of biological warfare. *Military Medicine, 166*, 27-28.

Office of the Press Secretary. (2010). Remarks by President Obama and President Zuma of South Africa before Bilateral Meeting. *The White House*. Retrieved February 4, 2011, from http://www.WhiteHouse.gov/the-press-office/remarks-President-Obama-and-President-Zuma-South-Africa-bilateral-meeting.

Ponniah, K., & Hollon, S. D. (2009). Empirically supported psychological treatments for adult acute stress disorder and posttraumatic stress disorder: A review. *Depress Anxiety, 26*, 1086-1109.

Project for Excellence in Journalism. (2011). The growing impact of the internet. *The Daily Source*. Retrieved March 28, 2004, from http://www.dailysource.org/about/impact.

Resick, P. A., Monson, C. M., & Chard, K. M. (2007). *Cognitive processing therapy: Veteran/military version*. Washington, DC: Department of Veterans Affairs.

Rodriguez, J. J., & Kohn, R. (2008). Use of mental health services among disaster survivors. *Current Opinion in Psychiatry, 21*, 370-378.

Roy, M. J. (2004). *A physician's guide to terrorist attack*. Totawa, NJ: Humana Press.

Saad, L. (2010). *Anti-Muslim feelings fairly common in US*. Princeton, MJ: The Gallup Poll. Retrieved August 13, 2010, from http://www.gallup.com/poll/24073/AntiMuslim-Sentiments-Fairly-Commonplace.aspx#1

Saul, J. (November 2002). *Learning from humanitarian crises: community recovery in Manhattan, post 9/11.* Presentation at the International Society for Traumatic Stress Studies Annual Meeting, Baltimore, MD.

Saul, J. (2004). Promoting community recovery in lower Manhattan after September 11, 2001. *Bulletin of the Royal Institute for Interfaith Studies, 5,* 1–16.

Schlenger, W. E., Caddell, J. M., Ebert, L., Jordan, B. K., Rourke, K. M., Wilson, D., . . . Kulka, R. A. (2002). Psychological reactions to terrorist attacks: Findings from the National Study of Americans' Reactions to September 11. *JAMA, 288,* 581–588.

Schmid, A. P., & Jongman, A. J. (1988). *Political terrorism: A new guide to actors, authors, concepts, data bases, theories and literature.* New Brunswick, NJ: Transaction Books.

Schuster, M. A., Stein, B. D., Jaycox, L., Collins, R. L., Marshall, G. N., Elliott, M. N., . . . Berry, S. H. (2001). A national survey of stress reactions after the September 11, 2001, terrorist attacks. *New England Journal of Medicine, 345,* 1507–1512.

Sheridan, L. P. (2006). Islamophobia pre- and post-September 11th, 2001. *Journal of Interpersonal Violence, 21,* 317–336.

Silver, R. C., Holman, E. A., McIntosh, D. N., Poulin, M., & Gil-Rivas, V. (2002). Nationwide longitudinal study of psychological responses to September 11. *JAMA, 288,* 1235–1244.

Stuart, J. A., Ursano, R. J., Fullerton, C. S., Norwood, A. E., & Murray, K. (2003). Belief in exposure to terrorist agents: Reported exposure to nerve or mustard gas by Gulf War veterans. *Journal of Nervous and Mental Disease, 191,* 431–436.

Stuart, J. A., Ursano, R. J., Fullerton, C. S., & Wessely, S. (2008). Belief in exposure to chemical and biological agents in Persian Gulf War soldiers. *Journal of Nervous and Mental Disease, 196,* 122–127.

Sunstein, C. R., & Vermeule, A. (2008). *Conspiracy theories (preliminary draft).* Harvard University Law School Public Law & Legal Theory Research Paper Series; University of Chicago Law School, Public Law & Legal Theory Research Paper Series, Paper No. 199; and University of Chicago Law School, Law & Economics Research Paper Series, Paper No. 387.

Swahn, M. H., Mahendra, R. R., Paulozzi, L. J., Winston, R. L., Shelley, G. A., Taliano, J., . . . Saul, J. R. (2003). Violent attacks on Middle Easterners in the United States during the month following the September 11, 2001 terrorist attacks. *Injury Prevention, 9,* 187–189.

Terrorism and Disaster Branch of the National Child Traumatic Stress Network and the National Center for PTSD. (2005). *Psychological first aid: Field operations guide.* The National Center for Child Traumatic Stress.

Tuchman, G., et al. (2011). Anxiety in Japan grows as rescue workers find more bodies. *CNN.Com.* Retrieved March 14, 2011, from http://www.azfamily.com/news/national/Anxiety-in-Japan-grows-as-rescue-workers-find-more-bodies-117931314.html

Vlahov, D., Galea, S., Resnick, H., Ahern, J., Boscarino, J. A., Bucavalas, M., . . . Kilpatrick, D. (2002). Increased use of cigarettes, alcohol, and marijuana among Manhattan, New York, residents after the September 11th terrorist attacks. *American Journal of Epidemiology, 155,* 988–996.

Walsh, F. (2007). Traumatic loss and major disasters: strengthening family and community resilience. *Family Process, 46,* 207–227.

Walsh, F., & McGoldrick, M. (2004). Loss and the family: A systemic perspective. In F. Walsh & M. McGoldrick (Eds.), *Living beyond loss: Death in the family* (2nd ed., pp. 3–26). New York: Norton.

Weisæth, L. (2001). Acute posttraumatic stress: Nonacceptance of early intervention. *Journal of Clinical Psychiatry, 62,* 35–40.

Weisæth, L., & Tønnessen, A. (2003). Responses of individuals and groups to consequences of technological disasters and radiation exposure. In R. J. Ursano, C. S. Fullerton, & A. E. Norwood (Eds.), *Terrorism and disaster: Individual and community mental health interventions* (pp. 209–235). New York: Cambridge University Press.

Wilkinson, P. (1997). The media and terrorism: A reassessment. *Terrorism and Political Violence, 9,* 51–64.

Zogby International. (2004). Half of New Yorkers believe US leaders had foreknowledge of impending 9–11 attacks and "consciously failed" To act. *IBOPE/Zogby International.* Retrieved January 15, 2008, from http://zogby.com/news/ReadNews.dbm?ID=855.

Zogby, J. (2001). Testimony of Dr. James J. Zogby, submission to the United States Commission on Civil Rights, October 12, 2001. *Arab American Institute Foundation.* Retrieved August 13, 2010, from http://www.humanitykingdom.com/library/general/arab-american.pdf

31

Key Concepts and Techniques for an Aging Workforce

SUSANNE M. BRUYÈRE, DEBRA A. HARLEY, CHARLENE M. KAMPFE, AND JOHN S. WADSWORTH

Older workers are one of the fastest growing subsets of the American workforce. The U.S. Bureau of Labor Statistics predicted that between 2002 and 2012, the number of workers 55 years and older will grow by 50%. The aging population is likely to result in an increasing number of people with disabilities in the workforce who may have difficulty staying employed. The U.S. Census Bureau (2004) estimated that the 45- to 54- and 55- to 64-year-old population in the United States would grow by nearly 44.2 million (17%) and 35 million (39%) in the next 10 years. By the year 2010, this group will account for nearly half (44%) of the working-age population (20–64 years), and the number of people with disabilities between the ages of 50 and 65 will almost double (Weathers, 2006).

Effective counseling practices must increasingly include attention to preparing both individuals and their workplaces for the impact of the aging process. Proactive education on ways to maximize the productivity of an aging workforce, effective case management, and workplace accommodations can significantly contribute to maximizing aging-worker retention.

Older persons frequently experience dehumanizing situations or attitudes. They are often devalued by society, discriminated against with regard to employment, discouraged from making their own decisions about a variety of aspects of their lives, and forced to make residential relocations into institutions that may not encourage or allow independence of thought or action. The professional counselor's philosophy is antithetical to these practices.

Employment is a key aspect of the current social effort to promote financial independence, emotional health, and physical wellness among the growing population of older individuals. Both the need for economic support and the personal and social benefits of work may be important for persons of all ages. Some baby boomers are not waiting until retirement age to stop working; more than 4 million already have left the workforce due to retirement or disability. However, many older workers will need to work longer for the income it brings.

THEORETICAL AND CLINICAL CONSIDERATIONS

The aging process is unique to every individual. Professional counselors have many opportunities to provide interventions that improve the quality of life for older persons. However, theoretical and philosophical models used in counseling older individuals are overwhelmingly grounded in the medical model, which emphasizes the identification and treatment of pathological physical changes that are associated with growing older. The medical model identifies a diagnosis, prescribes a protocol for intervention, and predicts a prognosis. As a dominant paradigm, this model asserts that the body is a physical mechanism that can be studied quantitatively through measurement of physiological function and can be treated as well at a strictly physical level. In many ways, the medical model disregards psychological concepts, emotional reactions, and subjective data. In addition, the medical model looks within the individual for a diagnosis of the problem, placing the physician above the person, and ignores the environment. This emphasis may lead counselors to anchor assessment results on biases against older adults. Ultimately, the medical model is too rigid, restrictive, and disempowering because it adheres to the notion that aging itself is a type of impairment that with appropriate treatment can be either cured or altered.

A better understanding of aging is more closely aligned with the developmental model (Erikson, 1959). Erickson described human life in terms of stages—sequential developmental occurrences in which individuals experience developmental crises (e.g., change in employment status, loss, and grief). He pointed out that old age is a time when people struggle to find meaning in the life they have lived, a sense of ego, integrity, and satisfaction with a life well spent. The stage of life designated as *old age* involves numerous transitions (e.g., retirement, loss of autonomy, and impaired health). The advantage for older people of the developmental model is its focus on wellness, planning for successful adaptations, and empowerment to realize the developmental goal and reach their full potential.

Developmental frameworks for counseling intervention have been reported to be successful in addressing a wide variety of concerns that impact older persons. Sexuality for older persons may be addressed through holistic and developmental frameworks that stress the potential for lifelong capacity to enjoy intimacy and sensual enjoyment. Career development may be presented as a lifelong, dynamic process that requires individuals to engage throughout their lifetime in the ongoing assessment, analysis, and synthesis of information about the world of work and self.

Persons who are aging successfully have a more integrative experience that includes acceptance of the past, resolution of conflicts, and reconciliation of reality with the ideal self than persons who utilize escape and obsessive reminiscence of the past. Life reviews may allow clients to integrate life experiences and create new meaning to promote the resolution of conflicts and reconciliation with others in preparation for life transitions and the termination of life. Life planning may assist older persons in clarifying transferable vocational or leisure skills, planning for age-related change, and setting goal.

Personal control is vital in maintaining mental health and life satisfaction. The ability to make decisions, self-regulate behavior, and control the environment is positively associated with psychological well-being. Paid work is recognized as an important source of well-being for older men and women because work provides a sense of independence and competence outside of immediate family networks. Counseling interventions that encourage personal control rather than focus on diagnosis and pathology may be more effective in promoting the well-being of older persons.

The aging population requires multiple services from various service professionals (e.g., counselors, health care providers, and employment human resource departments). To better facilitate positive outcomes for aging populations, interagency collaboration offers an opportunity for enhanced employment outcomes. Casework is the common denominator, which cuts across various service professionals and is relevant to deconstructing disincentives for either maintaining or returning to work. (See Harley, Donnell, & Rainey, 2003, for strategies and implications for functional integration collaboration for crossing professional borders.)

Counseling aids older adults in coping and meeting their needs in changing situations. However, fewer older adults than younger ones use mental health services and other related counseling services. Older individuals may associate counseling treatment with institutionalization or believe it is reserved for extremely disturbed individuals. They may also attribute emotional difficulties to the normal process of growing older, and they may believe that the inability to cope with difficulties is a sign of failure to age successfully.

Assessment may involve special considerations for older consumers. People with no recent experiences in standardized testing may find some assessments threatening and may require additional explanation to clarify what the test measures, its relevancy to the questions at hand, and the benefits of the actual results. Testing instruments must be chosen to be appropriate. Norms are not available on some instruments for age cohorts beyond 60 or 65 (e.g., Holland's *Self-Directed Search*; Holland, 1994). Even instruments that include older persons in the norm groups often only go to age 89 or 90 and thus would not necessarily be applicable to 100-year-olds (e.g., Wechsler Adult Intelligence Scales–Revised III [WAIS III]; Wechsler, 1997). Furthermore, the age range for older persons (e.g., 60–100 years) is great; there are very different functional levels, needs, and appropriate assessments within the age groups of 60 to 100. Test administrators need to assume responsibility for recognizing deficiencies of the instruments and selecting other appropriate instruments, if available.

Endurance must be a consideration in scheduling tests. People with sensory impairments, reduced energy levels, or disabling physical or mental conditions may benefit from accommodations during testing. Reflex speed typically decreases and sensory loss increases with age, so power tests may be more meaningful than speed tests. Abbreviated screening instruments may also be useful—shortened instruments to assess depression have been found to be as effective as longer ones, and a four-test short form of the WAIS III has been found as effective as the full form in determining intellectual functioning in persons over age 65. Situational assessments or job trials may be more relevant to older persons than paper-and-pencil testing. Behavioral assessment is an important adjunct.

Tests of functional level can be an important source of information in vocational assessments and can further assist in career planning with older adults who wish to return to work. Specific instruments have been developed to determine functional status of older persons. For example, the Instrumental Activities of Daily Living scale (Nourhashemi et al., 2001) has been effectively used with women aged 75 and older to assess independent living functioning and to predict successfully risk factors of frailty in older women who, at the time of the assessment, were healthy and living at home.

OPPORTUNITIES FOR OLDER WORKERS

In a society where careers and their role in society are a primary defining feature, the aging population, in a stage of development and that does not focus on employment, is displaced. However, the increased need to remain in the workforce longer is presenting the aging population with numerous barriers.

People who are older are more likely than younger people to be adapting to the effects of sensory loss; to see themselves as being closer to death; to have a loss of role models for social demands they encounter; to experience significant loss of cohort groups, long-term friendships, and family members; to experience role changes, role reversals, and alterations in role expectations; to perceive changes in social support; and to experience changes in perception of time. Counselors can assist with adjustment to these circumstances.

As people age, chronic conditions are more prevalent. These conditions often do not prevent people from working or impair their daily living skills. Lifestyle, coping abilities, activity accommodations, medical care, external supports, physical and social environments, therapeutic regimens, and rehabilitation may mediate the severity of functional limitations and subsequent development of disabilities.

Premorbid personality is an important component in adaptation to disability. The effects of endurance, resilience, energy level, and stress are important in rehabilitation planning for persons of all ages and even more important when chronic, multiple, and severe conditions are combined with effects of aging.

Older workers are most at risk of disability or additional disability related to changes in sensory acuity. Approximately 14% of all individuals in the general population experience a hearing impairment by age of 54. Visual impairments are also common, affecting approximately 15% of women and 12% of men over the age 65 (Hoyer & Roodin, 2003). Sensory impairments are a particularly significant source of functional limitation, regardless of chronological age, and these conditions often lead to a diminished ability to participate in everyday life. Employers are less familiar with accommodations for these types of impairments than for other disabilities and make them less frequently than they do other accommodations. This lack of experience lessens the likelihood that employers are prepared to deal with these disabilities. This barrier to continued productivity may affect older workers disproportionately.

People who are older experience the full range of disability, including mental illness and substance abuse. Approximately 15% to 20% of persons over age 65 have serious symptoms because of psychiatric disorders. Such symptoms may result from long-existing conditions such as personality disorders from more recent situations, such as severe depression related to medications, or may result from a combination of these. Older people are more likely than people from other age groups to experience primary depression, that is, depression resulting from physical causes or drug side effects.

Substance abuse in older individuals can be a continuation of a past addiction; a new coping strategy; an abuse of prescription medication; or a condition associated with anxiety, depression, or cognitive disorders. It may resemble conditions that are associated with aging such as chronic pain, fatigue, or depression. Once identified, however, those who have this disorder may benefit from treatment.

Information regarding various social norms imposed on older individuals within different cultures, including ethnic and racial minority groups (e.g., roles, status, and issues of respect), is needed. For example, older people from ethnic and racial minorities or Appalachian populations may rely heavily on informal networks and indigenous influence for intervention.

NEEDED PROACTIVE EMPLOYER RESPONSE

A major issue for aging workers and their employers is the work environment, and whether it might be unfriendly and perhaps even discriminatory toward older workers. A significant factor influencing the decision to retain or eject older workers is no doubt the culture of the workplace itself. Age-based stereotyping perpetuates discriminatory practices and discourages elderly workers from remaining in or returning to the workplace.

Keeping the senior worker not only preserves valuable institutional knowledge and memory but also creates beneficial diversity in the workplace. Incentives and workplace supports will be needed to encourage employers to retain older workers and to encourage older workers to remain in the workforce. Employers must create workplace policies and practices and effective intergenerational inclusion initiatives that support worker retention.

Research suggests that employers discriminate against older workers in the job application process. In addition, the stereotypes that younger workers have of their older peers can greatly influence workplace dynamics. Traditional stereotypes of older workers (e.g., being inflexible, sick, and unwilling to learn new technology) continue to persist at many levels. Such stereotypes have clearly had an influence on older workers' (particularly men) labor force participation in the past. Workers who experience age discrimination are more likely to leave their current employment setting and less likely to remain employed.

This may include adopting new management styles and work setting protocols that focus on an age-diverse workforce. Human resource policies and practices should reflect alternatives that will respond to the older workers' desire for flexible working hours, part-time positions, and the ability to choose what part of the day they work. Flexible workplace, telecommuting options, and flex-time agreements can help fill this need.

Benefit plans may also create disincentives for retaining older workers. Many plans can send mixed messages to older workers; some create incentives to retire while others encourage continued labor force activity. Some employers are creating health care and retirement policies that offer incentives to older workers to stay engaged in the workforce, such as phased retirement, "in demand" workforce for specialized consulting, senior staff mentors for new workers, casual/part-time workers' programs, discounts on pharmaceuticals, specialized health screenings, long-term care insurance, preretirement planning, and prorated benefits for employees on flexible work schedules.

COUNSELOR PRACTICE, TRAINING, AND RESEARCH IMPLICATIONS

The growing older population, with its increased levels of disability and its desire and need to work, creates the opportunity for counselors to provide services to older people. To be able to confront myths and stereotypes, counselors will need to have knowledge of the intellectual, social, and emotional well-being of older adults. Counselor educators can prepare counselors-in-training for this task by including aging issues in the counselor education curriculum.

Personal experiences with various groups of people and social learning experiences shape one's viewpoint toward a group. Counselors-in-training may have had prior exposure to negative stereotypes about persons with disabilities, have been repeatedly exposed to negative stereotypes about aging (ageism), have a prejudice against older persons (gerontophobia), have a fear of aging or of associating with older persons, or have other attitudinal barriers or misconceptions. Both personal and societal attitudes toward the aging process and older populations are appropriate to explore in psychosocial coursework. Inclusion of material on multicultural aspects of human relationships is intended to increase trainees' multicultural awareness, knowledge, and skills through developing an understanding of one's personal values, attitudes, motivations, and behaviors.

Retraining, adaptive devices, physical therapy, and occupational therapies can assist workers injured on the job, regardless of their ages. However, counselors should be aware that age-related changes in stamina and healing may require that older employees who do receive on-the-job injuries may need to be afforded additional time and extended therapy to fully restore optimal functioning.

Infusion of information regarding this population into existing counselor accreditation–approved curricula is vital if the counseling profession is to become a resource for the development of strategies to maintain the economic independence of older citizens. Such courses can also expose counselors-in-training to the issues and attitudes that impact the employment of older workers, particularly those with disabilities.

Research is needed on the issues of aging workers, such as training needs, career transition issues, and retirement planning. Research is also needed on which accommodations, workplace modifications, and changes to policies and practices positively impact the retention and continued productivity of an aging workforce. Counselor practitioners are in a unique position to contribute to needed research design conceptualization, metrics, and analyses, to test the multiplicity of interventions we will be exploring in the coming years to keep our aging workforce healthy and intellectually engaged in the employment environment. Counselors are experientially qualified to provide the needed services to keep this population productive and more fully engaged in their communities and continuing employment.

RESOURCES

National Organizations/Associations

Adult Development and Aging, Division 20 of the American Psychological Association: http://www.apa.org/about/division/div20.html
American Association of Geriatric Psychiatry: http://www.aagpgpa.org
American Association of Retired Persons (AARP): http://www.aagpgpa.org
Association for Adult Development and Aging, A Division of the American Counseling Association: http://www.aadaweb.org
The American Geriatrics Society: http://www.americangeriatrics.org
Council for Accreditation of Counseling Related Educational Programs (CACREP) Gerontological Counseling Standards: www.cacrep.org/2001standards.html

Related Articles

American Psychological Association. *Psychology and aging.* Retrieved July 11, 2008, from http://www.apa.org/journals/pag
Bruyère, S. M. (2006). Disability management: Key concepts and techniques for an aging workforce. *International Journal of Disability Management, 1,* 149–158.
Kampfe, C. M., Harley, D. B., Wadsworth, J. S., & Smith, S. M. (2007). Methods and materials for infusing aging issues into the rehabilitation curriculum. *Rehabilitation Education, 21,* 107–116.
Kampfe, C. M., Wadsworth, J. S., Smith, S. M., & Harley, D. A. (2005). The infusion of aging issues in the rehabilitation curriculum: A review of the literature. *Rehabilitation Education, 19,* 225–233.

REFERENCES

Erikson, E. H. (1959). *Identity and the life cycle: Psychological issues.* New York: International Universities Press.
Harley, D. A., Donnell, C., & Rainey, J. (2003). Interagency collaboration: Reinforcing professional bridges to serve aging populations with multiple service needs. *Journal of Rehabilitation, 69,* 32–37.
Holland, J. L. (1994). *Self-directed search.* Odessa, FL: Psychological Assessment Resources, Inc.
Hoyer, W. J., & Roodin, P. A. (2003). *Adult development and aging* (5th ed.). Boston: McGraw-Hill.
Nourhashemi, F., Andrieu, S., Gillette-Guyonnet, S., Vellas, B., Albarede, L., & Grandjean, H. (2001). Instrumental activities of daily living as a potential marker of frailty: A study of 7364 community-dwelling elderly women (the EPIDOS study). *The Journals of Gerontology, 56A,* M448–M453.
U.S. Census Bureau. (2004). *U.S. Census Bureau population projections.* Retrieved October 7, 2007, from http://www.census.gov/ipc/www/usinterimproj/.
Weathers, R. R. (2006). *Disability prevalence rates for an aging workforce.* Ithaca, NY: Cornell University, Rehabilitation Research and Training Center on Employment Policy.
Wechsler, D. (1997). *WAIS-III administration and scoring manual.* San Antonio, TX: The Psychological Corporation.

32

Reflections and Considerations

Part A: Reflections on the View From Here

Irmo Marini

Just over 30 years ago in the Northern Ontario city of Thunder Bay, I was in the middle of a game as a Lakehead University varsity hockey player; during the last minute of the second period, I was tripped up and collided headfirst into the end boards fracturing my neck at the C5 to C6 vertebral level. In the blink of an eye, I went from an all-around athlete, 13-year bodybuilder, to an almost totally dependent wheelchair user. The almost 11 months of hospitalization and rehabilitation began a long journey back mentally, physically, and philosophically. I emerged back into a world where not only I was viewing it differently from a seated position but also some people were viewing me differently with pity, curiosity, and sympathy. I needed to somehow make them see me as I was before—strong, independent, witty, disciplined, and emotionally stable. After all, I was still the same guy. For me, now being paralyzed from the chest down, it meant reinventing myself, turning what once was the physical discipline of bodybuilding and athletic prowess into exercising my brain and intellect to emerge with four academic degrees and ultimately becoming a professor in rehabilitation counseling.

Many of the chapters in this book are a reflection of not only some of my personal experiences but also the common lived experiences of others with various disabilities as found in the personal perspective stories at the end of each section and the appendices. Throughout this text, we have explored a variety of psychosocial issues related to chronic illness and disability. However, if this was all the book was about, it would be fairly straightforward and discipline-specific for rehabilitation counseling and related professionals. But unlike most of the social sciences, the complexities of human behavior, as we have discussed, are often reciprocally interdependent upon societal attitudes, environmental access or barriers, and social justice. In an era post the 2008 recession and economists' predictions that if corporate and Wall Street "business as usual" remains largely unregulated, the continuing ripple effect on Americans regarding cutbacks in Medicaid/Medicare, Social Security, and other social programs will negatively affect those most in need. Doomsday financial predictions abound regarding the U.S. debt ceiling, bankrupt federal and state governments, and the typical U.S. recoil reaction of drastically cutting programs leaves many lower-income individuals facing precarious futures (Reich, 2010).

In Chapter 1, Fox and Marini discussed the legal and blatant discrimination and exclusion of Americans with disabilities concerning the 1924 Immigration Act, involuntary sterilization, and forbidding some with disabilities to legally marry. Zanskas and Conduti in Chapter 29 elaborated on this and peered into the future regarding eugenics, euthanasia, and physician-assisted suicide. The ramifications of Social Darwinism regarding natural selection and the 20th-century mantra "survival of the fittest" have morphed into something else in 21st-century America. It has become increasingly apparent that we are in an era of "survival of the financially fittest." The social injustice inflicted on people with disabilities, especially minorities with disabilities who are uneducated and poor, is subconsciously and deniably ingrained in American social behavior. Although America strives for an egalitarian society ideal, Liu (2011) cites a plethora of literature painting a very different picture on the negative impact of social classism.

In Liu's book titled *Social Class and Classism in the Helping Professions*, he cites numerous studies exploring the discriminatory and deleterious impact of classism and oppression. Although rags-to-riches stories are often inspiring, the statistical reality of such instances is rare. For most people growing up in poverty, an often perpetuated and generational lineage occurs for numerous complex reasons, both individual and socio-structural. In other words, as we discussed in Chapter 24, positive psychology, the interrelationship between individual factors (e.g., intelligence, motivation, and resilience) and an individual's environment (e.g., societal attitudes, availability of health care, physical access, and family support and income) dictate potential successful adaptation or conversely succumb to one's circumstances. Liu argues that the fallout from classism and oppression stacks the deck against individuals and their children from ever climbing the social status ladder.

People with disabilities who are female and part of a minority represent the most disenfranchised population in America, but millions of other disabled and/or minorities face a number of socio-structural barriers that can overwhelm even the most resilient of individuals. The cascading cycle of poverty, poor education, poor health care, and poor living conditions exacerbates social injustice and "haves versus have nots." This vicious cycle of low income can be traced to the need to purchase less expensive, often more fat-laden food which can lead to obesity, subsequent poor health and disability (e.g., Type II diabetes), as well as sporadic employment. This stressful toll negatively impacts mental health and is often correlated with depression and anxiety (Garland et al., 2005; Marini, 2011; Minkler, Fuller-Thompson, & Guralnik, 2006; Schaefer-McDaniel, 2009). The less control individuals feel they have over their circumstances, the greater the feelings of hopelessness, learned helplessness, and psychological distress (Evans, 2004, 2006).

The growing economic and class disparity in America is unquestionably reaching a tipping point as it did during the Great Depression (Huffington, 2010; Reich, 2010). With America's middle class disappearing daily since even before the 2008 recession, American children living in poverty—and what *60 Minutes* calls the "motel generation"—indicates a child poverty rate of over 20% and growing (Kroft, 2011). Where will this leave people with disabilities and their families who are already living statistically at the lower end of the spectrum? Will the United States ever adopt universal health care as so many countries already have, or will corporatism, capitalism, and the "I am not my brother's keeper" mentality continue to force everyone to go down with the ship? Survival of the financially fittest will become meaningless if citizens revolt against the system as they have in other countries where all civility comes to a halt. How do rehabilitation counselors, educators, and related helping professionals even begin to address these seemingly insurmountable and arguably uncontrollable events? Are any of us even motivated to try?

SMALL STEPS AND THE POWER OF ALTRUISM

There needs to be a quantum shift in how we perceive the scope of our jobs, our ethical and moral responsibilities to our clients and ourselves, and the motivation to want to get out from behind our desks and do more. To pretend to ignore or simply remain ignorant of the changing realities conveys a laissez-faire attitude and/or violates the ethical principle of beneficence if we know we can do more for our clients but choose not to. In Chapter 24 by Marini and Chacon, regarding positive psychology, empirical evidence indicates the psychological rewards (e.g., subjective well-being, self-efficacy, and empathy toward others) of volunteering and helping others who are in need (Penner, 2004; Wilson, 2000). The American Counseling Association (ACA) has increasingly called upon professional counselors to voluntarily assist the Red Cross in working with survivors of natural disasters. Likewise, Surís and North in Chapter 30 discuss preparing mental-health workers for crisis intervention counseling following terrorist incidents.

Short of giving one's time to counsel individuals following such traumatic events, counselors and related professionals can also volunteer their time at the local level, assisting those in need by collecting for food banks, educational tutoring, clothing drives, and laboring for Habitat for Humanity, and so on. Offering free counseling services, which are generally offered at many nondenominational churches, is another excellent way of helping others during troubled times. Various fundraising activities by the local Masons, Centers for Independent Living, Easter Seals, March of Dimes, and other organizations are also frequently occurring.

At a more professional level, counselors can assist clients with disabilities by writing letters of complaint to businesses that are still not physically accessible to all. Teaching clients how to advocate for themselves and the fact that they have the power to implement change can be very empowering (Graf, Marini & Blankenship, 2009; Marini, Bhakta, & Graf, 2009). Clients can also be referred to Client Assistance Programs, which have the legal expertise in filing formal complaints with the Office of Civil Rights and filing lawsuits when needed. It is unfortunate that 21 years after the passage of the Americans with Disabilities Act, such lawsuits must still be pursued as observed by the thousands of ongoing new suits filed each year (Blackwell, Marini, & Chacon, 2001).

THE SOCIAL JUSTICE COUNSELOR

In view of ongoing societal oppression and classism toward many with disabilities and particularly those ethnic/racial minorities with disabilities, counselors could better serve this population not only by the status quo job duties of assisting the individual to live in an able-bodied world but also by affecting change in a socially unjust environment. To this end, the ACA officially recognized in its 2005 Code of Ethics revision that "when appropriate, counselors advocate at the individual, group, institutional, and societal levels to examine potential barriers and obstacles that inhibit access and/or growth and development of clients" (ACA, 2005, p. 5). The ACA now also recognizes a new subdivision of counseling: the Division for Counselors for Social Justice (CSJ). The CSJ defines social justice counseling on its website as follows:

> Social justice counseling represents a multifaceted approach to counseling in which practitioners strive to simultaneously promote human development and the common good through addressing challenges related to both individual and distributive justice. Social justice counseling includes empowerment of the individual as well as active confrontation of injustice and inequality in society as they impact clientele as well as those in their systemic contexts. In doing so, social justice counselors direct attention to the promotion of four critical principles that guide their work; equity, access, participation, and harmony. This work is done with a focus on the cultural, contextual, and individual needs of those served. (http://counselorsforsocialjustice.com)

Greenleaf and Williams (2009) note that the counseling profession has its roots and major influence from the medical model paradigm that focuses solely on treating the individual's impairments. Little or no consideration, other than lip service up until recently, has been paid to the holistic approach in working with people with disabilities. Medical and mental health professionals have traditionally taken a pathological orientation to diagnosis and treatment, focusing on what is wrong with the individual. However, as Peterson (Chapter 26) describes in outlining the International Classification of Functioning, it is the first mental health resource that holistically addresses environmental influences on individual mental and physical health. For years empirical research has shown that regardless of how strong or resilient someone is, an oppressive, dehumanizing and devaluing society can indeed negatively impact one's physical and mental health (Dohrenwend, 2000; Gee, 2002; Graf et al., 2009; Li & Moore, 1998; Liu, 2011; Rumbaut, 1994; Williams & Williams-Morris, 2000; Wright, 1988).

Dohrenwend (2000), for example, found that the ethnic/racial groups who perceived they had been prejudiced and discriminated against reported higher levels of psychological and physical stress-related illness including depression and anxiety. Perlow, Danoff-Burg, Swenson, and Pulgiano's (2004) similar observations that perceived discrimination can lead to believing one has no control over his or her circumstances, and that this can subsequently lead to feelings of hopelessness/helplessness and negatively affect one's health. The subsequent ripple and cyclical effect of oppression and discrimination on families was noted earlier (Eaton & Muntaner 1999; Kessler et al., 2003; Krieger, 1999).

I do not believe we can any longer afford to ignore the plight of those in need, not only because of the embarrassment it conveys about us as a society but also because of the social and economic ramifications of a morally and financially bankrupt society. Americans have been known to rise with great resilience and compassion at critical junctures of their history. As rehabilitation professionals, we must do our part to see the larger picture, to know the global and cultural issues, and to be more then just what our job description reads. Our piece of the puzzle is to assist people with disabilities, empower them, and educate society and advocate for social justice. Seligman (2002) in his book *Authentic Happiness* indicates that we can only be truly happy by giving and caring for others. The power of altruism is a reciprocal reward both to ourselves and to the recipients. Ultimately, when we are helping others, we are helping ourselves.

REFERENCES

American Counseling Association (2005). *ACA code of ethics.* Retrieved from http://www.counseling.org/ethics/feedback/ACA2005Code.pdf

Blackwell, T. M., Marini, I., & Chacon, M. (2001). The impact of the Americans with Disabilities Act on independent living. *Rehabilitation Education, 15*(4), 395–408.

Dohrenwend, B. P. (2000). The role of adversity and stress in psychopathology: Some evidence and its implications for theory and research. *Journal of Health and Social Behavior, 41,* 1–19.

Eaton, W. W., & Muntaner, C. (1999). Socioeconomic stratification and mental disorder. In A. V. Horwitz, & T. L. Scheid (Eds.). *A handbook for the study of mental health: Social contexts, theories, and systems* (pp. 259–283). Cambridge, UK: Cambridge University Press.

Evans, G. W. (2004). The environment of childhood poverty. *American Psychologist, 59,* 77–92.

Evans, G. W. (2006). Child development and the physical environment. *Annual Review of Psychology, 57,* 423–451.

Garland, A. F., Lau, A. S., Yeh, M., McCabe, K. M., Hough, R. L., & Landsverk, J. A. (2005). Racial and ethnic differences in utilization of mental health services among high-risk youths. *American Journal of Psychiatry, 162,* 1336–1343.

Gee, G. C. (2002). A multilevel analysis of the relationship between institutional racial discrimination and health status. *American Journal of Public Health, 5,* 109–117.

Graf, N. M., Marini, I., & Blankenship, C. (2009). 100 words about disability. *Journal of Rehabilitation, 75*(2), 25–34.

Greenleaf, A. T., & Williams, J. M. (2009). Supporting social justice advocacy: A paradigm shift toward an ecological perspective. *Journal for social Action in Counseling and Psychology, 2*(1), 1–12.

Huffington, A. (2010). *Third world America: How our politicians are abandoning the middle class and betraying the American dream.* New York: Crown.

Kessler, R. C., Berglund, P., Demler, O., Jin, R., Koretz, D., Merikangas, K. R., et al. (2003). The epidemiology of major depressive disorder: Results from the National Comorbidity Survey Replication. *Journal of the American Medical Association, 289,* 3095–3105.

Krieger, N. (1999). A review of concepts, measures, and methods for studying health consequences of discrimination. *Journal of Health Services, 29,* 295–352.

Kroft, S. (Writer). (2011). Hard Times Generation [Television series episode]. In Jeff Fager (Executive producer) *60 Minutes.* New York: CBS Broadcasting.

Li, L., & Moore, D., 1998. Acceptance of disability and its correlates. *Journal of Social Psychology, 138*(1), 13–25.

Liu, W. M. (2011). *Social class and classism in the helping professions: Research, theory, and practice.* Thousand Oaks, California: Sage.

Marini, I. (2011). The history of treatment toward persons with disabilities. In I. Marini, N. M. Graf, & M. J. Millington (Ed.). *Psychosocial aspects of disability: Insider perspectives and counseling strategies* (pp. 1–46). New York: Springer.

Marini, I., Bhakta, M. V., & Graf, N. (2009). A content analysis of common concerns of persons with physical disabilities. *Journal of Applied Rehabilitation Counseling, 40*(1), 44–49.

Minkler, M., Fuller-Thompson, E., & Guralnik, J. M. (2006). Gradient of disability across the socioeconomic spectrum in the Unites States. *New England Journal of Medicine, 355,* 695–703.

Penner, L. A. (2004). Volunteerism and social problem: Making things better or worse? *Journal of Social Issues, 60*(3), 645–666.

Perlow, H. M., Danoff-Burg, S., Swenson, R. R., & Pulgiano, D. (2004). The impact of ecological risk and perceived discrimination on the psychological adjustment of African American and European youth. *Journal of Community Psychology, 32,* 375–389.

Reich, R. B. (2010). *After shock: The next economy and America's future.* New York: Alfred A. Knopf.

Rumbaut, R. (1994). The crucible within: Ethnic identity, self-esteem, and segmented assimilation among children of immigrants. *International Migration Review, 28,* 748–794.

Schaefer-McDaniel, N. (2009). Neighborhood stressors, perceived neighborhood quality, and child mental health in New York City. *Health and Place, 15,* 148–155.

Seligman, M. E. (2002). *Authentic happiness: Using the new positive psychology to realize your potential for lasting fulfillment.* New York: Free Press.

Williams, D. R., & Williams-Morris, R. (2000). Racism and mental health: The African American experience. *Ethnicity and Health, 5,* 243–268.

Wilson, J. (2000). Volunteering. *Annual Review of Sociology, 26*(1), 215–241.

Wright, B. A. (1988). Attitudes and the fundamental negative bias: Conditions and Corrections. In H. E. Yuker (Ed.). *Attitudes toward persons with disabilities* (pp. 3–21). New York: Springer.

Part B: Reflections

MARK A. STEBNICKI

MY PERSONAL JOURNEY INTO THE HELPING PROFESSION

I started my career at a community rehabilitation center (sheltered workshop) around 1979 in a small rural town in southern Illinois. Besides doing work adjustment, job placement, and job coaching with these clients, I also drove the bus to pick them up for work and dropped them off at the end of the day. I got to know their family members and the psychosocial challenges of individuals with disabilities living in rural America. This was my introduction to working with people who had a variety of developmental, psychiatric, and physical disabilities. I remembered this as a very rewarding opportunity that helped launch my career, which has spanned over 30 years. In some ways, I never really left this community rehabilitation center despite working since then in a variety of vocational rehabilitation, substance abuse, consumer advocacy, neuro-rehabilitation, residential and outpatient rehabilitation, and mental health settings. The chapters presented in this text are an accurate description of the psychological, social, emotional, and vocational intricacies and problems confronting people with disabilities.

Despite being a rehabilitation counselor educator, I have always maintained a small counseling and forensic rehabilitation practice, which keeps me grounded in the reality of socio-political affairs, budget cuts, disability policy change, creative solutions to programs and services, and all other things that affect the psychosocial reaction of people that have chronic illnesses and disabilities. I have worked at the epicenter of catastrophic injury in acute rehabilitation settings, counseling people with drug and alcohol addictions and who have lost their health, home, jobs, and relationships; monitoring the care and feeding of elderly individuals living in deplorable nursing home conditions; advocating for people with psychiatric disabilities in locked state institutions where physical and chemical restraint is commonplace; and performing critical incident stress debriefings in school shootings, floods, hurricanes, tornados, and incidents of workplace violence. These experiences indeed have provided me with a personal–professional perspective of working with the immense psychosocial needs of individuals, groups, and family members that require assistance in getting back to balance.

BUILDING UPON THE GOOD WORKS OF FIVE PSYCHOSOCIAL EDITIONS

The previous five editions of Dell Orto and Marinelli and Dell Orto and Power's nationally recognized work, is a testament to documenting the experiences and insights of people living with disabilities in America. These authors' good works have also provided the perspective of professionals who deal with the psychosocial response to chronic illness and disability. The previous five editions signify the collaborative effort of many like-minded authors that have a passion and commitment to counselor education and training of the psychological and social impact that chronic illness and disability has on the individual from a holistic perspective. To this end, Irmo and I feel much gratitude and solace in knowing that Art, Bob, and Paul have entrusted to us this important work of carrying on their important work in psychosocial rehabilitation.

HISTORICAL SIGNIFICANCE

As the excellent work of many our authors point to, historically, the care, treatment, and attitudes toward people with physical and psychiatric disabilities in America have not been empowering. In fact, conditions have been unfavorable in attempting to achieve optimal living conditions, jobs and careers, healthy relationships, and overall mental and physical well-being. Issues of role-entrapment, women's issues, disempowerment, and inequality of programs and services across all life areas are a glaring example of why it is critical to advocate from a professional and political level for specific laws and policies that help "level the playing field."

As this text emphasizes, there is not one group or culture of "people with disabilities." Rather, from a multicultural perspective, there are individuals and within-group differences—all which have unique experiences, characteristics, attributes, and needs. Living optimally with a disability requires psychosocial adjustment throughout the life span, which has only a theoretical beginning and endpoint. In reality, one cannot "get closure" with a life-altering event that affects one's medical, physical, cognitive, mental, emotional, psychological, social, spiritual, career/vocational, environmental health, and independent living needs. Accordingly, the authors in this text suggest that there are multiple psychosocial responses, each of which is uniquely experienced and based on the individual and his or her life circumstances.

A PIVOTAL SHIFT IN THE HELPING PROFESSION

Despite the socio-political environment in some states that restrict the eligibility, licensure, insurance-reimbursement, and overall practice of some counseling professionals who work with the mental health needs of people with disabilities, the discipline of psychosocial rehabilitation lives on. In essence, working holistically with the psychosocial reactions of people with chronic illnesses and disabilities may be the most vital aspects of the individual's treatment and care.

Traditional models of vocational rehabilitation are challenged today by budget cuts and growing caseloads. People with psychiatric disabilities continue to be neglected from an appropriate array of services. Many individuals with psychiatric disabilities must be diagnosed as a "danger to self and others" and exhibit a psychiatric emergency before receiving inpatient treatment. Drug laws tend to punish rather than rehabilitate individuals. Within the dynamic ever-changing health care policies of the insurance industry, people with preexisting conditions are many times disqualified from obtaining coverage. Those fortunate enough to have access to health care coverage, pay substantially hirer premiums and co-pays than those without chronic health conditions and disabilities.

The list of challenges grows every year. Extraordinary times require extraordinary efforts for personal attention, advocacy, and cultivating personal growth and wellness, facilitating best practices in psychosocial services for people with disabilities. We should not wait around for new federal/state programs and services, entitlement programs, or policies and laws to change, for change happens within the individual. It requires a perception and attitude that can only be internally driven. This type of positive optimism and resilient way of being can become contagious and transferable to other individuals and groups. Perhaps, it is time to look back into the history of our respected leaders, organizers, and advocates that helped form the creative foundation of the rehabilitation counseling process for answers to more challenging questions.

FOUNDATIONS OF MIND, BODY, AND SPIRITUAL WELLNESS: THE FUTURE OF PSYCHOSOCIAL TREATMENT

This text emphasizes the importance of positive optimism, healthy coping abilities, and resiliency that the individual and professional helpers can cultivate across the life span. The type of personal growth and wellness required to transcend chronic illness and disability requires solution-focused approaches today as opposed to a focus on problem issues. Working with the holistic nature of people with disabilities requires approaches that consider the mind, body, and spirit as healing partners. Now, more than ever, there is a call for working with people in a dynamic, interactive, and interdependent way of being. Thus, optimal growth and wellness begins with the balance of one's mind, body, and spirit. This balance goes beyond improving the quality of life, trying to achieve higher levels of motivation, or hiring a life coach to help one get organized and focused. The dynamic nature of psychosocial adjustment and reaction to chronic illness and disability itself requires that the individual and professional give their highest level of attention to working within a true holistic framework. Herein lies what I believe to be the future of programs and services to providing services to people with disabilities.

The foundation of all wellness requires an understanding that our mind, body, and spirit are interconnected and interdependent upon self and others. It is an integral force in our healing. Let me invite you to be open to the idea that if helping professionals are truly dedicated to psychosocial change within a culturally centered practice, then we must pay attention to the care of our clients' mind, body, and spirit. This is in fact, working at the epicenter within one's cultural belief system, knowing how to treat the (1) mental–emotional–cognitive body (the mind); (2) physical health conditions (the body); and (3) parts of the soul that can only be experienced by rituals, beliefs, and/or folk practices (the spirit). To access this culturally centered system of health care, many individuals find it helpful to cultivate resiliency and hope, and place their faith in God, the Great Spirit, shamans, yogis, mystics, mediums, and/or spiritualists to gain optimal insight and awareness. Many medical and health care practitioners and rehabilitation and mental health professionals want to become part of this healing partnership.

As we have learned in positive psychology and resiliency research, it is essential to have faith in oneself to achieve optimal levels of mental, physical, and spiritual well-being. Paul Pederson once wrote that one of the most significant questions that all cultures have to ask is where we came from and where we will go after we pass on. Based on this statement, we can assume that humankind has struggled with this question since the beginning of time; the search for our ultimate creator or connecting with a divine source of energy. Accordingly, each individual possesses some degree of internal locus of control, has an inner spirit guide, therapist, or has the intuitive gift that can help cultivate personal resiliency and coping abilities. If individuals believe that they are an equal partner with their healing source or support system, then they may be empowered with to begin their healing journey. Accordingly, a good degree of faith, hope, and/or spiritual guidance should bring optimal knowledge, awareness, insight, and skill for transforming one's life.

THE FUTURE OF PSYCHOSOCIAL TREATMENT

Many who have struggled with and transcended issues related to addiction, chronic illness, life-threatening disease, disability, and other extraordinary stressful events have cultivated a personal wisdom in order to achieve optimal wellness and balance. The following list is based on a meta-analysis of principles, thoughts, and philosophies on mind, body, and spiritual wellness as found in the reading resource at the end of this chapter. This material is derived from counseling, psychology, theology, spirituality, complimentary, alternative, and integrated medicine resources. Some contain personal testimonials while others are based on the experiences of others who work extensively with people who have multiple and complex needs. This is not an all-inclusive manifesto, for this would be a chapter unto itself. Rather, this is based on some of the foundational principles, the collective wisdom, and universal thoughts of many writers. First, here are some generally recognized definitions of the mind, body, and spirit.

> *Mind*: consciousness, perceptions, philosophies, beliefs, thoughts, attitudes, feelings, and cognitions
> *Body*: physiological, cellular, and biological functioning of all body systems
> *Spirit*: (different from religiosity) that which cannot be seen but is made up of experiences of faith, hope, comfort, beliefs, philosophies, rituals, and a belief in a divine source of energy that guide our lives

- Achieving balance and wellness of your mind, body, and spirit is a journey not a goal. It requires constant mindfulness and attention to both your internal and external environment. There are multiple systems that one can use to help change their environment (e.g., laws governing accessibility, use of assistive technology).
- Heal the soul first; then healing of the mind and body will follow. For many people, their soul represents the shadow side or unconscious part of their personality and behaviors that cannot be accessed. To be enlightened, be aware, or develop insight requires that the individual open into a deeper or non-ordinary level of consciousness. The benefit of reaching one's soul then gives birth to new attitudes, perceptions, and life.
- Serious change first begins with a vision. A vision has potential to become reality. Einstein, through visualization, created the mathematical theory of relativity before he wrote it down on a chalk board; the Wright brothers had to visualize a flying machine before they left Ohio for their "first flight" from the Outer Banks of North Carolina; Dr. Martin Luther King, Jr. visualized or dreamed of civil rights before laws and enforcement powers of equality came into being; the Beatles had to visualize musical success in America before they departed England for their U.S. tour.
- Mindfulness simply means paying attention to your mind, body, and spirit at different levels of awareness in the present, here-and-now moment, in a nonjudgmental and unconditional way. This kind of attention nurtures and cultivates greater awareness, clarity, and acceptance of yourself day to day.
- It is possible to become a prisoner of your own past and buried alive in unhealthy thoughts, feelings, cognitions, addictions, and other dysfunctional patterns. Karma, which is the sum total of your life's direction, is created by your past actions, thoughts, and behaviors. Karma is often confused with a person's fixed destiny, but it is more of an accumulative pattern of actions, thoughts, and behaviors. You can change your Karma by choosing different thoughts, feelings, cognitions, and actions in the present moment. Thus, being mindful of matters relating to mind, body, and spirit can change your past and future; for living in the moment is empowering.
- Each new healthy thought, feeling, or experience you elicit has the potential to change your future. Once you have visualized the next moment, you are actually in a stage of action just by the mere act of thinking and feeling. A journey of a thousand miles begins with the first tumble, roll, step, or intentional movement.
- To attain balance and wellness of your mind, body, and spirit, look for the most parsimonious wisdom, knowledge, and practical approaches; ones that fit best with who

you are as a person and with your life, for many, solution-focused approaches work better than years of psychoanalysis.

- Recognize that you are a unique individual made up of different personalities, behaviors, emotions, philosophies, and beliefs and that you have acquired different levels of experience in your life.

- You are a unique individual because of your own DNA, mental, physical, and spiritual attributes. By virtue of this uniqueness, you can become your own best therapist and healer because you know yourself better than anyone. Becoming aware of who you are is paramount to the health and wellness of your mind, body, and spirit.

- There are not "good" and "bad;" "positive" and "negative;" or "acceptable" and "unacceptable" thoughts and feelings. It's okay to be who you are, because you are a unique individual. There are a range of human emotions, behaviors, and experiences we feel and communicate to ourselves and others throughout the day. Placing values, standards, or ideals on your thoughts, feelings, emotions, behaviors, and experiences can hinder growth and development of your mind, body, and spirit.

- Taking responsibility for your own mind, body, and spirit is essential to stay on the path of your journey. If you wait for others to take responsibility (e.g., the government, a family member, and disability benefits system), you could be waiting for a long time.

- You have the capacity to achieve higher states of mind, body, and spiritual well-being. Using the therapist within will provide opportunities for personal transformation living in optimal health and wellness.

- Strive for GOLD (Sha, 2010; gratitude, obedience, loyalty, devotion) toward your mind, body, and spirit. Cultivating more love and compassion toward yourself and others leaves less room for unwanted thoughts, feelings, and emotions, for this is true freedom from stress, anxiety, and depression.

- Becoming aware that you may be holding in, holding on, and holding out the true experience of your feelings, emotions, thoughts, cognitions, and other levels of consciousness requires higher states of consciousness. Reluctance or resistance to become enlightened and aware will not provide opportunities for optimal growth within your mind, body, and spirit.

- Awakening your mind, body, and spirit to optimal wellness requires active mindful participation in the present and being a passive observer of your past or future. Increased focus on the present moment leaves less time for worries about your past or what may or may not happen in the future.

COMPLEMENTARY AND INTEGRATED MEDICINE RESOURCES

Anderson, R. A. (2001). *Clinician's guide to holistic medicine.* New York: McGraw-Hill.

Braden, G. (2008). *The spontaneous healing of belief: Shattering the paradigm of false limits.* Carlsbad, CA: Hay House, Inc.

Brennan, B. A. (1987). *Hands of light: A guide to healing through the human energy field.* New York: Bantam Books.

Castaneda, C. (1968). *The teachings of Don Juan: A Yaqui way of knowledge.* Berkley: University of California Press.

Chopra, D. (1995). *The way of the wizard: Twenty spiritual lessons for creating the life you want.* New York: Harmony Books.

Dalai Lama (1999). *Ethics for the new millennium.* New York: Riverhead Books/Penguin Putnam, Inc.

Eliade, M. (1964). *Shamanism: Archaic techniques of ecstasy.* New York: Pantheon.

Elliott, W. (1996). *Tying rocks to clouds: Meetings and conversations with wise and spiritual people.* New York: Image Books/Doubleday.

Emoto, M. (2004). *The hidden messages in water.* Hillsboro, OR: Beyond Words Publishing, Inc.

Fanning, P., & McKay, M. (2000). *Family guide to emotional wellness: Proven self-help techniques and exercises for dealing with common problems and building crucial life skills.* Oakland, CA: New Harbinger Publications, Inc.

Foundation for Shamanic Studies (2010). Retrieved December 2, 2010 from http://www.shamanism.org/workshops/announcement.php?aid=1

Fox, M., & Sheldrake, R. (1996). *The physics of angels: Exploring the realm where science and spirit meets.* San Francisco: HarperSan Francisco.

Frankl, V. E. (1963). *Man's search for meaning.* New York: Pocket Books.

Goleman, D. (2003). *Healing emotions: Conversations with the Dalai Lama on mindfulness, emotions, and health.* Boston: Shambhala.

Harner, M. (1990). *The way of the shaman.* San Francisco: HarperSanFrancisco.

Ingerman, S. (1991). *Soul retrieval: Mending the fragmented self.* San Francisco: HarperSanFrancisco.

Institute of Noetic Sciences. (2010). Retrieved December 2, 2010, from www.ions.org

International Center for Reiki Training (2007). Southfield, MI. www.reiki.org.

Kabat-Zinn, J. (1990). *Full catastrophe living: Using the wisdom of your body and mind to face stress, pain, and illness.* New York: Dell Publishing.

Kabat-Zinn, J. (1994). *Wherever you go there you are: Mindfulness meditation in everyday life.* New York: Hyperion.

Kushner, H. S. (1980). *When bad things happen to good people.* New York: Avon Books.

Maslach, C. (2003). *Burnout: The cost of caring.* Cambridge, MA: Malor Books.

Mehl-Madrona, L. (1997). *Coyote medicine: Lessons from Native American healing.* New York: Fireside/Simon & Schuster.

Mitchell, K. K. (1994). *Reiki: A torch in daylight.* St.Charles, IL: Mind Rivers Publications.

Mijares, S. G. (2003) *Modern psychology and ancient wisdom: Psychological healing practices from the world's religious traditions.* New York: The Haworth Integrative Healing Press.

Moodly, R., & West, W. (2005). *Integrating traditional healing practices into counseling and psychotherapy.* Thousand Oaks, CA: Sage Publications.

Moore, T. (2004). *Dark nights of the soul: A guide to finding your way through life's ordeals.* New York: Penguin Group.

Seaward, B. L. (1997). *Stand like mountain flow like water: Reflections on stress and human spirituality.* Deerfield Beach, FL: Health Communications, Inc.

Seaward, B. L. (2006). *Essentials of managing stress.* Boston: Jones & Bartlett Publishers.

Sha, Z. G. (2010). *Tao I: The way of all life.* New York: Atria Books.

Siebert, A. (2005). *The resiliency advantage: Master change, thrive under pressure, and bounce back from setbacks.* San Francisco: Berrett-Koehler Publishers, Inc.

Stebnicki, M. A. (2008). *Empathy fatigue: Healing the mind, body, and spirit of professional counselors.* New York: Springer Publishing.

Swerdlow, J. L. (2000). *Nature's Medicine: Plants that heal.* Washington, DC: National Geographic.

Weil, A. (1995). *Spontaneous healing.* New York: Ballantine Publishing Group.

Weil, A. (2005). *Healthy aging: A lifelong guide to your physical and spiritual well-being.* New York: Alfred A. Knopf.

V

New Directions: Issues and Perspectives: Conclusion

DISCUSSION QUESTIONS

1. In your own life, what are the characteristics that may contribute to the perception of your own wellness?
2. Considering positive psychology, how might your self-esteem or sense of self-worth be affected if you were frequently surrounded by people without disabilities who ignored, devalued, and treated you like a child?
3. Can there be an objective standard for "successful aging," or is such a concept strictly a subjective belief, different for all of us?
4. What factor does Stebnicki discuss regarding empathy fatigue that all counselors should be aware of and self-monitor against, and what are some strategies to reduce it from occurring?
5. What are the economic, psychosocial, and medical implications as to why obesity is on the rise in the United States?
6. In what ways (cognitive, behavioral, and emotional) can counselors assist obese clients if requested to do so?
7. Why do you think rehabilitation professionals have been absent from the debate on euthanasia and physician-assisted suicide? Is it now possible to enter this conflictual discussion? Why?
8. How might you counsel persons nearing retirement with or without a disability? Specifically, what are the unique considerations for aging and/or retiring persons?
9. What are the unique concerns, and how would you best counsel persons with or without disabilities who are anxious and stressed about the continual threat of terrorist attacks?
10. In the final chapter, what are the current concerns Marini and Stebnicki have for the United States, and what specific strategies can you do or become involved in to reduce these potentially impending economic, psychosocial, and societal problems?

PERSONAL PERSPECTIVE: LIFE LESSONS TAUGHT TO ME BY MY DISABILITY

ALFRED H. DEGRAFF

At the age of 18, I dove off a pier on Martha's Vineyard island and experienced a cervical spinal cord injury. I became, and remain, a quadriplegic dependent on motorized wheelchair mobility, daily physical help from personal assistants (PAs), and enough prescription medications to make several pharmaceutical companies financially dependent on me.

That was almost 40 years ago. I'm convinced from experience that my severe physical disability becomes more valuable to me and to society with each passing year. While it initially takes a burst of courage and coping skills to acknowledge and "accept" a fresh disability in its infancy, the real test of skills is their adequacy to support and maintain one's disability lifestyle over the long haul, decade after decade. Does the person have the staying power to survive daily health crises, hundreds of whining and immature PAs, and for many, a chronic depression that makes addictions and suicide seem so attractive?

For some people, I'm convinced that the disability lifestyle is no longer viewed as a meaningless tragedy, but instead, as a meaningful gift teaching life lessons. People with disabilities encounter an endless stream of opportunities for unique experiences, learning, and growth.

My disability has gifted me with wisdom about humanity that I wouldn't have been able to realize, or realize in such detail and depth, had I been able bodied. This wisdom has given the disability a sense of worth. What follows is my "top ten" list of life lessons—my personal statement of what my disability has meant to me by way of personal experiences, learning, and growth. To many of my able-bodied peers without insightful experiences, these are nice clichés—the text of refrigerator magnets. Instead, for many of us with disabilities, these are lessons acquired from repeated experiences or crises. While coping with an active crisis, these lessons reveal themselves in response to our often-desperate plea to make sense of the situation, "Please show me what I'm to learn from this experience?"

I have learned that I have the choice of living this disability lifetime as a victor or a victim. While I attempt to live optimistically as a victor, I have found that no matter how deeply I might occasionally slip into the victim role, a return route is always made available to me.

Living with a life-long disability isn't easy. I have found that much of my success or failure has been dependent on how I view life. There is a big difference between whether I choose to be a victim or a victor. And I truly do always have a choice.

As a victim at various times, I have chosen to go through life in a semi-hopeless frame of mind. "Why me? I'll never get ahead, because I'm stuck in this wheelchair." Those who take up full-time residence as a victim erroneously believe they find comfort in wallowing in the anger, grief, sorrow, depression, and despair.

As a victor, I'm presented with the same rough times as the victim; however, I work hard at staying in control of my disability and the quality of my life. As a victim, the nucleus of my daily life is my disability, and my lifestyle becomes a consequence of what my disability permits. As a victor, my soul or spirit is my nucleus, and the disability, like other personal characteristics, is one of many electrons orbiting around my soul or spirit.

I have learned the importance of taking the time to formally grieve a loss, instead of unemotionally trivializing or dismissing it with denial.

Life with a disability is one with many losses. We have lots of opportunity and need to practice grieving. We repeatedly have the choice of grieving now, or grieving later—of paying now, or paying later. There are many factors, outside the scope of this essay, that give us no choice but to grieve later or grieve over a long duration in bite-size pieces.

When we delay, we are sometimes sentenced to carry the weight of the loss's baggage. Grief baggage can manifest itself in many forms, including sorrow, frustration, anger, and depression.

When possible, I try to grieve my losses soon, to defuse grieving of its depressing power, and to move on. The relative absence of unaddressed grief is one of the elements that can reward us with that desirable state we call inner peace.

I have learned that life does not randomly expose me to coincidences, accidents, or seemingly meaningless tragedies in life. Instead, I am routinely meant to encounter learning and growth opportunities that are sent to me in a variety of disguises.

The Rolling Stones have sung, "You can't always get what you want, but you get what you need." The Dalai Lama was articulate in countering with, "Remember that not getting what you want is sometimes a wonderful stroke of luck." More recently, there has been yet another outlook that states, "Be careful of what you ask for, you might receive it."

My personal experience has shown me that if I am open to recognizing and learning from life's lessons, and flowing with life's rhythms instead of fighting or fleeing from them, then a whole world of benefits can open up to me.

I have learned that if I were given the opportunity either to shed my disability and return to the experiences, knowledge, and values that I had at the time of my disabling injury, or to keep my current disability with the wisdom it has taught me, I would usually choose to retain my disability.

What about those unique experiences—some joyful and some painful—that I would not have encountered without my paralysis? I usually take full advantage of them. Regardless of whether they were good or bad memories, I have usually succeeded in learning and growing because of them.

I have had first-hand experience in needing, receiving, and then returning human compassion. My disability has also given me first-person insights into prejudice, bigotry, discrimination, injustice, poverty, caring, love, support, integrity, and many other human qualities and inequalities.

I'm not saying I enjoy having my disability; however, it has enabled me to learn much more about humanity and life than I could have learned in an able-bodied lifetime. It's now been almost 40 years of these specialized experiences, learning, and growth. Were I actually presented with the chance of walking away from my wheelchair—but also the need to leave behind the insights I've acquired—I really doubt I'd accept walking back to the starting line of wisdom.

I have learned that it is never appropriate for me to try to shift my responsibilities, that are rightfully mine and for which I am capable of managing, to others, and then to blame them when my needs aren't accommodated.

I learned that I should never blame any provider for not doing what I should be doing for myself. In addition, I am always ultimately responsible for an aide failing to do a task, or doing it incompletely. Most of the assistance an aide gives me is the face-to-face kind. I am right there, and have a continual responsibility to do QC, or quality control. If an aide has helped me get dressed, and I arrive at my downtown office to find that I am wearing shoes but no sox, is my morning aide to blame? I don't think so.

Sure, I am annoyed that the aide totally spaced out on where my socks were this morning, after remembering them for the previous seven months. However, I have decided that my responsibility to watch my help providers is more realistic than to attempt to hold anyone responsible for performing my help routine flawlessly with no mistakes. Indeed, I never hold a PA responsible for memorizing every detail of my routine. In the books I've written about PA management, I refer to working with an aide to be analogous to dancing. I expect each PA in each work shift to occasionally forget a detail—a dance step. As the PA and I dance through the routine's tasks, and I sense he or she has forgotten the next "step," it's my responsibility to subtly remind the PA of the next step so we can keep on dancing.

I have learned that I am the only valid source for my own joy, sorrow, and inner peace. My own inner peace most often occurs when my actions are in harmony and authentic with my perception of spiritual intentions.

Not only am I solely responsible for my own happiness, for answers to my own life questions, and for coordinating the help required to maintain my health, but no one else will care as much as I if I fail to reach my goals or permit my health to decline.

A rock star, who became addicted to drugs and then went through recovery, acknowledges that others can't be held responsible for his happiness or the consequences of not achieving happiness. This rock star believed that "we are who we choose to be" … "you've got to save yourself …" and "nobody knows what you want … and nobody will be as sorry if you don't get it."

I have learned that there is a difference between physical pain and emotional suffering. Physical pain is objective and physiological; emotional suffering is subjective and psychological. While I sometimes cannot control the physical pain, I usually do have the choice and ability to control the much more powerful suffering that is created in my mind.

There are psychological ways of alleviating many kinds of emotional suffering. What the mind has the power to create, it also has the power to take away. From many personal experiences, I have learned the difference between the different feelings of physical pain and emotional suffering. I can assure myself of my ability to control suffering, and this has saved my life several times.

I have learned about the powerful advantages and life-sustaining utility there are in making maximum use of mental discipline. I've participated in many workshops and seminars that taught me skills of self-hypnosis, healing mental imagery, and progressive relaxation. I had been routinely using these skills to consciously lower stress and relax, mindfully reduce constrictive asthma, and even attempt to image genital orgasms that I could no longer feel. My increasing skills at mind control had resulted in perhaps a 90% success rate for these varied objectives, while enabling me to occasionally reduce my need for prescription medications.

I have learned to live for today—in the present—because yesterday is gone and tomorrow might never happen. Today's events will never happen again, nor should they. Perhaps the predominate, daily challenge I have in living with my disability is in creating and maintaining a set of activities and goals that make life sufficiently interesting and important to merit my getting out of bed each morning.

When I first acquired my disability, I spent a lot of time living in the past. I would look at what I could no longer physically do and think back to the good old days when I was able-bodied and could do those things. This is, of course, a setup for depression—concentrating and aspiring to do what we cannot. If someone with diabetes lies in bed all day and thinks about hot fudge sundaes, he will get depressed. Crosby, Stills, and Nash, in the song "Judy Blue Eyes," sing "Don't let the past remind us of what we are not now."

People with disabilities should be cautious about reminiscing constantly about missing their able-bodied past or fantasizing about the shape of the future after their ship comes in (example, after they win the lottery) and how much better than their current lifestyle the future will be. Sometimes, when I repeatedly procrastinate about becoming involved in interesting events, I think of Stephen Levine. In his book *A Year to Live,* he cites one quite effective way to identify one's current life purpose is to vividly imagine that you are going to die exactly one year from today. Ask yourself what priorities you consequently have during this final year of your life!

I have learned the difference between my accepting my own disability and society accepting it. For my own acceptance, I should formally acknowledge it, accept my limitations, and then concentrate instead on living within my abilities. If I concentrate on limitations and loss, I will become depressed. For the social acceptance of my disability, I should mostly ignore it. If I speak mostly about my disability instead of my true personal self and interests, it is unfortunately my disability that people will most remember.

During my undergraduate years, I lived purposely in a campus residence hall to facilitate my socialization. Disability-related discussions would crop up occasionally, but for a tiny minority of time. I didn't deny I had a disability, or forbade my dorm mates "to talk about it;" instead, we had more important and interesting topics. One evening, a couple friends popped into my room and asked if I wanted to join them in casing out a new bar within walking distance from our living area. Out of curiosity, I asked if the entrance or interior had unavoidable steps. In response, they looked at each other and became very apologetic, "Oh, Al, we're so sorry, we forgot that was a concern." I grinned ear to ear and assured them they weren't guilty of anything. Indeed, they primarily invited me and my personal interests, and not the wheelchair. I felt quite honored that those were my friends' priorities!

So in conclusion to this essay, while I stay in continual communication with the physical and psychological aspects of my disability, it is essential that I concurrently transcend—rise above—this disability and its limitations. It is important that I be able to look beyond the limitations of the disability in order to see the benefits that it offers.

As my abilities decrease with progressing years and disability, it has become increasingly important for me to use my daily time, energy, and stamina as efficiently as possible. My daily aerobic workouts, my requirement for "smart food" quality nutrition, and other health measures are more important to me than to my able-bodied peers.

It has been said that freedom in life is not necessarily doing what one wishes, whenever one wishes to do so. Instead, true freedom is the ability to face, cope with, and successfully get through each of life's unpredictable crises. I believe that my disability and limitations have ironically taught me many lessons about freedom—wisdom that I would not have realized as an able-bodied person.

Appendix A: Perspective Exercises

We have selected six additional perspective exercises to prompt the reader to explore further the meaning of disability in one's life. These exercises enlarge the opportunity to personalize many of the disability-related issues explained in the text. Each one of the exercises challenges us to confront our personal beliefs when these beliefs are impacted by the disability experience.

PERSPECTIVE EXERCISE 1

Common Pain, Mutual Support

Perspective

A harsh reality of illness and disability is that individuals within a family are often abandoned, isolated, and left on their own. Group counseling and peer support can provide a helpful alternative for those challenged by a variety of illnesses, losses, and changes by providing structure, role models, perspective, support, and resources at a time of ongoing crisis. When thinking about group counseling and self-help alternatives, it is important to recognize that many individuals are not accustomed to sharing feelings with strangers and may resist the group counseling experience.

Exploration

1. List five ways group counseling or peer support could help a person with a disability adjust to living with the effects of the disability or other major life events.
2. If you had a disability, would you voluntarily enter a group? Why or why not?
3. What would be the most difficult aspect of group counseling for you as a group member?
4. Are there certain people with illnesses or disabilities you would not want to associate with?
5. List the characteristics of group members that make you uncomfortable.
6. If you could choose a group leader to lead a group for persons and families experiencing a major life changes, what would be the characteristics you would like this person to have?
7. What are the characteristics of a group leader or peer leader that would put you off?
8. Identify the most upsetting situation that could occur for you as a group member.
9. Should people with a disability and people without a disability be in the same group? Why or why not?
10. Should persons with a brain injury be in a group with individuals who are living with AIDS, spinal cord injury, or mental retardation?

PERSPECTIVE EXERCISE 2

Who Needs This Kind of Help?
Perspective

When families are in a state of crisis, they need to be listened to, responded to, and treated with sensitivity, caring, and respect. Often, the stress of health care and rehabilitation environments creates a situation in which professional and nonprofessional staff do not provide help but rather create pain by insensitive and nonhelpful remarks.

Exploration

1. List examples of how health care and human service professionals could be helpful in dealing with the impact of a disability.

Helpful responses:

(Example: It is not easy but we will be there to help.)

   a.
   b.

Not Helpful Responses:

(Example: After all, your daughter was an alcoholic who should not have been driving.)

   a.
   b.

PERSPECTIVE EXERCISE 3

Is the Person With a Disability More Important Than the Family?
Perspective

The occurrence of a severe disability often focuses all of the family's emotional resources on the person who has sustained the injury. Often this focusing is essential to contain the fallout from the injury and to stabilize the total family system. However, in order for families to realign their goals and to establish a different balance in their lives, they must make a transition. This transition should consider the individual needs of family members, the total needs of the family and the emerging, changing needs of the family and family member living with the opportunities, and problems, associated with an illness or disability.

Exploration

1. In coping with the demands of a disability in a family, how should the emotional resources be allocated? Financial resources?
2. Is it ever possible to regain balance in the family following an illness or disability? If so how?
3. How long is a long time?
4. Consider a severely disabled child with a grandparent with Alzheimer's disease and the other grandparent with a pre-existing psychiatric disorder. How should the emotional resources of a sibling be allocated?

PERSPECTIVE EXERCISE 4

Enough Is Enough

Perspective

An often overlooked factor in addressing the needs of the person with a disability and his or her family is the impact of additional illnesses on the patient, other family members, and/or primary caregivers. This can be a major issue because the resources of the support system can be greatly stressed. An example of this would be the following case overview.

June

June was a 54-year-old wife and mother of four children when she had a stroke. She had lived a very active, vigorous life and was the central figure in her family system. Caring for and managing was facilitated by the commitment of her husband, John, who felt it was a privilege to care for his wife and best friend. Although their children were living in the same town, they were able to maintain their separate lives due to the commitment and investment of their father. A major crisis occurred when their father suffered a severe heart attack and was in need of complete care himself. A temporary plan was to have an unmarried daughter move home to stabilize the situation. This worked for 3 weeks, until the daughter suffered a severe back injury while trying to lift her mother off of the floor.

Faced with a decision to either place the mother in a nursing home or have her move in with one of the children, the family was forced to realize that they had to become involved at a higher level of commitment and personal sacrifice. This decision never had to be made because both the mother and father died within 1 month. This case overview illustrates several points: (a) viable caregiving arrangements can suddenly change and (b) multiple illnesses can have a synergistic effect, overwhelming the resources of both caregiver and family.

Exploration

1. Having read the above case synopsis, list other additional factors that could have further complicated this case.
2. Consider a specific family challenged by a stroke that had to deal with the impact of multiple illnesses? What was the outcome? Were there any intergenerational issues? What would have been helpful?
3. What are some areas of competence that are important for family's caregiving for a family member who has a stroke?
4. What are the assets and limitations of being involved with a self-help group?
5. Do you think that families can ever be normal again after a stroke?
6. Identify those extended family members who would not be helpful to you or your immediate family. State why.

PERSPECTIVE EXERCISE 5

Fragile: Handle With Care

Perspective

When families are forced by reality to address the complexity and permanence of a disability, there is an urgent need for them to be listened to, appreciated, valued, and understood.

By listening, caring, and responding, the family is validated and given the opportunity to establish a communication process that is based on real issues, mutual respect and hope, based on reality and not on desperation.

Exploration

1. Develop a list of what is needed to maintain a sense of well-being and a positive quality of family life.

   a.

   b.

   c.

   d.

   e.

2. Develop a list of what is needed or would be needed to help negotiate the stress of a disability experience within the family.

   a.

   b.

   c.

   d.

   e.

PERSPECTIVE EXERCISE 6

I Am in Love With a Stranger

Perspective

Most relationships are based on common goals, mutual respect, interpersonal concerns, and emotional security. For those and a variety of other reasons, people choose to be with each other and enter a long-term relationship. Unfortunately, illness in general and disability in particular can introduce elements into a relationship that are stressful, challenging, and sometimes overwhelming. Some relationships can negotiate their challenges, whereas others struggle and are eroded away.

Exploration

1. Think of a couple you believe has an ideal relationship. How would this change if one of them acquired a disability? Who could cope the best as a caregiver? As a patient?
2. If you know a couple who has successfully experienced a major trauma, discuss what enabled them to survive.
3. If they did not do as well as they could have, what would they have needed?

Appendix B: Personal Perspectives

*A*vailable to the authors are the many dynamic stories of those who utilize different coping strategies to live and to grow despite a serious disability or illness. The
personal perspectives provided earlier in this volume are living illustrations of how to
be productive while experiencing significant life challenges. But we wish to include
some additional personal perspectives that can broaden the reader's understanding of
living with and beyond an illness or disability and also show that different perspectives
of coping and living only enrich an understanding of the dimensions of the total human
experience. These personal perspectives enlarge on Irving Kenneth Zola's conviction
clearly stated in the foreword of the third edition of *The Psychological and Social
Impact of Disability*: "Disability was not merely a personal problem to be solved by
individual effort ... as much a social problem created and reinforced by social attitudes
and prejudices whose solution would require governmental resources, protections, ad
interventions."

These additional personal statements also further emphasize and extend the implications of the disability-related issues identified in Parts I–V of this book. The personal
journeys of Robert Neumann and Tosca Appel illustrate both the material discussed by
Livneh and Antonak on psychological adaptation to chronic illness and disability and
the chapters in Part III on Family Issues in Illness and Disability. These family issues are
further highlighted by the narrative experiences of Judy Teplow, Karen's mother, and
both Chris and his mother. Paul Egan's poignant account brings to life many of the concepts identified in the chapters in Part II. With the description of David's experience,
all of these personal statements provide the reader with an opportunity to understand
the varied models of disability, discussed clearly in the chapter by Smart and Smart in
Part I.

CHRIS AND HIS MOTHER: HOPE AND HOME

CHRIS MOY

*The following personal perspective presents the often irrational life experience that can
test and strengthen the human mind, body, and spirit. A son and his mother share their
journey, as well as the hopes and dreams that had to be let go as well as aspired to.*

Reprinted from *Families Living with Chronic Illness and Disability*, by P. W. Power and A. E. Dell
   Orto, pp. 271–277, 2004. New York: Springer Publishing.

Chris's Perspective

Prior to my injury in July 1991, my family had endured its share of trials and tribulations. I guess you could say we were a typical middle-class family. At least we considered ourselves middle class. Actually, we were on the low-income end of middle class, but we were happy. We never felt deprived of anything; even though we didn't have a lot of money for clothes or extras, we never went without. My two older brothers and I shared many wonderful times with our parents. Everyone was always very close: church every Sunday, dinners together, and always discussions on how things were going. My parents, to my knowledge, never missed a sporting event or school function. Everyone was treated fairly, given the same opportunities, and encouraged to grow and learn by experiencing new things. We were always given the freedom to choose our activities, but we were expected not to quit halfway through. If we started something, we were always expected to give it a fair chance before deciding not to continue with it. I guess that's where I developed much of my determination.

My father and mother shared the responsibilities of keeping the household going. When my father lost his job, he took over all the household chores and my mother continued to work full time. Dad was always the athletic type, and he instilled in us the belief that hard work, determination, and self-confidence would not only help us athletically, but later in our lives as we began to go out into the world. Our friends were always welcome in our house. I'll never forget how my Dad would fix lunch every day for me and my best friend during our senior year. There aren't too many guys who would want to go home every day for lunch, but I always felt very comfortable with it.

Mom has always been the matriarch of the family. Being an optimist, she was able to see the good in everything. Although she's a petite woman, she had a quiet, gentle strength about her. I never tried to "pull one over on her," since she always had a way of finding things out. When one of us boys would do something we shouldn't have, mom always found out. This still amazes me.

My oldest brother was always quiet and kind of shy. Acting as a role model for me and my other brother, he worked hard in school and pursued extracurricular activities. At the time of my injury, he was out of school and living on his own. As the middle child, my other brother was more aggressive and outgoing. Striving for independence, he couldn't wait to be out on his own. As the youngest of the three boys, I was always on the go. I was very popular in school and gifted athletically. I had just graduated from high school and had secured a baseball scholarship at a nearby university. It had always been my dream to play professional ball. It seemed I had been preparing my whole life to play in the "big show." Little did I know that I was really preparing for the challenge of my life.

After graduating from high school, I was carefree and looked forward to a great future. I was planning on attending Walsh University, where I had been awarded the baseball scholarship, where I would major in business. I could not wait to start college, become independent, and meet new people. New challenges and new opportunities occupied my thoughts.

The summer after my graduation was a time I remember vividly. Playing 80-odd games in 6 weeks and enjoying my new freedom with friends, I thought I had it all. I figured as long as I had baseball, friends, and family, I had everything I would ever need. What I did not figure on was losing baseball, being separated from friends, and becoming almost completely dependent on my family.

On July 29, 1991, a friend and I went to the mall to do some school shopping. Afterward we decided to hang out at the local strip and see what was going on. We ran into two of our friends, Valerie and Bobby Joe. The four of us talked and cruised around enjoying the cool summer night. Around 10:30 p.m., we decided to stop off at Taco Bell to go to the restroom and get some drinks. When we entered the Taco Bell, I noticed nothing unusual so we proceeded to order. It was supposed to be a fun night out on the town, and it probably would have ended that way had the conclusion of the night not found me lying in a coma, fighting for my life.

As we were leaving the restaurant, I still hadn't noticed anything unusual. As I proceeded out the door a couple of steps behind my friends, I was struck in the face by a fist. Swinging around to see who had struck me, I was disoriented. As soon as I swung around, I felt a glass bottle shatter over my right temporal lobe. I immediately fell to the ground where I was kicked and beaten for what felt like an eternity, but was actually only a few minutes. Afterward, I slowly tried to regain consciousness. I was rushed to the hospital where I fell into a coma for a month.

Emerging from my coma was the greatest challenge of my life, a challenge I will never forget. It called for every resource I had if I were to breathe and walk again. It was like I was alone in a dense, thick fog groping for a familiar hand, yet unable to find anything concrete and strangely aware of a vast emptiness and solitude. This is a faint reflection of my coma. As I lay there, I experienced repeated flashes of light … my brain inevitably reacted. I wondered where the light came from! Had I really seen it or was it only a figment of my imagination? I convinced myself that the flash of light was real and thus my only hope of finding my way back home. From a great distance, I heard the distinct voices of my mother, father, and brothers, and Amy, the girl next door. Each time I heard their encouragement, I drew one step closer to the light. Although I felt like falling into despair, a word of love from God, my family, and my friends urged me forward. Without such love I would not have advanced even one step. Along with these words of love, I also heard the muffed voices of doctors and the high-pitched whispers of nurses as they wondered what they could do to help me. Eventually, they concluded that I would not make it. I was determined to prove them wrong.

Every day, I fought the coma with all of my might. Every day, I drew a little closer to the light. Finally, the day came when I opened my eyes and saw the heartbroken tears of the people I loved and longed to be with. Meanwhile, I could not move a single muscle in my body. I could not even talk. However, this did not bring my spirits down; somewhere deep within I knew that I had just answered the greatest challenge of all, the challenge of coming back from virtual death.

After awakening from my coma, I slowly began to realize what had happened. I went from a fully functional young adult to practically a vegetable in a blink of an eye. I was left totally immobile, not able to talk, and my world had seemed to crumble to dust. My family and friends were there to support me; if not for them, I think I would have died.

During the ensuing weeks, the doctors and nurses gave me little hope for recovery, but through persistent pleading, my mother convinced the doctors to give me time before decisions were made to institutionalize me. My family and I vowed to meet this brain injury head on and give it our best. I slowly regained mobility and could see gradual improvements. The doctors also saw my progress and decided to send me to a rehabilitation hospital to continue therapy.

It was at the rehabilitation hospital that my attitude and commitment to recovery preceded all other thoughts. My family, friends, therapist, nurses, and doctors were my team, and they were counting on me to bring them to victory. You see, it was the ninth inning, the game was tied, the bases were loaded, and I was at the plate facing a full count. It was the kind of situation I thrived on. It was do or die time. I could dig in, face the challenge, and try, or I could drop my bat, strike out, and die.

The choice was mine. What did I do? Well, I stepped up to the box, dug my feet in, and my mind focused on the pitcher, or in this case the injury. I saw the ball coming; it was like a balloon. I stepped toward the ball, made a smooth swing, and then I heard a crack. The ball ricocheted off my bat like a bullet from a gun. I just stood there and watched it soar high and long; I knew in an instant it was gone. As I touched each base, a part of my recovery passed, and before I knew it, I was home, starting school, and enjoying life again.

Although my recovery is not yet complete, I play a game every day in my head, and with every hit, catch, and stolen base, a part of my recovery passes. My next home run could be the one that brings me full circle. The pursuit of this dream is encompassed by the determination and hope that one day I will make it back to my ball field. All I can do is try and pray that everything will turn out right, and if it does not, I will still go on because I know I gave it my best.

The road to recovery has been long and wearisome, but I have already put many miles behind me and I know I will emerge completely triumphant. This experience has taught me many valuable lessons. Above all, it has convinced me that the human will can overcome obstacles that many consider insurmountable. I have walked through the valley of the shadow of death and have come out, not unscathed but undaunted. I am among the few people who can say that they have experienced near-death and were able to live and talk about it. I consider myself lucky and remain grateful to all who have helped me recover from this disaster. My experience has indisputably helped make me the person I am today.

Although many things helped my family overcome this catastrophe, the most helpful was first and foremost our faith in God and belief that He would make everything all right. Second, it was the overwhelming support we received from family and friends. How could we not make it with such kindness and compassion? The third thing was becoming knowledgeable about brain injury. This seemed to make us feel more in control of the situation, instead of relying on doctors and nurses for details of what was happening. Throughout the injury, we kept a positive outlook on life, knowing that we would pull through. The family, as a whole, had a kind of inner strength, which told each member things would work out in the end. Finally, we came to accept the situation and the consequences it has brought. The past cannot be changed, but the present and future can.

Intervention was never offered to my family. I often wonder why, but I guess no one ever thought to ask what the family needed. Intervention that would have been helpful to my family includes

- A team of doctors who would offer in-depth knowledge on the subject of head injury, or offer literature or reading material in lay-person's terms.
- Counseling for the family because just being able to talk to someone about what was happening would have helped. Information on support groups and meeting other families who have experienced such trauma would have been extremely soothing.
- Someone offering assistance with a list of attorneys, if needed, or other medical facilities better equipped and able to help patient progress.
- Someone who would have been able to structure a program that would have fit my family's needs, for example, phone numbers of groups or organizations that offer help, and if out of town, assistance with lodging, meals, churches, and so forth.

After reading and realizing the lack of professional help my family had, I have to wonder what really helped us get through this experience. It seemed that everything that was needed by the family, the family provided. I thank God for giving us the strength, courage, and wisdom to endure each day and for watching over us as we struggle through head injury.

His Mother's Perspective

I remember lying in bed the night we got the phone call. I was wondering why Chris was late. It was 10:30 p.m. He had gone school shopping at the mall with a friend. It wasn't like him not to call if he was going to stop somewhere else.

Just the weekend before, he had finished up a grueling summer baseball schedule, playing 80-odd games in 6 weeks. He had worked so hard on getting a scholarship, and we were very proud of him. I remember his last tournament game. When they lost, he quickly tossed his uniform, like only a ballplayer could, to get ready for the drive to Walsh University where he would be attending in the fall. It was orientation weekend, but he had come back to play his final game. His dad had said, "Well, Chris, that was your last game." A strange feeling passed through me, and I quickly added, "Until you get to college." As we later drove to the hospital that night, that conversation kept floating through my thoughts.

We really didn't know how bad things were until we arrived at the hospital. When they told us he was having seizures and would need immediate brain surgery, we were devastated. Some friends of ours had gone through a similar experience just the year before, so were all too aware of the seriousness of the situation. As friends and family gathered at the hospital to keep a constant vigil, the pain and devastation set in. So many questions kept going through our minds. Would he live? If he did, how would he be? Why was this happening to us? The nurses were very helpful and brought much needed comfort during the long weeks while he was in a coma. My husband and I could not bear to leave the hospital. The doctors did not seem to be educated enough to deal with the situation, so we finally had to make the agonizing decision to have him moved. All along we prayed to God to give us the strength, courage, and wisdom to make the right decisions.

My husband was offered a job, and the decision was made for him to go to work as I stayed with Chris. My husband quickly took over all the responsibilities of working and running the household, plus handling all the stacks of paperwork. I, on the other hand, was learning, right along with Chris, about therapy. Together we struggled to help him get better. For him, it was a matter of working relentlessly to make his body do what he wanted it to do. For me, it was the anguish of watching and being there for my child, but not really being able to make it all better. It was a feeling of helplessness. I was determined to learn everything I could about head injury. Somehow being more knowledgeable on the subject made me feel more in control. I always tried to keep a cheerful, encouraging face on for Chris even though my heart was breaking. My other two sons were great. The middle son remained at home with his father and did everything he could to help out. My oldest son visited Chris daily and opened his bachelor apartment, which he was sharing with two other guys, to me.

Although the outlook was bleak, we never gave up hope that Chris would return to normal. But as we've learned, nothing is ever normal. Our lives are constantly changing. As Chris begins to have more and more control over his body, he seems more content. When Chris started school again after his injury, I never imagined he would do this well or go this far. Having him transferred so far from home has been hard on the whole family, but he seems so happy that it's hard not to be happy for him. From the beginning, he was always accepted for who he was, not for what his body had trapped him into. The son we had was taken from us, but the son we were given back is even better in so many ways. Chris is a constant inspiration to all who come in contact with him. There is not a doubt in my mind that he will succeed in life.

As I reflect back, the pain and hurt will never go away, but I developed a tolerance for it. Life for all of us in this world is a challenge. You draw strength to meet those challenges through those around you. Things are so unpredictable, but would we really want to know how things will turn out? All we can hope for is to be surrounded by love and the courage to face what life has to offer. A Garth Brooks song better explains this point: "Yes my life is better left to chance. I could have missed the pain, but I'd had to miss the dance."

DISCUSSION QUESTIONS

1. If you were engaged and your fiancé had a traumatic brain injury, what would you do? What would your family suggest?
2. How would you respond if you or a family member were brain injured as a result of violence?
3. Discuss the athletic frame of reference that Chris had and how it was an asset in treatment, recovery, and rehabilitation.
4. Why was Chris's family able to rally in a time of crisis?
5. If your loved one were not expected to survive, what would you do if faced with the decision concerning the use of life supports?
6. After reading this personal perspective, would you consider rehabilitation at any cost?
7. What did Chris mean when he stated, "I know I gave it my best."
8. How can people learn to adapt to change as Chris and his family did?

KAREN—MY DAUGHTER FOREVER

Linda Stacey

Medical History: Karen

I am the mother of Karen. While it is she who must bear the trauma, the pain, and the limitations, it is I who suffers with her and sometimes, truthfully, because of her.

After writing Karen's brief medical history (below), I thought I would try to compute the hours spent in and traveling to and from hospitals. I found it impossible—the hours are uncountable. Which is worse, I think, life-or-death surgery with comparatively little follow-up or routine orthopedic surgery, which requires trips to Boston (20 miles one way), three times a week for physical therapy. It has been almost a year since the last surgery, and we are still making the trip twice a month. The exercises are never ending, the casts must be continually replaced, and trying to motivate acceptance of these responsibilities by Karen was, until recently, next to impossible.

She is mine forever, I sometimes think. I will never forget the doctor's response when I asked when all this would stop. His answer was to the point: "When her husband takes

Age	Medical Problem
4 weeks (4½ pounds)	Open-heart surgery
10½ months	Cerebral palsy diagnosed
2½ years	Brace on leg to allow for walking
6 years	Heel cord surgery
7 years	Open-heart surgery
10 years	Muscle transplant—arm

over." To him, she is not a person but an arm or a leg, depending on where the problems lay at the time.

I think back to her day of birth—thrilled with another girl. Karen was preemie weight but full term. Because she nursed well, she was allowed to come home with me. Symptoms began to appear within a few weeks, but nothing that seemed too unusual. A doctor who cared enough saw her once or twice a week to check and called me often when I didn't call him. Because he cared enough to keep a close watch, he was able to diagnose a congenital heart defect before it was too late—he saved her life. I had never dreamed of a problem of such magnitude.

The diagnosis was a septal defect in the heart. In other words, a hole in the heart that allowed oxygenated blood to mix with deoxygenated blood. Emergency surgery was needed to repair the defect. The doctors would not give us any odds on Karen's survival of the surgery, but she had no chance at all if surgery was not performed. Karen was, at the time, one of the smallest (although not the youngest) infants to survive this surgery. We thought our problems were over until we discovered (when she was 10½ months old) that Karen had cerebral palsy. It was years before I could say those last two words: cerebral palsy. I always said that she had damage to the motor area of the brain. Somehow that didn't seem so bad.

The cause will always remain unknown. It could be congenital, it could be due to a lack of oxygen before the corrective heart surgery, or it could have happened during the surgery at a time when techniques were not perfected for working on such a small child (she was hooked up to an adult sized heart-lung machine, for example). The cause is unimportant. It is the effects that we must deal with.

At first, the attention a family gets in these circumstances is unbelievable. You're special, everyone wants to help, and there is a certain amount of glory or martyrdom involved. "How do you manage?" they ask. They could never do it. Well, the answer to that is, you do it because you have to. There is no one else to do it for you. You only wonder how you managed after the latest crisis has passed. Then it's on to the next crisis—always another one to look forward to. It's almost as if this child will be mine forever—in the sense that I will always be responsible for her. While this may sound selfish, I can't imagine any parent wanting to keep their children with them for the rest of their lives. Cop out? Maybe it is, but I can't help it.

How do we feel about Karen? It was a long time before I could say that sometimes I hate her for all the problems she presents. A parent cannot easily voice this emotion regarding a child, especially a handicapped child—it's almost inhuman. Karen's sisters could say "hate" much easier—children's feelings are much closer to the surface than those of adults.

On the other hand, these same sisters who sometimes hate her will rise to her defense when they see that she is treated badly. She is not, however, an easy child to get along with. Although Karen functions well in school with a great deal of supportive help (resource room, counseling, etc.), she is socially immature and has no real friendships to rely on. It is we at home who care for her who must bear the brunt of her frustrations—acting out and generally behaving abominably.

Of course, we love Karen, but it is often difficult to show openly. A child of Karen's temperament can drain your emotions. The more affection and attention you give, the more she wants. I often feel as though I am bled dry. She is all-consuming.

Sometimes, I feel pity. What will she be able to do? Because she appears almost normal, people expect normalcy from her. For that matter, so do we, for I am always afraid of selling her short. We demand that she perform tasks that are within her capabilities—even

Reprinted from *Role of the family in the rehabilitation of the physically disabled,* by P. W. Power and A. E. Dell Orto, 1980. Baltimore: University Park Press.

more. If I tie her shoes for her now, who will do it when I'm not here? She needs to know how to tie shoes with one hand. She must learn in spite of herself.

Often I feel compassion. How do you console a child who has no "real" friends? What playmates she does have are not above tormenting her in insidious ways. What do you say when she tells you that the kids at school call her "mental"? How does it feel knowing that if someone comes to call for you, it is only because no one else can come out to play? Telling her not to pay attention is almost ludicrous. These things hurt us both, but it is very difficult to build self-image in a child who is "different" and intelligent enough to know it.

I always feel guilty—not because I've somehow done this to her, but because she is so much better off than other victims of cerebral palsy. Cerebral palsy can be devastating to the point of total immobility and retardation. Karen is neither. Why then should I complain? I guess I can only say that this is our problem, and it is we who must deal with it.

At night, I cry when I see her sleeping. She sleeps relaxed, the spasticity is gone, the cerebral palsy seems to have disappeared for 12 hours or so. But in the morning, Karen still limps, her hand is still misshapen, and she still has trouble with school work and social adjustment. I cry now.

What will Karen be when she grows up? My head knows that there's a place for her somewhere—my heart wonders if she'll find it.

Update: 30 years later, Karen is married and is working.

DISCUSSION QUESTIONS

1. What role do siblings play in the developmental process of a sibling who is disabled?
2. What role does birth order play in the area of sibling rivalry for an adolescent with a disability?
3. How can the family be a liability in the school-to-work transition for an adolescent with a disability?
4. How has the AIDS issue created additional concerns for families of adolescents with special needs?
5. How would you and your family feel if you had a child like Linda's child, and who was making great strides in managing the particular disability, but then was diagnosed with another debilitating disease?
6. What advice, help, or insight would you give a family member who may not stop focusing on what she or he has lost because of the caring demands associated with the severe disability of a child?

LIVING IN SPITE OF MULTIPLE SCLEROSIS

Tosca Appel

Multiple sclerosis (MS) was something I knew nothing about or even considered being part of my life. Even if I did, it was more an illness for those who were young adults. However, I was one of those rare cases of MS that occur before the age of 20—I was 11 years, 9 months old when my first symptom occurred.

My first attack of MS took the form of a lack of motor coordination of my right hand. I was unable to hold utensils, and my hand was turned inward. My parents in their concern rushed me to the emergency room of the hospital. The intern who saw me at the emergency room told my parents without any exam that I had a brain tumor. Needless to say, this shocked my parents because, other than this attack, limited to my right hand, I was otherwise normal and healthy. I was admitted to the hospital, where I stayed for 12 days.

Ten days after the initial attack, the symptoms abated. Two days later I was discharged from the hospital and was totally back to normal. The doctors had put the blame of the attack on a bad case of nerves. Before the attack, I was enrolled in Grove Lenton School of Boston. This was a very high-pressured school. From my A average in grammar school, my grades had dropped to roughly a B– average. I was worried, and I spent many sleepless nights crying myself back to sleep. I could not handle the pressure of going to a private school. Consequently, I transferred to a public junior high school. Without the pressure, my grades went up to an A– average. I was happier and everything was fine.

My second attack occurred when I was 16 years old and in the 11th grade. My mother and I were planning my Sweet-16 birthday party. My mother rented a room in a nightclub. I was all excited, planning who I was going to invite, what it was going to be, and what the room was going to be like. One day before the party, my history teacher asked me a question. I stood up to answer, and my speech came out all garbled. I was unable to string the words into a sentence. I was even unable to utter words. All that came out were sounds. I clutched my throat to help the words come out easier. At times they did, but at times it came out a garbled mess. I remembered the teacher's look. He looked at me in utter surprise and a little bit helplessly. In total utter shock, my attempts at speech sounded so ludicrous to me—so totally as if it did not belong to my head, and so totally foreign that I started laughing hysterically. I couldn't be serious about the sounds I was making. Again, my parents rushed me to the hospital where again another intern did his initial workup on me. However, the sounds that came out of me were so funny that I again started laughing almost hysterically, because I was well aware of what I wanted to say and I was also well aware that it was not coming out of my mouth right. The intern, in his wisdom, thought that this behavior was an attention-getter. He thought I was faking the whole thing.

After the first attack, my mother had decided that this time she would not let me be admitted to the hospital. I was then not admitted, but I was instead seen on an outpatient basis. The inability to speak lasted roughly 2 weeks. I had the party and had a good time. But pictures were taken during this time, and I hated them. Why? My smile came out cockeyed. I smiled with the left half of my mouth, without moving the right side. To me it was quite ugly. After my speech returned, the doctors said that the right side of my mouth and tongue were numb, paralyzed, thus making it very hard for me to talk. Overall, I do not remember the attack. Two weeks after this attack, I again went into complete remission.

In 1967, at the age of 19, I applied to and was accepted at Northeastern University. However, during the fall term, I started having trouble seeing. My father drove me to the train station so that I would be able to take the trolley to school. But after I got on the trolley, I took it beyond my stop, and went to the Massachusetts Eye and Ear Infirmary to have my eyes checked out. I did not tell my family about my concerns because I did not want to worry anybody. A doctor put me through a whole eye workup, and he said that he could not promise how much sight I would get back in my eye but that he would do all he could. Considering that I was an English major and I loved to read, this freaked me out. I asked him if glasses would help, and he said no, that he might be able to get all my sight back or none of it, but that he could not promise me anything. I had to call my mother after I left him. I first went into the restroom and cried. I controlled myself long enough to call my mother. I got off the phone with my mother as quickly as possible and left for school on the train.

During the ride, I was attempting to figure out if it would have been better to have been born blind and never have seen anything than to lose sight after having it and know what you are missing. As a result of this thinking process, I came to the conclusion that it would have been better for me to have been born blind, because I now knew the beauties

Reprinted from *Family interventions throughout chronic illness and disability,* by P. W. Power, A. E. Dell Orto, and M. Blechar-Gibbons, 1988. New York: Springer.

of a sunset, of reading, of a flower, of all the things that people who have sight take totally for granted. I do not know how I would rationalize it now.

When I got to school I went into the cafeteria, sat with my friends, and began crying. Once I stopped crying, I got it all out of my system and my friends and I decided that crying would not solve anything, and the best thing I could do was to go home, take some medication, and see if my sight returned. When I returned home, I did not initially tell my parents of what the doctor had said about the possibility that my sight might not return. I decided that my parents always got very nervous when something happened to me and that there was no need to worry them about me.

So, I did not say anything until my mother mentioned that she had spoken to my neurologist. At this time, unbeknownst to me, I was diagnosed as having MS. My neurologist had told my mother of the diagnosis and told her to tell me. My mother had refused. The doctor then told her that I would never forgive her if she did not tell me. She said that was something that she would have to deal with and did not want to tell me. Consequently, following my mother's wishes, the doctor naturally did not tell me.

The loss of sight in my left eye lasted 3 weeks, and then I went back to college and continued the daily routine of living. Still my mother had not told me about the MS. She bore it alone and did not tell anyone for 6 months after she knew. The only person she spoke to about my MS was my older sister, who is 6 years older than I am. When my mother would become depressed, she would call my sister and cry about the injustice of this happening to me rather than to herself.

My mother's rationale for not telling me was basically twofold. First, she felt that she should not burden me with the knowledge of my chronic degenerative disease because the knowledge of MS could deter me from doing what I wished to do. Second, when my mother saw me running out of the house to go on a date or to a party, she would get scared and sad, thinking about the day that I would not be able to go out and enjoy myself. My mother felt that the knowledge would hang like a cloud over my head, so she made it her responsibility that I was not to know.

However, this conspiracy of silence put my doctors in a difficult position when I went to see them. I would beg the doctor to tell me what was wrong, but he could not because of a promise made to my mother. Because I remembered when a doctor had told me I might have had a brain tumor, which was incorrect, I asked my neurologist if I was going to die of a brain tumor—to which he said, "You can only die of a brain tumor if you have a brain." This may have been a joke to him; it was not for me! The worry about the brain tumor was a preoccupation of mine. My fingers would tingle, or I would feel something go wrong with my balance, and I would be worried that it might be caused by a brain tumor. I was really worried about dying. I found no comfort in the silly remark that I would need a brain to have a brain tumor. At the time, I told the doctor that I was not kidding and that I was very worried. To that, he replied that they did not know what was wrong with me, but when they discovered a pill for it they would rush it to me. I left his office feeling very depressed, very alone, and not understood.

Finally, when my mother told me I had MS, I was sad and confused, but also very much relieved. Now there was a basis for my physical concerns. Because I had long periods of remission over the next 10 years, there were the low points of exacerbation but the long periods of life, living, and the pursuit of happiness. It was great to be a young adult who was living life and running ahead of the long-reaching shadow of MS.

At age 28, I reached a major crisis point in my life. I was faced with the reality of ongoing deterioration. My sight reached the point where I was not able to read the newspaper. In addition, I lost what functional use I had in my left hand. Although these losses may not seem to be catastrophic issues to the nondisabled, they were catastrophic to me. The reason was that they reaffirmed the reality that I had little control of my body and of what was happening to it.

The feeling intensified when I had to resign myself to the fact that I needed to use a wheelchair. To me, this was an admission of defeat and that my disease was getting the best of me. While I made the cognitive decision to continue to struggle, it was very difficult when the little physical control I had was slowly eroding away. As a result, I made the choice to live, rather than to deteriorate or die. Although this is easy to verbalize, it is often not easy to implement. I can choose to actualize myself, but I am limited by physical and emotional resources to follow through completely in that process.

My unique situation is that I was dependent upon my family, with whom I lived. I was also dependent upon my mother to provide me with the assistance I needed, such as cooking and partial dressing. Even though I wanted to live independently, I had to accept that I had a wonderful home life, caring parents, and a loyal brother.

The next major transition was when my father and mother died, both within the same year. While initially having to deal with the impact of the loss of people I care about, I also had to face the question of what would happen to me. Fortunately, when my parents became ill, I made the choice to get an apartment and to develop the independent-living support systems I would need. Another possibility for me was to extend the relationship with my boyfriend, to whom I was once engaged and whom I had been dating for 15 years. However, this possibility is questionable, for there were reasons we did not get married and they are still real concerns.

This is my response to the disease that has plagued me for 24 years and has altered the course of my life. I will not let it beat me. What motivates me is the memory of my parents and the knowledge of my heritage. My mother and father spent years in a concentration camp, and many of my other family members perished there. I feel the obligation to make the best of my situation and draw on the strength of those persons who suffered far more than I am suffering. As I see it, the key to my ability to survive is the memory, support, and encouragement of others. They have made the difference, accepting me as I am and helping me to resolve my feelings about not being what I was or could have been.

DISCUSSION QUESTIONS

1. What is your reaction to how Tosca was told about her MS?
2. What are the family issues with Tosca that helping professionals should be aware of?
3. After reading her personal perspective, if you were in Tosca's situation, would you consider marriage or having a child?
4. How do societal roles and expectations for women create stress for women with disabilities?
5. Do you think that the mental health needs of women with disabilities are different from those of men with disabilities? If so, please explain in what way(s)?
6. How would you feel if your parents decided, when you were 17 and had a crippling disability, to place you in another caring environment so that better care could be given to your sibling who also had a devastating illness?

SURVIVING AMYOTROPHIC LATERAL SCLEROSIS: A DAUGHTER'S PERSPECTIVE

JUDY TEPLOW

Betty Miller: Beloved Wife, Mother, and Grandmother, September 4, 1986, Age 70 Years

In the early spring, when the ground is soft, I will lay a marker on my mother's grave, a permanent marker to commemorate the life of a very special lady. The inscription will be short, impersonal, and incomplete—and somehow not befitting a woman who courageously struggled against a devastatingly cruel terminal illness.

I cannot inscribe her story in stone, but I can set it on paper as a lasting tribute. I hope it will be a comfort to those who are afflicted with a serious or terminal illness, and a help to the families and health professionals who are involved in their care and treatment.

It was going to be an unbearable, oppressive day, but my mother had no intention of sitting in her small, air-conditioned apartment. She set out early with her walking buddies on their 5-mile jaunt and, as usual, took the lead. She was amused that her companions, who towered over her 5-foot frame, could not keep up with her brisk pace.

Everything seemed to be going well for her and my dad. Retirement for them was not sedentary life, but rather one that was full and gratifying. In a few weeks, they would return to their apartment in Boston for 5 months of relief from Florida's intolerable heat.

But for now, Betty was enjoying her walk and thinking about how rich her life was. As she turned the bend, her thoughts were cutoff abruptly by a stiffening in her left leg— perhaps a cramp—but she did not have the pain associated with a cramp. Her gait slowed down considerably, and in a minute she found herself lying on her side. She was stunned by this unexpected interruption. She did not stumble over a rock or a crack in the roadside. What should she attribute this weakness to?

It took 5 months for the doctors to make an accurate diagnosis. An electromyogram was performed at the Brigham and Women's Hospital, and it was this test that ultimately determined that my mother had amyotrophic lateral sclerosis (ALS), Lou Gehrig's disease, a progressive, degenerative disease that is terminal. It is probably the most dreaded neurological disease and is one with no known cause or cure.

Within 1 year of the first visible symptom, Betty would be a virtual paraplegic, confined to a wheelchair, unable to talk or to feed herself. Breathing and swallowing would become progressively more difficult. At no time would the disease affect her mental faculties, and she would always be aware of the creeping paralysis.

My initial reaction to the diagnosis was one of disbelief, devastation, and helplessness. How could such an active and health-conscious person be stricken with such a catastrophic illness? I felt a sadness for my parents, and I had real concerns about my dad's health also. It was conceivable to me that this tragedy could destroy him as well, and I prepared myself for the worst.

The family and doctors were in total agreement as to how much to tell my mother. She had always been petrified of doctors and hospitals and was by nature very nervous and anxious. We knew that she could not cope with such outrageous news.

She was told that she had a chronic neuromuscular disease and that she would need intensive therapy. We did not offer her hope of a cure, nor did we inform her that she was terminally ill. She asked very few questions, wanted to know as little as possible about her disease, and became adept at tuning out whatever she was not ready to hear.

Like my mother, my aunt, my father, and my brother went to great lengths to avoid the truth. Denial became a protective measure they were to use effectively throughout the course of the illness. As much as I tried to beat through this barrier, I was met with resistance. It was this resistance that was to become a great source of frustration and anger for me. My aunt held out the longest, talking about the research, cures, and the possibility of people living several years. My brother, who never coped with adversity too well, did not become an integral part of the team, and his visits to the nursing home were often sporadic and brief.

Reprinted from *Families living with chronic illness and disability,* by P. W. Power and A. E. Dell Orto, pp. 229–233, 2004. NewYork: Springer.

I had to know all the medical aspects of the disease, so I asked a lot of questions and read many books on ALS, and on death and dying. Someone had to take charge, to plan, and to carry the family through this crisis.

From the Brigham and Women's Hospital, my mother was transferred to the Braintree Rehabilitation Hospital. It was there that she was put on a daily regimen of physical, speech, and occupational therapies. She was extremely tense and frightened, but the staff was very professional and experienced and knew how to respond to her emotional and physical needs. This was really not a time for rehabilitation as much as a time for enormous adjustment. It also allowed the family to make plans for home health care. I wished that my mother could stay at Braintree indefinitely, for I feared that the support systems at home would not be adequate.

My fears were well founded. She was not home 2 months when all systems began to breakdown. My mother required constant attention, and the Visiting Nurse's Association and private-home health professionals were not able to keep up with her demands. Oftentimes, my father was left without help, and he had to assume the role as primary caregiver. Tensions mounted and tempers began to flare, and what was once a very happy marriage now appeared to be very strained. My dad's health was deteriorating as well as my mother's, and they looked to me for a quick solution.

I knew that my mother required round-the-clock care in a skilled nursing facility, but I did not want to be responsible for initiating the search. I could not find it in my heart to do this to her, especially when she threatened to commit suicide before she would enter a nursing home. My grandmother had taken her own life because she could not cope with a painful illness, so I was worried about my mother's intentions. I began to get pressure from her sister, also, in defiance of any plan to move my mom from her home. We were in a crisis, and we needed help quickly.

I was fortunate to find a psychologist who would help me accept and confront problems that were difficult and painful. He helped me see issues more clearly when everything seemed overwhelming and confusing. It was through him that I began to understand the complexities surrounding chronic and terminal illnesses. His continued support and genuine concern were to sustain me through some very difficult times, the first of which was my mother's move to a nursing home.

The transition from the apartment to the nursing home was traumatic for the family. Ostensibly, the home was attractive and meticulous, with spacious rooms and beautiful furnishings. In sharp contrast to this orderliness was a picture of deterioration—of very old people in their 80s and 90s ravaged by debilitating diseases, marked with permanent deformities, hooked up to life-supporting machines, impaired by mental illness—there was an aura of sadness and loneliness, and a sense that many of these people were deserted by their families.

I wished that I could put blinders on my mother's eyes—to shut out a world that was so unreal, but yet only too real and disheartening. My mother was only 69 years old and looked 10 years younger. How could we do this to her! I knew that there was no alternative, but I was stricken with guilt, a guilt that was to stay with me for a long time. It took a good 3 months before I could walk into the nursing home without feeling sick—without feeling very, very shaken.

I don't think my mother ever adjusted to nursing-home life. I think she resigned herself to her fate. I know she often felt very sad, lonely, and misunderstood, but I do not think she felt abandoned. She knew that the family was there for her, and it was this prevailing sense of security that kept her from slipping into a deep depression.

A schedule was worked out wherein one or two family members would visit daily. This was arranged, mostly out of love, partly out of guilt, and out of an acute awareness that strangers would not minister to her needs the way family would. We also knew that if we were going to survive this ordeal, we would have to share the responsibilities, for each of us had a history of medical problems. Often, the burden of responsibility rested on my shoulders, and at times I felt overwhelmed. But I also felt that if my mother could cope with the effects of a very disabling disease, I could deal with any problems that arose.

I do not know how she endured all the suffering, and I do not understand what held her together. She certainly did not triumph over her disease—she did not write a book, or paint by mouth, or engage in anything that was extraordinary. She just tried to get through the day. There were many tears and many moments of anguish, but even in her despair, she insisted on getting up, getting dressed, and—above all—having her hair done weekly. Thank God there was a hairdresser on the premises, and thank God she still cared about her appearance. Throughout her illness, she never lost her sense of humor or her ability to smile and laugh. But the laughing was done for the staff, and most of the crying was done with the family.

We tried to maintain a sense of equilibrium, but it was difficult to keep control when all systems were failing. The disease was progressing at an alarming rate, and we knew she would need the strong support of the family and the specialized services of many health care professionals. Some services were effective, but most fell short. Many professionals were not familiar with or could not cope with the demands of ALS. They were uneasy in treating a terminally ill patient, or clearly had an attitude problem toward the sick and the elderly. I must acknowledge, though, that most people did try to help, and I cannot fault them for their human limitations in dealing with a very difficult case.

I also believe that my mother's inability to speak had a lot to do with the quality of care she received. This was a great source of frustration for her and for the health professionals who worked with her. The family members were the only ones who had the patience to make use of the communication boards. We acted as liaison between my mother and the staff, so our involvement in her care was crucial.

We also acted as her advocates and protectors. There were aspects of nursing-home care that were unsettling, but because we had a very good working relation with the staff, most of our grievances were worked out. I can only think of one incident that was offensive and repulsive, and it was due to a personality conflict between my mother and an aide. An aide had lost control and, out of anger and impatience, threw a sheet over my mother's head. This was a gross violation of my mother's right to be treated as a living human being until the day she died.

The only other situation that disturbed me occurred outside the home. A week before my mother died, her doctor was called to check on her deteriorating condition. To our dismay, we learned that the doctor was on vacation and had left instructions for the covering physician. Her doctor had promised to leave explicit directions regarding heroic measures. This was not an insignificant oversight. I had chosen this doctor because he had been highly recommended by another physician and was on staff at a hospital directly opposite the nursing home. Because of his close proximity, I thought that he would be accessible to my mother and the family, but unfortunately we found him to be very impersonal and distant.

Without the encouragement and concern of a handful of people, the experience would have been unbearable. There were three exceptionally caring people who made a great impact on my mother.

Janet, a nurse's aide, became my mother's guardian angel, and she was to watch over her and attend to all her needs while she was in the nursing home. There was such a strong attachment between them that on the day my mom died Janet was unable to work.

Margaret, the assistant director of nursing at the nursing home, had lost her mother to ALS, and she was familiar with the disease and its effects on the family. She was always available to us, and it was not unusual for her to interrupt a busy schedule to explain what comfort measures should be used. She was also instrumental in educating the staff about the nature of the disease. She was my inspiration and a great source of strength.

Bobby was a close friend of the family. He had experienced the loss of a loved one, so he was no stranger to personal tragedy. He attended many workshops with Elizabeth Kübler-Ross and was involved in hospice, and he knew how to relate to the terminally ill. Bobby showered my mother with gifts and flowers and made her feel very special. He was the only one who could talk to her about death and life after death and ultimately helped her accept her mortality. He was a good friend to me, also, and I was able to talk with him about my greatest fear—the use of life-support systems.

The issue of support systems was always a source of great pain and anguish for me. My anxiety was heightened by my mother's refusal to discuss these matters and the inability of family members to agree on a specific course of action. I personally believed that the use of heroic measures, in my mother's case, would be cruel and inhumane—a prolongation of inexorable suffering pain—and an interference with the natural order of things.

But I had to know where my mother stood on these issues for, ultimately, it was her life and her decision. Three months before her death, she began to make her wishes known. She slowly spelled out the word die every day. She made it quite clear to me that she could no longer tolerate living. She finally came to terms with her death, knew it was imminent, and had an urgency to express her grief and fears about dying. Once she accepted her death, she became more tranquil.

I did not want my mother to die in the arms of strangers, nor did I want her to experience death alone. I was fortunate to be with her at the final moment of death. My aunt and I sat by her side and held her hands, and except for a brief interruption by staff, this was a family affair. We exchanged a few words of support and comfort, but we were mostly caught up in remembering and recollecting. I wondered if my mother saw her life flashing before her, and if she were passing through the dark tunnel toward Omega, but I could not be sure.

DISCUSSION QUESTIONS

1. What aspects of Judy's mother's transition from the apartment to the nursing home were most traumatic for the family?
2. How does the slow deterioration of an elderly parent emotionally affect immediate members of his or her family?
3. What is the meaning of the statement: "My mother's inability to speak had a lot to do with the quality of care she received"? What is the relationship between those two factors?
4. Are there additional roles, other than advocate and protector, that an adult child of a chronically ill parent must play during the illness?
5. Of the three "exceptionally caring people who made a great impact on my mother," who would you choose if you could only select one to care for your own mother who may be chronically ill and needs caregiving efforts?
6. What would be your reaction if you were in a similar situation with an elderly, chronically ill parent, to the statement, "She made it quite clear to me that she could no longer tolerate living"?

MY LIFE WITH A DISABILITY: CONTINUED OPPORTUNITIES

Paul Egan

For me life began very comfortably over 57 years ago, in a then affluent suburb of Greater Boston. I was the third son of a prominent up-and-coming general contractor. I also had an older sister. A month before I was born, tragedy befell the family when the firstborn son, then aged 6, died of diphtheria. So, when I arrived healthy and sound, I was a most welcome addition to a grieving mother and father. Just before I turned 2, another brother was born.

In September 1944, I entered the U.S. Navy and, after completing boot camp, I was initially assigned to motor-torpedo boats in the Philippines. I was then assigned to a yard minesweeper with a team of 22 officers and men. Our assignment consisted of sweeping (dragging) the shipping channels and ports of the Philippine Islands. During this time, my job performance was classified as outstanding, and I received many promotions. However, my life suddenly came apart. While I was moving a keg of concentrated ammonia across the deck, it blew up in my face. The ammonia burned my eyes, the linings of my nose and throat, and also the skin around my facial area. I was rendered unconscious, and upon regaining consciousness 3 days later, the doctor told me that my eyes were badly burned and that I would have to be patient and pray for a miracle to take place.

One year, seven hospitals, and several operations later, vision returned to my right eye to the degree of 20/70 with corneal scarring. Other complications emerged as my head and my right hand became involved in a constant tremor. This ailment was incorrectly diagnosed as a nervous anxiety reaction. So I became a psychiatric bouncing ball. In May of 1947, I was discharged with a 70% Veterans Administration (VA) compensation.

I immediately went to work for a friend, pumping gas in a gas station. But I had greater ambitions, and I enrolled at Boston Business Institute in a business administration curriculum for 2 years. Shortly after returning to school, my mother developed cancer and passed away on December 15, 1947. This was a profound loss to all of us, as my mother was always on hand with her guidance and sense of fortitude. She was always there to listen, to encourage me to make the most of myself and to go back to school. In fact, in the initial stages of my readjustment to civilian life and to my own disability, it was mom's positive attitude, including her expectations for me, that inspired me to move forward. Her philosophy of making one's residual assets work for the fulfillment of goals is one that I have adopted in my own life.

In June 1948, I married Marietta, a girl I had known before I entered the service. Around this time, my father went on a trip to Newfoundland, his place of birth, and came back a few months later, married. He had married his brother's housekeeper, a plain-appearing woman who was 25 years younger than he was. They immediately isolated themselves from all family and friends for years to come.

In June 1949, I graduated from business school and started experimenting with the real world. Although I was very fortunate in not being unemployed for more than a month during the next 24 years, my choice of expanding my horizons was limited greatly by an uninformed business environment. Time after time when applying for positions for which I was qualified, ignorance, fear, stigmatizations, and prejudices were barriers I found most difficult to overcome.

During the next 20 years, my wife gave birth to five daughters, we moved to a larger house, and I was employed in various jobs. Shortly after the birth of our first daughter, I began a series of operations on my left eye. These operations climaxed with an unsuccessful corneal transplant, which resulted in the surgical removal of my left eyeball. Soon after the birth of our second daughter, I had a laminotomy. I understood this operation as involving the transaction of the thin layers of connective tissues around the optic nerve. The pain and suffering endured were the most excruciating of my life. But I was able to get through all of this because of the support of my wife. We didn't think about the past or about my other disabilities. We focused on the present, and together we often discussed our mutual concerns. This was a tremendous help to get through my own sufferings. But in 1968, my tremors got

From *Family interventions throughout chronic illness and disability,* by P. W. Power, A. E. Dell Orto, and M. Blechar-Gibbons, 1988. NY: Springer. Reprinted with permission.

worse, and I went into a VA hospital for a brain operation. After doing an encephalogram, the doctor thought the risks were too high. Instead of the operation, a new experimental drug was tried, but that increased the body involvement and was quickly discontinued.

Moreover, a trauma occurred in our family, when on a night in January 1970 when the temperature was 25 degrees below zero, our oil-burning furnace exploded, destroying our home and all of our possessions. All of our neighbors came to our support, and they held a fund-raising party for us that resulted in not only a substantial amount of money but also in donations of services in our efforts to rebuild. Another factor in our rebuilding effort was that after an absence of over 20 years, my father reappeared and lent us the remaining necessary funds to rebuild. After we had made a few repayments he said, "You've shown good faith," tore up the note, and then chose to go back into hibernation with his wife. I tried on numerous occasions to visit with him on his 90-acre farm, but he was always "out" or had to go some place in a hurry.

After getting settled into our new home in June 1970, our life returned to a semblance of normalcy until late in 1973 when I lost my job. My employment was not the only loss, however, for I also lost my sense of dignity and self-respect, and I drifted aimlessly in a sea of self-pity and depression for nearly 4 years. Though my family was very supportive of me during this time, I knew this was my own struggle and they themselves had to survive. My daughters were married, had their own families, but seemed to be there when I needed someone to share my feelings.

In June 1977 I was classified as blind. That November I entered the VA Blind Rehabilitation Center at West Haven, Connecticut, and from that time on life took on a new perspective. After 14 weeks of intensive training and guidance, I was again doing things for and by myself. The educational-testing evaluations done at the center indicated a potential for higher education. So in September 1978, I returned to school with the goal of becoming a social worker. In May 1982, I received my B.S. from Suffolk University, and then in 1984, I earned an M.S. from Boston University. In April of that year, I began a new career as a field representative and outreach-employment specialist with the Blind Veteran's Association. Yet as I look back now on all of these years of family life, of living with my disabilities, and then finally becoming blind, I often think of my own family, with their patience and understanding. They made the difference so often during my many rehabilitation efforts. Even when I became depressed, they urged me to continue, for somehow they appreciated what I could still do. Probably I would never have gone back to school without their encouragement. Even my father, who died in 1978 and who really never got over the shock of seeing his first financial empire disintegrate, was there one time when we really needed some assistance. To all of my family, I say thank you.

DISCUSSION QUESTIONS

1. After reading the personal perspective by Paul Egan, at what time during the progressive deterioration of his eyesight do you think that family intervention would have been most effective?
2. After reading the chapters in Part IV related to intervention approaches, what do you consider the role of spirituality and could it be applicable to Paul Egan's family?
3. If disability or a severe illness occurred in your own family, and considering Brodwin, Sui, and Cardoso's chapter of "The Use of Assistive Technology," how would you access the resources that could provide assistive technology?
4. Assuming that you have the opportunity for a meeting with Paul Egan and his wife at the time when he was discharged from the VA Blind Rehabilitation Center in 1977, design a

family-assessment approach utilizing the discussion in Pederson and Revenson's chapter in Part III.

5. Discuss the issues related to the following statement: "I really can't have any effective contact with a family that is living with a disability situation unless I have a degree in family counseling or family therapy."

FOR BETTER OR FOR WORSE

DAVID COLLINS

Growing up in a family as the youngest of three boys, competition and survival were natural qualities. Athletics followed and played an important part of my life. During high school, my time was spent practicing for the upcoming game and "getting by" in the classroom to maintain eligibility. In college, my priorities changed and academics were goals I pursued to stay out of the draft more than anything else. At 23, Valerie, the girl I met in college, and I walked down the church aisle and professed our love to those in attendance. Nine months and 3 days later, we welcomed an addition to our union. As a coach and teacher, my skills were enhanced at classes or clinics; parenting, I hoped, would be a natural talent. As Kerry started to grow and reach her second birthday, we were good pals. If she misbehaved, this coach would make her sit on her plastic chair and not get up—probably a theory I had read about from one of my coaching journals. As Kerry grew, so did Valerie. She was expecting our second child in April. After some thinking, I chose to give up coaching and go into real estate sales and tax work. With a family it was important to look to the future and be prepared. I would make my mark, and my family would enjoy the benefits. My planning was poor. After I played my last Christmas basketball game with fellow coaches, we convened at the local pub to review the game. After drinking beer and eating breakfast, I got in my car to drive home. Halfway home, I fell asleep and struck a utility pole while sitting atop my seatbelt. My life was instantaneously altered. As my pregnant wife entered the hospital emergency room at 4:00 a.m., the neurosurgeon blasted her about my high alcohol reading and poor prognosis. If I survived, I'd need constant attention.

The accident occurred on December 27. My first recollection was in March. I called my wife by her maiden name, asked if we had any children, and displayed not only confusion, but an indifference as well. I was not only brain injured, but I was a quadriplegic. At one point, I was convinced they had wheeled my bed up a floor to the obstetrics section, and I vividly remembered delivering a baby. My days were spent going to therapy and returning to bed and watching television. A young man started visiting and sharing his story. His name was Dave, and he had fallen out of a tree and broken his back 7 years earlier when he was 16 years old. He was very muscular as he wheeled around the halls and explained things like driving a car with hand controls, bowel and bladder control, and sexual activities with his dates. Dave got me out of my room and wheeling outside; he explained his life in graduate school to me and it was appealing. In time, I chose to attend graduate school at the University of Illinois, renowned for its accessible campus and wheelchair sports programs. After 6 months in the hospital, I was allowed to go home for weekends. My expectations upon returning home were that my relationship with my daughter and my wife would be as they were before. My foremost thought was to resume sexual activity with Valerie and provide for both our needs. At 27, I had serious doubts about being a person or a man and

From *Brain injury and the family—A life and living perspective, 2nd Edition,* by A. E. Dell Orto and P. W. Power, 2000. Boca Raton, FL: CRC Press. Reprinted with permission .

felt the only way to prove my virility was in the bedroom. Valerie was very patient and empathic to my needs. My hygiene was terrible, a tracheostomy was done on my throat, my bladder and bowel needed to be emptied prior to commencing intimacy, and there was always the chance of having an accident. To this day, I will always be indebted to her for allowing me to believe "I was a man." I told her she gave Oscar-winning performances when I needed them.

When I made it home permanently and reentered the family unit, it had become apparent that Kerry, our precocious 3-year-old, had taken my place. She had to be moved out of the king-size bed and back to her room. My adjustment to returning home, I had told Valerie, would be unnoticeable—or so I thought. My first morning home, I had forgotten to put my clothes next to my bed on the wheelchair (dressing is done prone on the bed). After 15 minutes of yelling for Valerie, I finally got, "Yeah what?" to which I requested she get my pants for me, which were on the floor. "I'm changing the baby and can't get back to you for 45 minutes," she said. I was livid. "Bullshit," I mumbled as I got in my chair, retrieved my trousers, and, getting back in bed, got dressed. Upon coming out to the kitchen and observing Valerie drinking coffee and reading a magazine, I let loose. "What in the hell is going on?!" I screamed. After 5 minutes of ranting, I stormed off. Today, Valerie and I use this story at workshops and seminars on coping to health care professionals and families. We refer to this as the "Pants Story," and the lesson we convey is that never again did I forget my pants. I'm sure it was hard for Valerie to hear my pleas and not give in, but the lesson we learned is it is a disservice to perform a task for an individual without his or her attempting the feat first.

As time progressed, I entered graduate school and due to the insight of my counselor, who suggested that only two courses be taken to start out, I succeeded. As I wheeled across the street on a campus of 45,000 students, my name was yelled out and I stopped. A fellow approached and asked, "Didn't you play basketball for Brother Rice in Chicago?" "Yeah," I said, and as we continued our discussion, I recognized him as a wide receiver for a rival high school in Chicago. He went on to tell me he was pursuing his PhD in therapeutic recreation/administration. He then asked if I would be interested in going out for the track team. The bewilderment on my face led him to explain therapeutic recreation and how the University of Illinois had wheelchair track, basketball, football, and a variety of other sports for those who are physically challenged. Practices were to start in 2 weeks. At my first practice, I was amazed to see the number of participants and their varying levels of function. I started to bring my daughter to practices and all of us seemed to enjoy ourselves. At various meets, my family would join me when ribbons were awarded and have their pictures taken—each of us was proud. The practices and the meets turned into family outings. Valerie coordinated things well by loading the car with the kids, a wheelchair, and me. I could sense my becoming less competitive with the girls.

As they became older, they became interested in playing sports. As a former coach, I had to use restraint as I cheered in from the sidelines at their t-ball games. One parent asked me if I would assist him in coaching the girls' basketball team that both our daughters were on. Reluctantly, I agreed, but again my daughters were proud of their dad sitting on the courtside bench. We truly began to communicate better and spoke about events that occurred in the practices or games.

I followed both girls as they progressed through the years. When they were younger, they didn't know that fathers in wheelchairs weren't cool. As they grew older, their parents knew less than they did, but I could tell that had nothing to do with my being in a wheelchair—just a normal reaction to parents. One time, as I pulled into a mall, Kerry asked, "Why do you park in wheelchair parking?" "Why not?" I replied. "You compete in 10K races and can wheel better than some of these older people can walk," she said. I thought for a few minutes and felt somewhat flattered and responded, "Yeah, I suppose you're right." "It sounds like a special favor you're taking advantage of," she said. "I'll remember that in the future" was my response.

It was August when both girls asked if I would drive them and their friends to an amusement park. Our group had about eight people waiting in a long line to ride the attraction. As we sweltered in 90° temperature, a woman who took tickets came up to me and asked, "Are you familiar with our wheelchair policy?" I said no, and she explained that any wheelchair patrons and their guests do not have to wait in line. They may go to the front and stay on the ride for a second time if they chose. I looked at my oldest daughter and said, "I don't know. It kind of sounds like a special favor to me. What do you think?" "Oh no, dad. This is okay this time." Later in the month, my wife offered to take the girls to the same amusement park to which they quickly responded, "Can Dad come?"

In my relationships with my spouse and daughters, I live by showing them that we all have choices—sometimes because of our behavior we must accept the consequences. We all have special qualities and are unique. When we speak to others, communication is stressed as very important. Times are difficult for a lot of people, and the key to my living is accepting and liking myself and taking it one day at a time.

During graduate school, I went to see the psychologist who worked at the rehabilitation center to inquire about what personal changes I might expect. His response stayed with me and makes a lot of sense: "If you were an S.O.B. before using a wheelchair, the chances are, post-trauma, you will be an S.O.B. in a wheelchair." The point is we usually don't plan bad things to happen to us: trauma, divorce, death, and so forth, but we still have the opportunity to change. Some are given a second chance, but that alone does not mean success. We are all individuals who need to work on our relationships within families and outside families. If we take one day at a time and keep a positive attitude, good things can result. In dealing with others, I clarify that my point is not to downplay or minimize trauma and its consequences. However, when one feels good about himself or herself, regardless of the circumstances, he or she can share routine feelings with others. Each of us has a choice—choice can never be taken away.

Allied health providers and all members in society must recognize each individual as unique and possess skills others don't have. No two people are alike—uniqueness in abilities is our gift to one another.

DISCUSSION QUESTIONS

1. What is lost/gained when a young athlete is faced with changes subsequent to a disability? Are there any inherent or positive traits an athlete may possess to aid the process of rehabilitation?

2. How can long-term goals be a source of stress for a person whose life is altered by a brain injury? How does this compare with the immediate stress related to hygiene, dressing, eating, and so forth?

3. Is a single person with a brain injury better off than a married person with young children?

4. Was the response of the neurosurgeon helpful to David's wife?

5. How would you respond if your spouse did not remember who you were and whether or not you had children?

6. How can exposure to role models be a positive or stressful experience? (e.g., having David meet with an active person who has mastered a disability)

7. How can the need for intimacy become a major priority for a person returning home from the hospital? How did Valerie facilitate the adjustment? What if the roles were reversed and Valerie had the injury? What issues could emerge?

8. How could re-entry into the family have been facilitated by creative discharge planning?
9. How would your spouse respond if he or she had to choose between your needs and those of a child?
10. Why were sports a critical element in David's adjustment to his family?
11. What does David mean when he states, "Each of us has a choice?"

EXPERIENCING SEXUALITY AS AN ADOLESCENT WITH RHEUMATOID ARTHRITIS

Robert J. Neumann

It was a walk I'd taken many times before, down to the train station of our town in suburban Chicago to watch the sleek yellow Milwaukee Road streamliners pass through. Usually it was nothing for the healthy 12-year-old kid that I was. Just seven or eight shady, tree-lined blocks— but today it felt like miles. With every step, my right knee was aching more, feeling more stiff.

My friend Terry was walking along with me. I gritted my teeth against the rising pain and struggled to maintain a steady gait. I didn't want Terry to know. I sensed that this was no ordinary ache, and I feared he would not understand. I was right on both counts.

Finally, I could stand it no longer. "You know, Terry, my right knee's feeling awfully stiff and sore," I said.

Without missing a beat, my horror-film-aficionado friend shot back, "Must be *rigor mortis!*"

Happily, *rigor mortis* it wasn't, just rheumatoid arthritis. Yet it would be 5 painful months before I and my family had even the small comfort of that diagnosis. But, in a way, Terry was right: It was the demise of the lifestyle I had known for my entire previous 12 years.

By my 12th birthday, I was just beginning to feel that things were going really well. I enjoyed getting out of the house by taking long rides on my bicycle; the guys were actually beginning to seek me out to play baseball with them; I was positively ecstatic when my parents allowed me to take my first long-distance train trip all alone to visit an aunt in Pittsburgh.

The arthritis changed all that. Literally within days my right knee became so stiff, swollen, and sore that it was all I could do to hobble from bedroom to bathroom to kitchen. I began seeing a bewildering succession of doctors who could not even arrive at a diagnosis, much less an effective treatment. They hypothesized tuberculosis or cancer of the bone. Their treatments were progressively more drastic aspiration of the knee, a leg brace, exploratory surgery. None accomplished much more than aggravating the condition physically and sending me emotionally even deeper into fear and depression. This was the late 1950s, and apparently in those days even the medical profession was less aware that rheumatoid arthritis can and does affect people of all ages, young and old.

Early in 1960, I went to the Mayo Clinic, where my arthritis was diagnosed at last and where more appropriate treatment was prescribed. Nonetheless, even this was not able to halt the progression of the disease to my other joints. First, it was my other knee, then my ankles, then my fingers, then my elbows, then my neck, then my hips, then. … With a sort of gallows humor, I'd say I had joined the Joint-of-the-Month Club. But behind this facade, I was terrified at how my body was progressively deteriorating before my eyes. Actually, I would avoid seeing it—or letting others see me—as much as possible. I would refuse all invitations to go to the beach or park for fear I would have to wear shorts that would expose my spindly, scarred legs. I would wear hot, long-sleeved shirts on even the most blistering summer days to avoid anyone's seeing my puny arms.

From *Family interventions throughout chronic illness and disability,* by P. W. Power, A. E. Dell Oreto, and M. Blechar-Gibbons, 1988. New York: Springer. Reprinted with permission.

One day, almost by chance, I could avoid it no longer. I caught a good look at myself in a full-length mirror and was appalled at what I saw. I had remembered myself as having an able body. The person I saw looking back at me had a face swollen from high doses of cortisone, hands with unnaturally bent fingers, and legs that could barely support his weight.

I felt devastated. But as I look back on it now, I believe that experience of seeing myself as I really was, was the first step in becoming comfortable with the person I am. Of course, what I did not realize then was that I was a victim, not just of a disease, but of that even more insidious social phenomenon that Beatrice Wright (1983) has identified as the idolization of the normal physique. As a society, we celebrate the body beautiful, the body whole. As Dion, Berscheid, and Walster's (1972) research has demonstrated, we believe that what is beautiful in conventional terms is good, and we equate physical attractiveness with greater intelligence, financial success, and romantic opportunities. Media images of all types reinforce the notion that being young, active, and attractive is the ticket to the good life. Lose that attractiveness, lose that physical perfection, the images imply, and gone as well are the chances for success in love and life. This is definitely not the type of foundation on which an adolescent's fragile self-concept is likely to develop a solid, confident base.

But, painful as it was, looking at myself in the mirror and seeing myself as I really was, was the prerequisite for self-acceptance. It was acknowledging the physical facts, if not liking them. It was not until years later when I was in graduate school that I attended a seminar given by a marvelous person named Jesse Potter, and came to understand our culture's body-beautiful emphasis is only one way—one narrow, constricting way—of viewing reality. She helped me redefine my experience and understand that a person's attractiveness, a person's value, depends on who one is, not on how one appears. Simple as it sounds, for me that was a revelation and a liberation to realize that in the words of the Velveteen Rabbit (Williams, 1975), "once you are real, you can't be ugly—except to those who don't understand."

If my rheumatoid arthritis was a trauma for me, its effects also extended to stress other members of the family. My mother was a quiet source of support and preferred to keep her feelings about the disease to herself. Often she would cry alone in her room; she told me this only years later. But nowhere were the effects of the disease more evident than on my father. A traveling salesman with stubborn ways and volatile temperament, my father would frequently return from business trips edgy, angry, and generally out of sorts. This in turn caused me to dread these homecomings because as an adolescent I had no way of predicting what mood he might be in or what might set him off. It was only after I had moved from home and was employed as a hospital-based psychologist that he felt free enough to tell me how he could do nothing but think of me at home while he was spending those long hours driving the expressways and lonely country roads, worried by how sick I was and frustrated by his own powerlessness to do anything about it. If only he had been able to express those feelings openly and directly 20 years earlier.

One subject my father was able to express himself directly on was the topic of education and my future. He put it in his customary unvarnished manner: "Bob, you don't have much of a body. But you got a good mind. If you're going to succeed, you've got to use it." And, as I was growing up, there never was any question I would succeed. It was simply assumed I would do well in school, go on to college, and get well-paid employment. Clearly, I internalized these expectations for academic success even more than my father intended. But there is no doubt his high expectations functioned as a self-fulfilling prophecy. In large measure, I owe the PhD after my name, the jobs I have had, and many of the wonderful people I have met to my father's simple belief that I could and would. And today, when I work with clients, it is a particular frustration to see how many parents needlessly limit their disabled children's life possibilities through well-intentioned but misguided protectionism or realism that lowers expectations for success by focusing on all the problems rather than on the potentials.

During my high school days, my social life was virtually nonexistent. Because I received physical therapy at home in the afternoon and because my stamina was poor in any event, I only attended school until about 1 p.m. This eliminated any possibility of interacting with peers in extracurricular activities. To complicate the situation further, because my life revolved around classes and studying, I routinely received unusually good grades and routinely broke the class curve, much to the animosity of those peers I did interact with. But perhaps most significantly, the school I attended was a Catholic, all-boy high school. This removed me from any contact whatsoever with the female part of the population at a time when my interest was anything but dormant. I literally had only one date, with the daughter of family friends, during my entire 4 years of high school. This situation bothered me enough that I eventually discussed it with my biology teacher. A layman, he suggested that things would be better when I got to college, a response that was only partially more reassuring and accurate than that of the priests who counseled cold showers when issues like these arose.

These less than satisfying experiences have led me to be a strong advocate of mainstreaming. From one perspective, I was fortunate to have experienced a limited form of mainstreaming in an era before the advent of Public Law 94–142. At least the interactions I had with male peers gave me a basic idea of how able-bodied adolescent males view the world. Unfortunately, neither the school authorities nor my parents understood how important it was to ensure that deficits in social skills would not develop through lack of informal, out-of-classroom socialization with male peers and the total lack of contact with any female ones. Meanwhile, I unsuspectingly continued to study and dream of the day I would start college and the active love life I had fantasized about for so long.

Finally, the big day arrived. Armed with a body of knowledge about women derived solely from TV, James Bond movies, and the *Playboy* magazines my younger brother smuggled in, I arrived at a small Midwestern college never dreaming I was, in reality, as green as the lovely pines that graced the campus.

It took only a short while before I noticed my actual accomplishments with women were falling far short, not only of my expectations, but also of the experiences of my friends and acquaintances. Within a few months, most of the people I knew, both men and women, had developed ongoing intimate relationships. Everywhere the couples were obvious: sitting together in classes, dining together in the cafeteria, partying together at dances, studying together, walking together, sleeping together. I, on the other hand, became frustratingly adept at performing all these activities alone.

Actually, I was quite good at developing nonsexual friendships with women, especially those who had other boyfriends. I could relate well to them because there was no need for me to do the mating dance, no need for me to call on sociosexual skills I had never learned. These friendships were a mixed blessing. They provided emotional support and the beginning of much-needed learning about the opposite sex. But inevitably there were many poignant moments when my friend would go off to her lover, and I would go off alone. As unpracticed as I was in picking up social cues, I continually confused friendship and romantic messages when meeting apparently available new women. A poem I wrote at that time unintentionally reflected the confusion:

> LOST
>
> I like you
>
> when we joked and laughed 'bout people that we knew. I wanted
>
> you

when you softly said

that you must have love too. I love you

then you took his hand, and oh, I knew, I knew.

It was a depressing pattern. A woman would express an incipient interest; I would misread the cues and respond inappropriately, then feel crushed when the relationship died. Rejection and depression became themes that were only too familiar. I became convinced I was unlovable.

Finally, my roommate Michael decided to do something about the situation. A self-styled ladies' man with the body and bravado of a Greek god, Michael appointed himself my teacher. My first assignment was to read a book he provided me with called *Scoremanship*. Once I had finished the book, Michael proclaimed me ready for field experience. It was late on Friday afternoon, and Michael and I were having an early supper in the cafeteria.

"Bob," he nudged me. "Isn't that that Jane over there you've been wanting to go out with?"

"Yeah," I responded dubiously, looking at a woman several tables from us. "Well, remember the book. Just go up and ask her to go to a movie tonight." "Tonight?" I nearly choked. "But it's too late. She's probably got ten dozen things to do."

"Self-defeating talk is unknown to the Scoreman," Michael smiled serenely. "Just go and do it!"

Michael would not let me back out, so I figured I had no alternative but go forward and experience my next rejection. Slowly I walked over to her table. "Oh, hi, Jane!" I said, as if I'd just noticed her. "You know, uh, seeing you here reminds me. I was thinking of going to a movie tonight. Would you like to come?" Listening to myself, I was sure she'd never buy this one. "Why I'd love to!" she enthused. "Pick me up at my dorm in a half hour!"

I could hardly believe it. I rushed back to our table. "My God! She actually said yes. She actually said yes! What do I do now?"

Michael gazed at me with a smile of patient superiority. "You take her to the movie. Then you bring her back to our room. I'll fix everything up. Don't you worry about a thing."

The date itself was fine. The movie was enjoyable, the conversation relaxed and friendly. She even agreed to come back to the room for a drink.

I put the key in the door. As I opened it, I discovered just how much fixing Michael had done. Out billowed clouds of incense. Inside the room, candles everywhere cast their flickering light on *Playboy* magazines that had been artfully strewn about and opened to the most suggestive pages. Clothes and books were piled high on all the furniture except my bed. (So she would have to sit right beside me, Michael later explained.) But the crowning touch came when I noticed that on the night table beside my bed, Michael had arranged a little altar, complete with candles, a small *Playboy* calendar, and an opened package of condoms. I could have died.

Needless to say, seeing all this, Jane instantly developed a headache that required her immediate return to her dorm. After she had set out for her dorm, and though Michael had been trying to be a friend, I was embarrassed and set out to find him and relate my feelings.

Obviously, my role models were not always the most appropriate. And being the only disabled person on that small campus meant I did not have the benefit of interacting with and learning from other disabled peers. Nonetheless, I was learning, observing which things I did worked and which did not. Over time, even I could see that I was gradually improving my relationships.

My senior year eventually arrived, and I celebrated my 21st birthday—still without ever having experienced a physical relationship. Chronologically, I had come of age, but emotionally I still felt insecure, lacking the physical experience that symbolized manhood. I assumed my disability was largely to blame, since by then I knew I could develop nonsexual friendships with ease. Increasingly I came to view my virginity as a barrier in need of being surmounted. But this was not just a matter of desire, a stirring of hormones. To me it was also a matter of self-worth and self-esteem. For as long as I was valued by others only for my companionship and intelligence, I still was not being related to as a whole person, a person with sexual dimensions and emotional, intellectual, and spiritual ones—and I feared for whether I ever would be a whole person.

As it happened, that doubt was soon to be laid to rest in a manner I could never have foreseen. It was a Saturday night, and my friend Justin and I had just finished viewing an on-campus theatrical production by the Garrick Players when we encountered Sarah in the foyer. Justin had been friends with her for some time, but I knew her only peripherally from having shared a class or two and an occasional meal in the cafeteria. Generally, Sarah traveled in a different circle than mine. But tonight she was alone, so after some discussion we three agreed it would be fun to drive to town to get a drink.

We stopped at the Nite-N-Gale, a popular campus hangout, and had a couple of glasses of wine. But mostly we just talked. The conversation was good: comfortable and convivial, a pleasant mix of the light-hearted and the more serious. After a while, we headed back to Sarah's room on campus and continued in the same vein. Midnight arrived, and Justin declared himself tired and left for his room, leaving Sarah and me alone.

The conversation turned more serious. She asked me what it was like to live with arthritis. I told her about the Joint-of-the-Month Club and looking in the mirror. She in turn shared some of the hurts she felt in growing up in poverty with parents in ill health. Finally, I noticed it was approaching 2 a.m. "Well, I guess it's time to go," I said.

"You don't sound too wild about it, Bob."

I was surprised she had picked up on a reluctance I thought I was not showing. "Yeah, you're right," I sighed. "It's just that when I get back to the room I'll find Michael there with his girlfriend. It's damn depressing. Hell, I met her before he did! I liked her too!"

For a long second, Sarah just stared at me. Then a smile, warm and tender like I had never before seen, began to cross her face. "Bob, you know you don't have to," she said.

I will never forget Sarah, perhaps more than most people will never forget their first. What we shared was physical, but also far more. With her, I did not have to worry about how to handle the issue of my disability because to my astonishment, she did not view my disability as an issue: The mere fact that our relationship was physical confirmed as nothing else could that this, too, was possible. The effect on my self-esteem was tremendous. As a disabled colleague once remarked, "When most of your problems have been on a physical level, it's on the physical level that you're most strongly reassured." That statement has always stayed with me, even though I would amend the thought somewhat. Self-esteem is most enhanced when one's positive expectations converge with the reality of one's experience. Lack one or the other, and the individual suffers. At any rate, I still recall how brilliantly the sun was shining the next day as Sarah and I walked across the campus.

REFERENCES

Dion, K., Berscheid, E., & Walster, E. (1972). What is beautiful is good. *Journal of Personality and Social Psychology, 24*, 285–290.

Williams, M. (1975). *The velveteen rabbit.* New York: Avon.

Wright, B. (1983). *Physical disability: A psychosocial approach* (2nd ed). New York: Harper & Row.

DISCUSSION QUESTIONS

1. What was your reaction to the statement by Neumann: "Self-esteem is most enhanced when one's positive expectations converge with the reality of one's experiences"?
2. Who should be responsible for sex education programs for adolescents coping with disabilities?
3. What role has society played in the formulation of attitudes toward the sexuality of persons with disabilities?
4. Would there be a significant difference in the critical issues with a young woman who has had an experience similar to that of Neumann as related in his personal perspective?
5. How is an adolescent's search for self-identity complicated by a serious, chronic disability?
6. What is the role of the health professional in working with parents concerned about the sexuality of their children?

Index